Classification of Lymphomas and Hematological Neoplasia in the Era of Genomic Research: A Themed Issue in Honor of Dr. Elaine S. Jaffe

Classification of Lymphomas and Hematological Neoplasia in the Era of Genomic Research: A Themed Issue in Honor of Dr. Elaine S. Jaffe

Editors

Alina Nicolae
Antonino Carbone

MDPI • Basel • Beijing • Wuhan • Barcelona • Belgrade • Manchester • Tokyo • Cluj • Tianjin

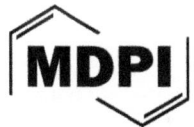

Editors
Alina Nicolae
Hautepierre Hospital
France

Antonino Carbone
National Cancer Institute
Italy

Editorial Office
MDPI
St. Alban-Anlage 66
4052 Basel, Switzerland

This is a reprint of articles from the Special Issue published online in the open access journal *Hemato* (ISSN 2673-6357) (available at: https://www.mdpi.com/journal/hemato/special_issues/TI_Elaine_Jaffe).

For citation purposes, cite each article independently as indicated on the article page online and as indicated below:

LastName, A.A.; LastName, B.B.; LastName, C.C. Article Title. *Journal Name* **Year**, *Volume Number*, Page Range.

ISBN 978-3-0365-5743-4 (Hbk)
ISBN 978-3-0365-5744-1 (PDF)

© 2022 by the authors. Articles in this book are Open Access and distributed under the Creative Commons Attribution (CC BY) license, which allows users to download, copy and build upon published articles, as long as the author and publisher are properly credited, which ensures maximum dissemination and a wider impact of our publications.
The book as a whole is distributed by MDPI under the terms and conditions of the Creative Commons license CC BY-NC-ND.

Contents

About the Editors vii

Preface to "Classification of Lymphomas and Hematological Neoplasia in the Era of Genomic Research: A Themed Issue in Honor of Dr. Elaine S. Jaffe" ix

Elaine S. Jaffe and Antonino Carbone
Evolution in the Definition of Follicular Lymphoma and Diffuse Large B-Cell Lymphoma: A Model for the Future of Personalized Medicine
Reprinted from: *Hemato* **2022**, *3*, 466–474, doi:10.3390/hemato3030032 1

Wing C. Chan and Javeed Iqbal
The Era of Genomic Research for Lymphoma: Looking Back and Forward
Reprinted from: *Hemato* **2022**, *3*, 485–507, doi:10.3390/hemato3030034 11

Sean Harrop, Costas Kleanthes Yannakou, Carrie Van Der Weyden and Henry Miles Prince
Epigenetic Modifications in Lymphoma and Their Role in the Classification of Lymphomas
Reprinted from: *Hemato* **2022**, *3*, 174–187, doi:10.3390/hemato3010015 35

Fina Climent, Joan Cid and Anna Sureda
Cold Agglutinin Disease: A Distinct Clonal B-Cell Lymphoproliferative Disorder of the Bone Marrow
Reprinted from: *Hemato* **2022**, *3*, 163–173, doi:10.3390/hemato3010014 49

Gioia Di Stefano, Francesca Magnoli, Massimo Granai, Federico Vittone, Raffaella Santi, Domenico Ferrara, Emanuela Boveri, Ada M. Florena, Falko Fend, Elena Sabattini, Marco Paulli, Maurilio Ponzoni, Stefano Lazzi, Stefano A. Pileri, Lorenzo Leoncini and the Italian Group of Hematopathology
B Lymphoproliferative Neoplasms of Uncertain Biological Significance: Report from the IV Workshop of the Italian Group of Hematopathology and Review of the Literature
Reprinted from: *Hemato* **2022**, *3*, 634–649, doi:10.3390/hemato3040043 61

Mark Roschewski and Dan L. Longo
The Clinical Impact of Precisely Defining Mantle Cell Lymphoma: Contributions of Elaine Jaffe
Reprinted from: *Hemato* **2022**, *3*, 508–517, doi:10.3390/hemato3030035 77

Cristina López, Pablo Mozas, Armando López-Guillermo and Sílvia Beà
Molecular Pathogenesis of Follicular Lymphoma: From Genetics to Clinical Practice
Reprinted from: *Hemato* **2022**, *3*, 595–614, doi:10.3390/hemato3040041 87

Miguel Alcoceba, María García-Álvarez, Jessica Okosun, Simone Ferrero, Marco Ladetto, Jude Fitzgibbon and Ramón García-Sanz
Genetics of Transformed Follicular Lymphoma
Reprinted from: *Hemato* **2022**, *3*, 615–633, doi:10.3390/hemato3040042 107

Marco Lucioni, Sara Fraticelli, Giuseppe Neri, Monica Feltri, Giuseppina Ferrario, Roberta Riboni and Marco Paulli
Primary Cutaneous B-Cell Lymphoma: An Update on Pathologic and Molecular Features
Reprinted from: *Hemato* **2022**, *3*, 318–340, doi:10.3390/hemato3020023 127

Stefan Nagel
The NKL- and TALE-Codes Represent Hematopoietic Gene Signatures to Evaluate Deregulated Homeobox Genes in Hodgkin Lymphoma
Reprinted from: *Hemato* **2022**, *3*, 122–130, doi:10.3390/hemato3010011 151

Sam M. Mbulaiteye and Susan S. Devesa
Burkitt Lymphoma Incidence in Five Continents
Reprinted from: *Hemato* **2022**, *3*, 434–453, doi:10.3390/hemato3030030 . . . . **161**

Emanuela Vaccher, Annunziata Gloghini, Chiara C. Volpi and Antonino Carbone
Lymphomas in People Living with HIV
Reprinted from: *Hemato* **2022**, *3*, 527–542, doi:10.3390/hemato3030037 . . . . **181**

Mark Bower and Antonino Carbone
KSHV/HHV8-Associated Lymphoproliferative Disorders: Lessons Learnt from People Living with HIV
Reprinted from: *Hemato* **2021**, *2*, 703–712, doi:10.3390/hemato2040047 . . . . **197**

Craig R. Soderquist and Govind Bhagat
Indolent T- and NK-Cell Lymphoproliferative Disorders of the Gastrointestinal Tract: Current Understanding and Outstanding Questions
Reprinted from: *Hemato* **2022**, *3*, 219–231, doi:10.3390/hemato3010018 . . . . **207**

Karthik A. Ganapathi, Kristin H. Karner and Madhu P. Menon
Peripheral T-Cell Lymphomas of the T Follicular Helper Type: Clinical, Pathological, and Genetic Attributes
Reprinted from: *Hemato* **2022**, *3*, 268–286, doi:10.3390/hemato3010020 . . . . **221**

About the Editors

Alina Nicolae

Alina Nicolae, MD, PhD, is an Associate Professor at the University of Strasbourg and is a hematopathologist in the Department of Pathology of the Hautepierre University Hospital. Before completing her residency program in Anatomic Pathology in Bucharest, Romania, she obtained a PhD scholarship supported by the Nogales Ortiz Memorial Grant of the University of Granada, Spain in 2009. It was the brightness and charismatic mentorship of Pr. Nogales that sparked her interest in academia. Given her similar interest in immunology, hematopathology was a natural step in her career. To gain more insights into diagnostic skills, she trained for seven months at the University of Bologna, Italy in the Hematopathology Unit directed by Pr. Stefano Pileri. To complement her training, she spent 4 years at the National Cancer Institute, US, as a research visiting fellow in the Hematopathology Section led by Dr. Elaine Jaffe. Since 2017, she has been the referee hematopathologist in Alsace for the French Lymphopath network, which offers expert pathological reviews for new lymphoma diagnoses. She is actively involved in hematopathology training in Romania, where she volunteered to teach. She perceives lymphomas as "caricatures" of the normal immune system. Therefore, her special interests gravitate around lymphomagenesis and lymphomas' microenvironment, more precisely around the pathogenesis of T-cell lymphomas and EBV-driven lymphoproliferative disorders. In addition, she is interested in molecular genetics and single-cell spatial biology. She has so far published 49 scientific papers and she is co-author of the 5th edition of the WHO Classification of Haematolymphoid Tumours and of the 3rd edition of Hematopathology by Jaffe ES et al.

Antonino Carbone

Professor Antonino Carbone is the former scientific director of the Centro di Riferimento Oncologico (CRO) and the former chairman of the Department of Pathology of the National Cancer Institute of Milano, Italy. He is internationally recognized for his diagnostic expertise and his many scholarly accomplishments in hematopathology. He is actively involved in the writing group of the WHO IARC Monograph Working Group on Biological Agents and Cancer and is the Chairman of the Italian TNM Staging Committee of the UICC. He has delivered many invited talks at various international conferences and schools (including, e.g., the second Digital Pathology Congress (London, UK, 2015) and the sixteenth Annual International Meeting of the Institute of Human Virology (Baltimora, USA, 2014)), in addition to more than 700 scientific papers, primarily in hematopathology, in international peer-reviewed journals (h-index: 81). Currently, he is the Editor-in-Chief of the new journal, Hemato. His main fields of interest are Hodgkin and non-Hodgkin lymphomas, HIV-associated lymphomas in particular. He contributed to the latter field of research, studying and improving the morphological classification of HIV-associated lymphomas and their viral association.

Preface to "Classification of Lymphomas and Hematological Neoplasia in the Era of Genomic Research: A Themed Issue in Honor of Dr. Elaine S. Jaffe"

This Special Issue is dedicated to a visionary woman in science, Dr. Elaine Jaffe. Her love of biology, dedication to disease discovery, and mentorship have shaped hematopathology over the last few decades. A singular lymphoma classification, with no differences on either side of the Atlantic, was sculpted by her remarkable work. In Dr. Jaffes's hands, the microscope served as a tool for lymphoma discovery. Through her eyes, multiple neoplasms of lymphoid tissue have been delineated. Through her voice, outstanding hematopathology teaching was spread. This distinguished investigator has advocated for the integration of basic research and clinical diagnosis in the day-to-day work of the hematopathologist. Through this intermingled clinical and investigational research, our understanding of malignant lymphomas' pathobiology and their relationship with the normal immune system has been enhanced. This has led to unprecedented advancements in the prognostication and management of patients with hematological malignancies.

In one of her earliest articles, a citation classic (N Engl J. Med 1974; 290: 813–819), Dr. Jaffe showed evidence of follicular lymphoma originating from normal follicular B cells. Since then, she has unveiled many pathologically and clinically relevant "guises and disguises" of follicular lymphoma. She described in situ follicular lymphoma, offering clues about the initial genetic changes in follicular lymphomagenesis. She identified histiocytic/dendritic cell tumors occurring with follicular lymphoma, providing the first piece of evidence for the lineage plasticity of mature lymphoid cells. Understanding the genetic and epigenetic events involved in mediastinal B cell lymphoma biology and, in particular, the mechanisms that cause a B cell to become a Hodgkin cell and the role of tumor cells' interaction with the microenvironment also engaged Dr. Jaffe's research interest.

The content of this Special Issue promises to be an outstanding "voyage through the eyes of a hematopathologist", aiming to carry the reader to follow and project the evolution of lymphoma classification, with the discovery of new clinicopathological entities, and achieving a better understanding of the molecular mechanisms involved in hematolymphoid neoplasms.

Alina Nicolae and Antonino Carbone
Editors

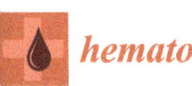

Review

Evolution in the Definition of Follicular Lymphoma and Diffuse Large B-Cell Lymphoma: A Model for the Future of Personalized Medicine

Elaine S. Jaffe [1,*] and Antonino Carbone [2]

[1] Laboratory of Pathology, Center for Cancer Research, National Cancer Institute, National Institutes of Health, Bethesda, MD 20892, USA
[2] Department of Pathology, Centro di Riferimento Oncologico di Aviano (CRO), Istituto di Ricovero e Cura a Carattere Scientifico (IRCCS), Via F. Gallini 2, I-33081 Aviano, Italy; acarbone@cro.it
* Correspondence: ejaffe@mail.nih.gov

Abstract: The definitions of follicular lymphoma (FL) and diffuse large B-cell lymphoma (DLBCL) are evolving in the era of personalized medicine. Early stages of the evolution of FL have been recognized. Two histological manifestations of early lesions are in situ follicular neoplasia and duodenal type FL. Additionally, FL frequently undergoes histological transformation, the most common form being DLBCL. High-grade B-cell lymphoma with double hit, with translocations involving BCL2 and MYC are important clinically. Rarer forms of transformation include classic Hodgkin lymphoma (CHL) and histiocytic sarcoma. In addition to conventional FL associated with the BCL2 translocation, alternative forms of BCL2-negative FL have been observed. These are heterogenous clinically and genetically. A distinctive group of B-cell lymphomas of follicle cell derivation arise in young patients and include pediatric type FL, testicular FL and a large B-cell lymphoma with IRF4 rearrangement. Historically DLBCL was separated into only two histological variants, centroblastic and immunoblastic. In 2017 the WHO classification recommended (1) the segregation of activated B cell and germinal center B cell derived DLBCL, (2) the identification of high-grade B-cell lymphoma with double hit, and (3) the recognition of an aggressive lymphoma that may resemble Burkitt lymphoma, currently designated in the International Consensus Classification as Large B-cell lymphoma with 11q aberration. Today we appreciate greater genomic complexity among aggressive B-cell lymphomas. Recent studies with NGS and mutational profiling have identified clinically significant genetic subgroups. It is hoped that these data ultimately will lead to targeted therapy based on the genetic profile.

Keywords: follicular lymphoma; in situ follicular neoplasia; FL transformation; FL in young patients; diffuse large B-cell lymphoma NOS; high grade B-cell lymphoma

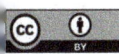

1. Introduction

The diagnosis of lymphoma is evolving in the era of personalized medicine. Indicative of these changes is the evolution that has occurred in the criteria and definition of follicular lymphoma (FL) and diffuse large B-cell lymphoma (DLBCL), two of the most common subtypes of B-cell lymphoma.

FL is a B cell malignancy that mimics normal follicles histologically and phenotypically. FL B-cells maintain the same state of differentiation as that of germinal centre (GC) B cells within the secondary lymphoid follicle [1,2]. Morphologically FL is a follicular proliferation of centrocytes and centroblasts associated with follicular dendritic cells (FDCs). The immunophenotypic profile of FL is CD20+, CD19+, CD79a+, CD10+, CD5−, Bcl-2+, Bcl-6+. The genetic alterations include JH/BCL2 rearrangement, t(14;18) and somatic mutations of VH. Most patients present with advanced stage disease, (IIIA–IV A), and with indolent, but generally incurable disease [1,2].

Diffuse large B-cell lymphoma NOS includes morphologic variants, i.e., centroblastic, immunoblastic, anaplastic and other rare variants. More recently, the subtypes of DLBCL have been related to the cell of origin, i.e., the germinal center B-cell (GCB) and activated B-cell (ABC) subtypes [3]. However, aggressive B-cell lymphomas are diverse and include many other specific clinico-pathologic entities; among these are T-cell histiocyte rich large B-cell lymphoma, EBV positive DLBCL NOS, primary mediastinal large B-cell lymphoma [4].

FL and DLBCL NOS are the most common forms of malignant lymphoma, with recent studies identifying much greater diversity than originally thought.

2. Evolving Spectrum of Follicular Lymphoma

The earliest stages in the evolution of FL have been explored (Figure 1). The classical model of FL lymphomagenesis is a multistage and progressive process, whereby t(14;18)(q32;q21) represents the founder event, and clinically significant disease results from a successive accumulation of genetic and epigenetic alterations. The discovery that non-neoplastic B cells that carry the t(14;18) in healthy individuals, later referred to as FL-like B-cells, influenced many aspects of FL research. FL like B cells are found in about 70% of individuals over the age of 50 [2].

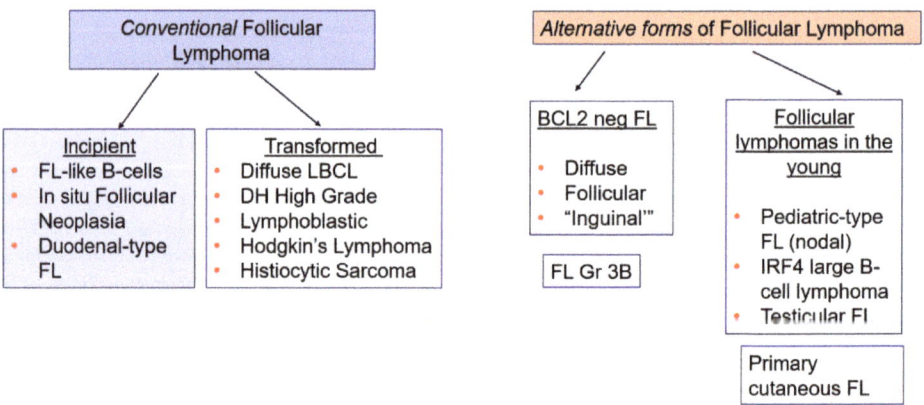

Figure 1. Evolving spectrum of follicular lymphoma.

In addition, the histological counterpart of this early lesion, is termed in situ follicular neoplasia (ISFN). It can be seen as an incidental finding in routine lymph node biopsies. ISFN is detected in 2–3% of routine lymph node biopsies. However, fewer than 5% of these patients will ever develop clinically significant FL. By array comparative genomic hybridization (CGH), ISFN has a very low level of genomic aberrations beyond the BCL2 translocation [5]. However, these early lesions may show mutations in CREBBP, EZH2, and TNFRSF14 [6]. Mutations in KMT2D appear to be a later event, associated with increased risk of progression.

Another early form of the disease is duodenal-type FL in which the BCL2 positive cells expand within the intestinal lymphoid tissue (Figure 2). All of these early lesions have a relatively low incidence of progression to clinically significant FL and this is especially rare in circulating FL-like B cells as found by sensitive PCR testing of normal peripheral blood [1,7].

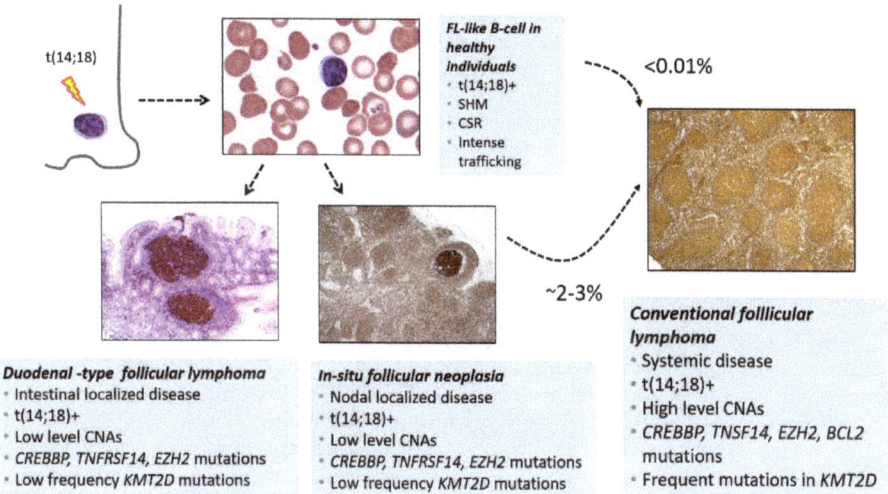

Figure 2. Incipient follicular lymphoma (FL) includes FL-like B cells found in the peripheral blood at low levels in normal individuals, most commonly after age 50. Tissue manifestations of incipient FL include in situ follicular neoplasia and duodenal-type FL. Abbreviations. CNAs, chromosomal numeric aberrations; SHM, somatic hypermutations; CSR: Class switch recombination. Reproduced with permission from Jaffe and Quintanilla-Martinez [7].

Similarly, knowledge of the diverse forms of histological transformation that may occur in FL has been expanded. The two most common forms of transformation are DLBCL and high-grade B-cell lymphoma with double hit (Figure 3) but other rarer forms of histologic transformation include classic Hodgkin lymphoma, and histiocytic sarcoma. Some cases of high grade B-cell lymphoma may be TdT-positive and resemble B lymphoblastic lymphoma leukemia (B-ALL/LBL) [8]. Most cases expressing TdT carry both MYC and BCL2 rearrangement. However, their mutational profile is distinct from B-ALL/LBL [9]. Thus, they are best considered a variant of double hit lymphoma.

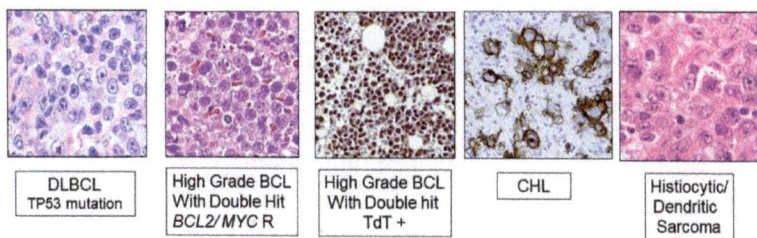

Figure 3. Transformed Follicular Lymphoma. All show clonal identity and retain the *BCL2* rearrangement.

Transformation to classic Hodgkin lymphoma and histiocytic sarcoma indicates the plasticity of the hematopoietic system. Histiocytic or dendritic cell sarcomas show loss of the B-cell program, most likely related to loss of expression of PAX5 [10]. Secondary histiocytic sarcomas share some of the molecular alterations of FL but also show evidence of evolution with acquisition of new mutations that are characteristic of primary histiocytic sarcoma with mutations in the RAS/RAF/MAPK pathway (Figure 3) [11,12].

Alternative forms of FL, so-called BCL2 negative FL, have been recognized (Figure 1). BCL2 negative FL are both clinically and pathologically heterogeneous and probably do not constitute a single disease entity. However, BCL2 negative FL should be segregated from BCL2 rearranged FL, as both clinical and biological differences exist [13]. A distinctive subgroup includes those cases presenting often with inguinal disease that tend to be low stage. These cases have a high frequency of STAT6 mutations, are frequently positive for CD23, a helpful feature in diagnosis. These cases are negative for BCL2R still carry some of the genetic alterations of BCL2 positive FL with frequent mutations in CREBBP [13]. The recent proposal from the International Consensus Classification (ICC) of lymphoid neoplasms proposed the terminology of BCL2-R negative, CD23-positive follicle center lymphoma for this lesion [14]. It is likely that this subtype of follicle center lymphoma is suitable for different management approaches [15].

B-cell lymphomas of follicle cell derivation occurring in young patients differ from those in adults. These include pediatric type FL, testicular FL and large B-cell lymphoma with IRF4 rearrangement [16]. Pediatric type FL (PTFL) has a low level of genomic complexity. Aberrations in MAP2K1 and 1p36/TNFRSF14 are the most common genetic changes in PTFL, each observed in 30–70% of the cases [17,18]. A recurrent loss-of-function mutation in IRF8, a tumor suppressor gene, was also reported more recently [19]. Recent work has shown that PTFL and the pediatric variant of nodal marginal zone lymphoma (PMZL) are morphological variants with a common molecular profile [19]. These cases typically present with localized disease, Stage I, and recurrence following simple surgical excision is rare. It is important to distinguish these cases from more aggressive B-cell lymphomas in young patients, as the management is entirely different [20].

IRF4 large B-cell lymphoma most commonly presents in young patients (Figures 1 and 4) with involvement of tonsil and Waldeyer's ring. In contrast to PTFL, which is mainly seen in young boys, IRF4 large B-cell lymphoma is seen equally in males and females. These cases can be follicular or diffuse and show co-expression of MUM1 associated with IRF4 rearrangement, are BCL6 positive and often CD10 positive. They are of germinal center B-cell derivation; and have a relatively good prognosis in contrast to other forms of diffuse large B-cell lymphoma seen in young patients [1,16,21].

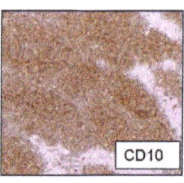
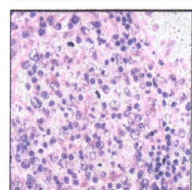

Pediatric type FL: Nodal, Usually Head and Neck, Stage I
M >>F; >10:1   CD10+, BCL6+, BCL2-, MUM1-
Mutations in *TNFRSF14*; loss of 1p36
Mutations in *MAP2K1* and MAPK pathway genes

IRF4 large B-cell lymphoma: Tonsil/ Waldeyer's ring;
May be follicular or diffuse; M=F
Co-expression of MUM1, BCL6, often CD10
Frequent *IRF4* breaks, FISH may be negative due to cryptic rearrangements

Testicular: Stage I, good prognosis
ChemoRx not required
CD10+, BCL6+, BCL2-, MUM-
Occasional BCL6 breaks

Figure 4. Follicular Lymphomas (FL) in young patients (<30 years) include pediatric type FL, IRF4 large B-cell lymphoma, testicular FL. Modified and adapted from Liu Q et al. [16].

Finally, there is testicular follicular lymphoma, which is a rare condition seen in young boys; these patients have a very good prognosis and in the vast majority of cases appear to be cured by simple orchiectomy [22,23]. Systemic chemotherapy is not required.

Another rare form of FL is primary cutaneous follicular lymphoma (Figure 1). It is negative for BCL2 rearrangement and negative for CD10 and has some of the genetic alterations that are observed in pediatric type FL with 1p36 deletions and mutations in TNFSR14. However, it is negative for most of the genetic alterations seen in classic nodal FL. This is an indolent disease that should be managed conservatively. However, if there is evidence of BCL2-R or BCL2 protein expressed, clinical evaluation is suggested to rule out secondary cutaneous involvement from a systemic FL [24–26].

In conclusion, FL is not a single disease but is a family of tumors derived from follicle center B cells. The therapeutic options vary widely from aggressive therapy to a minimal intervention.

3. Diffuse Large B-Cell Lymphoma NOS and Aggressive B-Cell Lymphomas

Historically DLBCL was separated based on the cytological appearance in routine H&E–stained sections. The two most common variants were centroblastic and immunoblastic. We now recognize that DLBCLs are a complex group of aggressive B-cell lymphomas [4]. Figure 5 shows a chart that outlines the major subtypes of aggressive B-cell lymphomas at the time of the 2016 WHO classification [3], which recommended the segregation of ABC and GCB derived diffuse large B-cell lymphoma, and the recognition of high-grade B-cell lymphomas with double hit. The most common and well characterized form of "double hit" lymphoma, is a tumor that has translocations involving BCL2 and c-MYC. Some of these tumors represent progression from follicular lymphoma. In addition, not all cases with a double hit involving MYC and BCL2 are detected by FISH. By gene expression profiling the identification of a double hit signature can uncover double hit high grade B cell lymphomas with genetic events that are cryptic to FISH analysis [27].

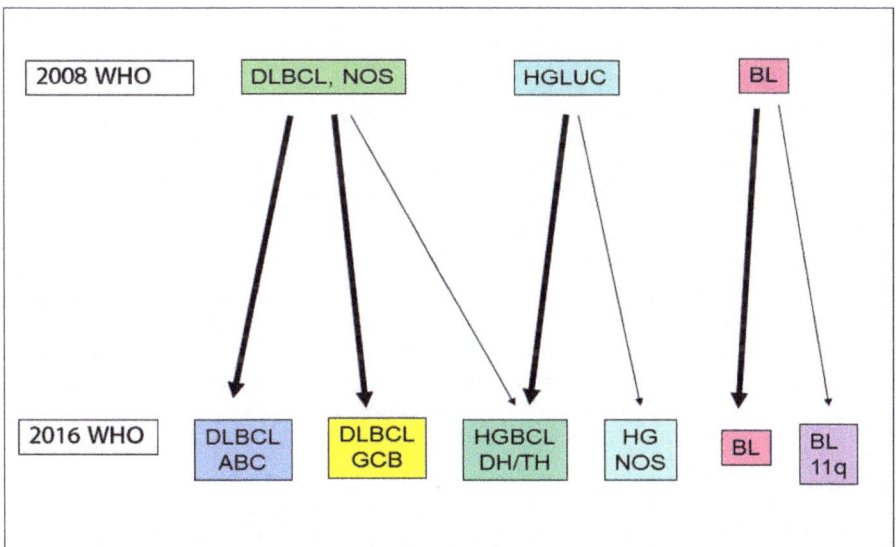

Figure 5. Aggressive B-cell lymphomas. Modified and adapted from Swerdlow et al. [3].

In 2017 the WHO bluebook also identified a rare variant of aggressive lymphoma, seen mainly in young patients, and most often presenting with nodal disease. This tumor was included as a provisional entity and the term "Burkitt-like lymphoma with 11q aberration" was proposed [28]. More recent studies have shown that these tumors lack the common mutational findings of Burkitt lymphoma, are more correctly considered a variant of GCB derived diffuse large B-cell lymphoma [29,30]. In the recently published report from the International Consensus Committee, the term large B-cell lymphoma with 11q aberration is offered as the preferred nomenclature for this lesion [14]. While clinically aggressive, it is not included among the "high-grade" B-cell lymphomas.

Figure 6 shows a flow chart for the diagnosis of aggressive B-cell lymphomas that provides a model for current clinical practice. The first step is biopsy of lymph node or extranodal lesion. At this stage one should consider any one of a group of specific entities, such as such as primary mediastinal large B-cell lymphoma, EBV positive large B-cell lymphoma and HHV8/KSHV associated lymphomas. FISH is still important to recognize high grade B-cell lymphomas with double hit and represents a valuable tool in the clinical setting.

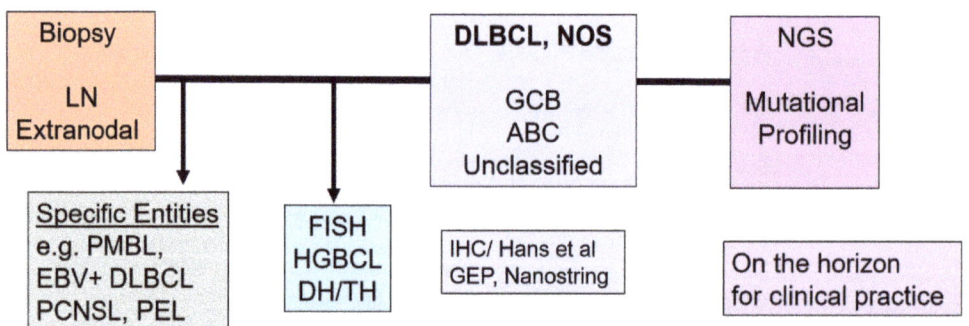

Figure 6. Flow Chart for the Diagnosis of Aggressive B-cell Lymphomas.

It is controversial as to whether aggressive B-cell lymphomas with dual translocations involving MYC and BCL6 should be retained in the "double hit" category [31,32]. These cases are heterogeneous at the gene expression level, and do not appear to have the very aggressive clinical behavior of the classic double hit lymphomas with MYC and BCL2. Further study of such cases is warranted to determine their proper place in the classification of aggressive B-cell lesions [14].

A new era is emerging with NGS and mutational profiling. This technology is on the horizon for clinical practice, although not currently required for the routine diagnosis of diffuse large B-cell lymphoma. However, there are many clinical settings in which NGS is commonly used in clinical practice.

Two major studies in the last few years showed that there is genetic heterogeneity in diffuse large B-cell lymphoma and that this heterogeneity can identify clinically significant genetic subgroups [33,34]. Variations in prognosis based on the mutational profile could be shown. The subtype termed MCD is based on the co-occurrence of the L265P mutation in MYD88 and mutations in CD79B. This subtype is highly enriched in primary central nervous system lymphoma, testicular diffuse large B-cell lymphoma, and other aggressive extranodal diffuse large B-cell lymphomas. The ICC group discussed the option of creating a separate category for extranodal DLBCL but deferred taking this step for the present time [14]. The subtype designated as BN2 is based on fusions involving BCL6 and mutations in NOTCH2. This subtype is heterogeneous in its gene expression profile and may represent an aggressive variant of marginal zone lymphoma. The prognosis of the BN2 group seems to be somewhat better than many of the other forms of diffuse large B-cell lymphoma [34]. Thus, it might represent marginal zone lymphoma with increased transformed cells.

In more recent work, even greater heterogeneity in the molecular classification of diffuse large B-cell lymphoma was observed [35]. New molecular variants were uncovered including a subset of aggressive lymphomas with a high degree of aneuploidy and a high frequency of p53 mutation and deletion [35]. The term A53 refers to these key features: p53 mutation and aneuploidy.

The historical cell of origin approach (ABC or activated B-cell; GCB or germinal center B-cell) for the classification of DLBCL can be integrated in part to the new data derived from genomic profiling based on NGS studies [36]. For example, the EZB and C4 subgroups are related to germinal center B cells. Mutations in EZB are common in germinal center derived neoplasms, including FL. The CD4 cluster, as designated by Chapuy et al. [33] includes the ST2 subset, as recognized by Wright et al. [35]. These cases are characterized by mutations in SGK1 and TET2 (hence ST2) and includes tumors with features of T-cell/histiocyte-rich large B-cell lymphoma related to nodular lymphocyte predominant B-cell lymphoma [14]. Tumors related to activated B-cells (ABC) are more heterogeneous, with the MCD group being a major subset. MCD tumors as noted above are almost always extranodal. N1, with mutations in NOTCH1 is ABC as well. The hope is that these data will be clinically relevant and lead to targeted therapy in the future based on the genetic profile [33,35–38]. A challenge will be to make this technology accessible for routine practice and diagnosis.

4. Pathology Provides a Roadmap for Disease Discovery and Treatment

Disease discovery and disease definition using routine diagnostic tools are critical first steps in elucidating the pathogenesis of lymphomas. Discovery of recurrent genetic alterations have usually followed on the heels of a precise description of the lymphoma entity based on clinical, morphological, or immunophenotypic grounds [39,40]. In other words, it starts with the microscope but insights from genetics, epigenetics, and knowledge of the cellular microenvironment, lead to refinement of diagnostic criteria, and ultimately appropriate therapy.

Author Contributions: E.S.J. designed the work, wrote the manuscript; A.C. wrote the manuscript. All authors have read and agreed to the published version of the manuscript.

Funding: This work was supported by the intramural research budget of the Center for Cancer Research, National Cancer Institute: ZIA SC 000550.

Institutional Review Board Statement: Not applicable.

Informed Consent Statement: Not applicable.

Data Availability Statement: Not applicable.

Conflicts of Interest: The authors declare no conflict of interest.

References

1. Jaffe, E.S.; Harris, N.L.; Swerdlow, S.H.; Ott, G.; Nathwani, B.N.; de Jong, D.; Yoshino, T.; Spagnolo, D.; Gascoyne, R.D. Follicular lymphoma. In *WHO Classification of Tumours of Haematopoietic and Lymphoid Tissues*, 4th ed.; Swerdlow, S.H., Campo, E., Harris, N.L., Jaffe, E.S., Pileri, S.A., Stein, H., Thiele, J., Eds.; IARC Press: Lyon, France, 2017; pp. 266–277.
2. Carbone, A.; Roulland, S.; Gloghini, A.; Younes, A.; von Keudell, G.; López-Guillermo, A.; Fitzgibbon, J. Follicular lymphoma. *Nat. Rev. Dis. Primers* **2019**, *5*, 83. (In English) [CrossRef]
3. Swerdlow, S.H.; Campo, E.; Pileri, S.A.; Harris, N.L.; Stein, H.; Siebert, R.; Advani, R.; Ghielmini, M.; Salles, G.A.; Zelenetz, A.D.; et al. The 2016 revision of the World Health Organization classification of lymphoid neoplasms. *Blood* **2016**, *127*, 2375–2390. (In English) [CrossRef] [PubMed]
4. Gascoyne, R.D.; Chan, J.K.C.; Campo, E.; Rosenwald, A.; Jaffe, E.S.; Stein, H.; Chan, W.C.; Swerdlow, S.H. Diffuse large B-cell lymphoma, NOS. In *WHO Classification of Tumours of Haematopoietic and Lymphoid Tissues*, 4th ed.; IARC, Ed.; IARC Press: Lyon, France, 2017; pp. 291–297.
5. Mamessier, E.; Song, J.Y.; Eberle, F.C.; Pack, S.; Drevet, C.; Chetaille, B.; Abdullaev, Z.; Adelaide, J.; Birnbaum, D.; Chaffanet, M.; et al. Early lesions of follicular lymphoma: A genetic perspective. *Haematologica* **2014**, *99*, 481–488. [CrossRef] [PubMed]
6. Schmidt, J.; Ramis-Zaldivar, J.E.; Bonzheim, I.; Steinhilber, J.; Muller, I.; Haake, A.; Yu, S.C.; Raffeld, M.; Fend, F.; Salaverria, I.; et al. CREBBP gene mutations are frequently detected in in situ follicular neoplasia. *Blood* **2018**, *132*, 2687–2690. (In English) [CrossRef]
7. Jaffe, E.S.; Quintanilla-Martinez, L. t(14;18)-positive B cells: Is it seed or soil? *Blood* **2018**, *132*, 1631–1632. (In English) [CrossRef]
8. Geyer, J.T.; Subramaniyam, S.; Jiang, Y.; Elemento, O.; Ferry, J.A.; de Leval, L.; Nakashima, M.O.; Liu, Y.C.; Martin, P.; Mathew, S.; et al. Lymphoblastic transformation of follicular lymphoma: A clinicopathologic and molecular analysis of 7 patients. *Hum. Pathol.* **2015**, *46*, 260–271. (In English) [CrossRef]
9. Bhavsar, S.; Liu, Y.C.; Gibson, S.E.; Moore, E.M.; Swerdlow, S.H. Mutational Landscape of TdT+ Large B-cell Lymphomas Supports Their Distinction From B-lymphoblastic Neoplasms: A Multiparameter Study of a Rare and Aggressive Entity. *Am. J. Surg. Pathol.* **2022**, *46*, 71–82. (In English) [CrossRef]

10. Feldman, A.L.; Arber, D.A.; Pittaluga, S.; Martinez, A.; Burke, J.S.; Raffeld, M.; Camos, M.; Warnke, R.; Jaffe, E.S. Clonally related follicular lymphomas and histiocytic/dendritic cell sarcomas: Evidence for transdifferentiation of the follicular lymphoma clone. *Blood* 2008, *111*, 5433–5439. (In English) [CrossRef]
11. Egan, C.; Lack, J.; Skarshaug, S.; Pham, T.A.; Abdullaev, Z.; Xi, L.; Pack, S.; Pittaluga, S.; Jaffe, E.S.; Raffeld, M. The mutational landscape of histiocytic sarcoma associated with lymphoid malignancy. *Mod. Pathol.* 2021, *34*, 336–347. (In English) [CrossRef]
12. Shanmugam, V.; Griffin, G.K.; Jacobsen, E.D.; Fletcher, C.D.M.; Sholl, L.M.; Hornick, J.L. Identification of diverse activating mutations of the RAS-MAPK pathway in histiocytic sarcoma. *Mod. Pathol.* 2019, *32*, 830–843. (In English) [CrossRef]
13. Nann, D.; Ramis-Zaldivar, J.E.; Müller, I.; Gonzalez-Farre, B.; Schmidt, J.; Egan, C.; Salmeron-Villalobos, J.; Clot, G.; Mattern, S.; Otto, F.; et al. Follicular lymphoma t(14;18)-negative is genetically a heterogeneous disease. *Blood Adv.* 2020, *4*, 5652–5665. (In English) [CrossRef] [PubMed]
14. Campo, E.; Jaffe, E.S.; Cook, J.R.; Quintanilla-Martinez, L.; Swerdlow, S.H.; Anderson, K.C.; Brousset, P.; Cerroni, L.; de Leval, L.; Dirnhofer, S.; et al. The International Consensus Classification of Mature Lymphoid Neoplasms: A Report from the Clinical Advisory Committee. *Blood*, 2022; in press. (In English). [CrossRef]
15. Katzenberger, T.; Kalla, J.; Leich, E.; Stocklein, H.; Hartmann, E.; Barnickel, S.; Wessendorf, S.; Ott, M.M.; Muller-Hermelink, H.K.; Rosenwald, A.; et al. A distinctive subtype of t(14;18)-negative nodal follicular non-Hodgkin lymphoma characterized by a predominantly diffuse growth pattern and deletions in the chromosomal region 1p36. *Blood* 2009, *113*, 1053–1061. Available online: http://www.ncbi.nlm.nih.gov/entrez/query.fcgi?cmd=Retrieve&db=PubMed&dopt=Citation&list_uids=18978208 (accessed on 1 July 2022). (In English) [PubMed]
16. Liu, Q.; Salaverria, I.; Pittaluga, S.; Jegalian, A.G.; Xi, L.; Siebert, R.; Raffeld, M.; Hewitt, S.M.; Jaffe, E.S. Follicular lymphomas in children and young adults: A comparison of the pediatric variant with usual follicular lymphoma. *Am. J. Surg. Pathol.* 2013, *37*, 333–343. (In English) [CrossRef]
17. Louissaint, A., Jr.; Schafernak, K.T.; Geyer, J.T.; Kovach, A.E.; Ghandi, M.; Gratzinger, D.; Roth, C.G.; Paxton, C.N.; Kim, S.; Namgyal, C.; et al. Pediatric-type nodal follicular lymphoma: A biologically distinct lymphoma with frequent MAPK pathway mutations. *Blood* 2016, *128*, 1093–1100. (In English) [CrossRef] [PubMed]
18. Schmidt, J.; Ramis-Zaldivar, J.E.; Nadeu, F.; Gonzalez-Farre, B.; Navarro, A.; Egan, C.; Montes-Mojarro, I.A.; Marafioti, T.; Cabecadas, J.; van der Walt, J.; et al. Mutations of MAP2K1 are frequent in pediatric-type follicular lymphoma and result in ERK pathway activation. *Blood* 2017, *130*, 323–327. (In English) [CrossRef] [PubMed]
19. Salmeron-Villalobos, J.; Egan, C.; Borgmann, V.; Müller, I.; Gonzalez-Farre, B.; Ramis-Zaldivar, J.E.; Nann, D.; Balagué, O.; Lopez-Guerra, M.; Colomer, D.; et al. PNMZL and PTFL: Morphological variants with a common molecular profile—A unifying hypothesis. *Blood Adv.* 2022; in press. (In English) [CrossRef]
20. Louissaint, A., Jr.; Ackerman, A.M.; Dias-Santagata, D.; Ferry, J.A.; Hochberg, E.P.; Huang, M.S.; Iafrate, A.J.; Lara, D.O.; Plukus, C.S.; Salaverria, I.; et al. Pediatric-type nodal follicular lymphoma: An indolent clonal proliferation in children and adults with high proliferation index and no BCL2 rearrangement. *Blood* 2012, *120*, 2395–2404. (In English) [CrossRef]
21. Ramis-Zaldivar, J.E.; Gonzalez-Farré, B.; Balagué, O.; Celis, V.; Nadeu, F.; Salmerón-Villalobos, J.; Andrés, M.; Martin-Guerrero, I.; Garrido-Pontnou, M.; Gaafar, A.; et al. Distinct molecular profile of IRF4-rearranged large B-cell lymphoma. *Blood* 2020, *135*, 274–286. (In English) [CrossRef]
22. Finn, L.S.; Viswanatha, D.S.; Belasco, J.B.; Snyder, H.; Huebner, D.; Sorbara, L.; Raffeld, M.; Jaffe, E.S.; Salhany, K.E. Primary follicular lymphoma of the testis in childhood. *Cancer* 1999, *85*, 1626–1635. Available online: http://www.ncbi.nlm.nih.gov/pubmed/10193956 (accessed on 1 July 2022).
23. Lones, M.A.; Raphael, M.; McCarthy, K.; Wotherspoon, A.; Terrier-Lacombe, M.J.; Ramsay, A.D.; Maclennan, K.; Cairo, M.S.; Gerrard, M.; Michon, J.; et al. Primary follicular lymphoma of the testis in children and adolescents. *J. Pediatr. Hematol. Oncol.* 2012, *34*, 68–71. (In English) [CrossRef]
24. Barasch, N.J.K.; Liu, Y.C.; Ho, J.; Bailey, N.; Aggarwal, N.; Cook, J.R.; Swerdlow, S.H. The molecular landscape and other distinctive features of primary cutaneous follicle center lymphoma. *Hum. Pathol.* 2020, *106*, 93–105. (In English) [CrossRef]
25. Gángó, A.; Bátai, B.; Varga, M.; Kapczár, D.; Papp, G.; Marschalkó, M.; Kuroli, E.; Schneider, T.; Csomor, J.; Matolcsy, A.; et al. Concomitant 1p36 deletion and TNFRSF14 mutations in primary cutaneous follicle center lymphoma frequently expressing high levels of EZH2 protein. *Virchows Arch.* 2018, *473*, 453–462. (In English) [CrossRef] [PubMed]
26. Lucioni, M.; Fraticelli, S.; Neri, G.; Feltri, M.; Ferrario, G.; Riboni, R.; Paulli, M. Primary Cutaneous B-Cell Lymphoma: An Update on Pathologic and Molecular Features. *Hemato* 2022, *3*, 318–340. Available online: https://www.mdpi.com/2673-6357/3/2/23 (accessed on 1 July 2022).
27. Hilton, L.K.; Tang, J.; Ben-Neriah, S.; Alcaide, M.; Jiang, A.; Grande, B.M.; Rushton, C.K.; Boyle, M.; Meissner, B.; Scott, D.W.; et al. The double-hit signature identifies double-hit diffuse large B-cell lymphoma with genetic events cryptic to FISH. *Blood* 2019, *134*, 1528–1532. (In English) [CrossRef] [PubMed]
28. Salaverria, I.; Martin-Guerrero, I.; Wagener, R.; Kreuz, M.; Kohler, C.W.; Richter, J.; Pienkowska-Grela, B.; Adam, P.; Burkhardt, B.; Claviez, A.; et al. A recurrent 11q aberration pattern characterizes a subset of MYC-negative high-grade B-cell lymphomas resembling Burkitt lymphoma. *Blood* 2014, *123*, 1187–1198. (In English) [CrossRef]
29. Gonzalez-Farre, B.; Ramis-Zaldivar, J.E.; Salmeron-Villalobos, J.; Balagué, O.; Celis, V.; Verdu-Amoros, J.; Nadeu, F.; Sábado, C.; Ferrández, A.; Garrido, M.; et al. Burkitt-like lymphoma with 11q aberration: A germinal center-derived lymphoma genetically unrelated to Burkitt lymphoma. *Haematologica* 2019, *104*, 1822–1829. (In English) [CrossRef]

30. Wagener, R.; Seufert, J.; Raimondi, F.; Bens, S.; Kleinheinz, K.; Nagel, I.; Altmuller, J.; Thiele, H.; Hubschmann, D.; Kohler, C.W.; et al. The mutational landscape of Burkitt-like lymphoma with 11q aberration is distinct from that of Burkitt lymphoma. *Blood* **2019**, *133*, 962–966. (In English) [CrossRef]
31. Moore, E.M.; Aggarwal, N.; Surti, U.; Swerdlow, S.H. Further Exploration of the Complexities of Large B-Cell Lymphomas with MYC Abnormalities and the Importance of a Blastoid Morphology. *Am. J. Surg. Pathol.* **2017**, *41*, 1155–1166. (In English) [CrossRef]
32. Pillai, R.K.; Sathanoori, M.; Van Oss, S.B.; Swerdlow, S.H. Double-hit B-cell lymphomas with BCL6 and MYC translocations are aggressive, frequently extranodal lymphomas distinct from BCL2 double-hit B-cell lymphomas. *Am. J. Surg. Pathol.* **2013**, *37*, 323–332. (In English) [CrossRef]
33. Chapuy, B.; Stewart, C.; Dunford, A.J.; Kim, J.; Kamburov, A.; Redd, R.A.; Lawrence, M.S.; Roemer, M.G.M.; Li, A.J.; Ziepert, M.; et al. Molecular subtypes of diffuse large B cell lymphoma are associated with distinct pathogenic mechanisms and outcomes. *Nat. Med.* **2018**, *24*, 679–690. (In English) [CrossRef]
34. Schmitz, R.; Wright, G.W.; Huang, D.W.; Johnson, C.A.; Phelan, J.D.; Wang, J.Q.; Roulland, S.; Kasbekar, M.; Young, R.M.; Shaffer, A.L.; et al. Genetics and Pathogenesis of Diffuse Large B-Cell Lymphoma. *N. Engl. J. Med.* **2018**, *378*, 1396–1407. (In English) [CrossRef]
35. Wright, G.W.; Huang, D.W.; Phelan, J.D.; Coulibaly, Z.A.; Roulland, S.; Young, R.M.; Wang, J.Q.; Schmitz, R.; Morin, R.D.; Tang, J.; et al. A Probabilistic Classification Tool for Genetic Subtypes of Diffuse Large B Cell Lymphoma with Therapeutic Implications. *Cancer Cell* **2020**, *37*, 551–568.e514. (In English) [CrossRef] [PubMed]
36. Ennishi, D.; Hsi, E.D.; Steidl, C.; Scott, D.W. Toward a New Molecular Taxonomy of Diffuse Large B-cell Lymphoma. *Cancer Discov.* **2020**, *10*, 1267–1281. [CrossRef] [PubMed]
37. Lacy, S.E.; Barrans, S.L.; Beer, P.A.; Painter, D.; Smith, A.G.; Roman, E.; Cooke, S.L.; Ruiz, C.; Glover, P.; Van Hoppe, S.J.L.; et al. Targeted sequencing in DLBCL, molecular subtypes, and outcomes: A Haematological Malignancy Research Network report. *Blood* **2020**, *135*, 1759–1771. (In English) [CrossRef] [PubMed]
38. Sha, C.; Barrans, S.; Cucco, F.; Bentley, M.A.; Care, M.A.; Cummin, T.; Kennedy, H.; Thompson, J.S.; Uddin, R.; Worrillow, L.; et al. Molecular High-Grade B-Cell Lymphoma: Defining a Poor-Risk Group That Requires Different Approaches to Therapy. *J. Clin. Oncol.* **2019**, *37*, 202–212. (In English) [CrossRef]
39. Jaffe, E.S.; Harris, N.L.; Stein, H.; Isaacson, P.G. Classification of lymphoid neoplasms: The microscope as a tool for disease discovery. *Blood* **2008**, *112*, 4384–4399. (In English) [CrossRef]
40. Carbone, A. Classification of Tumors of the Hematopoietic and Lymphoid Tissues. Discovering Diseases—Defining Their Features. *Hemato* **2020**, *1*, 7–9. Available online: https://www.mdpi.com/2673-6357/1/1/4 (accessed on 1 July 2022).

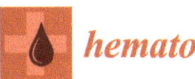 hemato · MDPI

Review

The Era of Genomic Research for Lymphoma: Looking Back and Forward

Wing C. Chan [1,*] and Javeed Iqbal [2]

[1] Department of Pathology, City of Hope National Medical Center, Duarte, CA 91101, USA
[2] Department of Pathology and Microbiology, University of Nebraska Medical Center, Omaha, NE 68198, USA
* Correspondence: jochan@coh.org

Abstract: Technological and informatics advances as well as the availability of well-annotated and reliable genomic data have ushered in the era of genomics research. We describe in this brief review how the genomics approach has impacted lymphoma research in the understanding of the pathogenesis and biology of lymphoma, in lymphoma diagnosis and in targeted therapy. Some exciting directions that could be explored in the future are also discussed.

Keywords: lymphoma; gene expression profiling; genetics; tumor microenvironment; diagnostics

Citation: Chan, W.C.; Iqbal, J. The Era of Genomic Research for Lymphoma: Looking Back and Forward. *Hemato* **2022**, *3*, 485–507. https://doi.org/10.3390/hemato3030034

Academic Editors: Alina Nicolae and Antonino Carbone

Received: 26 May 2022
Accepted: 29 July 2022
Published: 15 August 2022

Publisher's Note: MDPI stays neutral with regard to jurisdictional claims in published maps and institutional affiliations.

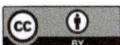

Copyright: © 2022 by the authors. Licensee MDPI, Basel, Switzerland. This article is an open access article distributed under the terms and conditions of the Creative Commons Attribution (CC BY) license (https://creativecommons.org/licenses/by/4.0/).

1. Introduction

Traditionally, laboratory research in cancers has been focused on hypothesis-driven investigation based on prior observations or experimental findings. With technological and informatics advances, it became possible to measure gene expression on a transcriptomic scale in the mid to late 1990s [1–4]. This raised the exciting possibility of measuring the gene expression profile of lymphomas and identifying the differences among different types of lymphomas and their putative normal counterparts, leading to a better understanding of the biology and pathogenesis of different types of lymphomas and perhaps a classification that is more biologically based. Initially, there was some skepticism regarding the accuracy and reproducibility of these global measurements and hence the usefulness of this approach [5–9]. However, with further refinement of the technology and analytical approaches and more experience gained in this type of study, it is now clear that this is a reliable, powerful approach that can lead to rapid advances in many aspects of lymphoma investigation and diagnosis [10,11].

Another major initiative starting at the beginning of this century is the sequencing of the human genome [12,13]. Only recently has the human genome sequence been completed [12], but the availability of drafts and near-complete versions has enabled and greatly enhanced various aspects of genomic research [14]. As neoplastic transformation is based on genetic alterations, it is important to identify key driver changes that contribute to the perturbation in gene expression. Moreover, with the human genome better characterized, it was possible to correct some of the annotation errors in the various array-based GEP platforms. One of the first applications of the human genome sequence was the study of genomic copy number abnormalities (gCNAs) which represented a major advance over the traditional comparative genomic hybridization [15–20]. Furthermore, as the sequence and location of the vast majority of coding genes, pseudogenes and non-coding sequences are known, it greatly facilities related genetic research that can utilize and build upon this known structural and sequence information.

The more recent development of next-generation sequencing has revolutionized genomic research and allowed individual laboratories to conduct cutting-edge research previously in the domain of genome centers. A vast array of genetic, epigenetic, transcriptomic, interactomic and other more specific investigations can be performed, frequently in collaboration with institutional core facilities. In this communication, how lymphoma research has been impacted in this omics age will be briefly reviewed, drawing mostly from the experience of a consortium of investigators in the Lymphoma/Leukemia Molecular Profiling Project (LLMPP) and their collaborators. Potential exciting developments with major implications on future research will also be discussed.

2. Gene Expression Profiling (GEP) Analysis
2.1. Diffuse Large B-Cell Lymphomas (DLBCLs)

GEP performed in a microarray format was developed in the 1990s. The probes on the array may consist of cDNA fragments or oligonucleotides [21–23]. Both of these may be spotted on the array, but oligonucleotides may also be synthesized in situ [24,25]. The initial arrays were generally not transcriptome-wide, but later commercial arrays such as the Affymetrix U133 arrays are close to whole transcriptome, and commercial arrays also tend to be more reproducibly manufactured with standard operating procedures and hence more comparable among studies than institution/lab-based ones [4]. The earliest microarray analysis of lymphoma was based on a cDNA array platform and is significant in demonstrating that different lymphoid malignancies tend to form unique clusters [26] (Figure 1). Furthermore, in diffuse large B-cell lymphomas (DLBCLs), two distinct clusters could be identified with one of them expressing many germinal center (GC) B-cell associated transcripts and hence having a GC B-cell differentiation program. The other cluster did not express the GC B-cell signature but expressed many transcripts associated with in vitro B-cell activation. The former was named GC B-cell like (GCB)-DLBCL, and the latter activated B-cell like (ABC)-DLBCL, which had worse survival independent of the international prognostic index (IPI) [26]. The findings were later confirmed in a follow-up study with a larger number of cases [27]. There was a group of cases that could not be classified into these two subtypes, initially called group 3, which was not a specific entity but a rather heterogeneous group of cases including some with low tumor content that precluded classification into the GCB or ABC subgroups. These earlier studies were performed on patients treated with CHOP chemotherapy, but a subsequent study on Rituximab (R)-CHOP treated patients confirmed that the ABC group has worse outcomes, even with R-CHOP treatment [28]. Since these two subtypes of cases have been validated to be biologically distinct and have different clinical outcomes [29], attempts have been made to reproduce the GEP-based classification with immunohistochemical (IHC) stains that can be readily performed on FFPE tissue and thus are applicable to routine clinical settings. The first published one, the "Hans algorithm", divided DLBCL into GCB and non-GCB (contained mostly ABC cases) subtypes based on three immunostains (CD10, BCL6 and MUM1) with a concordance rate to GEP-classified cases of >80% and demonstrated the more favorable prognosis of the GCB subtype [30]. The reproducibility of this algorithm has been quite variable with some laboratories unable to demonstrate a prognostic difference between GCB and non-GCB types. This may be related to the differences in the staining protocol, scoring, number of patients studied and even the composition of the patient populations. Several other IHC-based classification algorithms have been proposed, but the above-mentioned factors may still be major limitations [31,32]. A more recent attempt was made to transfer the original array-based diagnostic algorithm to another simpler transcript-based platform. The original diagnostic signature was condensed to 15 parameters with the assay performed on the NanoString platform [33]. This resulted in an assay with over 90% concordance with the original diagnosis, and the platform is highly reproducible in different laboratories [33].

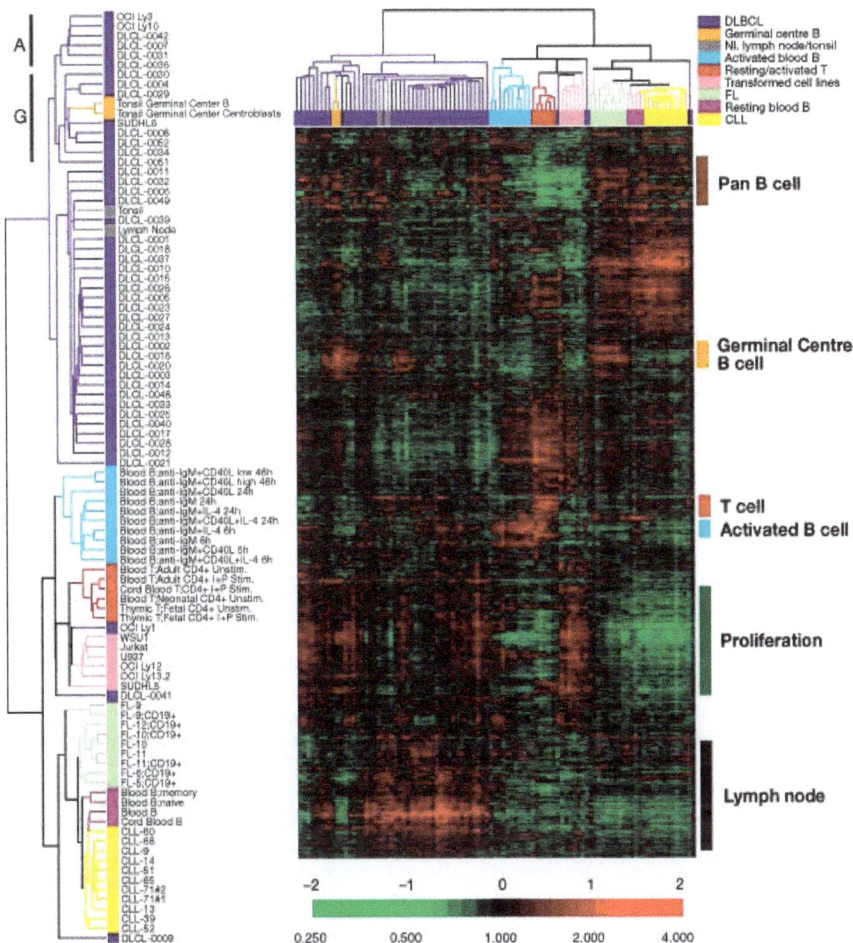

Figure 1. Hierarchical clustering of GEP data. Different lymphoid malignancies form distinct clusters based on their gene expression profile. Reproduced from Figure 1: Alizadeh AA et al. *Nature* volume 403, pages 503–511 (2000).

Several studies with global miRNA analysis demonstrated distinct miRNA signatures associated with DLBCL subtypes [34,35] and identified predictive miRNA biomarkers in DLBCL, including high expression of miR-155 and miRNA-363 [36], which is significantly associated with R-CHOP failure. miRNA-based studies are fewer than mRNA-based studies partly because of the rather late entry of miRNA into the field when many seminal studies were already reported. The advantage of using miRNA is the stability of the molecules and their good preservation in FFPE tissues.

The initial GEP studies were performed on DLBCL-NOS cases [26–28,37]. There are many other DLBCL subtypes that occur at rather low frequencies and likely have different biology and hence unique GE signatures. Some of these have been studied by GEP and demonstrated interesting findings. Among these is primary mediastinal large B-cell lymphoma (PMBL), which unexpectedly exhibited a signature similar to that of Hodgkin lymphoma (HL) cell lines [38,39]. It also characteristically had JAK/STAT pathway, IL13 and IL4, and NK-κB pathway activation [40]. Interestingly, later genetic studies also indicated overlaps of genetic alterations between these two diseases [41,42]. There is a study that examined the presence of PMBL signature in a series of "non-mediastinal DLBCL" with GEP studies [43]. A more detailed analysis of the clinical/radiological data indicated that most of the cases with this signature had evidence of mediastinal disease and morphology compatible with PMBL, indicating that the lymphoma most likely originated from the mediastinum, but there were rare cases with no apparent mediastinal involvement, suggesting that there may be PMBL-like DLBCL without clinical and radiological evidence of mediastinal disease. Most of the other types of DLBCL studied are non-GCB tumors with similarity to the ABC subtype (such as primary CNS, testicular, CD5+ and cutaneous diffuse large B-cell lymphoma-Leg type) or with more plasmablastic features (plasmablastic lymphoma and primary effusion lymphoma) [44–52].

There have been numerous attempts at identifying prognostically important biomarkers with the current standard R-CHOP therapy independent of the IPI [53,54]. Most of the single-parameter prognosticators described have not been reproducible. TP53 mutation [55], BCL2 expression in GCB-DLBCL [56] and high BCL2 expression in the ABC-DLBCL [57,58] appeared to be associated with worse outcome. It should be noted that BCL2 expression is controlled by different mechanisms in these two types of DLBCL. BCL2 expression is mainly associated with BCL2 rearrangement in the GCB-DLBCL while in ABC-DLBCL, it is regulated by NF-κB activation and/or 18q21 gain or amplification [57]. GEP-based prognosticators have also been developed including the one published by the LLMPP group [28]. These signatures still need to be independently validated and perhaps also examined in the context of genetic profiles, as discussed later.

2.2. Other B-Cell Lymphomas

Mantle cell lymphoma (MCL) was found to have a unique GEP that included high expression of cyclin D1 as expected, but also some transcripts not generally expressed in normal B-cells such as SOX11 [59]. Interestingly, there were some cases with strong MCL signature but lacking cyclin D1 expression and translocation. It was suspected that these cases may be initiated by translocation associated with other cyclin molecules, some of which were found to be overexpressed [60]. This is indeed the case as demonstrated by translocations involving cyclin D2 and cryptic insertion of Ig light chain enhancers near CCND2 and D3 [61]. The expression of SOX11 in classical MCL and also in these cyclin D1 negative cases makes it a useful marker for diagnosis [62]. A key prognosticator for MCL is the proliferation signature [62], and based on this finding, an assay (MCL35) has been developed using the NanoString platform that can be applied to FFPE tissues. This assay could be more objective and reproducible than the counting of Ki67 positive tumor cells in histological sections [63]. A unique group of MCL with indolent clinical course, non-nodal disease with blood involvement, small cell morphology and SOX11 negativity have been identified and under active investigation [64]. Aside from GEP studies, miRNA profiling studies also revealed a 19-miRNA classifier that was able to distinguish MCL from other B-cell lymphomas [65], and MCL patients with high expression of miRNAs from the polycistronic miR17-92 cluster and its prologues, miR-106a-363 and miR-106b-25, were associated with high proliferation gene signature and poor clinical outcome in further correlative observation [65].

Burkitt lymphoma (BL) with classical morphology, MYC rearrangement and IHC profile is generally readily distinguishable from other aggressive B-cell lymphomas [66]. There are, however, cases with more atypical features that makes it challenging to diagnose. Several groups, including LLMPP, had tried to derive a BL diagnostic signature that is highly sensitive and specific [67,68]. BL characteristically has a high MYC signature as expected, and a low level of expression of major-histocompatibility-complex class I genes and the NF-κB signature. It does express a GCB cell signature enriched in a subset of genes related to the dark zone of the GC [67,69]. The dark zone of the GC is normally largely devoid of MYC expression, but in the presence of MYC translocation, both a GC dark zone and a MYC signature are observed. However, even with GEP analysis, there are still cases that are difficult to classify. The utility of miRNA profiling has been studied, and BL also has a unique profile that can help distinguish it from DLBCL [34]. It is unclear whether combining these signatures would improve the diagnostic performance. Interestingly, the GEP signatures of pediatric and adult BL show remarkable similarity.

2.3. Follicular Lymphoma (FL) and Transformed FL (t-FL)

FL is a GC B cell-derived lymphoma and is therefore expected to express the GC B cell signature, which is clearly the case for the major group of FL with t(14;18) [70]. Higher grade cases tended to have a higher proliferation signature [71]. For the t(14;18) negative cases, there is an enrichment of ABC-like, NF-κB, post-GCB and T-cell signature [72,73]. Proliferation and cell cycle signatures also tend to be higher, which may be related to the observation of the frequent Grade 3A morphology in this type of FL. There is further heterogeneity within the t(14;18) negative group, such as pediatric-type FL, testicular FL and primary cutaneous follicular center lymphoma, that has been described and will not be further discussed here [74]. In the study by Dave et al. on prognosticators in FL, stromal signatures appear to be predictive of outcome [75]. There are generally many FL subclones in individual patients, and the clonal composition of the biopsied LN might be quite different from other lymphoma sites. It is possible the clone(s) that ultimately determine prognosis may not be well represented in the sample studied. This may explain why no specific tumor-related signature was identified as prognostic. The host response to the FL could be more uniform, and unique stromal responses could thus be more readily identified as prognosticators [76]. In the Dave study, factors specifically predictive of transformation were not investigated [75]. However, a gene expression signature predictive of FL prognosis when treated with R-CHOP was recently generated for tumor biopsies at the time of diagnosis [77]. In addition, miRNA studies identified upregulation of miR-193a-5p, 193b* and 663 downregulation of miR-17*, -30a, -33a, -106a) in FL [78] and a miRNAs profile associated with t(14;18) negative cases [79].

2.4. Peripheral T-Cell Lymphoma (PTCL)

PTCL constitutes only ~10–15% of all non-Hodgkin's lymphoma (NHL) in Western countries [80,81]. The current World Health Organization (WHO) classification recognizes many distinct PTCL subtypes, including angioimmunoblastic T-cell lymphoma (AITL), anaplastic large cell lymphoma (ALCL), adult T-cell leukemia/lymphoma (ATLL) and extra-nodal NK/T-cell lymphoma of nasal type (ENKTL) [74] as well as additional rare PTCLs that are mostly extra-nodal lymphomas [74]. Even for expert hematopathologists, the diagnosis and subtyping of PTCL is challenging [74,82], and 30–50% of PTCL cases are not classifiable with current approaches and are categorized as PTCL, not otherwise specified (PTCL-NOS) [74]. Thus, PTCL-NOS represents the most common group of PTCL with a broad morphological and immunophenotypic spectrum that does not correspond to any of the distinct T-cell entities in the WHO classification [83,84].

The study and understanding of the biology of PTCL has lagged behind that of their B-cell counterpart partly because of the relative rarity of PTCL [85]. A number of GEP studies have been reported for PTCL, but the number of cases is generally small and conclusions from these studies need to be validated [86–92]. Through extensive international collaborations, it was possible to perform several larger GEP studies on PTCL that led to the definition of robust molecular signatures for major subtypes of PTCL [93–95]. It validated previous reports suggesting a link between AITL and TFH cells [90,92]. Importantly, two novel biological and prognostic subgroups within PTCL-NOS with distinct GEP signatures were identified [95]. One subgroup, representing about a third of PTCL-NOS, is characterized by high expression of GATA3 and its target genes. GATA3 is the master transcriptional regulator in TH2 cell differentiation and regulates interleukin-4 (IL-4), IL-5 and IL-13 expression [96]. The other subgroup, representing about half of PTCL-NOS, has high expression of *TBX21* and its target genes. *TBX21* is a master regulator of TH1 cell differentiation and regulates the expression of IFNγ [97]. The "high GATA3" subgroup (designated as PTCL-GATA3) had poorer clinical outcomes, supported by an independent study [98]. The PTCL-GATA3 group had higher MYC and proliferation signatures, whereas NF-κB targets were enriched in the TBX21 subgroup. Further examination of the "TBX21" subgroup (designated as PTCL-TBX21) identifies a subset with a high cytotoxic signature including the expression of CD8 and cytotoxic molecules such as perforin, granzyme B, TIA1 and others. These cases have a poorer clinical outcome than the rest of the PTCL-TBX21 subgroup and may represent a separate cytotoxic subgroup of PTCL [94,95]. While these studies suggest the "cell-of-origin" of different subgroups of PTCL, it is unclear whether the tumors are derived from a certain subtype of T cells, or whether different genetic changes initiating/promoting the transformation may favor the polarization of the lymphocytes to a certain lineage. It is also uncertain how stable are the phenotypes and whether further genetic changes or the cytokine environment may re-polarize the cells either partially or completely due to the plasticity of T-cell differentiation [99]. There are little data on relapsed PTCL to address some of these questions.

While activation of distinct oncogenic pathways in these subgroups [94,95,100] and the observed clinical differences support the validity of the classification, recent genetic analysis including high-resolution genomic copy number abnormalities (gCNA) [101], and mutational analysis and even miRNA analysis [102], provided further evidence that PTCL-GATA3 and -TBX21 subgroups represent distinct diseases and exploit distinct genetic pathways for tumorigenesis [101], which will be elaborated on further in later sections.

Attempts have been made to use routine IHC assays to help to separate these two subtypes of PTCL, and it is possible to have a good concordance of around 80% with molecular classification using four immunostains (GATA3, CCR4, TBX21 and CXCR12) [103]. As IHC staining and scoring may not be readily standardized, a more objective and quantitative assay with high reproducibility is preferred. An assay based on the previous microarray data and adapted to the NanoString platform has been recently developed that can be performed using FFPE tissues and thus could be utilized in routinely processed biopsy materials [104]. This assay could benefit the classification of PTCL in clinical practice as well as in clinical trials for accurate stratification of patients.

Similar to B-cell lymphomas, GEP generates data that can be used for biological pathway and signature analysis, some of which could be correlated with clinical outcome or suggest response to targeted therapy. Thus, in ENKTCL, there is evidence for the activation of the aurora kinase A (AURKA) pathway and potential efficacy of a AURKAi [93,105,106]. A more extensive in vitro drug screening study independently confirmed that AURKAi was active against NK-lymphoma cell lines [107]. High NF-κB activation has been associated with worse prognosis in ALCL [108], while in AITL, a high B-cell signature is associated with better prognosis and a high macrophage/dendritic cell signature was associated with poorer outcome [94,95]. In the TBX21 PTCL, there is an inverse correlation between B-cell and cytotoxic signature and high B-cell signature is associated with better prognosis [95] while the reverse is true for the cytotoxic signature.

3. Global Genetic Analysis

The International Human Genome Sequencing Consortium announced on 14 April 2003, the successful completion of the Human Genome Project, and the sequence was published next year in *Nature* [13,109,110]. While the human genome was not completely sequenced and assembled until recently [12], the publication was an important landmark that ushered in the era of large-scale genomic research. The initial and subsequent cumulative published data on the human genome provide the information that has enabled numerous investigations to move forward. Subsequent development of massive parallel sequencing technology allows next generation sequencing (NGS) to be done in many facilities outside of the genome centers and further enables the rapid growth of genome-based research.

3.1. The Study of Genomic Copy Number Abnormalities (gCNAs)

One of the first applications in lymphoma research based on human genomic data is the study of genomic copy number abnormalities (gCNAs) that could be done using either SNP arrays or oligonucleotide arrays. A study by Lenz et al. on DLBCL revealed the common gCNAs and highlighted the different profiles between GCB and ABC DLBCL [111]. The simultaneous availability of GEP data further facilitated the identification of the potential driver genes associated with each of the gCNAs [111] such as *PRDM1* in 6q21 deletion, *BCL2*, *MALT1* and *TCF4* in 18q21 gain/amplification [112], *c-REL* and *BCL11A* in 2p14-16 gain/amplification. The selective requirement of a potential candidate genes to specific molecular subgroups could also be shown experimentally by the selective cytotoxic effect of knocking down of *SPIB* [19q telomeric gain/amp] [111] in ABC-DLBCL cell lines but not to GCB-DLBCL cell lines. Additionally, certain gCNAs or combinations appeared to be associated with prognosis as exemplified by the association with poor prognosis in ABC-DLBCL with del 9p21 (*CDKN2A and 2B*) and trisomy-3 [111]. Some common translocations also have differential distribution in the subtypes of DLBCL, such as the almost exclusive presence of *BCL2* translocation in GCB-DLCBL [113], and the more frequent *BCL6* translocation in ABC-DLBCL [114]. Methylation analysis also demonstrated distinct abnormal profiles in these two subtypes [115].

Several genome-wide DNA copy number studies on MCL identified recurrent deletions of tumor-suppressor genes, including TP53 (17p21), ATM (11q), RB1 (13q14.2) and CDKN2A, CDKN2B, MTAP (9p21.3), which provided insights into various deregulated pathways such as DNA damage repair (ATM) and cell cycle (TP53, RB1 and CDKN2A, CDKN2B) [116–118]. Somatic mutation and deletions/hypermethylation of TNFAIP3 (6q23.3) leading to NF-κB pathway activation have been observed [119,120]. Similarly, methylation analysis revealed a hypo-methylated genome in MCL; however, a subset of tumors with extensive CpG methylation, as well as an increased proliferation signature, were associated with poor prognosis [121]. Targeting the epigenome or specific aberrantly expressed genes (such as CD37) could be novel therapeutic options in MCL [122].

The genomic alteration in BL is generally much less complex compared with DLBCL, with far fewer numbers of gCNAs. In addition to the t(8;14) translocation or variant t(8;22) or t(2;8) translocations, BLs show recurrent gains involving a small locus in 13q31.3 encoding the miR17-92 cluster, recurrent gains of 1q localized to a minimal common region at 1q21.1 and 1q31.3, and frequent loss of 17p [123,124]; however, other observations are less consistent among studies [125,126]. Genomic aberrations (e.g., del13q14, del17p, gain8q24, and gain18q21) and effectors of chronic BCR–> NF-κB signaling were more associated with adult-mBL, and gain/amplification of MIR17HG and its paralogue are particularly frequent (present in 50%). BLs may be associated with EBV infection, particularly in those arising in endemic regions (>90%); recent studies have demonstrated differences in GEP as well as genetic landscape in EBV+ cases [127,128], notably the higher mutation burden due to increased AICDA activities but lower frequency of mutation in TP53, USP7 and TCF3/ID3 [129].

FL is associated with recurrent genetic alterations including chromosomal gains (7, 12, 18 and X) and deletions (6q and 1p) [130–134] and further refined to genetic loci del of 1p36.33-p36.31, 6q23.3-q24.1 and 10q23.1-q25.1 and gains of 2p16.1-p15, 8q24.13-q24.3 and 12q12-q13.13 with higher resolution techniques [135]. The transformation to aggressive lymphoma [136] is rarely associated with c-MYC rearrangement [136], but no specific changes are unique to transformation, although some genetic changes have been reported to be associated with transformation, including mutation of *p53* [137] and *BCL2* [138] and homozygous *9p21* deletions [139], and gains of 3q27.3-q28, 6p12-p21 and 17q21.33 [140]. Overall, genetic abnormalities associated with transformation impair immune surveillance, activate the NF-κB pathway and deregulate the cell cycle and B-cell transcription factors [135,141]. Of special interest are mutations and CNAs affecting S1P-activated pathways, which likely regulate lymphoma cell migration and survival outside of follicles [141]. Global methylation profiling of sequential FL and transformed-FL biopsies revealed a hypermethylated genome common to FL, and an over-representation of genes targeted for epigenetic repression by PRC2 within the hypermethylated gene set. Along with the similarity in hypermethylation pattern between paired biopsies, this suggested that the widespread methylation observed may represent an early event in lymphomagenesis [142].

3.2. Mutation Analysis: Example on DLBCL

Several driver mutations were identified before the era of NGS in DLBCL, such as *CD79b* affecting BCR signaling [143], *CARD11* activating the NF-κB pathway, TNFAIP3 mutation or loss dysregulating NF-κB and *MYD88* linking IL1/TLR pathway to NF-κB activation [144–147]. These mutations are far more common in the ABC-DLBCL, supporting the previous GEP finding of the importance of BCR signaling and NK-kB activation in this subtype of DLBCL [29]. Subsequent application of NGS in the study mutations in lymphoma leads to an explosive growth in mutations identified and the construction of the genomic landscape of several types of lymphoma including DLBCL [148–151], MCL [117,120,152], FL [153,154], BL [155,156] and marginal zone lymphomas [157–161]. As DLBCL is the most common lymphoma, it has also been most extensively studied, and genomic subgroups have been delineated. Using consensus clustering, Chapuy et al. [151] identified five genomics clusters based on mutation and gCNA analyses, and these clusters have biological and clinical implications. Schmitz et al. [150], using a different approach, identified four genetic subgroups, and three of these appear to overlap with three of the clusters reported by Chapuy et al. [151] (Table 1). These studies indicated there are genetic subgroups of DLBCL that could be robustly defined, and they could further refine the GCB vs. ABC distinction. In a subsequent analysis, Wright et al. [162] re-affirmed the previous findings by Schmitz et al. and reported an additional subgroup associated with TP53 abnormalities and another a small subgroup called ST2 that has a similar profile to T-cell rich B-cell lymphoma or DLBCL transformed from LPHL [163,164]. Whether ST2 tumors are de novo DLBCL or represent un-recognized transformation of LPHL is unclear. While mutation and gCNA data are critical in the defining of these genetic subgroups of DLBCL, other genetic information is also important such as BCL2, BCL6 or MYC rearrangement. Some of the genetic abnormalities may suggest the potential usefulness of targeted agents as pointed out by Wright et al. [162]. For example, DLBCL in the MCD group typically have mutations affecting MYD88 and CD79B and are associated with high response rate to ibrutinib. However, despite the apparent match of a putative driver mutation to a targeted drug, the effectiveness of the agent still needs to be determined by rigorous pre-clinical studies followed by well-designed clinical trials.

Table 1. Comparison of two genetic classification schemes for DLBCL.

Chapuy B. et al. Nat. Med. 2018	Schmitz R. et al. NEJM. 2018	COO Classification	Prognosis	Genetic Characteristics
Cluster 1	BN2	ABC or ABC + UC	F	BCL6 rearrangement; Notch pathway: Notch 2, SPEN, DTX1; NF-κB: A20, TNIP1, BCL10, PKCB; immune escape CD70, FAS, PDLI/L2
Cluster 2	N/C	Mixed	UF	TP53 biallelic abnormalities; CDKN2A/RB loss; miR17-92 gain; MCL1 gain
Cluster 3	EZB	GCB	UF	BCL2 translocation, EZH2 mutation, cRel amplification, TNFRSF14 alteration, MEF2B, and common chromatin modifier mutation: MLL2, CREBBP, EP300; SIPR2 pathway; STAT6; mTOR; MiR17-92; PTEN
Cluster 4	N/C	GCB	F	Histone core and linkers; immune evasion; GNA13, RHOA, SGK1; NF-κB; BRAF/STAT3
Cluster 5	MCD	ABC	UF	MYD88L265P, CD79B; 18p gain, PRDMI, CDKN2A, ETV6, BTG1/2, TBL1XR1; PIM1; immune editing, high cAID
N/C	N1	ABC	UF	NOTCH1 mutation; IRF4, 1D3, BCOR, A20; plasmacytic phenotype

F: favorable; UF: unfavorable.

3.3. Mutation and gCNA Analyses: Peripheral T-Cell Lymphoma

As with GEP studies, the genetic analysis of PTCL also lagged behind its B-cell counterpart, but a number of recent studies have provided important insights into the pathogenesis of several PTCLs [165–167]. One of the earliest mutations detected was *IDH2* mutation found in AITL [168]. Different from AML and glioblastoma, *IDH1* mutations were not found, and IDH2 R172 mutation was the only IDH2 mutation detected. Subsequently, *TET2* mutations were found to be very frequent in AITL, but surprisingly, *IDH2* mutation in AITL [100] almost always occurs together with TET2 mutation, distinct from their mutual exclusivity in AML. DNMT3A was also found to be frequently mutated, and again, it frequently co-occurs with TET2 mutations. This co-occurrence seems paradoxical as these genes have opposite functions in DNA methylation. Both TET2 and DNMT3A mutations are found in other PTCLs, being more frequent in the TBX21 than GATA3 subtype. There is a hotspot *DNMT3A* mutation affecting R882 that seems to be more frequently associated with tumors with the cytotoxic phenotype [169]. *IDH2R172* mutants acquire a neomorphic enzyme activity with the production of 2-hydroxyglutarate (HG) instead of alpha-ketoglutarate (aKG), resulting in the inhibition of all TET enzymes. However, 2HG inhibits a large group of dioxygenases, so there are functional alterations in addition to impaired DNA-demethylation. An interesting finding is that in some PTCL patients with *TET2* mutations, the same mutation was also found in a co-existing myeloid disorder, suggesting that the *TET2* mutation may be present in a hematopoietic stem cell (HSC) which gives rise to both the myeloid and T-cell disorders. There is evidence that AITL cases may also be associated with clonal hematopoiesis of undetermined potential (CHIP) [170] instead of an overt myeloid disorder and share the same *TET2* mutations. Thus, the mutational landscape in AITL is dominated by mutations that aberrantly modify the epigenome.

The other highly frequent mutation, present in about 70% of AITL, affects *RHOA*, which is a small GTPase important in a number of T-cell functions in addition to cytoskeleton organization and cellular motility/migration [171–173]. In AITL and PTCL with T_{FH} phenotype, the *RHOA* mutation is a unique G17V mutation resulting in an inability of the protein to associate with GTP or GDP and believed to be a dominant negative mutation. Other *RHOA* mutations have been described in other PTCLs, including some that are gain-of-function mutations such as *RHOA C16R and K118*. How these RHOA mutants contribute to T-cell transformation needs further investigation. As RHOA G17V mutation almost always occurs with TET2 mutation, their functional interaction is also intriguing. Another group of mutations in PTCL affects the proximal TCR signaling pathway [174–176]. They are much less common than the mutations just mentioned and affect signaling molecules including CD28, PI3K components, FYN, PCLG1 and VAV1. A number of fusion proteins have been described including CTLA4-CD28 [177], ICOS-CD28 [175], ITK-SYK [178], FYN-TRAF3IP2 [179,180] and VAV1 fusions [181], with a number of partners with deletion of the C-terminal autoregulatory SH3 domain of VAV1. These are generally activating mutations, but exactly how TCR signaling is altered to favor T-cell transformation is unclear. Another group of mutations affect the JAK/STAT pathway. JAK1 and JAK3 are the most commonly mutated with the mutation affecting most frequently the pseudo kinase domain. JAK fusions have also been described in ALK neg ALCL, which also contain a group of cases with DUSP22 rearrangement and rarely TP63 rearrangement with the former associated with good prognosis, while the latter with a very poor outcome [182,183]. Activated JAK may not only promote phosphorylation of the associated STATs, but may also phosphorylate other targets unrelated to STAT functions [184,185]. Of the STAT genes, STAT3 and STAT5B are the ones involved. Mutations occur mostly in the SH2 domain and affect the affinity and stability of the phosphorylated dimers, which persist much longer than the WT with increased target occupancy and changes in transcription [186] (Figure 2). STAT5B and STAT3 mutations have a different distribution profile, with STAT5B the dominant mutation in T-PLL [187], $\gamma\delta$-TCL and HSTCL [186] while STAT3 mutated is more frequent in ALCL and NK-cell lymphoma [188].

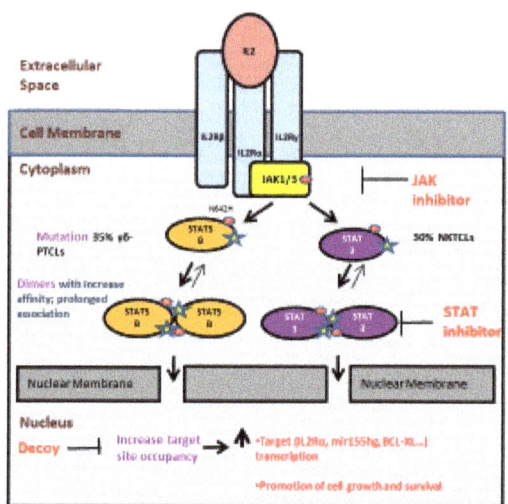

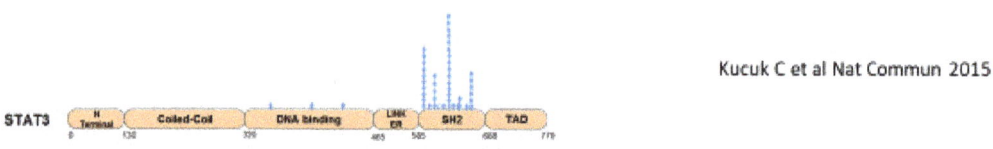

Figure 2. Biological effects of SH2 domain mutations in STAT3 and STAT5B (modified from Kucuk C et al. Nat Commun 2015 [186]).

gCNAs have been studied in AITL and several other PTCL, including the GATA3 and TBX21 subtypes, and they have distinctive profiles [101]. PTCL-GATA3 has the highest gCNAs, and there are highly frequent deletions of tumor suppressor genes (TSG) such as TP53, p16/19, RB, PRDM1 and PTEN, while there are gains including STAT3 and MYC [101]. An unusual feature is the co-occurrence of TP53 mutation/deletion and heterozygous loss of PTEN, rarely observed in lymphomas. These cases have similar genetic features to a cluster of cases identified in the study by Watatani Y et al. [189] that probably also represented mostly GATA3 cases. All these observations support the GEP classification of PTCL-GATA3 and TBX21 as unique entities.

The concept of T_{FH} cell-derived lymphoma has been expanded from AITL to tumors with T cells having similar immunophenotype but a follicular growth pattern (follicular T-cell lymphoma), and PTCL that would have been classified as PTCL-NOS except that the tumor T cells express two or more T_{FH} cell-associated markers, such as PD1, ICOS1, BCL6, CXCL13 and CD10 (PTCL-T_{FH}) [74,190]. PTCL-T_{FH}, as currently defined, is likely to be heterogeneous. Most of these cases appeared to have a stronger T_{FH} signature and AITL-like signature by GEP as well as mutations associated with AITL and thus likely to be part of the spectrum of T_{FH}-associated lymphoma [104,191]. However, there are also cases that appear to be unrelated to T_{FH} cells, and a more comprehensive study with more cases may be needed to further characterize this group of cases.

3.4. Cooperativity of Genetic Alterations

A mutation does not occur in isolation in a lymphoma; it co-operates with other alterations that could be genetic or epigenetic to mediate neoplastic transformation. *STAT3* is the most frequently mutated gene in ENKTCL and is often associated with PRDM1 deficiency, which is also a very common event in this lymphoma. A recent study examined the possible co-operation between these two abnormalities in normal NK-cells and found that STAT3 mutants can only mediate enhanced cell growth for a limited period of time. However, if *PRDM1* is knockout, the double mutant cells can undergo persistent proliferation which can be sustained using IL15 alone without other cytokines or the presence of feeder cells [188]. If the *STAT3* mutant was replaced with a common *STAT5B* mutant, *STAT5B N642H*, a co-operative effect with PRDM1 was not observed (unpublished observation). This co-operative event may partly explain the difference in *STAT* mutations observed in ENKTCL and γδ PTCL. Similar investigations in the future may unravel additional important co-operative events.

4. The Integration of Multiomics Data

With the ability of performing multiomics studies on the same biological samples, it is possible to obtain important complementary information that can lead to greater and more comprehensive understanding of the biological processes under investigation that may also provide novel leads to future investigations. This requires greater planning to obtain the requisite tissues and perform the necessary studies. The analyses and interpretation are more complex and require more expertise. An example of such an approach is the investigation of transcription factor binding and its functional consequences. Traditionally, ChIP analysis is performed and currently combined with NGS to identify binding sites. However, binding may not be associated with functional activities, which are now generally accessed by simultaneously determining chromatin accessibility and RNA expression. Some binding peaks occur in genomic regions without clear association with a particular gene. The availability of Hi-C data would be very helpful in identifying associations with specific genomic sequences with each of these peaks [192], thus allowing the prediction of the target of the TF when bound to specific DNA sequences.

5. The Tumor Microenvironment

It is quite clear from numerous studies that the TME is an integral and important component of the tumor which may be critical for tumor cell survival and in regulating the host/tumor interaction, particularly the immune reaction to the tumor, which could be especially relevant in this era of immunotherapy. It is notoriously difficult to derive cell lines from PTCL, clearly indicating the importance of TME in supporting the growth and survival of the tumor cells. In multiple lymphomas, TME signatures have been shown to be predictive of patient survival as mentioned above. In a bulk population, the GEP signature is a mixture of signals from multiple components, and it is challenging to decipher what components are present and their contributions to the GEP. Recent development in computational analysis such as the CiberSort approach [193,194] may help to deconvolute bulk GEP data to provide an estimate of the immune cell populations present in the TME. An extension of this approach includes the subtyping of tumor cells by GEP and defining their association with stromal elements to form unique tumor ecosystems that may provide further insight into tumor biology and clinical behavior [195]. It would be even more informative if these analyses are combined with immunophenotyping [196] to validate the computational findings and visualize the distribution and spatial relationship of the immune/tumor cells. Flow cytometry may be employed on isolated cells from the tissue, but spatial information is lost. Multiparameter immunophenotyping by multicolor fluorescence such as the Vectra Polaris (PerkinElmer) or CODEX (PhenoCycler, Akoya Biosciences) technology has been developed and has the advantage of maintained spatial relationship of the cells. The recent development of CyTOF technology [197–199] allows the determination of more markers than possible using fluorescence-based assays and tissue-based CyTOF assay. Imaging mass cytometry (IMC) is being developed to evaluate cellular populations in situ [200,201]. The drawback of IMC is the small area that can be examined and the limited panel of labeled antibodies available, often necessitating the labeling of antibodies by the user. The procedure is also destructive to the labeled tissues. The technical and analytical considerations of these high dimensional imaging approaches have been reviewed recently [202]. These are very promising tools for the study of the TME, but computational approaches [203,204] to fully exploit the data from these systems are challenging but critically needed.

Single-cell (sc) RNA-seq studies are now feasible, and the technology has been recently reviewed [205,206]. It has been employed recently to decipher the biological complexity of the tumor cells as well as the stromal cell populations [207–209]. When scRNA-seq is performed on isolated cells, spatial information is lost, and various artefacts may also be introduced. To overcome these barriers, techniques such as Slide-seq [210] that attempt to preserve the spatial information have been reported. Commercial platforms such as the 10X genomics (Visium) and NanoString platforms are now available for similar purposes and applicable for FFPE tissues. These platforms are not at true single cell resolution yet, and scRNA-seq has limitations such as high costs and low transcriptome coverage, but it is a valuable component of GEP analysis and can provide important insight into the functional states and activities of single cells, the heterogeneity of the tumor cell population, the potential interactions of neighboring cells and the possible trajectories of these interactions.

6. A New Diagnostic Platform

Traditionally, diagnosis is based on tissue biopsy and study of the tissue thus obtained, but a biopsy is an invasive procedure; yet, the biopsy obtained for diagnosis may not be the most diagnostic or representative. Lymphoma patients frequently relapse after therapy and usually a very limited needle biopsy or no biopsy is obtained, which is a tremendous impediment in the adequate characterization of relapsed disease even for clinical purposes. Thus, a new approach that addresses these major issues will have a powerful clinical impact. *Technological advances* have allowed the performance of sophisticated analysis on the small amounts of DNA and RNA present in cell-free plasma [211–213], an easily obtainable biospecimen that allows more frequent sampling without an invasive procedure. In addition, the plasma analytes represent the summation of the contribution from all tumor sites and provide a more global picture of the entire tumor content [212]. The successful development of the technology and implementation of it as a clinical assay would represent a major breakthrough in diagnostics, allowing molecular characterization of each patient at diagnosis and at different points of treatment to guide further actions. Circulating tumor DNA (ctDNA) also enables monitoring of tumor evolution and characterization of resistant clones [212,214]. The technology is applicable not only to lymphoma but also to other types of cancer [215]. In lymphoma, many of the studies had been focused on DLBCL using the Cancer Personalized Profiling by Deep Sequencing (CAPP-seq) approach [211], which used a pre-defined panel to capture the DNA from selected loci for deep sequencing. Another approach is to sequence the tumor to determine the mutations present and then design a custom panel for deep sequencing [216]. An exciting report on HL [217] has been published, demonstrating that it is possible to perform CAPP-seq successfully in liquid biopsy, even in a disease where the neoplastic cells may be as low as or lower than 1% of the cells in the tumor. Interestingly, their findings on the predictive value of early reduction in ctDNA on chemotherapy on treatment response and survival are quite similar to findings reported in DLBCL [218]. While ctDNA is the most frequently investigated analyte, other analytes include plasma miRNA and 5mC [219] and possibly 5hmC-modified DNA that may be assayed and may complement ctDNA information or constitute new assays. This is a rapidly evolving area with new technological and analytical developments [220]. Liquid biopsy may provide the platform for sensitive and specific molecular assays for multiple types of cancer and become the next-generation diagnostics for precision medicine [221,222]. However, much still needs to be done to determine various preanalytical variables, standardize the assay and platforms and validate the clinical characteristics and usefulness of the assays.

7. Perspectives

The last 22 years have seen an explosive growth in genomics data in lymphoid malignancies leading to a marked improvement in the understanding of their pathogenesis and biology. For the more common lymphomas, the genomic landscapes are fairly well defined, but the less common entities are still largely unexplored. A better understanding of the tumor/microenvironment interaction is crucial, and we have better tools to make significant discoveries in this area. Obtaining good, well-annotated tissue samples is particularly challenging in lymphoma, and samples collected often lack corresponding normal controls, making tissue availability a major barrier in future research. As mentioned above, multiomics investigations are important to more fully explore the omics data, but few studies have performed such investigations. In the future, the integration of omics and comprehensive TME findings, particularly with spatial information, would markedly improve our understanding of tumor biology and host/tumor interaction. The incorporation of single cell analysis will further provide essential information on tumor heterogeneity, clonal evolution and the diverse stromal components. While gaining genomic information is critical, painstakingly focused investigations are still necessary to understand the biological implications of specific findings. The information generated so far has suggested many potential drug targets against individual genes and/or pathways, which has led to many clinical trials. Further understanding of tumor biology and host/tumor interaction will no doubt lead to more novel targets, better stratification of patients for clinical studies and the elucidation of mechanisms of therapy resistance. This is true not only for traditional drug-based trials but also for immunotherapy. Plasma-based diagnostic platforms are rapidly advancing and could become the next-generation diagnostics that may vastly improve the monitoring of patients under treatment and on prognostication.

Author Contributions: W.C.C. and J.I. wrote and edited the manuscript. All authors have read and agreed to the published version of the manuscript.

Funding: W.C.C. acknowledges support from the Norman and Melinda Payson Professorship.

Institutional Review Board Statement: Not applicable.

Informed Consent Statement: Not applicable.

Data Availability Statement: Not applicable.

Acknowledgments: This review is a rather personal account of the authors on genomics research of lymphoma in the last two decades and not a comprehensive review of all aspects lymphoma research so many important studies have not been mentioned. We acknowledge the contributions of colleagues in LLMPP and many other colleagues in the exciting discoveries in lymphoma. The LLMPP and many of the reported studies with participation of the authors were or currently are supported by NCI UO1 CA 84967, U01-CA-114778, UO1 CA157581, UH3CA206127, R01 CA251412 and 1PO1CA229100 and grants from the LRF and LLS. We thank Yuping Li for assistance in the preparation of the manuscript.

Conflicts of Interest: The authors declare no conflict of interest.

References

1. Saluz, H.P.; Iqbal, J.; Gino, V.L.; Andre, R.; Wu, Z. Fundamentals of DNA-chip/array technology for comparative gene-expression analysis. *Curr. Sci.* **2002**, *83*, 829–833.
2. Freeman, W.M.; Robertson, D.J.; Vrana, K.E. Fundamentals of DNA hybridization arrays for gene expression analysis. *Biotechniques* **2000**, *29*, 1042–1046. [CrossRef] [PubMed]
3. Schena, M.; Shalon, D.; Davis, R.W.; Brown, P.O. Quantitative monitoring of gene expression patterns with a complementary DNA microarray. *Science* **1995**, *270*, 467–470. [CrossRef] [PubMed]

4. Lockhart, D.J.; Dong, H.; Byrne, M.C.; Follettie, M.T.; Gallo, M.V.; Chee, M.S.; Mittmann, M.; Wang, C.; Kobayashi, M.; Horton, H.; et al. Expression monitoring by hybridization to high-density oligonucleotide arrays. *Nat. Biotechnol.* **1996**, *14*, 1675–1680. [CrossRef] [PubMed]
5. Draghici, S.; Khatri, P.; Eklund, A.C.; Szallasi, Z. Reliability and reproducibility issues in DNA microarray measurements. *Trends Genet.* **2006**, *22*, 101–109. [CrossRef] [PubMed]
6. van Hijum, S.A.; de Jong, A.; Baerends, R.J.; Karsens, H.A.; Kramer, N.E.; Larsen, R.; den Hengst, C.D.; Albers, C.J.; Kok, J.; Kuipers, O.P. A generally applicable validation scheme for the assessment of factors involved in reproducibility and quality of DNA-microarray data. *BMC Genom.* **2005**, *6*, 77. [CrossRef] [PubMed]
7. McShane, L.M.; Radmacher, M.D.; Freidlin, B.; Yu, R.; Li, M.C.; Simon, R. Methods for assessing reproducibility of clustering patterns observed in analyses of microarray data. *Bioinformatics* **2002**, *18*, 1462–1469. [CrossRef] [PubMed]
8. Chen, J.J.; Hsueh, H.M.; Delongchamp, R.R.; Lin, C.J.; Tsai, C.A. Reproducibility of microarray data: A further analysis of microarray quality control (MAQC) data. *BMC Bioinform.* **2007**, *8*, 412. [CrossRef] [PubMed]
9. Yang, I.V.; Chen, E.; Hasseman, J.P.; Liang, W.; Frank, B.C.; Wang, S.; Sharov, V.; Saeed, A.I.; White, J.; Li, J.; et al. Within the fold: Assessing differential expression measures and reproducibility in microarray assays. *Genome Biol.* **2002**, *3*, research0062. [PubMed]
10. Iqbal, J.; d'Amore, F.; Hu, Q.; Chan, W.C.; Fu, K. Gene arrays in lymphoma: Where will they fit in? *Curr. Hematol. Malig. Rep.* **2006**, *1*, 129–136. [CrossRef]
11. Iqbal, J.; Liu, Z.; Deffenbacher, K.; Chan, W.C. Gene expression profiling in lymphoma diagnosis and management. *Best Pract. Res. Clin. Haematol.* **2009**, *22*, 191–210. [CrossRef] [PubMed]
12. Nurk, S.; Koren, S.; Rhie, A.; Rautiainen, M.; Bzikadze, A.V.; Mikheenko, A.; Vollger, M.R.; Altemose, N.; Uralsky, L.; Gershman, A.; et al. The complete sequence of a human genome. *Science* **2022**, *376*, 44–53. [CrossRef] [PubMed]
13. Lander, E.S.; Linton, L.M.; Birren, B.; Nusbaum, C.; Zody, M.C.; Baldwin, J.; Devon, K.; Dewar, K.; Doyle, M.; FitzHugh, W.; et al. Initial sequencing and analysis of the human genome. *Nature* **2001**, *409*, 860–921. [PubMed]
14. Schneider, V.A.; Graves-Lindsay, T.; Howe, K.; Bouk, N.; Chen, H.C.; Kitts, P.A.; Murphy, T.D.; Pruitt, K.D.; Thibaud-Nissen, F.; Albracht, D.; et al. Evaluation of GRCh38 and de novo haploid genome assemblies demonstrates the enduring quality of the reference assembly. *Genome Res.* **2017**, *27*, 849–864. [CrossRef]
15. Carter, N.P. Methods and strategies for analyzing copy number variation using DNA microarrays. *Nat. Genet.* **2007**, *39*, S16–S21. [CrossRef]
16. Coughlin, C.R.; Scharer, G.H., 2nd; Shaikh, T.H. Clinical impact of copy number variation analysis using high-resolution microarray technologies: Advantages, limitations and concerns. *Genome Med.* **2012**, *4*, 80. [CrossRef]
17. Zhang, F.; Gu, W.; Hurles, M.E.; Lupski, J.R. Copy number variation in human health, disease, and evolution. *Annu. Rev. Genom. Hum. Genet.* **2009**, *10*, 451–481. [CrossRef]
18. McCarroll, S.A.; Altshuler, D.M. Copy-number variation and association studies of human disease. *Nat. Genet.* **2007**, *39*, S37–S42. [CrossRef]
19. Hinds, D.A.; Kloek, A.P.; Jen, M.; Chen, X.; Frazer, K.A. Common deletions and SNPs are in linkage disequilibrium in the human genome. *Nat. Genet.* **2006**, *38*, 82–85. [CrossRef]
20. Chee, M.; Yang, R.; Hubbell, E.; Berno, A.; Huang, X.C.; Stern, D.; Winkler, J.; Lockhart, D.J.; Morris, M.S.; Fodor, S.P. Accessing genetic information with high-density DNA arrays. *Science* **1996**, *274*, 610–614. [CrossRef]
21. Lashkari, D.A.; DeRisi, J.L.; McCusker, J.H.; Namath, A.F.; Gentile, C.; Hwang, S.Y.; Brown, P.O.; Davis, R.W. Yeast microarrays for genome wide parallel genetic and gene expression analysis. *Proc. Natl. Acad. Sci. USA* **1997**, *94*, 13057–13062. [CrossRef] [PubMed]
22. Richter, A.; Schwager, C.; Hentze, S.; Ansorge, W.; Hentze, M.W.; Muckenthaler, M. Comparison of fluorescent tag DNA labeling methods used for expression analysis by DNA microarrays. *Biotechniques* **2002**, *33*, 620–628. [CrossRef]
23. DeRisi, J.; Penland, L.; Bittner, M.; Meltzer, P.; Ray, M.; Chen, Y.; Su, Y.; Trent, J. Use of a cDNA microarray to analyse gene expression. *Nat. Genet.* **1996**, *14*, 457–460. [PubMed]
24. Diehl, F.; Grahlmann, S.; Beier, M.; Hoheisel, J.D. Manufacturing DNA microarrays of high spot homogeneity and reduced background signal. *Nucleic Acids Res.* **2001**, *29*, E38. [CrossRef] [PubMed]
25. Lipshutz, R.J.; Fodor, S.P.; Gingeras, T.R.; Lockhart, D.J. High density synthetic oligonucleotide arrays. *Nat. Genet.* **1999**, *21*, 20–24. [CrossRef] [PubMed]
26. Alizadeh, A.A.; Eisen, M.B.; Davis, R.E.; Ma, C.; Lossos, I.S.; Rosenwald, A.; Boldrick, J.C.; Sabet, H.; Tran, T.; Yu, X.; et al. Distinct types of diffuse large B-cell lymphoma identified by gene expression profiling. *Nature* **2000**, *403*, 503–511. [CrossRef]
27. Rosenwald, A.; Wright, G.; Chan, W.C.; Connors, J.M.; Campo, E.; Fisher, R.I.; Gascoyne, R.D.; Muller-Hermelink, H.K.; Smeland, E.B.; Giltnane, J.M.; et al. The use of molecular profiling to predict survival after chemotherapy for diffuse large-B-cell lymphoma. *N. Engl. J. Med.* **2002**, *346*, 1937–1947. [CrossRef]
28. Lenz, G.; Wright, G.; Dave, S.S.; Xiao, W.; Powell, J.; Zhao, H.; Xu, W.; Tan, B.; Goldschmidt, N.; Iqbal, J.; et al. Stromal gene signatures in large-B-cell lymphomas. *N. Engl. J. Med.* **2008**, *359*, 2313–2323. [CrossRef]
29. Davis, R.E.; Brown, K.D.; Siebenlist, U.; Staudt, L.M. Constitutive nuclear factor kappaB activity is required for survival of activated B cell-like diffuse large B cell lymphoma cells. *J. Exp. Med.* **2001**, *194*, 1861–1874. [CrossRef]

30. Hans, C.P.; Weisenburger, D.D.; Greiner, T.C.; Gascoyne, R.D.; Delabie, J.; Ott, G.; Muller-Hermelink, H.K.; Campo, E.; Braziel, R.M.; Jaffe, E.S.; et al. Confirmation of the molecular classification of diffuse large B-cell lymphoma by immunohistochemistry using a tissue microarray. *Blood* **2004**, *103*, 275–282. [CrossRef]
31. Choi, W.W.; Weisenburger, D.D.; Greiner, T.C.; Piris, M.A.; Banham, A.H.; Delabie, J.; Braziel, R.M.; Geng, H.; Iqbal, J.; Lenz, G.; et al. A new immunostain algorithm classifies diffuse large B-cell lymphoma into molecular subtypes with high accuracy. *Clin. Cancer Res.* **2009**, *15*, 5494–5502. [CrossRef]
32. Meyer, P.N.; Fu, K.; Greiner, T.C.; Smith, L.M.; Delabie, J.; Gascoyne, R.D.; Ott, G.; Rosenwald, A.; Braziel, R.M.; Campo, E.; et al. Immunohistochemical methods for predicting cell of origin and survival in patients with diffuse large B-cell lymphoma treated with rituximab. *J. Clin. Oncol.* **2011**, *29*, 200–207. [CrossRef]
33. Scott, D.W.; Wright, G.W.; Williams, P.M.; Lih, C.J.; Walsh, W.; Jaffe, E.S.; Rosenwald, A.; Campo, E.; Chan, W.C.; Connors, J.M.; et al. Determining cell-of-origin subtypes of diffuse large B-cell lymphoma using gene expression in formalin-fixed paraffin-embedded tissue. *Blood* **2014**, *123*, 1214–1217. [CrossRef] [PubMed]
34. Iqbal, J.; Shen, Y.; Huang, X.; Liu, Y.; Wake, L.; Liu, C.; Deffenbacher, K.; Lachel, C.M.; Wang, C.; Rohr, J.; et al. Global microRNA expression profiling uncovers molecular markers for classification and prognosis in aggressive B-cell lymphoma. *Blood* **2015**, *125*, 1137–1145. [CrossRef] [PubMed]
35. Lim, E.L.; Trinh, D.L.; Scott, D.W.; Chu, A.; Krzywinski, M.; Zhao, Y.; Robertson, A.G.; Mungall, A.J.; Schein, J.; Boyle, M.; et al. Comprehensive miRNA sequence analysis reveals survival differences in diffuse large B-cell lymphoma patients. *Genome Biol.* **2015**, *16*, 18. [CrossRef] [PubMed]
36. Zhou, W.; Xu, Y.; Zhang, J.; Zhang, P.; Yao, Z.; Yan, Z.; Wang, H.; Chu, J.; Yao, S.; Zhao, S.; et al. MiRNA-363-3p/DUSP10/JNK axis mediates chemoresistance by enhancing DNA damage repair in diffuse large B-cell lymphoma. *Leukemia* **2022**, *36*, 1861–1869. [CrossRef] [PubMed]
37. Monti, S.; Savage, K.J.; Kutok, J.L.; Feuerhake, F.; Kurtin, P.; Mihm, M.; Wu, B.; Pasqualucci, L.; Neuberg, D.; Aguiar, R.C.; et al. Molecular profiling of diffuse large B-cell lymphoma identifies robust subtypes including one characterized by host inflammatory response. *Blood* **2005**, *105*, 1851–1861. [CrossRef]
38. Rosenwald, A.; Wright, G.; Leroy, K.; Yu, X.; Gaulard, P.; Gascoyne, R.D.; Chan, W.C.; Zhao, T.; Haioun, C.; Greiner, T.C.; et al. Molecular diagnosis of primary mediastinal B cell lymphoma identifies a clinically favorable subgroup of diffuse large B cell lymphoma related to Hodgkin lymphoma. *J. Exp. Med.* **2003**, *198*, 851–862. [CrossRef]
39. Savage, K.J.; Monti, S.; Kutok, J.L.; Cattoretti, G.; Neuberg, D.; De Leval, L.; Kurtin, P.; Dal Cin, P.; Ladd, C.; Feuerhake, F.; et al. The molecular signature of mediastinal large B-cell lymphoma differs from that of other diffuse large B-cell lymphomas and shares features with classical Hodgkin lymphoma. *Blood* **2003**, *102*, 3871–3879. [CrossRef] [PubMed]
40. Vigano, E.; Gunawardana, J.; Mottok, A.; Van Tol, T.; Mak, K.; Chan, F.C.; Chong, L.; Chavez, E.; Woolcock, B.; Takata, K.; et al. Somatic IL4R mutations in primary mediastinal large B-cell lymphoma lead to constitutive JAK-STAT signaling activation. *Blood* **2018**, *131*, 2036–2046. [CrossRef] [PubMed]
41. Green, M.R.; Monti, S.; Rodig, S.J.; Juszczynski, P.; Currie, T.; O'Donnell, E.; Chapuy, B.; Takeyama, K.; Neuberg, D.; Golub, T.R.; et al. Integrative analysis reveals selective 9p24.1 amplification, increased PD-1 ligand expression, and further induction via JAK2 in nodular sclerosing Hodgkin lymphoma and primary mediastinal large B-cell lymphoma. *Blood* **2010**, *116*, 3268–3277. [CrossRef] [PubMed]
42. Twa, D.D.; Chan, F.C.; Ben-Neriah, S.; Woolcock, B.W.; Mottok, A.; Tan, K.L.; Slack, G.W.; Gunawardana, J.; Lim, R.S.; McPherson, A.W.; et al. Genomic rearrangements involving programmed death ligands are recurrent in primary mediastinal large B-cell lymphoma. *Blood* **2014**, *123*, 2062–2065. [CrossRef] [PubMed]
43. Yuan, J.; Wright, G.; Rosenwald, A.; Steidl, C.; Gascoyne, R.D.; Connors, J.M.; Mottok, A.; Weisenburger, D.D.; Greiner, T.C.; Fu, K.; et al. Identification of Primary Mediastinal Large B-cell Lymphoma at Nonmediastinal Sites by Gene Expression Profiling. *Am. J. Surg. Pathol.* **2015**, *39*, 1322–1330. [CrossRef]
44. Klein, U.; Gloghini, A.; Gaidano, G.; Chadburn, A.; Cesarman, E.; Dalla-Favera, R.; Carbone, A. Gene expression profile analysis of AIDS-related primary effusion lymphoma (PEL) suggests a plasmablastic derivation and identifies PEL-specific transcripts. *Blood* **2003**, *101*, 4115–4121. [CrossRef]
45. Fan, W.; Bubman, D.; Chadburn, A.; Harrington, W.J., Jr.; Cesarman, E.; Knowles, D.M. Distinct subsets of primary effusion lymphoma can be identified based on their cellular gene expression profile and viral association. *J. Virol.* **2005**, *79*, 1244–1251. [CrossRef] [PubMed]
46. Kobayashi, T.; Yamaguchi, M.; Kim, S.; Morikawa, J.; Ogawa, S.; Ueno, S.; Suh, E.; Dougherty, E.; Shmulevich, I.; Shiku, H.; et al. Microarray reveals differences in both tumors and vascular specific gene expression in de novo CD5+ and CD5− diffuse large B-cell lymphomas. *Cancer Res.* **2003**, *63*, 60–66.
47. Karnan, S.; Tagawa, H.; Suzuki, R.; Suguro, M.; Yamaguchi, M.; Okamoto, M.; Morishima, Y.; Nakamura, S.; Seto, M. Analysis of chromosomal imbalances in de novo CD5-positive diffuse large-B-cell lymphoma detected by comparative genomic hybridization. *Genes Chromosomes Cancer* **2004**, *39*, 77–81. [CrossRef]
48. Jardin, F. Next generation sequencing and the management of diffuse large B-cell lymphoma: From whole exome analysis to targeted therapy. *Discov. Med.* **2014**, *18*, 51–65.
49. Choi, J.W.; Kim, Y.; Lee, J.H.; Kim, Y.S. MYD88 expression and L265P mutation in diffuse large B-cell lymphoma. *Hum. Pathol.* **2013**, *44*, 1375–1381. [CrossRef] [PubMed]

50. Ramis-Zaldivar, J.E.; Gonzalez-Farre, B.; Nicolae, A.; Pack, S.; Clot, G.; Nadeu, F.; Mottok, A.; Horn, H.; Song, J.Y.; Fu, K.; et al. MAPK and JAK-STAT pathways dysregulation in plasmablastic lymphoma. *Haematologica* **2021**, *106*, 2682–2693. [CrossRef] [PubMed]
51. Gandhi, M.K.; Hoang, T.; Law, S.C.; Brosda, S.; O'Rourke, K.; Tobin, J.W.D.; Vari, F.; Murigneux, V.; Fink, L.; Gunawardana, J.; et al. EBV-associated primary CNS lymphoma occurring after immunosuppression is a distinct immunobiological entity. *Blood* **2021**, *137*, 1468–1477. [CrossRef] [PubMed]
52. Pham-Ledard, A.; Prochazkova-Carlotti, M.; Andrique, L.; Cappellen, D.; Vergier, B.; Martinez, F.; Grange, F.; Petrella, T.; Beylot-Barry, M.; Merlio, J.P. Multiple genetic alterations in primary cutaneous large B-cell lymphoma, leg type support a common lymphomagenesis with activated B-cell-like diffuse large B-cell lymphoma. *Mod. Pathol.* **2014**, *27*, 402–411. [CrossRef]
53. Hans, C.P.; Weisenburger, D.D.; Greiner, T.C.; Chan, W.C.; Aoun, P.; Cochran, G.T.; Pan, Z.; Smith, L.M.; Lynch, J.C.; Bociek, R.G.; et al. Expression of PKC-beta or cyclin D2 predicts for inferior survival in diffuse large B-cell lymphoma. *Mod. Pathol.* **2005**, *18*, 1377–1384. [CrossRef]
54. Perry, A.M.; Mitrovic, Z.; Chan, W.C. Biological prognostic markers in diffuse large B-cell lymphoma. *Cancer Control* **2012**, *19*, 214–226. [CrossRef]
55. Young, K.H.; Leroy, K.; Moller, M.B.; Colleoni, G.W.; Sanchez-Beato, M.; Kerbauy, F.R.; Haioun, C.; Eickhoff, J.C.; Young, A.H.; Gaulard, P.; et al. Structural profiles of TP53 gene mutations predict clinical outcome in diffuse large B-cell lymphoma: An international collaborative study. *Blood* **2008**, *112*, 3088–3098. [CrossRef]
56. Iqbal, J.; Meyer, P.N.; Smith, L.M.; Johnson, N.A.; Vose, J.M.; Greiner, T.C.; Connors, J.M.; Staudt, L.M.; Rimsza, L.; Jaffe, E.; et al. BCL2 predicts survival in germinal center B-cell-like diffuse large B-cell lymphoma treated with CHOP-like therapy and rituximab. *Clin. Cancer Res.* **2011**, *17*, 7785–7795. [CrossRef]
57. Iqbal, J.; Neppalli, V.T.; Wright, G.; Dave, B.J.; Horsman, D.E.; Rosenwald, A.; Lynch, J.; Hans, C.P.; Weisenburger, D.D.; Greiner, T.C.; et al. BCL2 expression is a prognostic marker for the activated B-cell-like type of diffuse large B-cell lymphoma. *J. Clin. Oncol.* **2006**, *24*, 961–968. [CrossRef]
58. Fu, K.; Weisenburger, D.D.; Choi, W.W.; Perry, K.D.; Smith, L.M.; Shi, X.; Hans, C.P.; Greiner, T.C.; Bierman, P.J.; Bociek, R.G.; et al. Addition of rituximab to standard chemotherapy improves the survival of both the germinal center B-cell-like and non-germinal center B-cell-like subtypes of diffuse large B-cell lymphoma. *J. Clin. Oncol.* **2008**, *26*, 4587–4594. [CrossRef]
59. Rosenwald, A.; Wright, G.; Wiestner, A.; Chan, W.C.; Connors, J.M.; Campo, E.; Gascoyne, R.D.; Grogan, T.M.; Muller-Hermelink, H.K.; Smeland, E.B.; et al. The proliferation gene expression signature is a quantitative integrator of oncogenic events that predicts survival in mantle cell lymphoma. *Cancer Cell* **2003**, *3*, 185–197. [CrossRef]
60. Fu, K.; Weisenburger, D.D.; Greiner, T.C.; Dave, S.; Wright, G.; Rosenwald, A.; Chiorazzi, M.; Iqbal, J.; Gesk, S.; Siebert, R.; et al. Cyclin D1-negative mantle cell lymphoma: A clinicopathologic study based on gene expression profiling. *Blood* **2005**, *106*, 4315–4321. [CrossRef]
61. Salaverria, I.; Royo, C.; Carvajal-Cuenca, A.; Clot, G.; Navarro, A.; Valera, A.; Song, J.Y.; Woroniecka, R.; Rymkiewicz, G.; Klapper, W.; et al. CCND2 rearrangements are the most frequent genetic events in cyclin D1(-) mantle cell lymphoma. *Blood* **2013**, *121*, 1394–1402. [CrossRef]
62. Mozos, A.; Royo, C.; Hartmann, E.; De Jong, D.; Baro, C.; Valera, A.; Fu, K.; Weisenburger, D.D.; Delabie, J.; Chuang, S.S.; et al. SOX11 expression is highly specific for mantle cell lymphoma and identifies the cyclin D1-negative subtype. *Haematologica* **2009**, *94*, 1555–1562. [CrossRef]
63. Scott, D.W.; Abrisqueta, P.; Wright, G.W.; Slack, G.W.; Mottok, A.; Villa, D.; Jares, P.; Rauert-Wunderlich, H.; Royo, C.; Clot, G.; et al. New Molecular Assay for the Proliferation Signature in Mantle Cell Lymphoma Applicable to Formalin-Fixed Paraffin-Embedded Biopsies. *J. Clin. Oncol.* **2017**, *35*, 1668–1677. [CrossRef]
64. Clot, G.; Jares, P.; Gine, E.; Navarro, A.; Royo, C.; Pinyol, M.; Martin-Garcia, D.; Demajo, S.; Espinet, B.; Salar, A.; et al. A gene signature that distinguishes conventional and leukemic nonnodal mantle cell lymphoma helps predict outcome. *Blood* **2018**, *132*, 413–422. [CrossRef]
65. Iqbal, J.; Shen, Y.; Liu, Y.; Fu, K.; Jaffe, E.S.; Liu, C.; Liu, Z.; Lachel, C.M.; Deffenbacher, K.; Greiner, T.C.; et al. Genome-wide miRNA profiling of mantle cell lymphoma reveals a distinct subgroup with poor prognosis. *Blood* **2012**, *119*, 4939–4948. [CrossRef]
66. Sohani, A.R.; Hasserjian, R.P. Diagnosis of Burkitt Lymphoma and Related High-Grade B-Cell Neoplasms. *Surg. Pathol. Clin.* **2010**, *3*, 1035–1059. [CrossRef]
67. Dave, S.S.; Fu, K.; Wright, G.W.; Lam, L.T.; Kluin, P.; Boerma, E.J.; Greiner, T.C.; Weisenburger, D.D.; Rosenwald, A.; Ott, G.; et al. Molecular diagnosis of Burkitt's lymphoma. *N. Engl. J. Med.* **2006**, *354*, 2431–2442. [CrossRef]
68. Hummel, M.; Bentink, S.; Berger, H.; Klapper, W.; Wessendorf, S.; Barth, T.F.; Bernd, H.W.; Cogliatti, S.B.; Dierlamm, J.; Feller, A.C.; et al. A biologic definition of Burkitt's lymphoma from transcriptional and genomic profiling. *N. Engl. J. Med.* **2006**, *354*, 2419–2430. [CrossRef]
69. Victora, G.D.; Dominguez-Sola, D.; Holmes, A.B.; Deroubaix, S.; Dalla-Favera, R.; Nussenzweig, M.C. Identification of human germinal center light and dark zone cells and their relationship to human B-cell lymphomas. *Blood* **2012**, *120*, 2240–2248. [CrossRef]
70. Bouska, A.; Bagvati, S.; Iqbal, J.; William, B.; Chan, W. Follicular Lymphoma: Recent Advances. In *Cancer Growth and Progression*; Springer: Berlin/Heidelberg, Germany, 2012; pp. 21–42.

71. Glas, A.M.; Kersten, M.J.; Delahaye, L.J.; Witteveen, A.T.; Kibbelaar, R.E.; Velds, A.; Wessels, L.F.; Joosten, P.; Kerkhoven, R.M.; Bernards, R. Gene expression profiling in follicular lymphoma to assess clinical aggressiveness and to guide the choice of treatment. *Blood* 2005, *105*, 301–307. [CrossRef]
72. Nann, D.; Ramis-Zaldivar, J.E.; Muller, I.; Gonzalez-Farre, B.; Schmidt, J.; Egan, C.; Salmeron-Villalobos, J.; Clot, G.; Mattern, S.; Otto, F.; et al. Follicular lymphoma t(14; 18)-negative is genetically a heterogeneous disease. *Blood Adv.* 2020, *4*, 5652–5665. [CrossRef]
73. Leich, E.; Salaverria, I.; Bea, S.; Zettl, A.; Wright, G.; Moreno, V.; Gascoyne, R.D.; Chan, W.C.; Braziel, R.M.; Rimsza, L.M.; et al. Follicular lymphomas with and without translocation t(14;18) differ in gene expression profiles and genetic alterations. *Blood* 2009, *114*, 826–834. [CrossRef]
74. Swerdlow, S.H.; Campo, E.; Harris, N.L.; Jaffe, E.S.; Pileri, S.A.; Stein, H.; Thiele, J.; Vardiman, J.W. *WHO Classification: Pathology and Genetics of tumors of Haematopoietic and Lymphoid Tissues*, 4th ed.; WHO, Ed.; IARC Press: Lyon, France, 2008.
75. Dave, S.S.; Wright, G.; Tan, B.; Rosenwald, A.; Gascoyne, R.D.; Chan, W.C.; Fisher, R.I.; Braziel, R.M.; Rimsza, L.M.; Grogan, T.M.; et al. Prediction of survival in follicular lymphoma based on molecular features of tumor-infiltrating immune cells. *N. Engl. J. Med.* 2004, *351*, 2159–2169. [CrossRef]
76. Cerhan, J.R.; Wang, S.; Maurer, M.J.; Ansell, S.M.; Geyer, S.M.; Cozen, W.; Morton, L.M.; Davis, S.; Severson, R.K.; Rothman, N. Prognostic significance of host immune gene polymorphisms in follicular lymphoma survival. *Blood* 2007, *109*, 5439–5446. [CrossRef]
77. Huet, S.; Tesson, B.; Jais, J.P.; Feldman, A.L.; Magnano, L.; Thomas, E.; Traverse-Glehen, A.; Albaud, B.; Carrere, M.; Xerri, L.; et al. A gene-expression profiling score for prediction of outcome in patients with follicular lymphoma: A retrospective training and validation analysis in three international cohorts. *Lancet Oncol.* 2018, *19*, 549–561. [CrossRef]
78. Wang, W.; Corrigan-Cummins, M.; Hudson, J.; Maric, I.; Simakova, O.; Neelapu, S.S.; Kwak, L.W.; Janik, J.E.; Gause, B.; Jaffe, E.S.; et al. MicroRNA profiling of follicular lymphoma identifies microRNAs related to cell proliferation and tumor response. *Haematologica* 2012, *97*, 586–594. [CrossRef]
79. Leich, E.; Zamo, A.; Horn, H.; Haralambieva, E.; Puppe, B.; Gascoyne, R.D.; Chan, W.C.; Braziel, R.M.; Rimsza, L.M.; Weisenburger, D.D.; et al. MicroRNA profiles of t(14; 18)-negative follicular lymphoma support a late germinal center B-cell phenotype. *Blood* 2011, *118*, 5550–5558. [CrossRef]
80. Rudiger, T.; Weisenburger, D.D.; Anderson, J.R.; Armitage, J.O.; Diebold, J.; MacLennan, K.A.; Nathwani, B.N.; Ullrich, F.; Muller-Hermelink, H.K.; Non-Hodgkin's Lymphoma Classification Project. Peripheral T-cell lymphoma (excluding anaplastic large-cell lymphoma): Results from the Non-Hodgkin's Lymphoma Classification Project. *Ann. Oncol.* 2002, *13*, 140–149. [CrossRef]
81. Bellei, M.; Chiattone, C.S.; Luminari, S.; Pesce, E.A.; Cabrera, M.E.; de Souza, C.A.; Gabus, R.; Zoppegno, L.; Zoppegno, L.; Milone, J.; et al. T-cell lymphomas in South america and europe. *Rev. Bras. Hematol. Hemoter.* 2012, *34*, 42–47. [CrossRef]
82. Briski, R.; Feldman, A.L.; Bailey, N.G.; Lim, M.S.; Ristow, K.; Habermann, T.M.; Macon, W.R.; Inwards, D.J.; Colgan, J.P.; Nowakowski, G.S.; et al. The role of front-line anthracycline-containing chemotherapy regimens in peripheral T-cell lymphomas. *Blood Cancer J.* 2014, *4*, e214. [CrossRef]
83. Vose, J.; Armitage, J.; Weisenburger, D.; International TCLP. International peripheral T-cell and natural killer/T-cell lymphoma study: Pathology findings and clinical outcomes. *J. Clin. Oncol.* 2008, *26*, 4124–4130. [PubMed]
84. Sabattini, E.; Bacci, F.; Sagramoso, C.; Pileri, S.A. WHO classification of tumours of haematopoietic and lymphoid tissues in 2008: An overview. *Pathologica* 2010, *102*, 83–87.
85. Herek, T.A.; Iqbal, J. Molecular Classification of the Peripheral T-cell Lymphomas. In *The Peripheral T-Cell Lymphomas*; Wiley: New York, NY, USA, 2021; pp. 91–103.
86. Cuadros, M.; Dave, S.S.; Jaffe, E.S.; Honrado, E.; Milne, R.; Alves, J.; Rodriguez, J.; Zajac, M.; Benitez, J.; Staudt, L.M.; et al. Identification of a proliferation signature related to survival in nodal peripheral T-cell lymphomas. *J. Clin. Oncol.* 2007, *25*, 3321–3329. [CrossRef] [PubMed]
87. Miyazaki, K.; Yamaguchi, M.; Imai, H.; Kobayashi, T.; Tamaru, S.; Nishii, K.; Yuda, M.; Shiku, H.; Katayama, N. Gene expression profiling of peripheral T-cell lymphoma including gammadelta T-cell lymphoma. *Blood* 2009, *113*, 1071–1074. [CrossRef] [PubMed]
88. Ballester, B.; Ramuz, O.; Gisselbrecht, C.; Doucet, G.; Loi, L.; Loriod, B.; Bertucci, F.; Bouabdallah, R.; Devilard, E.; Carbuccia, N.; et al. Gene expression profiling identifies molecular subgroups among nodal peripheral T-cell lymphomas. *Oncogene* 2006, *25*, 1560–1570. [CrossRef]
89. Huang, Y.; de Reynies, A.; de Leval, L.; Ghazi, B.; Martin-Garcia, N.; Travert, M.; Bosq, J.; Briere, J.; Petit, B.; Thomas, E.; et al. Gene expression profiling identifies emerging oncogenic pathways operating in extranodal NK/T-cell lymphoma, nasal-type. *Blood* 2009, *115*, 1226–1237. [CrossRef]
90. de Leval, L.; Rickman, D.S.; Thielen, C.; Reynies, A.; Huang, Y.L.; Delsol, G.; Lamant, L.; Leroy, K.; Briere, J.; Molina, T.; et al. The gene expression profile of nodal peripheral T-cell lymphoma demonstrates a molecular link between angioimmunoblastic T-cell lymphoma (AITL) and follicular helper T (TFH) cells. *Blood* 2007, *109*, 4952–4963. [CrossRef] [PubMed]
91. Piccaluga, P.P.; Agostinelli, C.; Califano, A.; Rossi, M.; Basso, K.; Zupo, S.; Went, P.; Klein, U.; Zinzani, P.L.; Baccarani, M.; et al. Gene expression analysis of peripheral T cell lymphoma, unspecified, reveals distinct profiles and new potential therapeutic targets. *J. Clin. Investig.* 2007, *117*, 823–834. [CrossRef] [PubMed]

92. Piccaluga, P.P.; Agostinelli, C.; Califano, A.; Carbone, A.; Fantoni, L.; Ferrari, S.; Gazzola, A.; Gloghini, A.; Righi, S.; Rossi, M.; et al. Gene expression analysis of angioimmunoblastic lymphoma indicates derivation from T follicular helper cells and vascular endothelial growth factor deregulation. *Cancer Res.* **2007**, *67*, 10703–10710. [CrossRef] [PubMed]
93. Iqbal, J.; Weisenburger, D.D.; Chowdhury, A.; Tsai, M.Y.; Srivastava, G.; Greiner, T.C.; Kucuk, C.; Deffenbacher, K.; Vose, J.; Smith, L.; et al. Natural killer cell lymphoma shares strikingly similar molecular features with a group of non-hepatosplenic gammadelta T-cell lymphoma and is highly sensitive to a novel aurora kinase A inhibitor in vitro. *Leukemia* **2011**, *25*, 348–358. [CrossRef] [PubMed]
94. Iqbal, J.; Weisenburger, D.D.; Greiner, T.C.; Vose, J.M.; McKeithan, T.; Kucuk, C.; Geng, H.; Deffenbacher, K.; Smith, L.; Dybkaer, K.; et al. Molecular signatures to improve diagnosis in peripheral T-cell lymphoma and prognostication in angioimmunoblastic T-cell lymphoma. *Blood* **2010**, *115*, 1026–1036. [CrossRef] [PubMed]
95. Iqbal, J.; Wright, G.; Wang, C.; Rosenwald, A.; Gascoyne, R.D.; Weisenburger, D.D.; Greiner, T.C.; Smith, L.; Guo, S.; Wilcox, R.A.; et al. Gene expression signatures delineate biological and prognostic subgroups in peripheral T-cell lymphoma. *Blood* **2014**, *123*, 2915–2923. [CrossRef]
96. Tindemans, I.; Serafini, N.; Di Santo, J.P.; Hendriks, R.W. GATA-3 function in innate and adaptive immunity. *Immunity* **2014**, *41*, 191–206. [CrossRef]
97. Szabo, S.J.; Kim, S.T.; Costa, G.L.; Zhang, X.; Fathman, C.G.; Glimcher, L.H. A novel transcription factor, T-bet, directs Th1 lineage commitment. *Cell* **2000**, *100*, 655–669. [CrossRef]
98. Wang, T.; Feldman, A.L.; Wada, D.A.; Lu, Y.; Polk, A.; Briski, R.; Ristow, K.; Habermann, T.M.; Thomas, D.; Ziesmer, S.C.; et al. GATA-3 expression identifies a high-risk subset of PTCL, NOS with distinct molecular and clinical features. *Blood* **2014**, *123*, 3007–3015. [CrossRef] [PubMed]
99. O'Shea, J.J.; Paul, W.E. Mechanisms underlying lineage commitment and plasticity of helper CD4+ T cells. *Science* **2010**, *327*, 1098–1102. [CrossRef]
100. Wang, C.; McKeithan, T.W.; Gong, Q.; Zhang, W.; Bouska, A.; Rosenwald, A.; Gascoyne, R.D.; Wu, X.; Wang, J.; Muhammad, Z.; et al. IDH2R172 mutations define a unique subgroup of patients with angioimmunoblastic T-cell lymphoma. *Blood* **2015**, *126*, 1741–1752. [CrossRef] [PubMed]
101. Heavican, T.B.; Bouska, A.; Yu, J.; Lone, W.; Amador, C.; Gong, Q.; Zhang, W.; Li, Y.; Dave, B.J.; Nairismagi, M.L.; et al. Genetic drivers of oncogenic pathways in molecular subgroups of peripheral T-cell lymphoma. *Blood* **2019**, *133*, 1664–1676. [CrossRef] [PubMed]
102. Lone, W.; Bouska, A.; Sharma, S.; Amador, C.; Saumyaranjan, M.; Herek, T.A.; Heavican, T.B.; Yu, J.; Lim, S.T.; Ong, C.K.; et al. Genome-Wide miRNA Expression Profiling of Molecular Subgroups of Peripheral T-cell Lymphoma. *Clin. Cancer Res.* **2021**, *27*, 6039–6053. [CrossRef]
103. Amador, C.; Greiner, T.C.; Heavican, T.B.; Smith, L.M.; Galvis, K.T.; Lone, W.; Bouska, A.; D'Amore, F.; Pedersen, M.B.; Pileri, S.; et al. Reproducing the molecular subclassification of peripheral T-cell lymphoma-NOS by immunohistochemistry. *Blood* **2019**, *134*, 2159–2170. [CrossRef] [PubMed]
104. Amador, C.; Bouska, A.; Wright, G.; Weisenburger, D.D.; Feldman, A.L.; Smith, L.; Greiner, T.C.; Pileri, S.T.; Abanelli, V.; Ott, G.; et al. Gene expression signatures for the accurate diagnosis of peripheral T-cell lymphoma entities in the routine clinical practice. *J. Clin. Oncol.* **2022**; *in print*.
105. Ng, S.B.; Selvarajan, V.; Huang, G.; Zhou, J.; Feldman, A.L.; Law, M.; Kwong, Y.L.; Shimizu, N.; Kagami, Y.; Aozasa, K.; et al. Activated oncogenic pathways and therapeutic targets in extranodal nasal-type NK/T cell lymphoma revealed by gene expression profiling. *J. Pathol.* **2011**, *223*, 496–510. [CrossRef]
106. Iqbal, J.; Kucuk, C.; deLeeuw, R.J.; Srivastava, G.; Tam, W.; Geng, H.; Klinkebiel, D.; Christman, J.K.; Patel, K.; Cao, K.; et al. Genomic analyses reveal global functional alterations that promote tumor growth and novel tumor suppressor genes in natural killer-cell malignancies. *Leukemia* **2009**, *23*, 1139–1151. [CrossRef]
107. Dufva, O.; Kankainen, M.; Kelkka, T.; Sekiguchi, N.; Awad, S.A.; Eldfors, S.; Yadav, B.; Kuusanmaki, H.; Malani, D.; Andersson, E.I.; et al. Aggressive natural killer-cell leukemia mutational landscape and drug profiling highlight JAK-STAT signaling as therapeutic target. *Nat. Commun.* **2018**, *9*, 1567. [CrossRef] [PubMed]
108. Abate, F.; Todaro, M.; van der Krogt, J.A.; Boi, M.; Landra, I.; Machiorlatti, R.; Tabbo, F.; Messana, K.; Abele, C.; Barreca, A.; et al. A novel patient-derived tumorgraft model with TRAF1-ALK anaplastic large-cell lymphoma translocation. *Leukemia* **2015**, *29*, 1390–1401. [CrossRef] [PubMed]
109. International Human Genome Sequencing Consortium. Finishing the euchromatic sequence of the human genome. *Nature* **2004**, *431*, 931–945. [CrossRef]
110. She, X.; Jiang, Z.; Clark, R.A.; Liu, G.; Cheng, Z.; Tuzun, E.; Church, D.M.; Sutton, G.; Halpern, A.L.; Eichler, E.E. Shotgun sequence assembly and recent segmental duplications within the human genome. *Nature* **2004**, *431*, 927–930. [CrossRef] [PubMed]
111. Lenz, G.; Wright, G.W.; Emre, N.C.; Kohlhammer, H.; Dave, S.S.; Davis, R.E.; Carty, S.; Lam, L.T.; Shaffer, A.L.; Xiao, W.; et al. Molecular subtypes of diffuse large B-cell lymphoma arise by distinct genetic pathways. *Proc. Natl. Acad. Sci. USA* **2008**, *105*, 13520–13525. [CrossRef] [PubMed]
112. Jain, N.; Hartert, K.; Tadros, S.; Fiskus, W.; Havranek, O.; Ma, M.C.J.; Bouska, A.; Heavican, T.; Kumar, D.; Deng, Q.; et al. Targetable genetic alterations of TCF4 (E2-2) drive immunoglobulin expression in diffuse large B cell lymphoma. *Sci. Transl. Med.* **2019**, *11*, eaav5599. [CrossRef] [PubMed]

113. Iqbal, J.; Sanger, W.G.; Horsman, D.E.; Rosenwald, A.; Pickering, D.L.; Dave, B.; Dave, S.; Xiao, L.; Cao, K.; Zhu, Q.; et al. BCL2 translocation defines a unique tumor subset within the germinal center B-cell-like diffuse large B-cell lymphoma. *Am. J. Pathol.* **2004**, *165*, 159–166. [CrossRef]
114. Iqbal, J.; Greiner, T.C.; Patel, K.; Dave, B.J.; Smith, L.; Ji, J.; Wright, G.; Sanger, W.G.; Pickering, D.L.; Jain, S.; et al. Distinctive patterns of BCL6 molecular alterations and their functional consequences in different subgroups of diffuse large B-cell lymphoma. *Leukemia* **2007**, *21*, 2332–2343. [CrossRef] [PubMed]
115. Shaknovich, R.; Geng, H.; Johnson, N.A.; Tsikitas, L.; Cerchietti, L.; Greally, J.M.; Gascoyne, R.D.; Elemento, O.; Melnick, A. DNA methylation signatures define molecular subtypes of diffuse large B-cell lymphoma. *Blood* **2010**, *116*, e81–e89. [CrossRef] [PubMed]
116. Halldorsdottir, A.M.; Sander, B.; Goransson, H.; Isaksson, A.; Kimby, E.; Mansouri, M.; Rosenquist, R.; Ehrencrona, H. High-resolution genomic screening in mantle cell lymphoma—Specific changes correlate with genomic complexity, the proliferation signature and survival. *Genes Chromosomes Cancer* **2011**, *50*, 113–121. [CrossRef] [PubMed]
117. Hartmann, E.M.; Campo, E.; Wright, G.; Lenz, G.; Salaverria, I.; Jares, P.; Xiao, W.; Braziel, R.M.; Rimsza, L.M.; Chan, W.C.; et al. Pathway discovery in mantle cell lymphoma by integrated analysis of high-resolution gene expression and copy number profiling. *Blood* **2010**, *116*, 953–961. [CrossRef] [PubMed]
118. de Leeuw, R.J.; Davies, J.J.; Rosenwald, A.; Bebb, G.; Gascoyne, R.D.; Dyer, M.J.; Staudt, L.M.; Martinez-Climent, J.A.; Lam, W.L. Comprehensive whole genome array CGH profiling of mantle cell lymphoma model genomes. *Hum. Mol. Genet.* **2004**, *13*, 1827–1837. [CrossRef]
119. Honma, K.; Tsuzuki, S.; Nakagawa, M.; Tagawa, H.; Nakamura, S.; Morishima, Y.; Seto, M. TNFAIP3/A20 functions as a novel tumor suppressor gene in several subtypes of non-Hodgkin lymphomas. *Blood* **2009**, *114*, 2467–2475. [CrossRef] [PubMed]
120. Bea, S.; Valdes-Mas, R.; Navarro, A.; Salaverria, I.; Martin-Garcia, D.; Jares, P.; Gine, E.; Pinyol, M.; Royo, C.; Nadeu, F.; et al. Landscape of somatic mutations and clonal evolution in mantle cell lymphoma. *Proc. Natl. Acad. Sci. USA* **2013**, *110*, 18250–18255. [CrossRef] [PubMed]
121. Enjuanes, A.; Albero, R.; Clot, G.; Navarro, A.; Bea, S.; Pinyol, M.; Martin-Subero, J.I.; Klapper, W.; Staudt, L.M.; Jaffe, E.S.; et al. Genome-wide methylation analyses identify a subset of mantle cell lymphoma with a high number of methylated CpGs and aggressive clinicopathological features. *Int. J. Cancer* **2013**, *133*, 2852–2863.
122. Leshchenko, V.V.; Kuo, P.Y.; Shaknovich, R.; Yang, D.T.; Gellen, T.; Petrich, A.; Yu, Y.; Remache, Y.; Weniger, M.A.; Rafiq, S.; et al. Genomewide DNA methylation analysis reveals novel targets for drug development in mantle cell lymphoma. *Blood* **2010**, *116*, 1025–1034. [CrossRef]
123. Boerma, E.G.; Siebert, R.; Kluin, P.M.; Baudis, M. Translocations involving 8q24 in Burkitt lymphoma and other malignant lymphomas: A historical review of cytogenetics in the light of todays knowledge. *Leukemia* **2009**, *23*, 225–234. [CrossRef]
124. Scholtysik, R.; Kreuz, M.; Klapper, W.; Burkhardt, B.; Feller, A.C.; Hummel, M.; Loeffler, M.; Rosolowski, M.; Schwaenen, C.; Spang, R.; et al. Detection of genomic aberrations in molecularly defined Burkitt's lymphoma by array-based, high resolution, single nucleotide polymorphism analysis. *Haematologica* **2010**, *95*, 2047–2055. [CrossRef]
125. Schiffman, J.D.; Lorimer, P.D.; Rodic, V.; Jahromi, M.S.; Downie, J.M.; Bayerl, M.G.; Sanmann, J.N.; Althof, P.A.; Sanger, W.G.; Barnette, P.; et al. Genome wide copy number analysis of paediatric Burkitt lymphoma using formalin-fixed tissues reveals a subset with gain of chromosome 13q and corresponding miRNA over expression. *Br. J. Haematol.* **2011**, *155*, 477–486. [CrossRef] [PubMed]
126. Salaverria, I.; Zettl, A.; Bea, S.; Hartmann, E.M.; Dave, S.S.; Wright, G.W.; Boerma, E.J.; Kluin, P.M.; Ott, G.; Chan, W.C.; et al. Chromosomal alterations detected by comparative genomic hybridization in subgroups of gene expression-defined Burkitt's lymphoma. *Haematologica* **2008**, *93*, 1327–1334. [CrossRef] [PubMed]
127. Abate, F.; Ambrosio, M.R.; Mundo, L.; Laginestra, M.A.; Fuligni, F.; Rossi, M.; Zairis, S.; Gazaneo, S.; De Falco, G.; Lazzi, S.; et al. Distinct Viral and Mutational Spectrum of Endemic Burkitt Lymphoma. *PLoS Pathog.* **2015**, *11*, e1005158. [CrossRef] [PubMed]
128. Navari, M.; Fuligni, F.; Laginestra, M.A.; Etebari, M.; Ambrosio, M.R.; Sapienza, M.R.; Rossi, M.; De Falco, G.; Gibellini, D.; Tripodo, C.; et al. Molecular signature of Epstein Barr virus-positive Burkitt lymphoma and post-transplant lymphoproliferative disorder suggest different roles for Epstein Barr virus. *Front. Microbiol.* **2014**, *5*, 728. [CrossRef]
129. Grande, B.M.; Gerhard, D.S.; Jiang, A.; Griner, N.B.; Abramson, J.S.; Alexander, T.B.; Allen, H.; Ayers, L.W.; Bethony, J.M.; Bhatia, K.; et al. Genome-wide discovery of somatic coding and noncoding mutations in pediatric endemic and sporadic Burkitt lymphoma. *Blood* **2019**, *133*, 1313–1324. [CrossRef]
130. Horsman, D.E.; Connors, J.M.; Pantzar, T.; Gascoyne, R.D. Analysis of secondary chromosomal alterations in 165 cases of follicular lymphoma with t(14;18). *Genes Chromosomes Cancer* **2001**, *30*, 375–382. [CrossRef]
131. Cheung, K.J.; Delaney, A.; Ben-Neriah, S.; Schein, J.; Lee, T.; Shah, S.P.; Cheung, D.; Johnson, N.A.; Mungall, A.J.; Telenius, A.; et al. High resolution analysis of follicular lymphoma genomes reveals somatic recurrent sites of copy-neutral loss of heterozygosity and copy number alterations that target single genes. *Genes Chromosomes Cancer* **2010**, *49*, 669–681. [CrossRef]
132. Ross, C.W.; Ouillette, P.D.; Saddler, C.M.; Shedden, K.A.; Malek, S.N. Comprehensive analysis of copy number and allele status identifies multiple chromosome defects underlying follicular lymphoma pathogenesis. *Clin. Cancer Res.* **2007**, *13*, 4777–4785. [CrossRef]

133. Hoglund, M.; Sehn, L.; Connors, J.M.; Gascoyne, R.D.; Siebert, R.; Sall, T.; Mitelman, F.; Horsman, D.E. Identification of cytogenetic subgroups and karyotypic pathways of clonal evolution in follicular lymphomas. *Genes Chromosomes Cancer* **2004**, *39*, 195–204. [CrossRef]
134. d'Amore, F.; Chan, E.; Iqbal, J.; Geng, H.; Young, K.; Xiao, L.; Hess, M.M.; Sanger, W.G.; Smith, L.; Wiuf, C.; et al. Clonal evolution in t(14;18)-positive follicular lymphoma, evidence for multiple common pathways, and frequent parallel clonal evolution. *Clin Cancer Res.* **2008**, *14*, 7180–7187. [CrossRef]
135. Bouska, A.; McKeithan, T.W.; Deffenbacher, K.E.; Lachel, C.; Wright, G.W.; Iqbal, J.; Smith, L.M.; Zhang, W.; Kucuk, C.; Rinaldi, A.; et al. Genome-wide copy-number analyses reveal genomic abnormalities involved in transformation of follicular lymphoma. *Blood* **2014**, *123*, 1681–1690. [CrossRef] [PubMed]
136. Yano, T.; Jaffe, E.S.; Longo, D.L.; Raffeld, M. MYC rearrangements in histologically progressed follicular lymphomas. *Blood* **1992**, *80*, 758–767. [CrossRef] [PubMed]
137. Sander, C.A.; Yano, T.; Clark, H.M.; Harris, C.; Longo, D.L.; Jaffe, E.S.; Raffeld, M. p53 mutation is associated with progression in follicular lymphomas. *Blood* **1993**, *82*, 1994–2004. [CrossRef]
138. Matolcsy, A.; Casali, P.; Warnke, R.A.; Knowles, D.M. Morphologic transformation of follicular lymphoma is associated with somatic mutation of the translocated Bcl-2 gene. *Blood* **1996**, *88*, 3937–3944. [CrossRef] [PubMed]
139. Pinyol, M.; Cobo, F.; Bea, S.; Jares, P.; Nayach, I.; Fernandez, P.L.; Montserrat, E.; Cardesa, A.; Campo, E. p16(INK4a) gene inactivation by deletions, mutations, and hypermethylation is associated with transformed and aggressive variants of non-Hodgkin's lymphomas. *Blood* **1998**, *91*, 2977–2984. [CrossRef]
140. Martinez-Climent, J.A.; Alizadeh, A.A.; Segraves, R.; Blesa, D.; Rubio-Moscardo, F.; Albertson, D.G.; Garcia-Conde, J.; Dyer, M.J.; Levy, R.; Pinkel, D.; et al. Transformation of follicular lymphoma to diffuse large cell lymphoma is associated with a heterogeneous set of DNA copy number and gene expression alterations. *Blood* **2003**, *101*, 3109–3117. [CrossRef]
141. Bouska, A.; Zhang, W.; Gong, Q.; Iqbal, J.; Scuto, A.; Vose, J.; Ludvigsen, M.; Fu, K.; Weisenburger, D.D.; Greiner, T.C.; et al. Combined copy number and mutation analysis identifies oncogenic pathways associated with transformation of follicular lymphoma. *Leukemia* **2017**, *31*, 83–91. [CrossRef]
142. O'Riain, C.; O'Shea, D.M.; Yang, Y.; Le Dieu, R.; Gribben, J.G.; Summers, K.; Yeboah-Afari, J.; Bhaw-Rosun, L.; Fleischmann, C.; Mein, C.A.; et al. Array-based DNA methylation profiling in follicular lymphoma. *Leukemia* **2009**, *23*, 1858–1866. [CrossRef]
143. Davis, R.E.; Ngo, V.N.; Lenz, G.; Tolar, P.; Young, R.M.; Romesser, P.B.; Kohlhammer, H.; Lamy, L.; Zhao, H.; Yang, Y.; et al. Chronic active B-cell-receptor signalling in diffuse large B-cell lymphoma. *Nature* **2010**, *463*, 88–92. [CrossRef]
144. Lenz, G.; Davis, R.E.; Ngo, V.N.; Lam, L.; George, T.C.; Wright, G.W.; Dave, S.S.; Zhao, H.; Xu, W.; Rosenwald, A.; et al. Oncogenic CARD11 mutations in human diffuse large B cell lymphoma. *Science* **2008**, *319*, 1676–1679. [CrossRef]
145. Phelan, J.D.; Young, R.M.; Webster, D.E.; Roulland, S.; Wright, G.W.; Kasbekar, M.; Shaffer, A.L., 3rd; Ceribelli, M.; Wang, J.Q.; Schmitz, R.; et al. A multiprotein supercomplex controlling oncogenic signalling in lymphoma. *Nature* **2018**, *560*, 387–391. [CrossRef] [PubMed]
146. Ngo, V.N.; Young, R.M.; Schmitz, R.; Jhavar, S.; Xiao, W.; Lim, K.H.; Kohlhammer, H.; Xu, W.; Yang, Y.; Zhao, H.; et al. Oncogenically active MYD88 mutations in human lymphoma. *Nature* **2011**, *470*, 115–119. [CrossRef] [PubMed]
147. Pasqualucci, L.; Neumeister, P.; Goossens, T.; Nanjangud, G.; Chaganti, R.S.; Kuppers, R.; Dalla-Favera, R. Hypermutation of multiple proto-oncogenes in B-cell diffuse large-cell lymphomas. *Nature* **2001**, *412*, 341–346. [CrossRef]
148. Morin, R.D.; Johnson, N.A.; Severson, T.M.; Mungall, A.J.; An, J.; Goya, R.; Paul, J.E.; Boyle, M.; Woolcock, B.W.; Kuchenbauer, F.; et al. Somatic mutations altering EZH2 (Tyr641) in follicular and diffuse large B-cell lymphomas of germinal-center origin. *Nat. Genet.* **2010**, *42*, 181–185. [CrossRef]
149. Reddy, A.; Zhang, J.; Davis, N.S.; Moffitt, A.B.; Love, C.L.; Waldrop, A.; Leppa, S.; Pasanen, A.; Meriranta, L.; Karjalainen-Lindsberg, M.L.; et al. Genetic and Functional Drivers of Diffuse Large B Cell Lymphoma. *Cell* **2017**, *171*, 481–494.e15. [CrossRef] [PubMed]
150. Schmitz, R.; Wright, G.W.; Huang, D.W.; Johnson, C.A.; Phelan, J.D.; Wang, J.Q.; Roulland, S.; Kasbekar, M.; Young, R.M.; Shaffer, A.L.; et al. Genetics and Pathogenesis of Diffuse Large B-Cell Lymphoma. *N. Engl. J. Med.* **2018**, *378*, 1396–1407. [CrossRef] [PubMed]
151. Chapuy, B.; Stewart, C.; Dunford, A.J.; Kim, J.; Kamburov, A.; Redd, R.A.; Lawrence, M.S.; Roemer, M.G.M.; Li, A.J.; Ziepert, M.; et al. Molecular subtypes of diffuse large B cell lymphoma are associated with distinct pathogenic mechanisms and outcomes. *Nat. Med.* **2018**, *24*, 679–690. [CrossRef] [PubMed]
152. Zhang, J.; Jima, D.; Moffitt, A.B.; Liu, Q.; Czader, M.; Hsi, E.D.; Fedoriw, Y.; Dunphy, C.H.; Richards, K.L.; Gill, J.I.; et al. The genomic landscape of mantle cell lymphoma is related to the epigenetically determined chromatin state of normal B cells. *Blood* **2014**, *123*, 2988–2996. [CrossRef]
153. Bodor, C.; Grossmann, V.; Popov, N.; Okosun, J.; O'Riain, C.; Tan, K.; Marzec, J.; Araf, S.; Wang, J.; Lee, A.M.; et al. EZH2 mutations are frequent and represent an early event in follicular lymphoma. *Blood* **2013**, *122*, 3165–3168. [CrossRef] [PubMed]
154. Pasqualucci, L.; Khiabanian, H.; Fangazio, M.; Vasishtha, M.; Messina, M.; Holmes, A.B.; Ouillette, P.; Trifonov, V.; Rossi, D.; Tabbo, F.; et al. Genetics of follicular lymphoma transformation. *Cell Rep.* **2014**, *6*, 130–140. [CrossRef]
155. Richter, J.; Schlesner, M.; Hoffmann, S.; Kreuz, M.; Leich, E.; Burkhardt, B.; Rosolowski, M.; Ammerpohl, O.; Wagener, R.; Bernhart, S.H.; et al. Recurrent mutation of the ID3 gene in Burkitt lymphoma identified by integrated genome, exome and transcriptome sequencing. *Nat. Genet.* **2012**, *44*, 1316–1320.

156. Schmitz, R.; Young, R.M.; Ceribelli, M.; Jhavar, S.; Xiao, W.; Zhang, M.; Wright, G.; Shaffer, A.L.; Hodson, D.J.; Buras, E.; et al. Burkitt lymphoma pathogenesis and therapeutic targets from structural and functional genomics. *Nature* **2012**, *490*, 116–120. [CrossRef] [PubMed]
157. Arribas, A.J.; Campos-Martin, Y.; Gomez-Abad, C.; Algara, P.; Sanchez-Beato, M.; Rodriguez-Pinilla, M.S.; Montes-Moreno, S.; Martinez, N.; Alves-Ferreira, J.; Piris, M.A.; et al. Nodal marginal zone lymphoma: Gene expression and miRNA profiling identify diagnostic markers and potential therapeutic targets. *Blood* **2012**, *119*, e9–e21. [CrossRef]
158. Spina, V.; Khiabanian, H.; Messina, M.; Monti, S.; Cascione, L.; Bruscaggin, A.; Spaccarotella, E.; Holmes, A.B.; Arcaini, L.; Lucioni, M.; et al. The genetics of nodal marginal zone lymphoma. *Blood* **2016**, *128*, 1362–1373. [CrossRef]
159. Vela, V.; Juskevicius, D.; Dirnhofer, S.; Menter, T.; Tzankov, A. Mutational landscape of marginal zone B-cell lymphomas of various origin: Organotypic alterations and diagnostic potential for assignment of organ origin. *Virchows Arch.* **2022**, *480*, 403–413. [CrossRef]
160. Tu, P.H.; Giannini, C.; Judkins, A.R.; Schwalb, J.M.; Burack, R.; O'Neill, B.P.; Yachnis, A.T.; Burger, P.C.; Scheithauer, B.W.; Perry, A. Clinicopathologic and genetic profile of intracranial marginal zone lymphoma: A primary low-grade CNS lymphoma that mimics meningioma. *J. Clin. Oncol.* **2005**, *23*, 5718–5727. [CrossRef] [PubMed]
161. Moody, S.; Thompson, J.S.; Chuang, S.S.; Liu, H.; Raderer, M.; Vassiliou, G.; Wlodarska, I.; Wu, F.; Cogliatti, S.; Robson, A.; et al. Novel GPR34 and CCR6 mutation and distinct genetic profiles in MALT lymphomas of different sites. *Haematologica* **2018**, *103*, 1329–1336. [CrossRef]
162. Wright, G.W.; Huang, D.W.; Phelan, J.D.; Coulibaly, Z.A.; Roulland, S.; Young, R.M.; Wang, J.Q.; Schmitz, R.; Morin, R.D.; Tang, J.; et al. A Probabilistic Classification Tool for Genetic Subtypes of Diffuse Large B Cell Lymphoma with Therapeutic Implications. *Cancer Cell* **2020**, *37*, 551–568.e14. [CrossRef]
163. Song, J.Y.; Egan, C.; Bouska, A.C.; Zhang, W.; Gong, Q.; Venkataraman, G.; Herrera, A.F.; Chen, L.; Ottesen, R.; Niland, J.C.; et al. Genomic characterization of diffuse large B-cell lymphoma transformation of nodular lymphocyte-predominant Hodgkin lymphoma. *Leukemia* **2020**, *34*, 2238–2242. [CrossRef]
164. Hartmann, S.; Schuhmacher, B.; Rausch, T.; Fuller, L.; Doring, C.; Weniger, M.; Lollies, A.; Weiser, C.; Thurner, L.; Rengstl, B.; et al. Highly recurrent mutations of SGK1, DUSP2 and JUNB in nodular lymphocyte predominant Hodgkin lymphoma. *Leukemia* **2016**, *30*, 844–853. [CrossRef]
165. Iqbal, J.; Wilcox, R.; Naushad, H.; Rohr, J.; Heavican, T.B.; Wang, C.; Bouska, A.; Fu, K.; Chan, W.C.; Vose, J.M. Genomic signatures in T-cell lymphoma: How can these improve precision in diagnosis and inform prognosis? *Blood Rev.* **2016**, *30*, 89–100. [CrossRef]
166. Iqbal, J.; Naushad, H.; Bi, C.; Yu, J.; Bouska, A.; Rohr, J.; Chao, W.; Fu, K.; Chan, W.C.; Vose, J.M. Genomic signatures in B-cell lymphoma: How can these improve precision in diagnosis and inform prognosis? *Blood Rev.* **2016**, *30*, 73–88. [CrossRef]
167. Iqbal, J.; Amador, C.; McKeithan, T.W.; Chan, W.C. Molecular and Genomic Landscape of Peripheral T-Cell Lymphoma. *Cancer Treat. Res.* **2019**, *176*, 31–68.
168. Cairns, R.A.; Iqbal, J.; Lemonnier, F.; Kucuk, C.; de Leval, L.; Jais, J.P.; Parrens, M.; Martin, A.; Xerri, L.; Brousset, P.; et al. IDH2 mutations are frequent in angioimmunoblastic T-cell lymphoma. *Blood* **2012**, *119*, 1901–1903. [CrossRef]
169. Herek, T.A.; Bouska, A.; Lone, W.; Amador, C.; Heavican, T.B.; Sharma, S.; Greiner, T.C.; Smith, L.; Pileri, S.; Feldman, A.L.; et al. DNMT3A mutation defines a unique biological and prognostic subgroup in PTCL-NOS. *Blood*, **2022**; in print.
170. Cheng, S.; Zhang, W.; Inghirami, G.; Tam, W. Mutation analysis links angioimmunoblastic T-cell lymphoma to clonal hematopoiesis and smoking. *eLife* **2021**, *10*, e66395. [CrossRef]
171. Palomero, T.; Couronne, L.; Khiabanian, H.; Kim, M.Y.; Ambesi-Impiombato, A.; Perez-Garcia, A.; Carpenter, Z.; Abate, F.; Allegretta, M.; Haydu, J.E.; et al. Recurrent mutations in epigenetic regulators, RHOA and FYN kinase in peripheral T cell lymphomas. *Nat. Genet.* **2014**, *46*, 166–170. [CrossRef]
172. Manso, R.; Sanchez-Beato, M.; Monsalvo, S.; Gomez, S.; Cereceda, L.; Llamas, P.; Rojo, F.; Mollejo, M.; Menarguez, J.; Alves, J.; et al. The RHOA G17V gene mutation occurs frequently in peripheral T-cell lymphoma and is associated with a characteristic molecular signature. *Blood* **2014**, *123*, 2893–2894. [CrossRef]
173. Sakata-Yanagimoto, M.; Enami, T.; Yoshida, K.; Shiraishi, Y.; Ishii, R.; Miyake, Y.; Muto, H.; Tsuyama, N.; Sato-Otsubo, A.; Okuno, Y.; et al. Somatic RHOA mutation in angioimmunoblastic T cell lymphoma. *Nat. Genet.* **2014**, *46*, 171–175. [CrossRef]
174. Lee, S.H.; Kim, J.S.; Kim, J.; Kim, S.J.; Kim, W.S.; Lee, S.; Ko, Y.H.; Yoo, H.Y. A highly recurrent novel missense mutation in CD28 among angioimmunoblastic T-cell lymphoma patients. *Haematologica* **2015**, *100*, e505–e507. [CrossRef]
175. Rohr, J.; Guo, S.; Huo, J.; Bouska, A.; Lachel, C.; Li, Y.; Simone, P.D.; Zhang, W.; Gong, Q.; Wang, C.; et al. Recurrent activating mutations of CD28 in peripheral T-cell lymphomas. *Leukemia* **2016**, *30*, 1062–1070. [CrossRef] [PubMed]
176. Vallois, D.; Dobay, M.P.; Morin, R.D.; Lemonnier, F.; Missiaglia, E.; Juilland, M.; Iwaszkiewicz, J.; Fataccioli, V.; Bisig, B.; Roberti, A.; et al. Activating mutations in genes related to TCR signaling in angioimmunoblastic and other follicular helper T-cell-derived lymphomas. *Blood* **2016**, *128*, 1490–1502. [CrossRef]
177. Kataoka, K.; Nagata, Y.; Kitanaka, A.; Shiraishi, Y.; Shimamura, T.; Yasunaga, J.; Totoki, Y.; Chiba, K.; Sato-Otsubo, A.; Nagae, G.; et al. Integrated molecular analysis of adult T cell leukemia/lymphoma. *Nat. Genet.* **2015**, *47*, 1304–1315. [CrossRef]
178. Wartewig, T.; Kurgyis, Z.; Keppler, S.; Pechloff, K.; Hameister, E.; Ollinger, R.; Maresch, R.; Buch, T.; Steiger, K.; Winter, C.; et al. PD-1 is a haploinsufficient suppressor of T cell lymphomagenesis. *Nature* **2017**, *552*, 121–125. [CrossRef] [PubMed]

179. Debackere, K.; Marcelis, L.; Demeyer, S.; Vanden Bempt, M.; Mentens, N.; Gielen, O.; Jacobs, K.; Broux, M.; Verhoef, G.; Michaux, L.; et al. Fusion transcripts FYN-TRAF3IP2 and KHDRBS1-LCK hijack T cell receptor signaling in peripheral T-cell lymphoma, not otherwise specified. *Nat. Commun.* **2021**, *12*, 3705. [CrossRef]
180. Moon, C.S.; Reglero, C.; Cortes, J.R.; Quinn, S.A.; Alvarez, S.; Zhao, J.; Lin, W.W.; Cooke, A.J.; Abate, F.; Soderquist, C.R.; et al. FYN-TRAF3IP2 induces NF-kappaB signaling-driven peripheral T cell lymphoma. *Nat. Cancer* **2021**, *2*, 98–113. [CrossRef]
181. Abate, F.; da Silva-Almeida, A.C.; Zairis, S.; Robles-Valero, J.; Couronne, L.; Khiabanian, H.; Quinn, S.A.; Kim, M.Y.; Laginestra, M.A.; Kim, C.; et al. Activating mutations and translocations in the guanine exchange factor VAV1 in peripheral T-cell lymphomas. *Proc. Natl. Acad. Sci. USA* **2017**, *114*, 764–769. [CrossRef]
182. Crescenzo, R.; Abate, F.; Lasorsa, E.; Tabbo, F.; Gaudiano, M.; Chiesa, N.; Di Giacomo, F.; Spaccarotella, E.; Barbarossa, L.; Ercole, E.; et al. Convergent mutations and kinase fusions lead to oncogenic STAT3 activation in anaplastic large cell lymphoma. *Cancer Cell* **2015**, *27*, 516–532. [CrossRef]
183. Parrilla Castellar, E.R.; Jaffe, E.S.; Said, J.W.; Swerdlow, S.H.; Ketterling, R.P.; Knudson, R.A.; Sidhu, J.S.; Hsi, E.D.; Karikehalli, S.; Jiang, L.; et al. ALK-negative anaplastic large cell lymphoma is a genetically heterogeneous disease with widely disparate clinical outcomes. *Blood* **2014**, *124*, 1473–1480. [CrossRef] [PubMed]
184. Rui, L.; Emre, N.C.; Kruhlak, M.J.; Chung, H.J.; Steidl, C.; Slack, G.; Wright, G.W.; Lenz, G.; Ngo, V.N.; Shaffer, A.L.; et al. Cooperative epigenetic modulation by cancer amplicon genes. *Cancer Cell* **2010**, *18*, 590–605. [CrossRef]
185. Yan, J.; Li, B.; Lin, B.; Lee, P.T.; Chung, T.H.; Tan, J.; Bi, C.; Lee, X.T.; Selvarajan, V.; Ng, S.B.; et al. EZH2 phosphorylation by JAK3 mediates a switch to noncanonical function in natural killer/T-cell lymphoma. *Blood* **2016**, *128*, 948–958. [CrossRef]
186. Kucuk, C.; Jiang, B.; Hu, X.; Zhang, W.; Chan, J.K.; Xiao, W.; Lack, N.; Alkan, C.; Williams, J.C.; Avery, K.N.; et al. Activating mutations of STAT5B and STAT3 in lymphomas derived from gammadelta-T or NK cells. *Nat. Commun.* **2015**, *6*, 6025. [CrossRef] [PubMed]
187. Kiel, M.J.; Velusamy, T.; Rolland, D.; Sahasrabuddhe, A.A.; Chung, F.; Bailey, N.G.; Schrader, A.; Li, B.; Li, J.Z.; Ozel, A.B.; et al. Integrated genomic sequencing reveals mutational landscape of T-cell prolymphocytic leukemia. *Blood* **2014**, *124*, 1460–1472. [CrossRef]
188. Dong, G.; Liu, X.; Wang, L.; Yin, W.; Bouska, A.; Gong, Q.; Shetty, K.; Chen, L.; Sharma, S.; Zhang, J.; et al. Genomic profiling identifies distinct genetic subtypes in extra-nodal natural killer/T-cell lymphoma. *Leukemia* **2022**, *36*, 2064–2075. [CrossRef]
189. Watatani, Y.; Sato, Y.; Miyoshi, H.; Sakamoto, K.; Nishida, K.; Gion, Y.; Nagata, Y.; Shiraishi, Y.; Chiba, K.; Tanaka, H.; et al. Molecular heterogeneity in peripheral T-cell lymphoma, not otherwise specified revealed by comprehensive genetic profiling. *Leukemia* **2019**, *33*, 2867–2883. [CrossRef]
190. Laurent, C.; Fazilleau, N.; Brousset, P. A novel subset of T-helper cells: Follicular T-helper cells and their markers. *Haematologica* **2010**, *95*, 356–358. [CrossRef]
191. Dobay, M.P.; Lemonnier, F.; Missiaglia, E.; Bastard, C.; Vallois, D.; Jais, J.-P.; Scourzic, L.; Dupuy, A.; Fataccioli, V.; Pujals, A.; et al. Integrative clinicopathological and molecular analyses of angioimmunoblastic T-cell lymphoma and other nodal lymphomas of follicular helper T-cell origin. *Haematologica* **2017**, *102*, e148–e151. [CrossRef] [PubMed]
192. Golloshi, R.; Sanders, J.T.; McCord, R.P. Iteratively improving Hi-C experiments one step at a time. *Methods* **2018**, *142*, 47–58. [CrossRef]
193. Newman, A.M.; Liu, C.L.; Green, M.R.; Gentles, A.J.; Feng, W.; Xu, Y.; Hoang, C.D.; Diehn, M.; Alizadeh, A.A. Robust enumeration of cell subsets from tissue expression profiles. *Nat. Methods* **2015**, *12*, 453–457. [CrossRef] [PubMed]
194. Chen, B.; Khodadoust, M.S.; Liu, C.L.; Newman, A.M.; Alizadeh, A.A. Profiling Tumor Infiltrating Immune Cells with CIBERSORT. *Methods Mol. Biol.* **2018**, *1711*, 243–259.
195. Steen, C.B.; Luca, B.A.; Esfahani, M.S.; Azizi, A.; Sworder, B.J.; Nabet, B.Y.; Kurtz, D.M.; Liu, C.L.; Khameneh, F.; Advani, R.H.; et al. The landscape of tumor cell states and ecosystems in diffuse large B cell lymphoma. *Cancer Cell* **2021**, *39*, 1422–1437.e10. [CrossRef] [PubMed]
196. Mansfield, J.R. Phenotyping Multiple Subsets of Immune Cells In Situ in FFPE Tissue Sections: An Overview of Methodologies. *Methods Mol. Biol.* **2017**, *1546*, 75–99.
197. Trapecar, M.; Khan, S.; Roan, N.R.; Chen, T.H.; Telwatte, S.; Deswal, M.; Pao, M.; Somsouk, M.; Deeks, S.G.; Hunt, P.W.; et al. An Optimized and Validated Method for Isolation and Characterization of Lymphocytes from HIV+ Human Gut Biopsies. *AIDS Res. Hum. Retrovir.* **2017**, *33*, S31–S39. [CrossRef]
198. Scurrah, C.R.; Simmons, A.J.; Lau, K.S. Single-Cell Mass Cytometry of Archived Human Epithelial Tissue for Decoding Cancer Signaling Pathways. *Methods Mol. Biol.* **2019**, *1884*, 215–229.
199. Yao, Y.; Liu, R.; Shin, M.S.; Trentalange, M.; Allore, H.; Nassar, A.; Kang, I.; Pober, J.S.; Montgomery, R.R. CyTOF supports efficient detection of immune cell subsets from small samples. *J. Immunol. Methods* **2014**, *415*, 1–5. [CrossRef]
200. Giesen, C.; Wang, H.A.; Schapiro, D.; Zivanovic, N.; Jacobs, A.; Hattendorf, B.; Schuffler, P.J.; Grolimund, D.; Buhmann, J.M.; Brandt, S.; et al. Highly multiplexed imaging of tumor tissues with subcellular resolution by mass cytometry. *Nat. Methods* **2014**, *11*, 417–422. [CrossRef]
201. Chang, Q.; Ornatsky, O.I.; Siddiqui, I.; Loboda, A.; Baranov, V.I.; Hedley, D.W. Imaging Mass Cytometry. *Cytom. A* **2017**, *91*, 160–169. [CrossRef]
202. Fincham, R.E.A.; Bashiri, H.; Lau, M.C.; Yeong, J. Editorial: Multiplex Immunohistochemistry/Immunofluorescence Technique: The Potential and Promise for Clinical Application. *Front. Mol. Biosci.* **2022**, *9*, 831383. [CrossRef]

203. Spagnolo, D.M.; Gyanchandani, R.; Al-Kofahi, Y.; Stern, A.M.; Lezon, T.R.; Gough, A.; Meyer, D.E.; Ginty, F.; Sarachan, B.; Fine, J.; et al. Pointwise mutual information quantifies intratumor heterogeneity in tissue sections labeled with multiple fluorescent biomarkers. *J. Pathol. Inform.* **2016**, *7*, 47. [CrossRef]
204. Norton, S.; Kemp, R. Computational Analysis of High-Dimensional Mass Cytometry Data from Clinical Tissue Samples. *Methods Mol. Biol.* **2019**, *1989*, 295–307.
205. Hedlund, E.; Deng, Q. Single-cell RNA sequencing: Technical advancements and biological applications. *Mol. Asp. Med.* **2018**, *59*, 36–46. [CrossRef]
206. Camara, P.G. Topological methods for genomics: Present and future directions. *Curr. Opin. Syst. Biol.* **2017**, *1*, 95–101. [CrossRef] [PubMed]
207. Aoki, T.; Chong, L.C.; Takata, K.; Milne, K.; Hav, M.; Colombo, A.; Chavez, E.A.; Nissen, M.; Wang, X.; Miyata-Takata, T.; et al. Single-Cell Transcriptome Analysis Reveals Disease-Defining T-cell Subsets in the Tumor Microenvironment of Classic Hodgkin Lymphoma. *Cancer Discov.* **2020**, *10*, 406–421. [CrossRef]
208. Rindler, K.; Jonak, C.; Alkon, N.; Thaler, F.M.; Kurz, H.; Shaw, L.E.; Stingl, G.; Weninger, W.; Halbritter, F.; Bauer, W.M.; et al. Single-cell RNA sequencing reveals markers of disease progression in primary cutaneous T-cell lymphoma. *Mol. Cancer* **2021**, *20*, 124. [CrossRef]
209. Ysebaert, L.; Quillet-Mary, A.; Tosolini, M.; Pont, F.; Laurent, C.; Fournie, J.J. Lymphoma Heterogeneity Unraveled by Single-Cell Transcriptomics. *Front. Immunol.* **2021**, *12*, 597651. [CrossRef]
210. Rodriques, S.G.; Stickels, R.R.; Goeva, A.; Martin, C.A.; Murray, E.; Vanderburg, C.R.; Welch, J.; Chen, L.M.; Chen, F.; Macosko, E.Z. Slide-seq: A scalable technology for measuring genome-wide expression at high spatial resolution. *Science* **2019**, *363*, 1463–1467. [CrossRef] [PubMed]
211. Newman, A.M.; Bratman, S.V.; To, J.; Wynne, J.F.; Eclov, N.C.; Modlin, L.A.; Liu, C.L.; Neal, J.W.; Wakelee, H.A.; Merritt, R.E.; et al. An ultrasensitive method for quantitating circulating tumor DNA with broad patient coverage. *Nat. Med.* **2014**, *20*, 548–554. [CrossRef] [PubMed]
212. Murtaza, M.; Dawson, S.J.; Pogrebniak, K.; Rueda, O.M.; Provenzano, E.; Grant, J.; Chin, S.F.; Tsui, D.W.; Marass, F.; Gale, D.; et al. Multifocal clonal evolution characterized using circulating tumour DNA in a case of metastatic breast cancer. *Nat. Commun.* **2015**, *6*, 8760. [CrossRef] [PubMed]
213. Dawson, S.J.; Tsui, D.W.; Murtaza, M.; Biggs, H.; Rueda, O.M.; Chin, S.F.; Dunning, M.J.; Gale, D.; Forshew, T.; Mahler-Araujo, B.; et al. Analysis of circulating tumor DNA to monitor metastatic breast cancer. *N. Engl. J. Med.* **2013**, *368*, 1199–1209. [CrossRef]
214. Murtaza, M.; Dawson, S.J.; Tsui, D.W.; Gale, D.; Forshew, T.; Piskorz, A.M.; Parkinson, C.; Chin, S.F.; Kingsbury, Z.; Wong, A.S.; et al. Non-invasive analysis of acquired resistance to cancer therapy by sequencing of plasma DNA. *Nature* **2013**, *497*, 108–112. [CrossRef]
215. Bratman, S.V.; Newman, A.M.; Alizadeh, A.A.; Diehn, M. Potential clinical utility of ultrasensitive circulating tumor DNA detection with CAPP-Seq. *Expert Rev. Mol. Diagn.* **2015**, *15*, 715–719. [CrossRef]
216. McDonald, B.R.; Contente-Cuomo, T.; Sammut, S.J.; Odenheimer-Bergman, A.; Ernst, B.; Perdigones, N.; Chin, S.F.; Farooq, M.; Mejia, R.; Cronin, P.A.; et al. Personalized circulating tumor DNA analysis to detect residual disease after neoadjuvant therapy in breast cancer. *Sci. Transl. Med.* **2019**, *11*, eaax7392. [CrossRef]
217. Spina, V.; Bruscaggin, A.; Cuccaro, A.; Martini, M.; Di Trani, M.; Forestieri, G.; Manzoni, M.; Condoluci, A.; Arribas, A.; Terzi-Di-Bergamo, L.; et al. Circulating tumor DNA reveals genetics, clonal evolution, and residual disease in classical Hodgkin lymphoma. *Blood* **2018**, *131*, 2413–2425. [CrossRef]
218. Kurtz, D.M.; Scherer, F.; Jin, M.C.; Soo, J.; Craig, A.F.M.; Esfahani, M.S.; Chabon, J.J.; Stehr, H.; Liu, C.L.; Tibshirani, R.; et al. Circulating Tumor DNA Measurements As Early Outcome Predictors in Diffuse Large B-Cell Lymphoma. *J. Clin. Oncol.* **2018**, *36*, 2845–2853. [CrossRef]
219. Henriksen, S.D.; Thorlacius-Ussing, O. Cell-Free DNA Methylation as Blood-Based Biomarkers for Pancreatic Adenocarcinoma-A Literature Update. *Epigenomes* **2021**, *5*, 8. [CrossRef]
220. Lauer, E.M.; Mutter, J.; Scherer, F. Circulating tumor DNA in B-cell lymphoma: Technical advances, clinical applications, and perspectives for translational research. *Leukemia* **2022**, *6*, 1–14. [CrossRef]
221. Kurtz, D.M.; Esfahani, M.S.; Scherer, F.; Soo, J.; Jin, M.C.; Liu, C.L.; Newman, A.M.; Duhrsen, U.; Huttmann, A.; Casasnovas, O.; et al. Dynamic Risk Profiling Using Serial Tumor Biomarkers for Personalized Outcome Prediction. *Cell* **2019**, *178*, 699–713.e19. [CrossRef]
222. Rossi, D.; Kurtz, D.M.; Roschewski, M.; Cavalli, F.; Zucca, E.; Wilson, W.H. The development of liquid biopsy for research and clinical practice in lymphomas: Report of the 15-ICML workshop on ctDNA. *Hematol. Oncol.* **2020**, *38*, 34–37. [CrossRef] [PubMed]

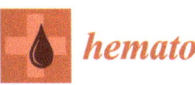 *hemato*

Review

Epigenetic Modifications in Lymphoma and Their Role in the Classification of Lymphomas

Sean Harrop [1,*], Costas Kleanthes Yannakou [2], Carrie Van Der Weyden [1] and Henry Miles Prince [1,2,3]

1. Peter MacCallum Cancer Center, Melbourne, VIC 3000, Australia; carrie.vanderweyden@petermac.org (C.V.D.W.); miles.prince@petermac.org (H.M.P.)
2. Epworth HealthCare, East Melbourne, VIC 3002, Australia; costas.yannakou@epworth.org.au
3. Sir Peter MacCallum Department of Oncology, University of Melbourne, Parkville, VIC 3052, Australia
* Correspondence: sean.harrop@petermac.org

Abstract: The characterisation of the lymphoma epigenome has provided insight into mechanisms involved in lymphomagenesis. Multiple lymphoma subtypes demonstrate recurrent mutations in key epigenetic regulators that have been utilised to define clinicogenetic groups that can predict clinical behaviour in these heterogenous entities. The high frequency of mutations in epigenetic regulators provides rationale to incorporate these in the classification of some subtypes of lymphoma. In addition, their recurrent nature provides a rationale to target such mutations, or the relevant pathway, for treatment. In this review, we summarised the available literature on epigenetic dysregulation in lymphoma and how it has been utilised in diagnosis and classification.

Keywords: lymphomagenesis; methylation; histone modification

1. Introduction

Epigenetics describes the modification of the transcription of genetic code independent of the DNA sequence. This is usually via the regulation of DNA methylation and histone modification, which controls gene expression and plays a critical role in normal cellular differentiation and growth. The epigenome is important for normal lymphocyte development and plays a role in the normal immune response [1]. Beyond normal development, the deregulation of the epigenome is frequently observed in human cancers and is thought to play a key role in oncogenesis through the silencing of tumour suppressor genes, as well as through changes in the tumor microenvironment (TME) and immune response [2].

With respect to lymphoma, epigenetic alterations are frequently observed across many subtypes. Indeed, the development of rapid and accurate gene sequencing technologies, such as next generation sequencing (NGS), has led to the use of mutational profiling as an integral component of lymphoma classification; mutations of epigenetic genes are frequently encountered. The detection of these epigenetic aberrancies may be useful diagnostically, as certain mutational profiles are supportive of a particular diagnosis. This is particularly relevant in the T-cell lymphomas, such as angioimmunoblastic T-cell lymphoma (AITL), where histological diagnosis can be challenging.

There is an emerging recognition that patterns of epigenetic dysregulation, which are often reflective of the underlying stage of differentiation, can be prognostically relevant; specific epigenetic mutations have now been incorporated into prognostic scores [3]. Certain lymphoma subtypes, such as follicular lymphoma (FL), have a significant degree of epigenetic dysregulation, which likely drives lymphomagenesis and disease progression. These mutations have proven to be therapeutically exploitable [4].

In this review, we highlight the progress that has been made in characterising the epigenetic landscape of different subtypes of lymphoma, with a particular focus on how epigenetic dysregulation contributes to the evolving classification of lymphoma.

Citation: Harrop, S.; Yannakou, C.K.; Van Der Weyden, C.; Prince, H.M. Epigenetic Modifications in Lymphoma and Their Role in the Classification of Lymphomas. *Hemato* **2022**, *3*, 174–187. https://doi.org/10.3390/hemato3010015

Academic Editor: Jude Fitzgibbon

Received: 26 January 2022
Accepted: 16 February 2022
Published: 21 February 2022

Publisher's Note: MDPI stays neutral with regard to jurisdictional claims in published maps and institutional affiliations.

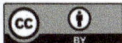

Copyright: © 2022 by the authors. Licensee MDPI, Basel, Switzerland. This article is an open access article distributed under the terms and conditions of the Creative Commons Attribution (CC BY) license (https://creativecommons.org/licenses/by/4.0/).

2. Key Epigenetic Regulators Involved in Lymphomagenesis

Epigenetic dysregulation occurs through a complex interplay of different mechanisms, including somatic mutations in key proteins involved in DNA methylation and histone acetylation, deacetylation, and methylation. These alterations influence gene transcription, leading to either the activation or repression of key tumour suppressor genes, DNA repair proteins and cell cycle regulators. Some of the most frequent, recurrently mutated key regulators in lymphoma are described below.

EZH2: The Enhancer of zeste homolog 2 (*EZH2*) encodes the catalytic subunit of the polycomb repressive complex 2 that mediates histone methylation, leading to transcriptional silencing. Expression of mutant *EZH2* impairs germinal center differentiation, driving aberrant proliferation by silencing genes such as *IRF4* and *PRDM1* [5]. Tumours that lack MHCI and MHCII are enriched for *EZH2* mutations, supporting the role of epigenetic regulation in immune evasion [6]. *EZH2* was one of the first recurrently mutated epigenetic regulators identified in FL and has provided a novel therapeutic target [7].

KMT2: The histone lysine methyltransferase 2 (*KMT2*) proteins, previously known as mixed lineage leukaemia (*MLL*), form complexes that methylate lysine 4 on histone H3 (H3K4). Mutations in *KMT2* are seen across all types of human cancers; they are the most frequently detected mutations in FL, where they have a tumour suppressor function by impeding B-cell differentiation [8].

CREBBP: CREB binding protein (*CREBBP*) has histone acetyltransferase activity and is structurally and functionally similar to *EP300*. Loss-of-function mutations in *CREBBP* have been demonstrated to cooperate with *BCL2* and to lead to a reduction in histone acetylation affecting germinal center development and B-cell signalling pathways [9,10]. In vitro disruption of *CREBBP* has been demonstrated to promote lymphomagenesis via accelerated cellular growth and MHCII downregulation, providing evidence of the tumour suppressor role that these pathways play in addition to altering the TME to favour malignant proliferation [9].

ARID1A: AT-rich interactive domain-containing protein 1A (*ARID1A*) promotes the formation of SWI/SNF nucleosome remodelling complexes containing BRG1 or BRM, which catalyse disruption of DNA-histone contacts, thereby, controlling chromatin condensation and DNA accessibility. *ARID1A* is critical for maintaining haematopoiesis, with differentiation of both myeloid and lymphoid lineages impaired in *ARID1A* knockout mice [11].

DNMT3A: DNA methyltransferase 3A (*DNMT3A*) functions as a DNA methyltransferase catalysing cytosine methylation of CpG islands in promoters, leading to transcriptional silencing. *DNMT3A is critical for hematopoietic stem cell differentiation*; mutations in this gene are thought to be early events in lymphoid malignancies [12].

TET2: The ten eleven translocation 2 (*TET2*) gene encodes an alpha-ketoglutarate dependent dioxygenase that regulates DNA hydroxymethylation by converting 5-methylcytosine (5mC) to 5-hydroxymethylcytosine (5 hmC), which promotes DNA methylation. The interaction between mutated *DNMT3A* and *TET2*, which leads to a reduction and increase in global DNA methylation, respectively, creates a complex methylation landscape [13].

IDH2: Isocitrate dehydrogenase 2 (*IDH2*) converts isocitrate to a-ketoglutarate, a key co-factor in the oxidative demethylase reactions that remove methyl-groups from DNA. Mutant *IDH2* converts isocitrate to 2-hydroxyglutarate, which is an oncogenic metabolite that cannot function as an obligatory cofactor of TET catalytic functions. Mutations in *IDH2* and *TET2* reduce 5hmC levels due to global hypermethylation of promoters and CpG, islands resulting in transcriptional repression [14].

3. The B-Cell Lymphomas

The B-cell lymphomas are genetically heterogenous malignancies derived from mature B-lymphocytes and characterised by a broad range of clinical features. The genetic processes that lead to lymphomagenesis include large chromosomal changes, classically chromosomal translocations involving the immunoglobulin heavy chain locus, copy number aberrancies and somatic mutations in key regulators of intracellular pathways. These genetic events result in hyperproliferative and anti-apoptotic activity and are recognised as key to the development of malignancy. Chromosomal translocations, while often entity defining, are, alone, mostly insufficient to lead to lymphomagenesis and are seen in the lymphocytes of healthy individuals. Age-related non-random genetic mosaicism has been associated with the development of lymphoid malignancy [15–17]. Epigenetic dysregulation leads to lymphomagenic alteration of gene expression required for germinal center development and post germinal center differentiation. FL and diffuse large B-cell lymphoma (DLBCL), in particular, are enriched for mutations of histone modifiers, while, in other subtypes, methylation profiles can be reflective of disease biology; epigenetic mutations have been shown to contribute to clinical behaviour.

3.1. Follicular Lymphoma

FL is a malignancy of germinal center B cells that share the cellular architecture of the normal lymphoid follicle. There is recognition that, beyond classical FL, there is a range of mature B-cell neoplasms with a follicular growth pattern, such as diffuse variant of FL and paediatric nodal FL, that differ in their clinical behaviour and genetic mutation repertoire. Conventional FL is defined by the hallmark t(14:18) translocation that juxtaposes the IGH and *BCL2* loci, leading to anti-apoptotic activity. Despite this early and disease-defining event, there is an appreciation that additional genetic aberrancies that alter normal germinal cell differentiation and the tumour microenvironment are required for the development of lymphoma. This is supported by the identification of the translocation in healthy individuals' lymphocytes often years prior to diagnosis, where a high prevalence of t(11:14) predicts the eventual development of FL [18].

The accumulation of further molecular lesions in these lymphocytes is thought to be needed for progression to overt FL; there is an enrichment of epigenetic dysregulation that is seen in almost all cases of conventional FL (>85%). NGS has identified frequent mutations in epigenetic regulators *KMT2D* (80%), *CREBBP* (33–68%), *EZH2* (25%), *ARID1A* (14%), and *EP300* (9%), which result in gene repression via histone modification. Moreover, there is often the presence of multiple epimutations within a single tumour—at least 50% of cases have both *KMT2D* and *CREBBP* mutations. The implications of the resultant histone modifications for lymphomagenesis are yet to be fully understood but suggest a state of transcriptional repression [6,14,15].

Epigenetic pathway alterations are thought to be an early clonal event. In-situ follicular neoplasia is a collection of clonal B-cells within a lymph node that carries the *BCL2* rearrangement and is recognised as a precursor state to FL. These early clonal lesions can harbour mutations in *CREBBP* and *EZH2*, while mutations in *KMT2D* are also seen but less commonly supporting increasing epigenetic complexity as a key driver of oncogenesis [16,17]. The cumulative result of this complex dysregulation is the promotion of differentiation block at the germinal center stage of development, the loss of key tumour suppressors and an alteration in the tumour microenvironment that promotes and sustains lymphomagenesis.

The clinicogenetic risk model M7-FLIPI combined mutations in seven key genes, including epigenetic regulators *EZH2*, *ARID1A*, *CREBBP* and *EP300* with the follicular international prognostic index (FLIPI) and Eastern Cooperative Oncology Group (ECOG) performance status; it was validated in the GALLIUM cohort [3,19]. The model stratifies patients into "low-risk" and "high risk" cohorts by M7-FLIPI score. Mutations in *EZH2* and *ARID1A* convey better outcomes, while *CREBBP/EP300* are associated with a worse prognosis. In comparison to the conventional FLIPI score, the M7-FLIP is more accurate in predicting progression of disease within 24 months (POD24) and discriminating between low- and high-risk patients [20]. The predictive power of M7-FLIPI, however, may be limited to patients treated with chemotherapy-based regimens [3,21].

Somatic mutations in *EZH2* have been demonstrated to have significantly longer progression free survival and less early relapse [22]. *EZH2* is essential for normal GC differentiation; alterations have been demonstrated to alter the TME by reducing tumour dependence on T-follicular helper cells, allowing for the persistence of tumour cells in the germinal center. This change in the microenvironment is reflected in a reduction in the number of tumour-infiltrating lymphocytes in lymphomas with *EZH2* mutation [6]. Single-amino acid changes at Y641 in the catalytic SET domain are the most frequently seen *EZH2* mutations in FL and result in higher levels of trimethylation at H3K27 (H3K27Me3) on the histone tail. *EZH2* mutations are of clinical interest, as they have proven to be therapeutically vulnerable [4,7].

Primary cutaneous follicle center lymphomas (pcFCL) are indolent B-cell lymphomas that are distinct from secondary cutaneous involvement by systemic FL. They have similar histological features but tend to have weaker CD10 expression and are negative for BCL2 expression. Clinicopathologically, it can be difficult to differentiate pcFCL from skin restricted FL at diagnosis; however, comprehensive genomic assessment by whole exome sequencing (WES) and for copy number aberrancies has demonstrated that alterations in chromatin modifying genes are infrequent when compared to FL. Indeed, cases of 'pcFCL' with mutations in the chromatin modifiers were more likely to progress to systemic involvement and, perhaps, were biologically 'conventional-systemic' FL. Zhou et al. proposed a criterion that incorporated the presence of mutations in chromatin modifying genes (*EZH2, KMT2D, CREBBP, EP300*) along with BCL2 gene rearrangement and a high proliferative index (Ki-67 > 30%) for distinguishing between pcFCL and cutaneous involvement of FL [23].

Diffuse variant of FL (dFL) is a rare variant of FL that also lacks the t(14:18) translocation, has low-grade histology and a typically favourable prognosis. Mutations in *CREBBP* are seen in >90% of cases and are frequently bi-allelic and co-exist with *STAT6* mutations, suggestive of a level of cooperativity. The transcription factor *STAT6* is frequently mutated in primary mediastinal B-cell lymphoma but not germinal center B-cell (GCB)-subtype DLCBL. The BCL2-like antiapoptotic protein BCL-xL/BCL2L1 is a key target of STAT6 [24–26]. Epigenetic mutations are typically lacking in another rare variant of t(14;18)-negative FL, paediatric type nodal FL, which has a very favourable prognosis and is characterised by recurrent mutations in *MAPK* pathway signalling [27].

3.2. Diffuse Large B-Cell Lymphoma

DLBCL has remarkable genetic heterogeneity. Gene expression profiling (GEP) via DNA microarray has been utilised to identify molecular subtypes of DLCBL, leading to the 'cell of origin (COO)' classification, which broadly divides DLBCL into GCB and activated B-cell (ABC) type, leaving 10% unclassifiable [28]. Despite this broad division, DLBCL tumours have one of the highest tumour mutational burdens (TMB) of any malignancy, with somatic mutations recognized in over 700 genes [29]. The GCB subtype has similar genetic lesions to FL, with frequent expression of *EZH2*, while the ABC subtype is enriched with mutations of B-cell receptor signalling pathways [30].

There are various immunohistochemistry-based algorithms that approximate the GEP-derived cell-of-origin classification. The most widely used is the Hans algorithm, which can be used to divide DLCBL into GCB and non-GCB, mostly ABC subtype, and which has a high concordance with GEP (80%) [31]. The Hans algorithm uses expression of CD10, BCL6 and MUM1 to assign the subtype, while newer algorithms utilize further immunostains to improve accuracy. Expression of these immunostains appears to be independent of epigenetic aberrancies. Indeed, expression of EZH2 appears to not be restricted to COO subtype, with high levels seen regardless of *EZH2* mutation status [32,33]. These algorithms are imperfect classifications with substantial heterogeneity within each group. In part, this may be because the COO classification provides a phenotypic description of the lymphoma cell and does not necessarily fully reflect the complex, dysregulated biological pathways involved.

Genome-wide methylation studies have demonstrated that, as in many other cancers, disrupted methylation is frequent in DLCBL and higher levels of aberrant DNA methylation are associated with a poorer prognosis [34]. Epigenetic dysregulation provides a permissive transcriptional environment that promotes germinal center development, while silencing tumour suppressors and suppressing terminal differentiation. A pivotal paper by Morin et al. reported frequent mutations in epigenetic regulatory genes in 32% of patients with DLBCL with enrichment of these alterations seen in the GCB subtype [7]. A similar mutational profile, including sequence variants of *EZH2*, *CREBBP* and *EP300*, among others, was seen across patients with FL (89% of patients) analysed in the same study, highlighting the genetic similarity between FL and the GCB subtype of DLCBL, where epigenetic disruption appears to play a key role in the lymphomagenesis in both entities [7,35].

As mentioned, DLBCL has been associated with many somatic mutations [29]. Clustering of recurrent somatic mutations within subtypes was reported by Schmitz et al., who utilised WES, targeted sequencing, and copy number analysis to characterise the genomic landscape of DLBCL [36]. An algorithm used key mutations to converge on four clinicogenetic subtypes MCD (MYD88/CD79B), BN2 (BCL6/NOTCH2), N1 (NOTCH1), and EZB (EZH2/BCL2) (Table 1). The MCD and N1 subtypes overlapped genetically with ABC subtype, while the EZB subtype shared the genetic hallmarks of GCB. Genetic alterations in epigenetic regulatory genes were seen across the GCB-ABC 'spectrum' but were enriched in the GCB subtype. *EZH2* mutations were almost exclusive to the GCB-subtype, as were loss-of-function mutations in the tumour suppressor *CREBBP*, which cooperates with *BCL2* overexpression to promote lymphomagenesis [10].

Epigenetic aberrancy was enriched in, but not exclusive to, the EZB subtype. SET domain containing 1B (*SETD1B*), also known as *KMT2G* and part of the KMT2 histone lysine methyltransferase family, was incorporated in the MCD subtype and was seen in 25% of ABC DLBCL. Mutations in *SETD1B* are also frequently seen in DLBCL subtypes in which ABC type predominates, such as primary CNS lymphoma and intravascular lymphoma, a rare extranodal lymphoma of small blood vessels with lymphadenopathy, where *SETD1B* mutants are seen in approximately 50% of cases [37,38].

TET2 was the most frequently seen mutation in the "unclassifiable" subtype. *TET2* somatic mutations occur recurrently in approximately 10% of DLBCL. Intact *TET2* promotes DNA methylation via the oxidization of 5-methylcytosine to 5-hydroxymethylcytosine (5 hmC) and is required for germinal center B cells to undergo plasma cell differentiation. TET2-deficient germinal center B cells cannot up-regulate the plasma cell master regulator PRDM1 due to reduction in 5 hmC [39]. Genome-wide methylation profiling has demonstrated a distinct methylation profile in *TET2* mutated DLBCL; however, there does not appear to be a clinically relevant difference in patients with *TET2* mutant versus wild-type DLBCL [40].

Similar comprehensive genetic analysis was performed by Chapuy et al. who described five distinct genetic clusters (C1, C2, C3, C4 and C5). The C3 cluster, which is genetically similar to the previously described EZB subtype, had frequent mutations in *KMT2D*, *CREBBP* and *EZH2* and had substantial genetic overlap with GCB. There was a particularly high incidence of *CREBBP* mutations (53%). The C4 cluster, which is also mostly GCB subtype and which has a distinctly favourable prognosis, lacked the chromatin modifier mutations seen in the C3 subtype; however, recurrent mutations in histone linker genes were seen [41].

Genetic clustering methodology was further refined with the LymphGen classification system, which divided DLBCL into six genetically defined subgroups (EZB, ST2, BN2, A53, N1, MCD) based on prevalent hallmark mutations [42]. The EZB subtype is, again, defined by epigenetic dysregulation, which is a defining attribute of EZB due to loss-of-function mutations of several epigenetic regulators (*KMT2D*, *CREBBP*, *EP300*, *ARID1A*) and gain-of-function of *EZH2*. The ST2 subtype is characterized by recurrent loss-of-function *TET2* mutations suggestive of tumour-suppressor function.

Table 1. Corresponding Diffuse Large B-cell Lymphoma subtypes based on genetic mutations * Epigenetic regulatory gene.

Genetic Subtype [36]	Genetic Cluster [41]	LymphGen Classification [42]	Cell of Origin	Characteristic Mutations	5-Year OS
BN2	Cluster 1	BN2	ABC, GCB, unclassified	BCL6, NOTCH2, TNFAIP3	36–79%
-	Cluster 2	A53	ABC, GCB	TP53	33–62%
EZB	Cluster 3	EZB	GCB	BCL2, EZH2 *, CREBBP *, KMT2D *	48–68%
-	Cluster 4	ST2	GCB	TET2 *, SGK1, DUSP2, ITPKB, NFKBIA	72–84%
MCD	Cluster 5	MCD	ABC	MYD88, CD79B, CDKN2A, ETV6, SPIB	26–54%
N1	-	N1	ABC	NOTCH1, IRF2BP2	22–27%

Early attempts to utilise the burden of epigenetic mutations in DLBCL led to the development of the "EpiScore" by Szablewski et al. Utilizing GEP, they demonstrated that the level of expression of epigenetic regulators *DNMT3A*, *DOT1L*, and *SETD8* was an independent predictor of survival with high levels of expression associated with a poorer prognosis [43]. Further work is needed, but the "EpiScore" or similar models may identify DLBCL patients, who may benefit from epigenetic-targeted therapies.

A molecular high-risk group of high-grade B-cell lymphoma (HGBCL) has been defined by Sha et al. using GEP [44]. This poor prognosis group with *MYC* and *BCL2* and/or *BCL6* rearrangement (otherwise known as double-hit or triple-hit lymphomas) had recurrent mutations demonstrated via targeted sequencing in epigenetic genes such as *EZH2* and *KMT2D*. Recurrent loss-of-function *CREBBP* mutations are also frequently (80% of cases) seen in HGBCL [44,45]. The contribution of epigenetic dysregulation to the aggressive disease behaviour is unclear; however, epigenetic regulatory genes appear to be more frequently mutated in HGBCL than in GCB DLBCL.

These molecular classification schemas are yet to be recognised by the World Health Organization (WHO) classification of aggressive lymphomas, which still relies on the GEP-defined 'cell-of-origin' subtypes. The prognostic and potential therapeutic implications of mutation-defined subgroups within DLBCL, with the incorporation of high throughput sequencing, such as NGS, into routine clinical practice may change this. Frequent mutations in chromatin modifiers and other epigenetic regulators seen in certain mutation-defined subtypes may provide therapeutic rationale for harnessing therapies targeting epigenetic dysregulation as well as risk-adapted treatment strategies based on genomic classification.

3.3. Mantle Cell Lymphoma

Mantle cell lymphoma (MCL) is defined by t(11;14)(q13;q32) leading to cyclin D1 overexpression and, generally, a poor overall survival rate and high rates of relapse.

High degrees of global epigenetic dysregulation are associated with more aggressive clinical behaviour. Genome wide methylation analyses have demonstrated heterogeneous patterns of DNA methylation in MCL with frequent hypermethylation of tumour suppressor genes, leading to transcriptional repression. A subset of MCL tumours have extensive CpG methylation that is associated with highly proliferative disease and a poorer prognosis [46,47].

There is a nodal variant that commonly involves the gastrointestinal tract and that requires early treatment, while the non-nodal leukemic variant usually demonstrates indolent clinical behaviour. *SOX11* encodes for a transcription factor that is overexpressed in nodal MCL, with low levels seen in patients with the non-nodal leukemic variant. *SOX11* expression is under epigenetic control and may, in part, be responsible for the differing clinical phenotypes [46,48].

Loss of function mutations in the methyltransferase *KMT2D* appear to be relatively common, seen in 12–32% of cases, and may be associated with poorer outcome. NGS of a cohort of young MCL patients in the Fondazione Italiana Linfomi MCL0208 phase 3 trial (lenalidomide vs. observation post autologous transplantation) demonstrated loss of function of *KMT2D* in 13.4% of patients (25/186), which was associated with a poorer 4-year progression-free-survival (33.2% vs. 63.7%) and overall survival (62.3% vs. 86.8%). The authors proposed the addition of *KMT2D* mutation to a prognostic index, the 'MIPI-genetic' score [49–51]. *EZH2* expression may predict for a poorer prognosis in MCL. In a retrospective series of 166 patients, 57 patients (38%) stained positive for EZH2 by immunohistochemistry. This finding was associated with a median overall survival of 4.6 years, compared to 9.6 years for those without EZH2 staining. EZH2 expression was also associated with aggressive histology and p53 overexpression (43% vs. 2%) [52].

3.4. Chronic Lymphocytic Leukaemia/Small Lymphocytic Leukaemia

A clinically heterogeneous disease, there are two distinct clinicobiologic subtypes of CLL based on the presence or absence of somatic mutations in the variable region of the immunoglobulin heavy-chain gene (IGHV). IGHV mutated CLL has a more favourable outcome and arises from the post-germinal center B cell, while IGHV unmutated CLL arises from the pre-germinal center B cell and typically has a poorer outcome.

The putative cell of origin is reflected in the epigenetic signature, with genome wide methylation studies revealing differences in the DNA methylation patterns of the two molecular subtypes [53]. Queirós et al. reported on the methylation status of five CpGs islands and identified three distinct groups, naive B-cell-like CLL (n-CLL), memory B-cell-like CLL (m-CLL) and intermediate CLL. The n-CLL and m-CLL group were closely associated with unmutated and mutated IGHV, respectively, and mirrored their biological behaviour. These epigenetic marks, representative of the cellular origin, were shown to be robust predictors of outcome [54]. Evolutions of methylation patterns have also been demonstrated during therapy, suggesting a dynamic epigenetic tumour response [55].

The chromatin modifier chromodomain helicase DNA binding protein 2 (*CHD2*) is one of the most recurrently mutated genes in IGHV mutated CLL (5% of cases) and is thought to be a driver of malignancy [56]. However, the overall contribution of epigenetic dysregulation to CLL leukemogenesis is poorly defined.

3.5. Marginal Zone Lymphoma

Marginal zone lymphoma (MZL) is a relatively rare indolent lymphoma with three recognised subtypes, splenic MZL, extranodal MZL and nodal MZL. Recurrent mutations in epigenetic regulators, such as *KMT2D* and *CREBBP*, are seen across all subtypes [57–59]. Epigenetic dysregulation has been demonstrated to play a role in the clinical behaviour of splenic MZL, with higher degrees of promotor hypermethylation leading to inferior outcomes, possibly due to repression of key tumour suppressor genes such as *KLF4* and *CDKN2A* [60].

3.6. Classical Hodgkin's Lymphoma

Classical Hodgkin's lymphoma (cHL) is derived from postgerminal center B cells and is usually composed of a small number of Hodgkin cells (multinucleated Reed–Sternberg cells) residing in an extensive inflammatory background. In contradistinction to other B-cell lymphomas, the malignant cells lack the expression of almost all B-cell markers, such as CD19, CD20 and CD79a. This downregulation has been demonstrated in vivo to be mediated, at least in part, by epigenetic silencing via hypermethylation of the promoter regions of these genes [61]. WES and NGS have demonstrated a heterogenous genetic landscape, with key signalling pathways, such as NF-κB and JAK/STAT, playing an important role. Frequent amplification of 9p24.1 is likely the basis for the response to PD-1/PD-L1 immune checkpoint inhibitors [62]. Recurrent mutations in epigenetic regulators, particularly *CREBBP* and *EP300*, have been demonstrated; however, the role that these play in lymphomagenesis and disease progression is unclear [63].

4. The T-Cell Lymphomas

T-cell lymphomas are rarer than their B-cell counterparts, comprising around 15% of all non-Hodgkin lymphomas. They are subdivided into the peripheral T-cell lymphomas (PTCL) and cutaneous T-cell lymphomas (CTCL). Although mutations in genes affecting chromatin structure and histone post-translational modification are frequent, as in B-cell lymphomas, the T-cell lymphomas are also enriched with sequence variants of genes that modulate DNA methylation, leading to a highly dysregulated epigenome in certain subtypes.

4.1. Peripheral T-Cell Lymphoma—TFH Phenotype

PTCL-NOS is the most common type of PTCL comprising around 25% of new diagnoses. There is clinicogenetic heterogeneity and epigenetic mutations are less frequent than in other subtypes, such as angioimmunoblastic T-cell lymphoma (AITL). Previously classified under PTCL-NOS, peripheral T-cell lymphoma with T follicular helper phenotype (PTCL-TFH) was recognised by the WHO in 2016 as a distinct subtype and warrants special mention [64]. There is considerable overlap between PTCL-TFH and AITL with a shared COO and mutation profile. There is a recognition that these two entities may represent different ends of the spectrum of the same disorder, which is supported by their molecular characterisation. Frequent *TET2* coding mutations in PTCL-TFH was demonstrated in an early series. The presence of *TET2* mutations in this cohort was associated with advanced-stage disease and shorter PFS [65]. Subsequent targeted sequencing of PTCL-TFH revealed mutations in genes frequently mutated in AITL, such as *TET2*, *DNMT3A* and *RHOA* G17V [66]. Furthermore, PTCL-TFH demonstrates responsiveness to therapy that targets the epigenome with retrospective data supporting the use of histone deacetylase inhibitors in this subtype [67].

4.2. Angioimmunoblastic Lymphoma

AITL is a prototypical epigenetic disorder characterised by a homogenous genetic landscape with hallmark mutations in *TET2*, *IDH2* and *RHOA* leading to widespread aberrant DNA methylation. *TET2* is the most commonly mutated gene in AITL and is reported in up to 80% of AITL while *IDH2* mutations are identified in about a third of AITL cases [68]. The *IDH2* R172 variant appears unique to AITL among lymphoma and generates 2HG, which can inhibit the TET2 enzyme. Given this, co-existent mutations would not be expected; however, most cases with *IDH2* mutants also have *TET2* mutation [69,70]. Mutations in *TET2* and *IDH2* are strongly associated with the *RHOA* G17V mutation, which is seen exclusively in the context of *TET2* mutations with or without *IDH2* mutations in 70% of AITL patients [71]. *DNMT3* loss of function mutation is reported in 10–25% of cases of AITL, of which 80% also have *TET2* mutations. While these mutations in key epigenetic regulators contribute to the aberrant epigenome that leads to lymphomagenesis, it is not yet clear whether specific mutations alter prognosis. *IDH2* mutations, for example, are commonly seen in acute myeloid leukaemia, where they are associated with a poorer prognosis. Despite this, they do not appear to be a prognostic biomarker in AITL [72]. This epigenetic dysregulation has been exploited therapeutically; therapies that target the epigenome have proven particularly beneficial in this disease entity [73].

4.3. Mycosis Fungoides and Sezary Syndrome

Mycosis fungoides (MF) is the most common CTCL variant and is related to the rare leukemic variant, Sézary syndrome (SS). Alterations in epigenetic regulators and cellular growth signalling pathways are frequent and oncogenic in these conditions. There is recurrent loss of function mutations in epigenetic regulators such as *ARID1A* (62%) and *DNMT3A* (42%) [74,75]. The degree of methylation aberrancy in CTCL is higher than many other malignancies, suggestive of the key role of the altered epigenome in pathogenesis [76]. CTCL tumour cells display widespread hypermethylation of CpG islands in promotor regions of tumour suppressor genes such as *CDKN2A* [77]. This hypermethylation involves the *CMTM2* gene, which encodes a chemokine-like factor and appears to be distinct to SS. Furthermore, many of the highly expressed genes identified in SS, such as *CD158*, *DNMT3* and *PLS3*, have large CpG islands, suggesting that changes in methylation may be a mechanism of hyper-expression [78]. Despite a highly dysregulated epigenome, it is currently unclear if clinically relevant subgroups can be delineated using methylation patterns or mutational profiling.

5. Conclusions

Dysregulation of the epigenome is a hallmark of human cancer and is frequent in lymphoid malignancies, where the epigenetic mechanisms that regulate lymphoid cell development are disrupted. Clearly, epigenetic changes that alter DNA transcription—whether that be through modification of function (i.e., hyperacetylation of histones) or through direct mutations of genes known to modify the epigenome—impact on the development and behaviour of various lymphoma types (Table 2). This review has focused on key genes that influence behaviour; there is no doubt that the detection of epigenetic alterations alters outcome, such that they are already being incorporated into prognostic algorithms, such as the M7-FLIPI for follicular lymphoma. Moreover, epigenetic mutations have already entered the WHO classification system for T cell lymphomas, defining the nodal PTCL with TFH phenotype. At this stage, it is probably too early to use epigenetic changes to re-define B cell lymphomas beyond the existing WHO classification that centers around the cell of origin concept, although EZB-DLBCL has to be a front-runner. Nonetheless, for all lymphomas, recognition of epigenetic changes is going to become increasingly important as we develop more complex prognostic tools.

Table 2. Utility of epigenetic dysregulation to classification and prognostication in lymphoma subtypes.

Lymphoma Type	Epigenetic Dysregulation	Classification and Prognostic Utility
Follicular Lymphoma	Frequent mutations in regulators including *KMT2D*, *CREBBP*, *EZH2*, *ARID1A* and *EP300*	*EZH2*, *ARID1A*, *CREBBP* and *EP300* mutations contribute to clinicogenetic risk model m7-FLIPI. *EZH2* mutations identify prognostically favourable subset of patients. Distinct epigenetic mutation clustering between FL subtypes
Diffuse Large B-cell Lymphoma	Frequent mutations in regulatory genes with enrichment seen in the GCB subtype. A similar mutational profile to FL, with sequence variants of *EZH2*, *CREBBP* and *EP300*	Clustering of mutations in epigenetic regulatory genes define prognostically relevant subtypes of DLBCL. Higher levels of aberrant DNA methylation are associated with a poorer prognosis
Marginal Zone Lymphoma	Recurrent mutations in *KMT2D* and *CREBBP* are seen across all subtypes	Higher degrees of promotor hypermethylation have been demonstrated to lead to inferior outcomes
Mantle Cell Lymphoma	Frequent hypermethylation of tumour suppressor genes leading to transcriptional repression. Recurrent mutations in *KMT2D*	Extensive CpG methylation associated a poorer prognosis. Loss-of-function mutations in *KMT2D* may be associated with poorer prognosis. Epigenetic regulation of *SOX11* expression
Classical Hodgkin's Lymphoma	Recurrent mutations in epigenetic regulators seen, particularly *CREBBP* and *EP300*	Unclear role for epigenetic dysregulation in prognosis or subclassification

Table 2. Cont.

Lymphoma Type	Epigenetic Dysregulation	Classification and Prognostic Utility
Chronic Lymphocytic Leukaemia	Recurrent mutations in chromodomain helicase DNA binding protein 2 (CHD2)	Methylation status of CpGs islands identifies distinct groups with differing prognosis
Peripheral T-cell lymphoma TFH	Frequent mutations in TET2, DNMT3A and RHOA G17V	Mutational profile of epigenetic regulators distinguishes this subtype from prior classification of PTCL-NOS TET2 mutations may be associated with poor prognosis
Angioimmunoblastic T-cell Lymphoma	Frequent hallmark mutations in TET2, IDH2 and RHOA Recurrent loss-of-function mutations in DNMT3A	Increasingly defined by presence of epigenetic regulatory mutations Unclear effect on prognosis of specific mutations
Mycosis Fungoides/Sezary Syndrome	Higher degree of methylation aberrancy compared to other malignancies Widespread hypermethylation of CpG islands in promotor regions of tumour suppressor genes such CDKN2A Recurrent loss of function mutations in ARID1A and DNMT3A.	Unclear role for epigenetic dysregulation in prognosis or subclassification despite high dysregulated epigenome

Funding: This research received no external funding.

Informed Consent Statement: Not applicable.

Conflicts of Interest: The authors declare no conflict of interest.

References

1. Shaknovich, R.; Cerchietti, L.; Tsikitas, L.; Kormaksson, M.; De, S.; Figueroa, M.E.; Ballon, G.; Yang, S.N.; Weinhold, N.; Reimers, M.; et al. DNA methyltransferase 1 and DNA methylation patterning contribute to germinal center B-cell differentiation. *Blood* **2011**, *118*, 3559–3569. [CrossRef] [PubMed]
2. Marks, D.L.; Olson, R.L.; Fernandez-Zapico, M.E. Epigenetic control of the tumor microenvironment. *Epigenomics* **2016**, *8*, 1671–1687. [CrossRef] [PubMed]
3. Pastore, A.; Jurinovic, V.; Kridel, R.; Hoster, E.; Staiger, A.M.; Szczepanowski, M.; Pott, C.; Kopp, N.; Murakami, M.; Horn, H.; et al. Integration of gene mutations in risk prognostication for patients receiving first-line immunochemotherapy for follicular lymphoma: A retrospective analysis of a prospective clinical trial and validation in a population-based registry. *Lancet Oncol.* **2015**, *16*, 1111–1122. [CrossRef]
4. Morschhauser, F.; Tilly, H.; Chaidos, A.; McKay, P.; Phillips, T.; Assouline, S.; Batlevi, C.L.; Campbell, P.; Ribrag, V.; Damaj, G.L.; et al. Tazemetostat for patients with relapsed or refractory follicular lymphoma: An open-label, single-arm, multicentre, phase 2 trial. *Lancet Oncol.* **2020**, *21*, 1433–1442. [CrossRef]
5. Béguelin, W.; Popovic, R.; Teater, M.; Jiang, Y.; Bunting, K.L.; Rosen, M.; Shen, H.; Yang, S.N.; Wang, L.; Ezponda, T.; et al. EZH2 is required for germinal center formation and somatic EZH2 mutations promote lymphoid transformation. *Cancer Cell* **2013**, *23*, 677–692. [CrossRef] [PubMed]
6. Ennishi, D.; Takata, K.; Béguelin, W.; Duns, G.; Mottok, A.; Farinha, P.; Bashashati, A.; Saberi, S.; Boyle, M.; Meissner, B.; et al. Molecular and Genetic Characterization of MHC Deficiency Identifies EZH2 as Therapeutic Target for Enhancing Immune Recognition. *Cancer Discov.* **2019**, *9*, 546. [CrossRef] [PubMed]
7. Morin, R.D.; Johnson, N.A.; Severson, T.M.; Mungall, A.J.; An, J.; Goya, R.; Paul, J.E.; Boyle, M.; Woolcock, B.W.; Kuchenbauer, F.; et al. Somatic mutations altering EZH2 (Tyr641) in follicular and diffuse large B-cell lymphomas of germinal-center origin. *Nat. Genet.* **2010**, *42*, 181–185. [CrossRef]
8. Zhang, J.; Dominguez-Sola, D.; Hussein, S.; Lee, J.-E.; Holmes, A.B.; Bansal, M.; Vlasevska, S.; Mo, T.; Tang, H.; Basso, K.; et al. Disruption of KMT2D perturbs germinal center B cell development and promotes lymphomagenesis. *Nat. Med.* **2015**, *21*, 1190–1198. [CrossRef]
9. Hashwah, H.; Schmid, C.A.; Kasser, S.; Bertram, K.; Stelling, A.; Manz, M.; Müller, A. Inactivation of CREBBP expands the germinal center B cell compartment, down-regulates MHCII expression and promotes DLBCL growth. *Proc. Natl. Acad. Sci. USA* **2017**, *114*, 9701. [CrossRef]
10. García-Ramírez, I.; Tadros, S.; González-Herrero, I.; Martín-Lorenzo, A.; Rodríguez-Hernández, G.; Moore, D.; Ruiz-Roca, L.; Blanco, O.; López, D.A.; Rivas, J.D.L.; et al. Crebbp loss cooperates with Bcl2 overexpression to promote lymphoma in mice. *Blood* **2017**, *129*, 2645–2656. [CrossRef]

11. Han, L.; Madan, V.; Mayakonda, A.; Dakle, P.; Teoh, W.W.; Shyamsunder, P.; Nordin, H.B.M.; Cao, Z.; Sundaresan, J.; Lei, I.; et al. ARID1A Is Critical for Maintaining Normal Hematopoiesis in Mice. *Blood* **2018**, *132* (Suppl. 1), 3833. [CrossRef]
12. Challen, G.A.; Sun, D.; Jeong, M.; Luo, M.; Jelinek, J.; Berg, J.S.; Bock, C.; Vasanthakumar, A.; Gu, H.; Xi, Y.; et al. Dnmt3a is essential for hematopoietic stem cell differentiation. *Nat. Genet.* **2011**, *44*, 23–31. [CrossRef] [PubMed]
13. Couronné, L.; Bastard, C.; Bernard, O.A. TET2 and DNMT3A mutations in human T-cell lymphoma. *N. Engl. J. Med.* **2012**, *366*, 95–96. [CrossRef] [PubMed]
14. François, L.; Elsa, P.; Aurélie, D.; Lucile, C.; Nadine, M.; Laurianne, S.; Fataccioli, V.; Bruneau, J.; Cairns, R.A.; Mak, T.W.; et al. Loss of 5-hydroxymethylcytosine is a frequent event in peripheral T-cell lymphomas. *Haematologica* **2018**, *103*, e115–e118.
15. Schüler, F.; Dölken, L.; Hirt, C.; Kiefer, T.; Berg, T.; Fusch, G.; Weitmann, K.; Hoffmann, W.; Fusch, C.; Janz, S.; et al. Prevalence and frequency of circulating t(14;18)-MBR translocation carrying cells in healthy individuals. *Int. J. Cancer* **2009**, *124*, 958–963. [CrossRef]
16. Hirt, C.; Schüler, F.; Dölken, L.; Schmidt, C.A.; Dölken, G. Low prevalence of circulating t(11;14)(q13;q32)–positive cells in the peripheral blood of healthy individuals as detected by real-time quantitative PCR. *Blood* **2004**, *104*, 904–905. [CrossRef]
17. Machiela Mitchell, J.; Zhou, W.; Sampson Joshua, N.; Dean Michael, C.; Jacobs Kevin, B.; Black, A.; Chang, I.-S.; Chen, C.; Chen, C.; Chen, K.; et al. Characterization of Large Structural Genetic Mosaicism in Human Autosomes. *Am. J. Hum. Genet.* **2015**, *96*, 487–497. [CrossRef]
18. Roulland, S.; Kelly, R.S.; Morgado, E.; Sungalee, S.; Solal-Celigny, P.; Colombat, P.; Jouve, N.; Palli, D.; Pala, V.; Tumino, R.; et al. t(14;18) Translocation: A Predictive Blood Biomarker for Follicular Lymphoma. *J. Clin. Oncol.* **2014**, *32*, 1347–1355. [CrossRef]
19. Jurinovic, V.; Passerini, V.; Oestergaard, M.Z.; Knapp, A.; Mundt, K.; Araf, S.; Richter, J.; FitzGibbon, J.; Klapper, W.; Marcus, R.E.; et al. Evaluation of the m7-FLIPI in Patients with Follicular Lymphoma Treated within the Gallium Trial: EZH2 mutation Status May be a Predictive Marker for Differential Efficacy of Chemotherapy. *Blood* **2019**, *134* (Suppl. 1), 122. [CrossRef]
20. Jurinovic, V.; Kridel, R.; Staiger, A.M.; Szczepanowski, M.; Horn, H.; Dreyling, M.H.; Rosenwald, A.; Ott, G.; Klapper, W.; Zelenetz, A.D.; et al. Clinicogenetic risk models predict early progression of follicular lymphoma after first-line immunochemotherapy. *Blood* **2016**, *128*, 1112–1120. [CrossRef]
21. Lockmer, S.; Ren, W.; Brodtkorb, M.; Østenstad, B.; Wahlin, B.E.; Pan-Hammarström, Q.; Kimby, E. M7-FLIPI is not prognostic in follicular lymphoma patients with first-line rituximab chemo-free therapy. *Br. J. Haematol.* **2020**, *188*, 259–267. [CrossRef] [PubMed]
22. Huet, S.; Xerri, L.; Tesson, B.; Mareschal, S.; Taix, S.; Mescam-Mancini, L.; Sohier, E.; Carrère, C.; Lazarovici, J.; Casasnovas, R.-O.; et al. EZH2 alterations in follicular lymphoma: Biological and clinical correlations. *Blood Cancer J.* **2017**, *7*, e555. [CrossRef] [PubMed]
23. Zhou, X.A.; Yang, J.; Ringbloom, K.G.; Martinez-Escala, M.E.; Stevenson, K.E.; Wenzel, A.T.; Fantini, D.; Martin, H.K.; Moy, A.P.; Morgan, E.A.; et al. Genomic landscape of cutaneous follicular lymphomas reveals 2 subgroups with clinically predictive molecular features. *Blood Adv.* **2021**, *5*, 649–661. [CrossRef]
24. Xian, R.R.; Xie, Y.; Haley, L.M.; Yonescu, R.; Pallavajjala, A.; Pittaluga, S.; Jaffe, E.S.; Duffield, A.S.; McCall, C.M.; Gheith, S.M.F.; et al. CREBBP and STAT6 co-mutation and 16p13 and 1p36 loss define the t(14;18)-negative diffuse variant of follicular lymphoma. *Blood Cancer J.* **2020**, *10*, 69. [CrossRef] [PubMed]
25. Aronica, M.A.; Goenka, S.; Boothby, M. IL-4-dependent induction of BCL-2 and BCL-X(L)IN activated T lymphocytes through a STAT6- and pi 3-kinase-independent pathway. *Cytokine* **2000**, *12*, 578–587. [CrossRef]
26. Ritz, O.; Rommel, K.; Dorsch, K.; Kelsch, E.; Melzner, J.; Buck, M.; Leroy, K.; Papadopoulou, V.; Wagner, S.; Marienfeld, R.; et al. STAT6-mediated BCL6 repression in primary mediastinal B-cell lymphoma (PMBL). *Oncotarget* **2013**, *4*, 1093–1102. [CrossRef]
27. Schmidt, J.; Gong, S.; Marafioti, T.; Mankel, B.; Gonzalez-Farre, B.; Balagué, O.; Mozos, A.; Cabeçadas, J.; van der Walt, J.; Hoehn, D.; et al. Genome-wide analysis of pediatric-type follicular lymphoma reveals low genetic complexity and recurrent alterations of TNFRSF14 gene. *Blood* **2016**, *128*, 1101–1111. [CrossRef]
28. Rosenwald, A.; Wright, G.; Chan, W.C.; Connors, J.M.; Campo, E.; Fisher, R.I.; Gascoyne, R.D.; Muller-Hermelink, H.K.; Smeland, E.B.; Giltnane, J.M.; et al. The use of molecular profiling to predict survival after chemotherapy for diffuse large-B-cell lymphoma. *N. Engl. J. Med.* **2002**, *346*, 1937–1947. [CrossRef]
29. Chalmers, Z.R.; Connelly, C.F.; Fabrizio, D.; Gay, L.; Ali, S.M.; Ennis, R.; Schrock, A.; Campbell, B.; Shlien, A.; Chmielecki, J.; et al. Analysis of 100,000 human cancer genomes reveals the landscape of tumor mutational burden. *Genome Med.* **2017**, *9*, 34. [CrossRef]
30. Alizadeh, A.A.; Eisen, M.B.; Davis, R.E.; Ma, C.; Lossos, I.S.; Rosenwald, A.; Boldrick, J.C.; Sabet, H.; Tran, T.; Yu, X.; et al. Distinct types of diffuse large B-cell lymphoma identified by gene expression profiling. *Nature* **2000**, *403*, 503–511. [CrossRef]
31. Hans, C.P.; Weisenburger, D.D.; Greiner, T.C.; Gascoyne, R.D.; Delabie, J.; Ott, G.; Müller-Hermelink, H.K.; Campo, E.; Braziel, R.M.; Jaffe, E.S.; et al. Confirmation of the molecular classification of diffuse large B-cell lymphoma by immunohistochemistry using a tissue microarray. *Blood* **2004**, *103*, 275–282. [CrossRef]
32. Choi, W.W.L.; Weisenburger, D.D.; Greiner, T.C.; Piris, M.A.; Banham, A.H.; Delabie, J.; Braziel, R.M.; Geng, H.; Iqbal, J.; Lenz, G.; et al. A New Immunostain Algorithm Classifies Diffuse Large B-Cell Lymphoma into Molecular Subtypes with High Accuracy. *Clin. Cancer Res.* **2009**, *15*, 5494. [CrossRef]
33. Zhou, Z.; Gao, J.; Popovic, R.; Wolniak, K.; Parimi, V.; Winter, J.N.; Licht, J.D.; Chen, Y.-H. Strong expression of EZH2 and accumulation of trimethylated H3K27 in diffuse large B-cell lymphoma independent of cell of origin and EZH2 codon 641 mutation. *Leuk. Lymphoma* **2015**, *56*, 2895–2901. [CrossRef]

34. Chambwe, N.; Kormaksson, M.; Geng, H.; De, S.; Michor, F.; Johnson, N.A.; Morin, R.; Scott, D.W.; Godley, L.A.; Gascoyne, R.D.; et al. Variability in DNA methylation defines novel epigenetic subgroups of DLBCL associated with different clinical outcomes. *Blood* **2014**, *123*, 1699–1708. [CrossRef]
35. Morin, R.D.; Mendez-Lago, M.; Mungall, A.J.; Goya, R.; Mungall, K.L.; Corbett, R.D.; Johnson, N.A.; Severson, T.M.; Chiu, R.; Field, M.; et al. Frequent mutation of histone-modifying genes in non-Hodgkin lymphoma. *Nature* **2011**, *476*, 298–303. [CrossRef]
36. Schmitz, R.; Wright, G.W.; Huang, D.W.; Johnson, C.A.; Phelan, J.D.; Wang, J.Q.; Roulland, S.; Kasbekar, M.; Young, R.M.; Shaffer, A.L.; et al. Genetics and Pathogenesis of Diffuse Large B-Cell Lymphoma. *N. Engl. J. Med.* **2018**, *378*, 1396–1407. [CrossRef]
37. Shimada, K.; Yoshida, K.; Suzuki, Y.; Iriyama, C.; Inoue, Y.; Sanada, M.; Kataoka, K.; Yuge, M.; Takagi, Y.; Kusumoto, S.; et al. Frequent genetic alterations in immune checkpoint–related genes in intravascular large B-cell lymphoma. *Blood* **2021**, *137*, 1491–1502. [CrossRef]
38. Yoshida, K.; Nakamoto-Matsubara, R.; Chiba, K.; Okuno, Y.; Kakiuchi, N.; Shiraishi, Y.; Sato, Y.; Suzuki, H.; Yoshizato, T.; Shiozawa, Y.; et al. Genetic Basis of Primary Central Nervous System Lymphoma. *Blood* **2015**, *126*, 2687. [CrossRef]
39. Rosikiewicz, W.; Chen, X.; Dominguez, P.M.; Ghamlouch, H.; Aoufouchi, S.; Bernard, O.A.; Melnick, A.; Li, S. TET2 deficiency reprograms the germinal center B cell epigenome and silences genes linked to lymphomagenesis. *Sci. Adv.* **2020**, *6*, eaay5872. [CrossRef]
40. Fazila, A.; Vasu, P.; Jesper, C.; Marianne, T.P.; Anja, P.; Anders, B.N.; Hother, C.; Ralfkiaer, U.; Brown, P.; Ralfkiaer, E.; et al. Genome-wide profiling identifies a DNA methylation signature that associates with TET2 mutations in diffuse large B-cell lymphoma. *Haematologica* **2013**, *98*, 1912–1920.
41. Chapuy, B.; Stewart, C.; Dunford, A.J.; Kim, J.; Kamburov, A.; Redd, R.A.; Lawrence, M.S.; Roemer, M.G.M.; Li, A.J.; Ziepert, M.; et al. Molecular subtypes of diffuse large B cell lymphoma are associated with distinct pathogenic mechanisms and outcomes. *Nat. Med.* **2018**, *24*, 679–690. [CrossRef] [PubMed]
42. Wright, G.W.; Huang, D.W.; Phelan, J.D.; Coulibaly, Z.A.; Roulland, S.; Young, R.M.; Wang, J.Q.; Schmitz, R.; Morin, R.; Tang, J.; et al. A Probabilistic Classification Tool for Genetic Subtypes of Diffuse Large B Cell Lymphoma with Therapeutic Implications. *Cancer Cell* **2020**, *37*, 551–568.e14. [CrossRef] [PubMed]
43. Szablewski, V.; Bret, C.; Kassambara, A.; Devin, J.; Cartron, G.; Costes-Martineau, V.; Moreaux, J. An epigenetic regulator-related score (EpiScore) predicts survival in patients with diffuse large B cell lymphoma and identifies patients who may benefit from epigenetic therapy. *Oncotarget* **2018**, *9*, 19079. [CrossRef] [PubMed]
44. Sha, C.; Barrans, S.; Cucco, F.; Bentley, M.A.; Care, M.A.; Cummin, T.; Kennedy, H.; Thompson, J.S.; Uddin, R.; Worrillow, L.; et al. Molecular High-Grade B-Cell Lymphoma: Defining a Poor-Risk Group That Requires Different Approaches to Therapy. *J. Clin. Oncol.* **2019**, *37*, 202–212. [CrossRef]
45. Evrard, S.M.; Péricart, S.; Grand, D.; Amara, N.; Escudié, F.; Gilhodes, J.; Bories, P.; Traverse-Glehen, A.; Dubois, R.; Brousset, P.; et al. Targeted next generation sequencing reveals high mutation frequency of CREBBP, BCL2 and KMT2D in high-grade B-cell lymphoma with MYC and BCL2 and/or BCL6 rearrangements. *Haematologica* **2019**, *104*, e154–e157. [CrossRef]
46. Queiros, A.; Beekman, R.; Vilarrasa-Blasi, R.; Duran-Ferrer, M.; Clot, G.; Merkel, A.; Raineri, E.; Russiñol, N.; Castellano, G.; Beà, S.; et al. Decoding the DNA Methylome of Mantle Cell Lymphoma in the Light of the Entire B Cell Lineage. *Cancer Cell* **2016**, *30*, 806–821. [CrossRef]
47. Enjuanes, A.; Albero, R.; Clot, G.; Navarro, A.; Bea, S.; Pinyol, M.; Martin-Subero, J.I.; Klapper, W.; Staudt, L.M.; Jaffe, E.S.; et al. Genome-wide methylation analyses identify a subset of mantle cell lymphoma with a high number of methylated CpGs and aggressive clinicopathological features. *Int. J. Cancer* **2013**, *133*, 2852–2863. [CrossRef]
48. Nadeu, F.; Martin-Garcia, D.; Clot, G.; Díaz-Navarro, A.; Duran-Ferrer, M.; Navarro, A.; Vilarrasa-Blasi, R.; Kulis, M.; Royo, R.; Gutiérrez-Abril, J.; et al. Genomic and epigenomic insights into the origin, pathogenesis, and clinical behavior of mantle cell lymphoma subtypes. *Blood* **2020**, *136*, 1419–1432. [CrossRef]
49. Simone, F.; Davide, R.; Andrea, R.; Alessio, B.; Valeria, S.; Christian, W.E.; Evangelista, A.; Moia, R.; Kwee, I.; Dahl, C.; et al. KMT2D mutations and TP53 disruptions are poor prognostic biomarkers in mantle cell lymphoma receiving high-dose therapy: A FIL study. *Haematologica* **2020**, *105*, 1604–1612.
50. Zhang, J.; Jima, D.; Moffitt, A.; Liu, Q.; Czader, M.; Hsi, E.D.; Fedoriw, Y.; Dunphy, C.H.; Richards, K.L.; Gill, J.I.; et al. The genomic landscape of mantle cell lymphoma is related to the epigenetically determined chromatin state of normal B cells. *Blood* **2014**, *123*, 2988–2996. [CrossRef]
51. Jeong, S.; Park, Y.J.; Yun, W.; Lee, S.-T.; Choi, J.R.; Suh, C.; Jo, J.-C.; Cha, H.J.; Jeong, J.-Y.; Chang, H.; et al. Genetic heterogeneity and prognostic impact of recurrent ANK2 and TP53 mutations in mantle cell lymphoma: A multi-centre cohort study. *Sci. Rep.* **2020**, *10*, 13359. [CrossRef]
52. Martinez-Baquero, D.; Sakhdari, A.; Mo, H.; Kim, D.H.; Kanagal-Shamanna, R.; Li, S.; Young, K.H.; O'Malley, D.P.; Dogan, A.; Jain, P.; et al. EZH2 expression is associated with inferior overall survival in mantle cell lymphoma. *Mod. Pathol.* **2021**, *34*, 2183–2191. [CrossRef]
53. Kulis, M.; Heath, S.; Bibikova, M.; Queirós, A.C.; Navarro, A.; Clot, G.; Martínez-Trillos, A.; Castellano, G.; Brun-Heath, I.; Pinyol, M.; et al. Epigenomic analysis detects widespread gene-body DNA hypomethylation in chronic lymphocytic leukemia. *Nat. Genet.* **2012**, *44*, 1236–1242. [CrossRef]

54. Queiros, A.; Villamor, N.; Clot, G.; Martineztrillos, A.; Kulis, M.; Navarro, A.; Penas, E.M.M.; Jayne, S.; Majid, A.M.S.A.; Richter, J.A.; et al. A B-cell epigenetic signature defines three biologic subgroups of chronic lymphocytic leukemia with clinical impact. *Leukemia* **2015**, *29*, 598–605. [CrossRef]
55. Tsagiopoulou, M.; Papakonstantinou, N.; Moysiadis, T.; Mansouri, L.; Ljungström, V.; Duran-Ferrer, M.; Malousi, A.; Queirós, A.C.; Plevova, K.; Bhoi, S.; et al. DNA methylation profiles in chronic lymphocytic leukemia patients treated with chemoimmunotherapy. *Clin. Epigenetics* **2019**, *11*, 177. [CrossRef]
56. Rodríguez, D.; Bretones, G.; Quesada, V.; Villamor, N.; Arango, J.R.; López-Guillermo, A.; Ramsay, A.J.; Baumann, T.; Quiros, P.M.; Navarro, A.; et al. Mutations in CHD2 cause defective association with active chromatin in chronic lymphocytic leukemia. *Blood* **2015**, *126*, 195–202. [CrossRef]
57. Pillonel, V.; Juskevicius, D.; Ng, C.K.Y.; Bodmer, A.; Zettl, A.; Jucker, D.; Dirnhofer, S.; Tzankov, A. High-throughput sequencing of nodal marginal zone lymphomas identifies recurrent BRAF mutations. *Leukemia* **2018**, *32*, 2412–2426. [CrossRef]
58. Jung, H.; Yoo, H.Y.; Lee, S.H.; Shin, S.; Kim, S.C.; Lee, S.; Ko, Y.H. The mutational landscape of ocular marginal zone lymphoma identifies frequent alterations in TNFAIP3 followed by mutations in TBL1XR1 and CREBBP. *Oncotarget* **2017**, *8*, 17038–17049. [CrossRef]
59. Parry, M.; Rose-Zerilli, M.; Ljungström, V.; Gibson, J.; Wang, J.; Walewska, R.; Parker, H.; Parker, A.; Davis, Z.; Gardiner, A.; et al. Genetics and Prognostication in Splenic Marginal Zone Lymphoma: Revelations from Deep Sequencing. *Clin. Cancer Res. Off. J. Am. Assoc. Cancer Res.* **2015**, *21*, 4174–4183. [CrossRef]
60. Arribas, A.J.; Rinaldi, A.; Mensah, A.A.; Kwee, I.; Cascione, L.; Robles, E.F.; Martinez-Climent, J.A.; Oscier, D.; Arcaini, L.; Baldini, L.; et al. DNA methylation profiling identifies two splenic marginal zone lymphoma subgroups with different clinical and genetic features. *Blood* **2015**, *125*, 1922–1931. [CrossRef]
61. Ushmorov, A.; Leithäuser, F.; Sakk, O.; Weinhaüsel, A.; Popov, S.W.; Möller, P.; Wirth, T. Epigenetic processes play a major role in B-cell-specific gene silencing in classical Hodgkin lymphoma. *Blood* **2006**, *107*, 2493–2500. [CrossRef]
62. Roemer, M.G.M.; Ligon, A.H.; Engert, A.; Younes, A.; Santoro, A.; Zinzani, P.L.; Timmerman, J.M.; Ansell, S.; Armand, P.; Fanale, M.A.; et al. Chromosome 9p24.1/PD-L1/PD-L2Alterations and PD-L1 Expression and Treatment Outcomes in Patients with Classical Hodgkin Lymphoma Treated with Nivolumab (PD-1 Blockade). *Blood* **2016**, *128*, 2923. [CrossRef]
63. Mata, E.; Díaz-López, A.; Martín-Moreno, A.M.; Sánchez-Beato, M.; Varela, I.; Mestre, M.J.; Santonja, C.; Burgos, F.; Menárguez, J.; Estévez, M.; et al. Analysis of the mutational landscape of classic Hodgkin lymphoma identifies disease heterogeneity and potential therapeutic targets. *Oncotarget* **2017**, *8*, 111386. [CrossRef]
64. Swerdlow, S.H.; Campo, E.; Pileri, S.A.; Harris, N.L.; Stein, H.; Siebert, R.; Advani, R.; Ghielmini, M.; Salles, G.A.; Zelenetz, A.D.; et al. The 2016 revision of the World Health Organization classification of lymphoid neoplasms. *Blood* **2016**, *127*, 2375–2390. [CrossRef]
65. Lemonnier, F.; Couronné, L.; Parrens, M.; Jaïs, J.P.; Travert, M.; Lamant, L.; Tournillac, O.; Rousset, T.; Fabiani, B.; Cairns, R.A.; et al. Recurrent TET2 mutations in peripheral T-cell lymphomas correlate with TFH-like features and adverse clinical parameters. *Blood* **2012**, *120*, 1466–1469. [CrossRef]
66. Watatani, Y.; Sato, Y.; Miyoshi, H.; Sakamoto, K.; Nishida, K.; Gion, Y.; Nagata, Y.; Shiraishi, Y.; Chiba, K.; Tanaka, H.; et al. Molecular heterogeneity in peripheral T-cell lymphoma, not otherwise specified revealed by comprehensive genetic profiling. *Leukemia* **2019**, *33*, 2867–2883. [CrossRef]
67. Ghione, P.; Faruque, P.; Mehta-Shah, N.; Seshan, V.; Ozkaya, N.; Bhaskar, S.; Yeung, J.; Spinner, M.A.; Lunning, M.; Inghirami, G.; et al. T follicular helper phenotype predicts response to histone deacetylase inhibitors in relapsed/refractory peripheral T-cell lymphoma. *Blood Adv.* **2020**, *4*, 4640–4647. [CrossRef]
68. Odejide, O.; Weigert, O.; Lane, A.A.; Toscano, D.; Lunning, M.A.; Kopp, N.; Kim, S.S.; Van Bodegom, D.; Bolla, S.; Schatz, J.; et al. A targeted mutational landscape of angioimmunoblastic T-cell lymphoma. *Blood* **2014**, *123*, 1293–1296. [CrossRef]
69. Cairns, R.A.; Iqbal, J.; Lemonnier, F.; Kucuk, C.; de Leval, L.; Jais, J.-P.; Parrens, M.; Martin, A.; Xerri, L.; Brousset, P.; et al. IDH2 mutations are frequent in angioimmunoblastic T-cell lymphoma. *Blood* **2012**, *119*, 1901–1903. [CrossRef]
70. Figueroa, M.E.; Abdel-Wahab, O.; Lu, C.; Ward, P.S.; Patel, J.; Shih, A.; Li, Y.; Bhagwat, N.; VasanthaKumar, A.; Fernandez, H.F.; et al. Leukemic IDH1 and IDH2 mutations result in a hypermethylation phenotype, disrupt TET2 function, and impair hematopoietic differentiation. *Cancer Cell* **2010**, *18*, 553–567. [CrossRef]
71. Nguyen, P.N.; Tran, N.T.B.; Nguyen, T.P.X.; Ngo, T.N.M.; Lai, D.V.; Deel, C.D.; Hassellf, L.A.; Vuong, H.G. Clinicopathological Implications of RHOA Mutations in Angioimmunoblastic T-Cell Lymphoma: A Meta-analysis: RHOA mutations in AITL. *Clin. Lymphoma Myeloma Leuk.* **2021**, *21*, 431–438. [CrossRef] [PubMed]
72. Wang, C.; McKeithan, T.W.; Gong, Q.; Zhang, W.; Bouska, A.; Rosenwald, A.; Gascoyne, R.D.; Wu, X.; Wang, J.; Muhammad, Z.; et al. IDH2R172 mutations define a unique subgroup of patients with angioimmunoblastic T-cell lymphoma. *Blood* **2015**, *126*, 1741–1752. [CrossRef] [PubMed]
73. Zhang, P.; Zhang, M. Epigenetic alterations and advancement of treatment in peripheral T-cell lymphoma. *Clin. Epigenetics* **2020**, *12*, 169. [CrossRef]
74. Weinstein, J.N.; Collisson, E.A.; Mills, G.B.; Shaw, K.R.; Ozenberger, B.A.; Ellrott, K.; Shmulevich, I.; Sander, C.; Stuart, J.M. The Cancer Genome Atlas Pan-Cancer analysis project. *Nat. Genet.* **2013**, *45*, 1113–1120. [CrossRef] [PubMed]

75. Kiel, M.J.; Sahasrabuddhe, A.A.; Rolland, D.C.M.; Velusamy, T.; Chung, F.; Schaller, M.; Bailey, N.G.; Betz, B.L.; Miranda, R.N.; Porcu, P.; et al. Genomic analyses reveal recurrent mutations in epigenetic modifiers and the JAK–STAT pathway in Sézary syndrome. *Nat. Commun.* **2015**, *6*, 8470. [CrossRef] [PubMed]
76. Choi, J.; Goh, G.; Walradt, T.; Hong, B.S.; Bunick, C.G.; Chen, K.; Bjornson, R.D.; Maman, Y.; Wang, T.; Tordoff, J.; et al. Genomic landscape of cutaneous T cell lymphoma. *Nat. Genet.* **2015**, *47*, 1011–1019. [CrossRef] [PubMed]
77. van Doorn, R.; Slieker, R.C.; Boonk, S.E.; Zoutman, W.H.; Goeman, J.J.; Bagot, M.; Michel, L.; Tensen, C.P.; Willemze, R.; Heijmans, B.T.; et al. Epigenomic Analysis of Sézary Syndrome Defines Patterns of Aberrant DNA Methylation and Identifies Diagnostic Markers. *J. Investig. Dermatol.* **2016**, *136*, 1876–1884. [CrossRef]
78. Michel, L.; Jean-Louis, F.; Begue, E.; Bensussan, A.; Bagot, M. Use of PLS3, Twist, CD158k/KIR3DL2, and NKp46 gene expression combination for reliable Sézary syndrome diagnosis. *Blood* **2013**, *121*, 1477–1478. [CrossRef]

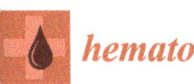

Review

Cold Agglutinin Disease: A Distinct Clonal B-Cell Lymphoproliferative Disorder of the Bone Marrow

Fina Climent [1,*], Joan Cid [2] and Anna Sureda [3]

1. Department of Pathology, Hospital Universitari de Bellvitge, IDIBELL, L'Hospitalet de Llobregat, 08907 Barcelona, Spain
2. Apheresis & Cellular Therapy Unit, Department of Hemotherapy and Hemostasis, ICMHO, IDIBAPS, Hospital Clínic, University of Barcelona, 08036 Barcelona, Spain; jcid@clinic.cat
3. Department of Hematology, Institut Català d'Oncologia, IDIBELL, L'Hospitalet de Llobregat, Universitat de Barcelona, 08907 Barcelona, Spain; asureda@iconcologia.net
* Correspondence: fcliment@bellvitgehospital.cat

Abstract: Cold agglutinin disease (CAD) is a distinct clinicopathologic entity characterized by clonal B-cell lymphoproliferative disorder in the bone marrow. B-cell gene mutations affect NF-KB as well as chromatin modification and remodeling pathways. Clonal immunoglobulins produced by B cells bind to red cells (RBCs) at cold temperatures causing RBC aggregation, complement cascade activation and cold-autoantibody autoimmune hemolytic anemia (cAIHA). The clinical picture shows cold-induced symptoms and cAIHA. Therapeutic options include "wait and watch", rituximab-based regimens, and complement-directed therapies. Steroids must not be used for treating CAD. New targeted therapies are possibly identified after recent molecular studies.

Keywords: autoimmune hemolytic anemia; cold agglutinin; B-cell lymphoproliferative disorder

Citation: Climent, F.; Cid, J.; Sureda, A. Cold Agglutinin Disease: A Distinct Clonal B-Cell Lymphoproliferative Disorder of the Bone Marrow. *Hemato* **2022**, *3*, 163–173. https://doi.org/10.3390/hemato3010014

Academic Editors: Antonino Carbone and Alina Nicolae

Received: 23 January 2022
Accepted: 10 February 2022
Published: 13 February 2022

Publisher's Note: MDPI stays neutral with regard to jurisdictional claims in published maps and institutional affiliations.

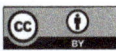

Copyright: © 2022 by the authors. Licensee MDPI, Basel, Switzerland. This article is an open access article distributed under the terms and conditions of the Creative Commons Attribution (CC BY) license (https://creativecommons.org/licenses/by/4.0/).

1. History

As early as 1529, a case of anemia after the exposure to cold was described by Johannes Actuarius, although Dressler is generally credited with being the first person to give a clear description of an autoimmune hemolytic anemia (AIHA), probably paroxysmal cold hemoglobinuria (PCH), in 1854 [1]. Nowadays, it is surprising to us that PCH was the first described AIHA in the latter part of the nineteenth century, given that PCH is the least common type of AIHA. However, its early recognition is due to the fact that hemoglobinuria is a striking symptom and it is also true that PCH was much more common in the past, due its association with late-stage syphilis or congenital syphilis. In the early years of the twentieth century, a distinction of congenital and acquired forms of hemolytic anemias was well defined, though the underlying mechanism was not well understood [2]. The description of the antiglobulin test by Coombs, Mourant, and Race in 1945 was a sight for sore eyes [3]. The direct antiglobulin test (DAT) not only distinguished between the familial and acquired forms of hemolytic anemia, but also demonstrated a difference in their etiology. Finally, in 1951, Young et al. were the first to coin the term AIHA [4]. Those authors theorized that the production of an autoantibody leads to autoimmunization.

Cold agglutinins (CA) were recognized in 1903 by Landsteiner in animal blood and in human blood by Mino in 1924. Their role in human disease was not recognized until 1943 when Stats and Wasserman published a review in which they stated that CAs could be innocuous in the great majority of cases, although in some cases cold hemagglutination was of pathogenetic significance [2]. In 1953, Schubothe introduced the term *cold hemagglutinin disease* to separate the disorder from other acquired hemolytic anemias [5]. With regard to the red blood cell (RBC) specificity of CAs, the serum of patients with CAs was said to contain "anti-I" ("I" for individuality) by Wiener et al. after testing a serum derived from a patient against 22,964 RBC samples [6]. More recently, when methods of immunoelectrophoresis became available, the nature of CAs was identified as monoclonal M-type immunoglobulin (IgM) [7].

The terminology used for describing patients with AIHA is confusing [8]. The traditional classification of AIHA based on the results obtained with the DAT must be updated as follows (Table 1). Cold AIHAs have traditionally been classified as primary or "idiopathic" and secondary to viral infections or malignant diseases. However, nowadays, the primary or "idiopathic" form of cold agglutinin syndrome (CAS) is a well-defined clinicopathological entity and should be called a disease, not a syndrome.

Table 1. Classification of autoimmune hemolytic anemias (AIHA).

Warm AIHA	Cold AIHA	Atypical AIHA
Idiopathic	Primary: cold agglutinin disease (CAD)	Warm and cold
Secondary	Secondary: cold agglutinin syndrome (CAS)Paroxysmal cold hemoglobinuria (PCH)	DAT-negative AIHA

2. Definition of Cold Agglutinin Disease (CAD)

CAD is a designation used for a form of an acquired AIHA caused by a bone marrow lymphoproliferative disorder (LPD). The clonal B-cell lymphocytes produce monoclonal immunoglobulins (Ig), usually IgM-kappa that recognizes its own antigens located on the RBC membrane [9]. By far, the most common RBC antigen recognized by CAs is "I", a small minority recognize the "i" antigen and a few antibodies react with antigens other than I and i. The recognition of RBC antigens, particularly below core body temperature, provokes RBC agglutination in the acral circulation and acrocyanosis may appear. Extravascular hemolytic anemia is driven by classical pathway complement activation (Figure 1). Finally, thromboembolic risk is increased in CAD patients when compared with controls [10].

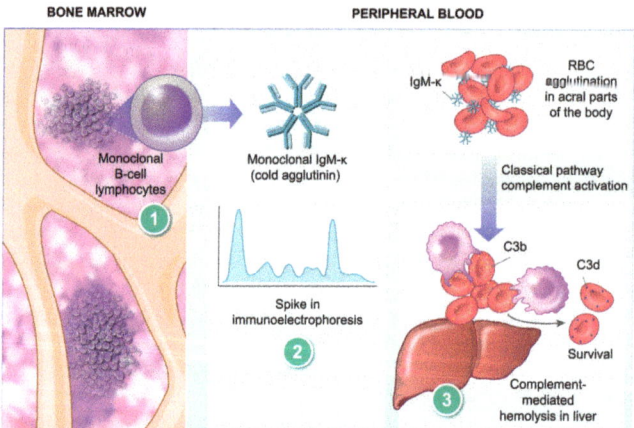

Figure 1. Cold agglutinin disease (CAD) is a form of acquired autoimmune hemolytic anemia (AIHA) caused by a bone marrow lymphoproliferative disorder (1). The clonal B-cell lymphocytes produce monoclonal immunoglobulin (Ig), usually IgM-kappa (2). IgM-κ acts as a cold autoantibody that recognizes its own red blood cells (RBC) producing RBC agglutination at low temperatures during passage through the acral parts of the circulation (3). Binding of IgM-κ to RBC antigens is a potent complement activator by the classical pathway from C1q to C3b. On rewarming to 37 °C in the central circulation, IgM-κ is detached and C3b-opsonized RBCs undergo phagocytosis in the liver, known as extravascular hemolysis. On the surviving cells, surface-bound C3b is degraded into C3d (3).

3. Epidemiology

It is usually said that cold AIHAs account for 15% of all AIHAs, the incidence rate of CAD is 1 case per million inhabitants per year, and the prevalence is 16 cases per million inhabitants. However, the majority of authors agree that these figures must be underestimated because the data come from small retrospective series [7,11]. A recent multinational, observational study was undertaken to improve knowledge of the epidemiological findings in CAD. Authors collected data from 232 patients in 5 countries (Norway, Italy, the U.K., Finland, and Denmark). Notwithstanding, they used data from Norway and Italy because the identification procedure of patients was considered to be population-based. For the first time, authors demonstrated a marked association of climate and incidence and prevalence of CAD. The incidence and prevalence of CAD was 1.9 cases/million per year and 20 cases/million, respectively, in Norway, with 0.48 cases/million per year and 5 cases/million, respectively, in Italy. They found a four-fold difference between cold and warm climates [12].

CAD affects middle-aged or elderly women, according to data obtained from an old and small-scale study [13]. This statement is confirmed by the previous population-based study in which authors found a male-to-female ratio of 0.56, with a mean age (range) at disease onset and at disease diagnosis of 67 years (32–94) and 68 years (33–96), respectively [12].

4. Pathogenesis of CAD

Cold reactive antibodies bind to the antigen at temperatures of 0–4 °C. CAs are cold autoantibodies that react with their own RBC antigens and produce RBC agglutination. The thermal amplitude of CAs is the highest temperature at which RBC agglutination occurs and CAs with thermal amplitude higher than 28–30 °C are pathogenic.

As stated before, nowadays we know that CAD is produced by a clonal LPD localized in the bone marrow that can be difficult to recognize and it remains a challenging diagnosis for pathologists [14]. For this reason, an expert central review of bone marrow biopsies is encouraged to increase the correct identification of this CA-associated LPD by hematopathologists [12]. Moreover, a centralized review offers promise for the clinician, the pathologist, and the patient [15].

The LPD found in the bone marrow in patients with CAD was previously classified into several entities of low-grade LPD, such as LPL or MZL [11]. A detailed histopathological study of 54 patients with CAD showed a homogenous lymphoid infiltration that has been termed CA-associated LPD [16]. The lymphoid infiltration usually consists of intraparenchymal nodular B-cell aggregates composed of small lymphoid cells and plasma cells. Infiltration can vary between 5% and 80% of the intertrabecular space. The immunophenotype of B cells shows CD20+, CD19+, CD22+, CD200+, IgMs+, and IgDs+. CD5 might be positive in less than half of the cases. CD10 and CD23 are negative. Immunoglobulin κ light chain is observed in 90% of cases. Mature plasma cells are seen surrounding the lymphoid nodular aggregates and throughout the marrow in between. The plasma cells have the same heavy and light chain restriction as the B-cells. The histological pattern does not display features typically found in LPL, such as paratrabecular infiltrates, fibrosis, lymphoplasmacytoid cell morphology, or infiltration by mast cells [17]. Bone marrow infiltration mimics that of MZL by morphology, immunophenotype, and molecular features [16]. However, CAD patients do not have an extramedullary MZL. These data suggest that CA-associated LPD, although exclusively present in the bone marrow, might be related to MZL. The transformation to large B-cell lymphoma is uncommon, probably occurring in less than 4% of the patients over 8 years [12].

Chromosome instability is one of the hallmarks of cancer. Malecka et al. studied 13 patients with CAD using cytogenetic microarrays and exome sequencing, and detected complete or partial gain of chromosome 3 (+3 or +3q) in all samples, barring one. Moreover, most cases showed either a gain of chromosome 12 or 18. These chromosome gains were mutually exclusive [18]. However, gains of chromosomes 3, 12, and 18 are not a specific feature of CAD because they are also found in patients with MZL [19,20]. Similar to MZL [21], a gain of chromosomes 12 and 18 might be a predictor of therapy outcome [18].

The mutational landscape of CAD studied by whole exome sequencing and targeted sequencing showed mutations in genes known to be involved in lymphoma development [22]. Four genes showed nonsynonymous mutations in more than 20% of patients: KMT2D (67%), IGLL5 (61%), CARD11 (33%), and CXCR4 (28%). All patients with either CARD11 or CXCR4 mutations, or both, had concurrent KMT2D mutations, and these patients presented lower hemoglobin levels at diagnosis compared to patients with an absence of the KMT2D mutation or patients with KMT2D mutations without CARD11 or CXCR4 mutations. Gene mutations observed in CAD affected the NF-KB pathway as well as chromatin modification or organization [22]. Importantly, the MYD88 L265P mutation, present in over 90% of cases of lymphoplasmacytic lymphoma (LPL), was not found in any of the CAD cases. CXCR4 mutations, described in up to 40% of LPL cases, tended to have a more aggressive disease at diagnosis [23].

Monoclonal B-cell lymphocytes produce monoclonal Ig, usually IgM-κ, and at molecular level, the IGHV4-34 gene is the most frequent gene that encodes for the IgM heavy chain molecule found in CAD (more than 85%). Framework region 1 (FR1) of the heavy gene variable region is essential for recognition of the I antigen on the RBC membrane. It would appear that affinity and specificity for I antigen binding also depends upon the heavy chain complementarity determining region 3 (CDR3) and the light chain variable region [10]. The IG light chain is encoded by the IGKV3-20 and IGKV3-15 genes in more than 80% of patients, indicating that the light chain equally contributes to I antigenbinding [24].

Table 2 shows a summary of the main characteristics in order to differentiate among CA-associated LPD, LPL, and MZL.

Table 2. Differential diagnosis of CA-associated LPD, lymphoplasmacytic lymphoma (LPL), and marginal zone lymphoma (MZL).

Characteristic	CA-Associated LPD	LPL	MZL
Histology	Intraparenchymal nodules	Interstitial, nodular, paratrabecular, and intrasinusoidal infiltrates	Intraparenchymal nodules and/or intrasinusoidal infiltrates (splenic)
Cytology	Small lymphoid cells, plasma cells	Small lymphocytes, lymphoplasmacytoid cells, and plasma cells	Small lymphocytes with abundant, pale cytoplasm and few admixed plasma cells
Cytogenetics	+3, +12, +18	del(6q), gain(6p), +18	+3, +12, +18
IGHV gene	IGHV4-34	IGHV3, IGHV3-23, IGHV3-7	IGHV1-2 (splenic), IGHV3-4 (nodal)
MYD88 L265P	Absent	Present (>90% cases)	Present (10% cases)
KMT2D	67%	Absent	34%
CARD11	33%	Absent	8%
CXCR4	28%	40%	Absent
Transformation to large B-cell lymphoma	Rare (3.4%)	Yes (5–13%)	Yes (15%)

5. Clinical Presentation

CAD should be considered in an elderly patient with unexplained chronic hemolytic anemia, with or without cold-induced symptoms and/or thromboembolic complications.

5.1. Fatigue

Fatigue is usually considered a common symptom in patients with CAD and it is attributed to different factors, such as chronic anemia and underlying conditions. However, this symptom is poorly reported in the previous published literature. In a retrospective analysis of 89 patients at the Mayo Clinic, it was found that fatigue was reported at diagnosis and throughout the course of the disease in 21% and 40% of patients with CAD, respectively [7]. More detailed data about the level of fatigue can be found in a recent multicenter, open-label, single-group study that was conducted to assess the efficacy and safety of a new drug for patients with CAD and a recent history of blood transfusion [25]. The authors included 24 patients in the study, and a secondary end point was to assess quality of life with the use of the Functional Assessment of Chronic Illness Therapy (FACIT) fatigue scale (scores range from 0 to 52, with a higher score indicating less fatigue). Patients with CAD had a mean baseline score on the FACIT fatigue scale of 32.5, a value similar to that reported in patients with advanced cancer or rheumatoid arthritis [25].

5.2. Anemia

Symptoms related to chronic anemia are not only very common in patients with CAD, but also vary greatly from patient to patient [13]. More than 90% of patients had anemia with a median (range) hemoglobin value of 92 g/L (45–153) [12]. Severe (hemoglobin <80 g/L), moderate (hemoglobin 80–100 g/L), and mild anemia (hemoglobin >100 g/L) was observed in 27%, 35%, and 38% of cases, respectively [11]. All series describing the clinical picture of patients with CAD include a number of cases with compensated hemolysis, thus, anemia is not detected [7,11,12]. This variability depends on the thermal range of the CAs as well as cold weather [13]. Nowadays, this assumption is challenged by a recent observational study, in which the authors have shown that hemolysis can persist throughout the year, although they confirmed that the variability of disease severity across patients is vast [26].

5.3. Cold-Induced Symptoms

As mentioned in the previous definition section, CAs recognize RBC antigens at low temperatures, which can be attained in the superficial skin vessels of acral parts of the body, such as the hands, feet, nose, and ears [13]. The result of RBC agglutination is pain, along with distal ischemia and the appearance of blue to deep purple in the extremities [27]. The thermal range of the CA is more important than the agglutination titer in explaining the severity of the symptoms. It is important to point out that skin manifestations in patients with CAD are the result of physical RBC agglutination and the use of Raynaud's phenomena to describe these symptoms are, strictly speaking, incorrect. Raynaud's disease is the consequence of vasoconstriction and Raynaud's phenomena are, in reality, three consecutive phenomena: first, the affected part becomes white and perhaps numb; secondly, it becomes swollen, stiff, and livid; and thirdly, vasoconstriction passes off and the part becomes red due to hyperemia [2]. Interestingly, the authors who published the largest series of patients with CAD classified them into 3 clinical phenotypes: type 1 (69% of cases) were patients with hemolytic anemia without cold-induced symptoms or only acrocyanosis; type 2 (21% of cases) were patients with hemolytic anemia with more severe acrocyanosis interfering with daily living or even gangrene or ulcerations; and type 3 (10% of cases) were patients with cold-induced symptoms and compensated hemolysis [12].

5.4. Thromboembolic Complications

An increased risk of thromboembolic events (TEs) in patients with many types of RBC hemolysis was noted in the past, although this was supported by low quality and a limited amount of data [13]. Nowadays, more data coming from three different studies are available. First, Ungprasert et al. conducted a systematic review and meta-analysis of four observational studies (three retrospective cohort studies and one cross-sectional study) comprising 13,036 patients with AIHA who had 472 venous thromboembolisms (VTE) [28]. The pooled risk ratio (RR) of VTE of patients with AIHA versus the control group was 2.63 (95% CI: 1.37 to 5.05). However, the statistical heterogeneity was high with an I^2 of 97%. To investigate this high heterogeneity, the authors performed a sensitivity analysis by excluding the cross-sectional study, which is generally considered a lower-quality design compared with cohort studies. After excluding this study, the I^2 was 0% and the pooled RR was 3.74 (95% CI: 3.39 to 4.13). Second, Bylsma et al. identified 72 patients with CAD between 1999 and 2013 in the Danish National Patient Registry and matched them to a general population comparison cohort of 720 individuals [29]. The risk of TEs was higher in the CAD patient cohort than in the comparison cohort: 1 year (7.2% vs. 1.9%), 3 years (9% vs. 5.3%), and 5 years (11.5% vs. 7.8%) after the index date. Third, Broome et al. identified

608 patients with CAD in the U.S.A. between 2006 and 2016 in the Optum Claims Clinical data set and matched them with 5873 patients without CAD [30]. Authors found that the overall risk of having a TE was 1.9 times higher in patients with CAD than in the patients without CAD during the study period. To summarize, although limitations exist in the previous data with regard to the previous three study designs, it seems clear that CAD is associated with an increased risk of TEs when compared with the general population [9].

6. Diagnosis

A direct antiglobulin test (DAT) must be ordered to demonstrate autoimmune pathogenesis when a hemolytic anemia is suspected in a patient, because of the presence of anemia with other signs of hemolysis (high LDH, high indirect bilirubin, high reticulocyte count, and low haptoglobin) [31]. It is important to note that the blood sample used for performing not only DAT, but also other laboratory parameters in a patient with suspected CAs should be kept warm (at 37–38 °C) after collection to avoid RBC agglutination. Prewarming at 37 °C for up to 2 h or a short preheating at 41 °C for 1 min may be tried to overcome the problems with the obtention of hemoglobin values and blood cell counts. Once plasma or serum is separated from the blood cells, the sample can be handled at room temperature [10,32].

6.1. Principles of DAT

DAT is a simple, quick, and inexpensive test with a good predictive value if it is performed when immune-hemolysis is suspected [33,34], and a blood sample is collected in a tube containing ethylenediaminetetraacetic acid (EDTA) as anticoagulant. In a physiological state, without hemolysis or anemia, it is known that RBCs can be opsonized with 100–500 molecules of IgG and/or 400–1000 molecules of complement (C3). However, under normal circumstances, RBCs contained in a sample collected in an EDTA tube do not autoagglutinate, due to the fact that their electrostatic charge causes them to mutually repel in solution (zeta potential). When RBC autoantibodies or C3 molecules are attached to RBC membrane (RBC sensitization), two main situations can occur. If RBCs are sensitized with IgG or C3, even with higher quantities than previously cited, they are incapable of overcoming the electrostatic repulsive force and antihuman globulin antisera (Coombs' reagent) is necessary to bridge the distance between RBCs sensitized with IgG and/or C3. In contrast, when RBCs are sensitized with as low as 50 molecules of IgM, this 1 million Daltons molecule is capable of spanning the intercellular distance between RBCs, and agglutination is visible to the naked eye after RBCs are incubated at low temperature (4 °C) [33].

6.2. Methods of Performing DAT

As with other basic procedures in immunohematology, the DAT principle is to detect an antigen–antibody reaction. Traditionally, the evidence of the formation of this reaction in vitro has been the visualization of agglutinates or the presence of hemolysis within the tube test. Nowadays, manual tube tests have been replaced by automated systems, such as the column agglutination method. The sensitivity limit of the routine tube method or the column agglutination method is almost 200 and 100 IgG molecules/RBC, respectively [35]. Although automation within a laboratory has a considerable number of advantages, when DAT is performed with this new technology, one must have in mind that the final accuracy of the test is different when compared with old, manual tube agglutination tests. Barcellini et al. compared the DAT results obtained with these two methods and they observed a sensitivity and specificity of tube test of 43% and 87%, respectively. The sensitivity and specificity of the microcolumn test was 70% and 65%, respectively [36]. The authors confirmed that the DAT tube test was the gold standard in diagnosing AIHA, although they also found that some negative results with the DAT tube test were identified with microcolumn test, reflecting the different accuracy of these laboratory tests to detect the low quantity of IgG bound on the RBC membrane [37]. More sensitive techniques can be used to detect less than 100 IgG molecules/RBC, such as flow cytometry [38] or immunoradiometric assays. In one study using radioimmunoassay, the lowest limit to detect RBC-bound IgG was 78.5 IgG molecules/RBC [39].

6.3. Results of DAT in CAD and Further Characterization

CAs are suspected after obtaining a positive DAT for C3. The next steps must be undertaken to define thermal amplitude, specificity and titer of CAs (Table 3). Thermal amplitude is the highest temperature at which the CA will bind to its antigen. Specificity is the antigenic determinant recognized by the CA. The CA titer is the inverse value of the highest serum dilution at which agglutination can be detected.

Table 3. Immunohematologic study when CAD is suspected.

Study	Results
Direct antiglobulin test	Positive for C3 (negative or weakly positive for IgG)
Titration	≥ 64
Specificity	I, i
Thermal amplitude	>4 °C

After the characterization of CAs, serum monoclonal IgM-κ with electrophoresis and immunofixation is detected in more than 90% of patients [40]. Only 7% of cases show λ light chain restriction and IgG class is observed in less than 5% of cases [10,11].

Finally, a bone marrow biopsy is mandatory to discover the specific bone marrow histopathological pattern previously detailed and termed as "CA-associated LPD".

7. Treatment

All treatment should aim at an improved quality of life. Therefore, each patient must be carefully assessed in order to guide therapy decisions depending upon his/her main complaint. As stated before, fatigue, anemia, cold-induced symptoms, and TE complications are common in patients with CAD. If patients have no relevant symptoms or problems, a "watch and wait" decision is appropriate. General measures, such as folic acid and B12 vitamin supplementation, avoiding low temperatures, and early treatment of bacterial infections can be used to manage these patients. When a patient needs a more specific therapeutic approach, physicians should consider the availability of clinical trials at all stages of treatment.

Glucocorticoids, other active therapies in patients with warm AIHA, and splenectomy must not be used to treat patients with CAD because response rates are low and the liver is the dominant site of destruction of C3-sensitized RBCs [41]. Moreover, patients who respond to steroids need a high dose of medication to maintain remission with an unacceptable number of adverse events [9,42].

7.1. Fatigue and Anemia

Thanks to a clinical trial performed in patients with CAD and a recent history of blood transfusion, we are now aware that a clinically meaningful reduction in fatigue occurred very fast (within one week) after starting treatment with sutimlimab [25]. Sutimlimab is a humanized monoclonal antibody that selectively targets the C1s protein. By acting at this juncture, classical pathway complement activation is stopped. The authors hypothesized that fatigue, in addition to anemia, could be related to the inactivation of complement pathway or hemolytic activity, or both. However, as authors stated, the open-label design of the study makes the interpretation of these results difficult. Another study with sutimlimab administered to patients who suffered CAD without a recent history of blood transfusion has just finished, and the results are keenly awaited (Clinicaltrials.gov number NCT03347422).

7.2. Cold-Induced Symptoms and TE Complications

Acrocyanosis is common in patients with CAD, but it is rarely an indication for starting treatment. However, descriptive studies have shown that up to 80% of patients have received pharmacological treatment [7,11]. Thermal protection is enough to manage this symptom, and only when severe cold-induced symptoms appear is it necessary to perform other therapeutic approaches with the aim of removing IgM from the circulation [27]. New treatments aimed at inhibiting classical pathway complement activation are not useful for treating acrocyanosis, because this clinical manifestation is due to the binding of Cas to RBC antigen. With regard to TE complications, it is unclear whether treatment of the hemolytic process itself could reduce the risk of VTE. Thus, thromboprophylaxis is recommended in acute exacerbations or for chronic disease in risk situations [40].

7.3. Emergency Situations

When an acute trigger develops a severe or life-threatening anemia, urgent therapy is necessary to remove Cas from circulation [27]. Plasma exchange can be an excellent approach, given the fact that most of the IgM is located in intravascular space and plasma exchange is highly efficient in removing intravascular molecules [43]. In fact, severe CAD is considered a category II (second line treatment) indication for performing plasma exchange in the evidence-based guidelines published by the American Society for Apheresis (ASFA) [44]. However, this apheresis procedure has to be considered part of a whole treatment strategy consisting in removing IgM with plasma exchange and blocking the production of new CAs with an associated treatment, such as rituximab. This approach was used by our group for treating patients with not only severe AIHAs [45,46], but also with different severe autoimmune diseases [47–49]. A meta-analysis published in 2020 found that the use of plasma exchange may yield a 22% increase in the incidence of AIHA remission compared to no plasma exchange, and that plasma exchange may also increase the incidence of adverse events by 12% compared to the control group, although this increase was not statistically significant [50]. The authors concluded that plasma exchange may be beneficial for short-term control of AIHA. However, it should be noted that the authors could not establish the efficacy of plasma exchange in warm and cold AIHA subgroups, due to a lack of subgroup data.

7.4. Current Recommendations

A treatment directed to deplete the B-cell clone located in the bone marrow seems to be a reasonable approach to treat patient with CAD [9]. There are no prospective, randomized trials in this setting, but different prospective, non-randomized, and "real life" observational studies support the use of different chemoimmunotherapy regimens. Table 4 summarizes that rituximab, alone or in combination with bendamustine, shows a beneficial effect with low toxicity.

Table 4. Current recommended treatments for patients with CAD.

Reference	Therapy	n	Overall Response	Response Duration	Toxicity
[51]	Rituximab	37	54%	11 months	Low
[52]	Rituximab+bendamustine	45	71%	>32 months	Low
[53]	Rituximab+fludarabine	29	76%	>66 months	Significant
[54]	Bortezomib	19	32%	216 months	Low

When these previous treatments are not effective, a small series suggests that ibrutinib, a Bruton's tyrosine kinase inhibitor, could be effective [55]. Finally, new drugs under development, such as sutimlimab [25], as previously cited, and pegcetacoplan [41], are directed to inhibit the classical pathway complement activation.

8. Conclusions

CAD is an acquired form of AIHA caused by a distinct B-cell LPD in the bone marrow named CA-associated LPD. Monoclonal B-cell lymphocytes produce monoclonal IgMκ, with the ability to bind to I antigen on the RBC membrane at low temperatures. Restrictions, not only in *IGHV* but also in immunoglobulin light chain *V*, contribute to I antigen-binding on the RBC membrane. RBCs agglutinate in the acral parts of the body causing acrocyanosis, while the classical pathway complement activation by CAs is responsible for extravascular hemolysis in the liver of C3b-sensitized RBCs. The accurate diagnosis of CA-associated LPD is a challenge for pathologists and hematologists, and it highlights the importance of integrating clinical, analytical, and pathological data.

Author Contributions: Conceptualization, F.C., J.C. and A.S.; Writing—original draft preparation, F.C. and J.C.; Writing—review and editing, A.S. All authors have read and agreed to the published version of the manuscript.

Funding: This research received no external funding.

Acknowledgments: Authors acknowledge Alison Schroeer (www.illustratingscience.com; last accessed date 11 February 2022) for drawing Figure 1. This text was revised by David Kennedy (MCIL), Member of the United Kingdom's Chartered Institute of Linguists.

Conflicts of Interest: The authors declare no conflict of interest.

References

1. Mack, P.; Freedman, J. Autoimmune hemolytic anemia: A history. *Transfus. Med. Rev.* **2000**, *14*, 223–233. [CrossRef]
2. Petz, L.D.; Garratty, G. Historical concepts of immune hemolytic anemias. In *Immune Hemolytic Anemias*, 2nd ed.; Petz, L.D., Garratty, G., Eds.; Churchill Livingstone: Philadelphia, PA, USA, 2004; Volume 1, pp. 1–31.
3. Coombs, R.R. Historical note: Past, present and future of the antiglobulin test. *Vox Sang.* **1998**, *74*, 67–73. [CrossRef] [PubMed]
4. Young, L.E.; Miller, G.; Christian, R.M. Clinical and laboratory observations on autoimmune hemolytic disease. *Ann. Intern. Med.* **1951**, *35*, 507–517. [CrossRef] [PubMed]
5. Schubothe, H. The cold hemagglutinin disease. *Semin. Hematol.* **1966**, *3*, 27–47. [PubMed]
6. Wiener, A.S.; Unger, L.J.; Cohen, L.; Feldman, J. Type-specific cold auto-antibodies as a cause of acquired hemolytic anemia and hemolytic transfusion reactions: Biologic test with bovine red cells. *Ann. Intern. Med.* **1956**, *44*, 221–240. [CrossRef]
7. Swiecicki, P.L.; Hegerova, L.T.; Gertz, M.A. Cold agglutinin disease. *Blood* **2013**, *122*, 1114–1121. [CrossRef]
8. Hill, Q.A.; Hill, A.; Berentsen, S. Defining autoimmune hemolytic anemia: A systematic review of the terminology used for diagnosis and treatment. *Blood Adv.* **2019**, *3*, 1897–1906. [CrossRef]
9. Berentsen, S.; Barcellini, W. Autoimmune Hemolytic Anemias. *N. Engl. J. Med.* **2021**, *385*, 1407–1419. [CrossRef]
10. Berentsen, S. New Insights in the Pathogenesis and Therapy of Cold Agglutinin-Mediated Autoimmune Hemolytic Anemia. *Front. Immunol.* **2020**, *11*, 590. [CrossRef]
11. Berentsen, S.; Ulvestad, E.; Langholm, R.; Beiske, K.; Hjorth-Hansen, H.; Ghanima, W.; Sorbo, J.H.; Tjonnfjord, G.E. Primary chronic cold agglutinin disease: A population based clinical study of 86 patients. *Haematologica* **2006**, *91*, 460–466.
12. Berentsen, S.; Barcellini, W.; D'Sa, S.; Randen, U.; Tvedt, T.H.A.; Fattizzo, B.; Haukas, E.; Kell, M.; Brudevold, R.; Dahm, A.E.A.; et al. Cold agglutinin disease revisited: A multinational, observational study of 232 patients. *Blood* **2020**, *136*, 480–488. [CrossRef] [PubMed]
13. Petz, L.D.; Garratty, G. Classification and clinical characteristics of autoimmune hemolytic anemias. In *Immune Hemolytic Anemias*, 2nd ed.; Petz, L.D., Garratty, G., Eds.; Churchill Livingstone: Philadelphia, PA, USA, 2004; Volume 1, pp. 61–131.
14. Campbell, A.; Podbury, B.; Yue, M.; Mollee, P.; Bird, R.; Hapgood, G. The Role of a Routine Bone Marrow Biopsy in Autoimmune Hemolytic Anemia for the Detection of an Underlying Lymphoproliferative Disorder. *Hemasphere* **2022**, *6*, e674. [CrossRef] [PubMed]
15. Jaffe, E.S. Centralized review offers promise for the clinician, the pathologist, and the patient with newly diagnosed lymphoma. *J. Clin. Oncol.* **2011**, *29*, 1398–1399. [CrossRef] [PubMed]
16. Randen, U.; Troen, G.; Tierens, A.; Steen, C.; Warsame, A.; Beiske, K.; Tjonnfjord, G.E.; Berentsen, S.; Delabie, J. Primary cold agglutinin-associated lymphoproliferative disease: A B-cell lymphoma of the bone marrow distinct from lymphoplasmacytic lymphoma. *Haematologica* **2014**, *99*, 497–504. [CrossRef]
17. Garcia-Reyero, J.; Martinez Magunacelaya, N.; Gonzalez de Villambrosia, S.; Gomez Mediavilla, A.; Urquieta Lam, M.; Insunza, A.; Tonda, R.; Beltran, S.; Gut, M.; Gonzalez, A.; et al. Diagnostic value of bone marrow core biopsy patterns in lymphoplasmacytic lymphoma/Waldenstrom macroglobulinaemia and description of its mutational profiles by targeted NGS. *J. Clin. Pathol.* **2020**, *73*, 571–577. [CrossRef]

18. Malecka, A.; Delabie, J.; Ostlie, I.; Tierens, A.; Randen, U.; Berentsen, S.; Tjonnfjord, G.E.; Troen, G. Cold agglutinin-associated B-cell lymphoproliferative disease shows highly recurrent gains of chromosome 3 and 12 or 18. *Blood Adv.* **2020**, *4*, 993–996. [CrossRef]
19. Bertoni, F.; Rossi, D.; Zucca, E. Recent advances in understanding the biology of marginal zone lymphoma. *F1000Research* **2018**, *7*, 406. [CrossRef]
20. Van den Brand, M.; van Krieken, J.H. Recognizing nodal marginal zone lymphoma: Recent advances and pitfalls. A systematic review. *Haematologica* **2013**, *98*, 1003–1013. [CrossRef]
21. Krugmann, J.; Tzankov, A.; Dirnhofer, S.; Fend, F.; Wolf, D.; Siebert, R.; Probst, P.; Erdel, M. Complete or partial trisomy 3 in gastro-intestinal MALT lymphomas co-occurs with aberrations at 18q21 and correlates with advanced disease stage: A study on 25 cases. *World J. Gastroenterol.* **2005**, *11*, 7384–7385. [CrossRef]
22. Malecka, A.; Troen, G.; Delabie, J.; Malecki, J.; Ostlie, I.; Tierens, A.; Randen, U.; Berentsen, S.; Tjonnfjord, G.E. The mutational landscape of cold agglutinin disease: CARD11 and CXCR4 mutations are correlated with lower hemoglobin levels. *Am. J. Hematol.* **2021**, *96*, E279–E283. [CrossRef]
23. Kaiser, L.M.; Hunter, Z.R.; Treon, S.P.; Buske, C. CXCR4 in Waldenstrom's Macroglobulinema: Chances and challenges. *Leukemia* **2021**, *35*, 333–345. [CrossRef] [PubMed]
24. Malecka, A.; Troen, G.; Tierens, A.; Ostlie, I.; Malecki, J.; Randen, U.; Berentsen, S.; Tjonnfjord, G.E.; Delabie, J.M. Immunoglobulin heavy and light chain gene features are correlated with primary cold agglutinin disease onset and activity. *Haematologica* **2016**, *101*, e361–e364. [CrossRef] [PubMed]
25. Roth, A.; Barcellini, W.; D'Sa, S.; Miyakawa, Y.; Broome, C.M.; Michel, M.; Kuter, D.J.; Jilma, B.; Tvedt, T.H.A.; Fruebis, J.; et al. Sutimlimab in Cold Agglutinin Disease. *N. Engl. J. Med.* **2021**, *384*, 1323–1334. [CrossRef] [PubMed]
26. Roth, A.; Fryzek, J.; Jiang, X.; Reichert, H.; Patel, P.; Su, J.; Morales Arias, J.; Broome, C.M. Complement-mediated hemolysis persists year round in patients with cold agglutinin disease. *Transfusion* **2021**, *62*, 51–59. [CrossRef]
27. Linz, W.J.; Tauscher, C.; Winters, J.L.; Gastineau, D.A.; Moore, B. Transfusion medicine illustrated: Cold agglutinin disease. *Transfusion* **2003**, *43*, 1185. [CrossRef]
28. Ungprasert, P.; Tanratana, P.; Srivali, N. Autoimmune hemolytic anemia and venous thromboembolism: A systematic review and meta-analysis. *Thromb. Res.* **2015**, *136*, 1013–1017. [CrossRef]
29. Bylsma, L.C.; Gulbech Ording, A.; Rosenthal, A.; Ozturk, B.; Fryzek, J.P.; Arias, J.M.; Roth, A.; Berentsen, S. Occurrence, thromboembolic risk, and mortality in Danish patients with cold agglutinin disease. *Blood Adv.* **2019**, *3*, 2980–2985. [CrossRef]
30. Broome, C.M.; Cunningham, J.M.; Mullins, M.; Jiang, X.; Bylsma, L.C.; Fryzek, J.P.; Rosenthal, A. Increased risk of thrombotic events in cold agglutinin disease: A 10-year retrospective analysis. *Res. Pr. Thromb. Haemost.* **2020**, *4*, 628–635. [CrossRef]
31. Cid, J.; Ortin, X.; Beltran, V.; Escoda, L.; Contreras, E.; Elies, E.; Martin-Vega, C. The direct antiglobulin test in a hospital setting. *Immunohematology* **2003**, *19*, 16–18. [CrossRef]
32. Berentsen, S.; Roth, A.; Randen, U.; Jilma, B.; Tjonnfjord, G.E. Cold agglutinin disease: Current challenges and future prospects. *J. Blood Med.* **2019**, *10*, 93–103. [CrossRef]
33. Petz, L.D.; Garratty, G. The diagnosis of hemolytic anemia. In *Immune Hemolytic Anemias*, 2nd ed.; Petz, L.D., Garratty, G., Eds.; Churchill Livingstone: Philadelphia, PA, USA, 2004; Volume 1, pp. 33–60.
34. Kaplan, H.S.; Garratty, G. Predictive value of direct antiglobulin test results. *Diagn. Med.* **1985**, *8*, 29–33.
35. Kamesaki, T.; Kajii, E. A Comprehensive Diagnostic Algorithm for Direct Antiglobulin Test-Negative Autoimmune Hemolytic Anemia Reveals the Relative Ratio of Three Mechanisms in a Single Laboratory. *Acta Haematol.* **2018**, *140*, 10–17. [CrossRef] [PubMed]
36. Barcellini, W.; Revelli, N.; Imperiali, F.G.; Villa, M.A.; Manera, M.C.; Paccapelo, C.; Zaninoni, A.; Zanella, A. Comparison of traditional methods and mitogen-stimulated direct antiglobulin test for detection of anti-red blood cell autoimmunity. *Int. J. Hematol.* **2010**, *91*, 762–769. [CrossRef] [PubMed]
37. Kamesaki, T. Diagnostic algorithm for classification and characterization of direct antiglobulin test-negative autoimmune hemolytic anemia with 1-year clinical follow-up. *Transfusion* **2021**, *62*, 205–216. [CrossRef] [PubMed]
38. Alvarez, A.; Rives, S.; Montoto, S.; Sanz, C.; Pereira, A. Relative sensitivity of direct antiglobulin test, antibody's elution and flow cytometry in the serologic diagnosis of immune hemolytic transfusion reactions. *Haematologica* **2000**, *85*, 186–188.
39. Kamesaki, T.; Oyamada, T.; Omine, M.; Ozawa, K.; Kajii, E. Cut-off value of red-blood-cell-bound IgG for the diagnosis of Coombs-negative autoimmune hemolytic anemia. *Am. J. Hematol.* **2009**, *84*, 98–101. [CrossRef]
40. Jager, U.; Barcellini, W.; Broome, C.M.; Gertz, M.A.; Hill, A.; Hill, Q.A.; Jilma, B.; Kuter, D.J.; Michel, M.; Montillo, M.; et al. Diagnosis and treatment of autoimmune hemolytic anemia in adults: Recommendations from the First International Consensus Meeting. *Blood Rev.* **2020**, *41*, 100648. [CrossRef]
41. Berentsen, S.; Hill, A.; Hill, Q.A.; Tvedt, T.H.A.; Michel, M. Novel insights into the treatment of complement-mediated hemolytic anemias. *Ther. Adv. Hematol.* **2019**, *10*, 2040620719873321. [CrossRef]
42. Berentsen, S. How I treat cold agglutinin disease. *Blood* **2021**, *137*, 1295–1303. [CrossRef]
43. Reeves, H.M.; Winters, J.L. The mechanisms of action of plasma exchange. *Br. J. Haematol.* **2014**, *164*, 342–351. [CrossRef]
44. Padmanabhan, A.; Connelly-Smith, L.; Aqui, N.; Balogun, R.A.; Klingel, R.; Meyer, E.; Pham, H.P.; Schneiderman, J.; Witt, V.; Wu, Y.; et al. Guidelines on the Use of Therapeutic Apheresis in Clinical Practice—Evidence-Based Approach from the Writing Committee of the American Society for Apheresis: The Eighth Special Issue. *J. Clin. Apher.* **2019**, *34*, 171–354. [CrossRef] [PubMed]

45. Rovira, J.; Cid, J.; Gutierrez-Garcia, G.; Pereira, A.; Fernandez-Aviles, F.; Rosinol, L.; Martinez, C.; Carreras, E.; Urbano, A.; Rovira, M.; et al. Fatal immune hemolytic anemia following allogeneic stem cell transplantation: Report of 2 cases and review of literature. *Transfus. Med. Rev.* **2013**, *27*, 166–170. [CrossRef] [PubMed]
46. Garcia-Garcia, I.; Cid, J.; Palomino, A.; Gine, E.; Alvarez-Larran, A.; Cibeira, M.T.; Lozano, M. Role of therapeutic plasma exchanges in refractory severe warm autoimmune hemolytic anemia: Presentation of two case reports. *Transfusion* **2020**, *60*, 2753–2757. [CrossRef] [PubMed]
47. Pons-Estel, G.J.; Salerni, G.E.; Serrano, R.M.; Gomez-Puerta, J.A.; Plasin, M.A.; Aldasoro, E.; Lozano, M.; Cid, J.; Cervera, R.; Espinosa, G. Therapeutic plasma exchange for the management of refractory systemic autoimmune diseases: Report of 31 cases and review of the literature. *Autoimmun. Rev.* **2011**, *10*, 679–684. [CrossRef] [PubMed]
48. Cid, J.; Carbasse, G.; Andreu, B.; Baltanas, A.; Garcia-Carulla, A.; Lozano, M. Efficacy and safety of plasma exchange: An 11-year single-center experience of 2730 procedures in 317 patients. Transfus. *Apher. Sci.* **2014**, *51*, 209–214. [CrossRef]
49. Cid, J.; Perez-Valencia, A.I.; Torrente, M.A.; Avarez-Larran, A.; Diaz-Ricart, M.; Esteve, J.; Lozano, M. Successful management of three patients with autoimmune thrombotic thrombocytopenic purpura with paradigm-changing therapy: Caplacizumab, steroids, plasma exchange, rituximab, and intravenous immunoglobulins (CASPERI). Transfus. *Apher. Sci.* **2021**, *60*, 103011. [CrossRef]
50. Deng, J.; Zhou, F.; Wong, C.Y.; Huang, E.; Zheng, E. Efficacy of therapeutic plasma exchange for treatment of autoimmune hemolytic anemia: A systematic review and meta-analysis of randomized controlled trials. *J. Clin. Apher.* **2020**, *35*, 294–306. [CrossRef]
51. Berentsen, S.; Ulvestad, E.; Gjertsen, B.T.; Hjorth-Hansen, H.; Langholm, R.; Knutsen, H.; Ghanima, W.; Shammas, F.V.; Tjonnfjord, G.E. Rituximab for primary chronic cold agglutinin disease: A prospective study of 37 courses of therapy in 27 patients. *Blood* **2004**, *103*, 2925–2928. [CrossRef]
52. Berentsen, S.; Randen, U.; Oksman, M.; Birgens, H.; Tvedt, T.H.A.; Dalgaard, J.; Galteland, E.; Haukas, E.; Brudevold, R.; Sorbo, J.H.; et al. Bendamustine plus rituximab for chronic cold agglutinin disease: Results of a Nordic prospective multicenter trial. *Blood* **2017**, *130*, 537–541. [CrossRef]
53. Berentsen, S.; Randen, U.; Vagan, A.M.; Hjorth-Hansen, H.; Vik, A.; Dalgaard, J.; Jacobsen, E.M.; Thoresen, A.S.; Beiske, K.; Tjonnfjord, G.E. High response rate and durable remissions following fludarabine and rituximab combination therapy for chronic cold agglutinin disease. *Blood* **2010**, *116*, 3180–3184. [CrossRef]
54. Rossi, G.; Gramegna, D.; Paoloni, F.; Fattizzo, B.; Binda, F.; D'Adda, M.; Farina, M.; Lucchini, E.; Mauro, F.R.; Salvi, F.; et al. Short course of bortezomib in anemic patients with relapsed cold agglutinin disease: A phase 2 prospective GIMEMA study. *Blood* **2018**, *132*, 547–550. [CrossRef] [PubMed]
55. Jalink, M.; Berentsen, S.; Castillo, J.J.; Treon, S.P.; Cruijsen, M.; Fattizzo, B.; Cassin, R.; Fotiou, D.; Kastritis, E.; De Haas, M.; et al. Effect of ibrutinib treatment on hemolytic anemia and acrocyanosis in cold agglutinin disease/cold agglutinin syndrome. *Blood* **2021**, *138*, 2002–2005. [CrossRef] [PubMed]

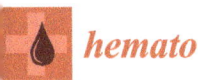

Review

B Lymphoproliferative Neoplasms of Uncertain Biological Significance: Report from the IV Workshop of the Italian Group of Hematopathology and Review of the Literature

Gioia Di Stefano [1,2], Francesca Magnoli [3], Massimo Granai [4], Federico Vittone [5], Raffaella Santi [1], Domenico Ferrara [2], Emanuela Boveri [6], Ada M. Florena [7], Falko Fend [4], Elena Sabattini [8], Marco Paulli [9], Maurilio Ponzoni [10,11], Stefano Lazzi [2], Stefano A. Pileri [12], Lorenzo Leoncini [2,*] and the Italian Group of Hematopathology [†]

1. Pathology Section, Department of Health Sciences, University of Florence, 50100 Florence, Italy
2. Section of Pathology, Department of Medical Biotechnologies, University of Siena, 53100 Siena, Italy
3. Department of Pathology, University Hospital, 21100 Varese, Italy
4. Institute of Pathology and Neuropathology, Tübingen University Hospital and Comprehensive Cancer Center Tübingen-Stuttgart, 72070 Tübingen, Germany
5. Department of Pathology, Ivrea Hospital ASLTO4, Piazza Credenza 2, 10015 Ivrea, Italy
6. Department of Pathology, IRCCS Fondazione Policlinico San Matteo, 27100 Pavia, Italy
7. Anatomic Pathology, Department of Sciences for the Promotion of Health and Mother and Child Care, University of Palermo, 90127 Palermo, Italy
8. Haematopathology Unit, Department of Experimental Diagnostic and Specialty Medicine, S. Orsola-Malpighi Hospital, University of Bologna, 40138 Bologna, Italy
9. Unit of Anatomic Pathology, Department of Molecular Medicine, Fondazione IRCCS Policlinico San Matteo and Università degli Studi di Pavia, 27100 Pavia, Italy
10. Faculty of Medicine, Vita-Salute San Raffaele University, 20100 Milan, Italy
11. Pathology Unit, Ospedale San Raffaele Scientific Institute, 20100 Milan, Italy
12. Division of Hematopathology, European Institute of Oncology, IRCCS, 20100 Milan, Italy
* Correspondence: lorenzo.leoncini@dbm.unisi.it
† "Italian Group of Hematopathology" (GIE) is the group of italian pathologist interested in Hematopathology in the Italian society of Pathology (SIAPEC) and organizing several tutorial and WS for the society.

Abstract: Lymphoproliferative neoplasms of uncertain biological significance are increasingly encountered due to widespread usage of immunophenotypic and molecular techniques. Considering that clearer biological criteria and patient management have been established for B-cell lymphoproliferative diseases of undetermined significance occurring in the peripheral blood, many issues are still obscure for early lesions detected in lymphoid tissues. Regardless that some categories of lymphoproliferative neoplasms of uncertain biological significance have been recognized by the 4th edition of the WHO, other anecdotal early lymphoproliferative lesions still remain fully undefined. Some early lesions frequently originate from the germinal center, including atypical germinal centers BCL2-negative, an early pattern of large B-cell lymphoma with *IRF4* rearrangement, and "in situ" high-grade B lymphomas. Moreover, other early lymphoproliferative lesions arise outside the germinal center and include those developing within the setting of monocytoid B-cell hyperplasia, but they also can be directly or indirectly associated with chronic inflammations. This review aims to summarize the concepts discussed during the IV Workshop organized by the Italian Group of Hematopathology, focus on the state-of-the-art on B-cell lymphoproliferative neoplasms of uncertain biological significance, and offer operative insights to pathologists and clinicians in routine diagnostics.

Keywords: lymphoproliferative neoplasms of uncertain biological significance; monoclonal B-cell lymphocytosis; "in situ" follicular neoplasia; "in situ" mantle cell neoplasia; atypical germinal centers; large B-cell lymphoma with *IRF4* rearrangement; "in situ" high-grade B lymphomas; non-Hodgkin lymphoma; Hodgkin lymphoma

1. Introduction

The IV Workshop, organized by the Italian Group of Hematopathology, focused on lymphoproliferative neoplasms of uncertain biological significance. The long-standing concept of in situ/early neoplasia has been already established in epithelial tumors; the same approach is not so readily applicable to lymphoid proliferative disorders, due to the fact that lymphocytes are usually circulating and not sessile cells. Indeed, in this context, early lesions are often an incidental finding that partially/minimally involve an otherwise reactive-appearing lymph node and never progress in most instances. Along with the historical recognition of monoclonal immunoglobulins in the serum, namely monoclonal gammopathy of undetermined significance (MGUS), a clear conceptual definition of peripheral blood B-cell lymphoproliferative diseases of undetermined significance (monoclonal B-cell lymphocytosis) is well-established [1]. A series of early lesions histologically detected in lymphoid tissues, also in view of their uncertain risk of progression, are actually still seeking a biological determination. The early lesions within the lymphoid tissue accepted by the 4th edition of the World Health Organization (WHO) Classification of Tumors of Hematopoietic and Lymphoid Tissues are "in situ" follicular neoplasia and "in situ" mantle cell neoplasia [2] that could actually be considered as the tissue counterpart of circulating elements with t(14;18) and t(11;14) rearrangements (Table 1). "In situ" follicular neoplasia (ISFN) is defined as partial or total colonization of germinal centers by clonal B cells carrying the *BCL2* translocation characteristic of follicular lymphoma (FL) in a lymph node where the overall architecture is preserved [3,4]. ISFN is characterized by lack of polarization, closely packed centrocytes with very few, if present, centroblasts, although it is not commonly recognizable in routine H&E-stained sections [3]; this condition is frequently identified by an intense immunoreactivity for germinal center markers (e.g., CD10) and aberrant positivity for BCL2, along with a low proliferation index. ISFN must be distinguished from partial involvement by follicular lymphoma (pFL), where an architectural distortion is observed. The risk of progression of ISFN is very low (<5%) [5], and it does not seem to be influenced by the number of follicles involved within a single lymph node [5,6]. "In situ" mantle cell neoplasia (ISMCN) is defined as the occurrence of Cyclin D1 expressing B cells in nonexpanded mantle zones of otherwise morphologically reactive-appearing lymph nodes [4,7,8]. The clinical outcome has not been completely clarified; the progression into an overt mantle cell lymphoma (MCL) is uncommon [7], although ISMCN or minimal accumulations of Cyclin D1-positive B cells can sometimes be detected several years before developing an overt MCL [9]; additionally, it has been reported that ISMCN with expression of SOX11 has a higher chance to progress [7].

In cases of ISFN and ISMCN, it is necessary to proceed to a complete staging workup to exclude an overt lymphoma in another site. Additionally, a composite form, namely ISFN and ISMCN, can be associated with another overt lymphoma, as presented in the first three cases of the Workshop.

Other anecdotal early lymphoproliferative lesions with uncertain biological significance have been previously published and are not present in the 4th edition of the WHO Classification (Table 1). They mostly originate from the germinal centers and encompass atypical BCL2-negative germinal centers, an early pattern of large B-cell lymphoma (LBCL) with *IRF4* rearrangement, and "in situ" high-grade B lymphomas. Nybakken et al. published a case series of atypical germinal centers in reactive/non-neoplastic lymph nodes characterized by isolated follicles with germinal centers substantially composed of aggregates of large centroblasts showing atypical mitoses without centrocytes [10]. These atypical follicles do not express BCL2 by immunohistochemistry and show the absence of *BCL2/IGH* translocation by FISH [10]: the differential diagnoses include a focal involvement by diffuse large B-cell lymphoma (DLBCL) or grade 3B, BCL2-negative FL, or a reactive follicular hyperplasia with unusual morphologic features.

Table 1. Lymphoproliferative neoplasms of uncertain biological significance.

	GC Involvement	Non-GC Involvement	Histologic Characteristics	Suggested Procedures When Lymphoproliferative Neoplasms of Uncertain Biological Significance Are Encountered
Entities accepted in the 4th WHO edition				
"In situ" follicular neoplasia (ISFN)	Yes	No	Lack of polarization, closely packed centrocytes with few centroblast.	Exclude pFL and a composite form with appropriate immunohistochemistry. Suggest a complete staging workup to rule out an overt lymphoma in another site.
"In situ" mantle cell neoplasia (ISMCN)	No	Yes	Cyclin D1-expressing B-cells in non-expanded mantle zones of otherwise morphologically reactive lymph node.	Exclude a MCLGP and composite form with appropriate immunohistochemistry. Suggest a complete staging workup to rule out an overt lymphoma in another site.
Entities not included in the in the 4th WHO edition				
Atypical GC BCL2-negative	Yes	No	Isolated follicles with GC composed of aggregates of large centroblast with atypical mitosis without centrocytes and *BCL2* negative by immunohistochemistry and FISH analysis.	Apply immunohistochemestry to confirm the presence of follicular dendritic networks and the GC origin of the B cell population. Occurrence of strong and diffuse immunoreactivity for IRF4, BCL2, and c-MYC must be assessed. In addition, FISH analysis for *IRF4, BCL2, c-MYC* rearrangements is advisable. Exclusion of an overt disease with a complete staging workup is mandatory.
Early pattern of large B-cell lymphoma (LBCL) with *IRF4* rearrangement	Yes	No	Atypical GC enriched with centroblasts, without tingible body macrophages or polarization with strong IRF4 positivity and *IRF4* rearrangement.	
Single extranodal involvement of "double hit" Follicular lymphoma (DH-FL)	Yes	No	Atypical GC B-cell population with follicular dendritic networks and *BCL-2 + c-MYC* rearrangements.	
Early Burkitt lymphoma (BL)	No	Yes	Aggregates composed of medium-sized lymphoid cells morphologically and phenotypically consistent with BL cells along with mitotic figures and apoptotic bodies	Apply immunohistochemical analysis to characterize the medium size population with BL features added to FISH to identify *c-MYC* rearrangement
Early classic Hodgkin lymphoma (cHL)	No	Yes	Presence of RS and HL cells in perifollicular areas with preserved lymph node architecture.	Evaluation of the preserved lymph node architecture. Investigate the scattered atypical RS- and HL-cells by immunohistochemistry. Exclusion of an overt disease with a complete staging workup is mandatory.

Early LBL with *IRF4* rearrangement has been reported in one case with predominant follicular hyperplasia that exhibited single atypical germinal centers enriched with centroblasts without accompanying tingible body macrophages displaying expression of CD20, CD10, BCL6, IRF4/MUM1, lambda immunoglobulin light chain restriction, and a gain and rearrangement of the *IRF4* gene detected by FISH [11].

Two cases of so-called "in situ" high-grade B lymphomas with *c-MYC* rearrangement have been previously reported [12] as well. By definition, a very low tumor burden was noticed in contrast to other overt B-cell lymphomas with *MYC* gene rearrangements; this feature may suggest that these early "double hit" lesions may require additional genetic hits to progress [12,13]. From a practical perspective, these lymphoproliferations have to be assessed in the context of all clinical findings and accompanied by a strict-follow-up to rule out any possible evolution.

Some operative considerations arise from the previously reported situations. In routine practice, whenever we face potential atypical germinal centers, the immunohistochemical confirmation of the presence of follicular dendritic networks, the germinal center origin of the B cell population, and the occurrence of strong and diffuse immunoreactivity for IRF4, BCL2, and c-MYC must be assessed. In addition, FISH analysis for *IRF4*, *BCL2*, and *c-MYC* rearrangements is advisable. This approach will enable in most instances to rule out, focal area(s) of diffuse large B-cell lymphoma/high-grade B-cell lymphoma "double hit", partial involvement by grade 3B BCL2-negative FL, and early LBCL with *IRF4* rearrangement, respectively. Following the examples of ISFN and ISMCN, the exclusion of an overt disease with a complete staging workup is mandatory in all these cases.

Another niche where early lesions have been described beside the germinal center is monocytoid B-cell hyperplasia [14,15]. Monocytoid B cells (MBCs) were described for the first time by Karl Lennert as immature sinus histiocytosis, representing cells closely related to marginal zone hyperplasia [16]. Morphologically, MBCs measure one-and-a-half to three times the size of small lymphocytes, display round, oval, or indented nuclei with a slightly clumped to vesicular chromatin structure, small and inconspicuous (when present) nucleoli, and abundant pale cytoplasm. These cells can be arranged in perifollicular clusters within and around sinuses and are commonly admixed with scattered neutrophils. Unlike marginal zone B-lymphocytes, MBCs are negative for BCL2 [17]. Reactive MBCs are frequently associated with follicular hyperplasia and epithelioid macrophages [18] and have been recognized occurring in association with lymphoproliferative diseases, like classic Hodgkin lymphomas (cHL) [19,20]. More recently, clusters of Burkitt cells have been reported with MBC hyperplasia in both immunocompromised and immunocompetent patients [14,15]. In immunocompromised patients, it has been proven that these early lesions carry the risk of progression into an overt Burkitt lymphoma with a worse outcome [14,15].

Different non-Hodgkin lymphomas have been associated with chronic inflammation, either infectious or not. In cases of chronic infection due to non-lymphotropic agents, the pathogen's role in establishing the proliferation and progression towards overt lymphoma radically differs from other lymphotropic agents. Moreover, IgG4-related disease (IgG4-RD) represents an important topic, as confirmed by the occurrence of a ISFN associated with this condition and presented during the Workshop. IgG4-RD is a fibroinflammatory disorder of uncertain etiology which affects almost any organ [21]. Although most patients with IgG4-RD do not present an association with lymphomas, some cases have been reported to develop concomitant or metachronous low- and high-grade lymphomas [22–28], suggesting that a potential pathogenetic link may lie in the context of a shared chronic antigenic stimulation [22,29,30]. This hypothesis is confirmed by cases #7 and #8 of the Workshop. On these grounds, a practical consideration is that monoclonal rearrangements can be demonstrated in a nonmalignant, antigen-driven proliferation of B cells, such as autoimmune disorders; accordingly, additional criteria of malignancy must be fulfilled to efficiently differentiate neoplastic proliferations from reactive conditions in this setting [31].

2. Submitted Cases of ISFN and ISMCN Associated with Overt Lymphoma

2.1. Case n. 1

Dr. Magnoli presented the previously published case [32] of a 75-year-old woman with multiple and bilateral lymphadenopathies that underwent an excisional biopsy of a right cervical lymph node. Morphological and immunohistochemical findings allowed to conclude for a diagnosis of a composite lymphoma encompassing FL, grade 1 to 2, "in situ" mantle cell neoplasia (ISMCN), and MCL with mantle zone growth pattern (MCLGP). A stage IVA was assessed, and the patient was treated with eight cycles of R-CVP (Rituximab plus a combination of Cyclophosphamide, Vincristine, and Prednisone) regimen, obtaining a complete remission. After two years, diffuse lymphadenopathy appeared, and the subsequent biopsy revealed a low-grade FL without any signs of a neoplastic mantle cell component, and after four years of "watch and wait", a progression of the disease was documented; the patient died of lymphoma after being treated with a new line of chemotherapy with eight cycles of Chlorambucil chemotherapy, followed by a steroid-based support therapy. Karyotype and Spectral Karyotyping (SKY) FISH analyses on metaphases performed on the first biopsy tissue sample confirmed different cell clones. The neoplastic clone carrying the t(11;14) translocation involving *CCND1* did not show additional cytogenetic abnormalities, whereas the neoplastic cell population with the t(14;18) translocation involving *BCL2* was characterized by a triploid karyotype with several additional alterations, including also the rearrangement of *BCL6*. In this context, the observations led the authors to suggest that the progressively aggressive behavior of this B-cell lymphoma was determined by the complex karyotype of the overt FL [32]. On the contrary, the ISMCN did not harbor additional genetic abnormalities, nevertheless not affecting the clinical outcome [32]. Therefore, the following case confirms that the occurrence of additional genetic aberrations may drive progression and clinical outcomes.

2.2. Case n. 2

Dr. Granai discussed the case of a 45-year-old male who underwent the excisional biopsy of an enlarged axillary lymph node following the diagnosis of MCL of the appendix. The lymph node architecture was replaced by a diffuse proliferation of small monotonous lymphocytes with round nuclei and scant cytoplasm surrounding hyperplastic follicles with regularly structured germinal centers (Figure 1). Immunohistochemical investigations demonstrated the presence of two distinct lymphoid populations. The interfollicular cells were immunoreactive for CD20, CD5, CD23, and LEF1 (Figure 2). Cyclin D1 and SOX11 were expressed by reduced mantle zones surrounding reactive lymphoid follicles and absent in the interfollicular areas. Accordingly, a composite ISMCN and small lymphocytic lymphoma (SLL) diagnosis was made. IgH rearrangement confirmed the existence of two clonally unrelated B-cell neoplastic populations. The present case describes the well-known combination of ISMCN and SLL [33], exemplifies the concept that "in situ" lymphoma might be observed in association with overt MCL in distant sites, and highlights that the significance of the early lesion remains uncertain, thus suggesting that the clinical evaluation for evidence of overt lymphoma is highly recommended.

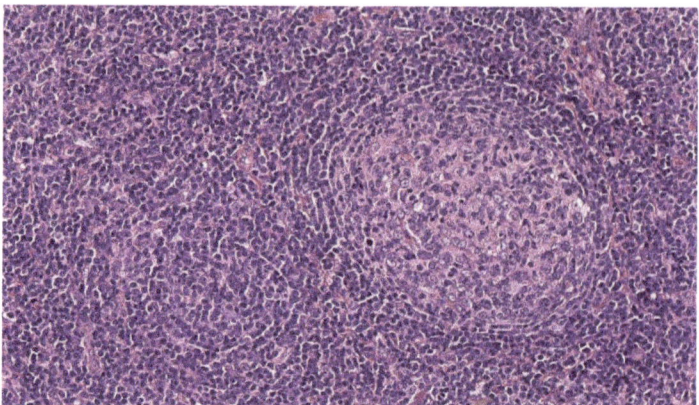

Figure 1. H&E original magnification 20×. The lymph node architecture is replaced by a diffuse, interfollicular monotonous proliferation of small lymphocytes with round nuclei and scant cytoplasm surrounding hyperplastic follicles with regularly structured germinal centers.

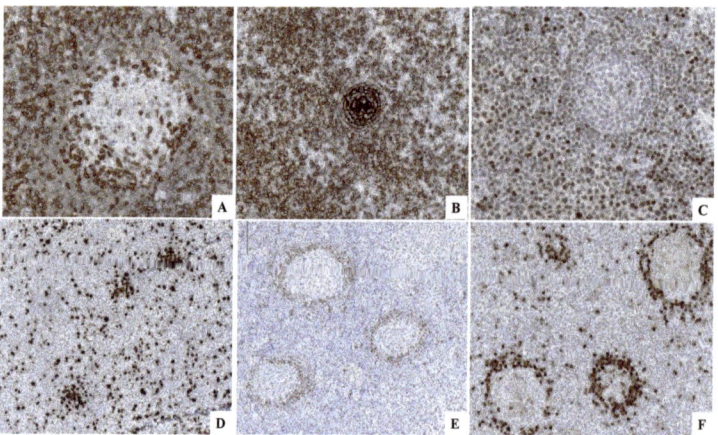

Figure 2. (**A**) CD5+ in both components. (**B**) CD23+ in the SLL component. (**C**) LEF1+ in the SLL component. (**D**) Ki-67 highlights the proliferation centers. (**E**) Cyclin D1+ in the ISMCN. (**F**) SOX11+ in the ISMCN.

2.3. Case n. 3

Dr. Di Stefano submitted the case of a 45-year-old male patient that received a diagnosis of chronic lymphocytic leukemia (CLL) with atypical phenotype according to a bone marrow biopsy and the flow cytometric analysis results. The bone marrow biopsy showed a diffuse interstitial infiltrate of small B lymphocytes with a round nucleus and scant cytoplasm, immunoreactive for CD20, BCL2, and CD5 and negative for CD23, Cyclin D1, SOX11, CD10, and BCL6. A few weeks later, the patient underwent an excisional biopsy of three small cervical lymph nodes. The lymph node architecture was effaced by a small-to-medium-sized population with an immunophenotypic profile consistent with CLL with an atypical phenotype [34,35]. Two residual follicular structures were present, and their germinal centers showed a strong immunoreactivity for CD10 and BCL2 with a low proliferation index. The final diagnosis was CLL with an atypical phenotype and ISFN. In the present case, it is also confirmed that ISFN can be associated with other forms of overt lymphoma such as CLL. In such an event, it is necessary to always report the early lesion to guarantee appropriate clinical management.

3. Submitted Cases of Early Lymphoproliferative Lesions Originating from the Germinal Center Other Than ISFN and ISMCN

3.1. Case n. 4

Dr. Lazzi submitted the case of a 77-year-old male patient that underwent radical prostatectomy with bilateral lymphadenectomy for prostatic adenocarcinoma. Within one of the right iliac-obturator lymph nodes, two isolated follicles (Figure 3A–C) displayed germinal centers with atypical features such as the absence of polarization and enrichment of centroblasts. The atypical follicles were positive for B-cell and germinal center-related markers but negative for BCL2 by immunohistochemistry and for *BCL2* translocation by FISH analysis (Figure 3D–F). An overt FL grade 3A was found in a contralateral lymph node (Figure 3G,H), which was negative for BCL2, as well both by immunohistochemistry and FISH; therefore, the final diagnosis was of FL, grade 3A with focal localization on the contralateral lymph node. The histologic interpretation of isolated atypical germinal centers can be challenging, but an overt FL helped achieve the correct diagnosis. A Next-Generation Sequencing (NGS) analysis was performed using an Illumina custom 80-gene-targeted NGS panel for B-cell lymphomas and revealed genetic variants in *TNFAIP3* and *NOTCH2*.

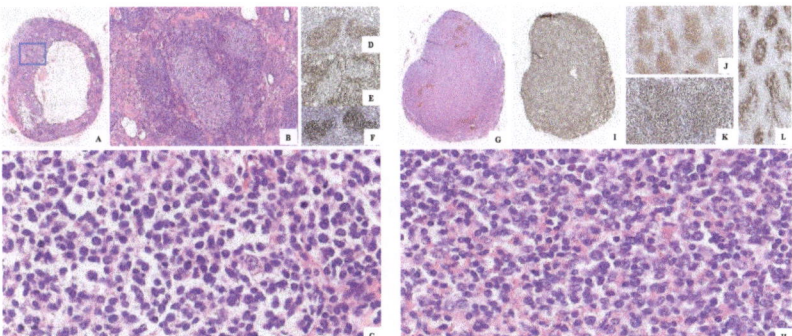

Figure 3. (**A**) H&E original magnification 2× of the right iliac-obturator lymph node displaying two atypical follicles highlighted in the blue rectangle. (**B**) H&E original magnification 10× of the atypical follicles. (**C**) H&E original magnification 40× of the atypical germinal centers with the absence of polarization and enrichment in centroblasts. (**D**) CD10+, (**E**) BCL2-, and (**F**) Ki67 immunostains. (**G**) H&E original magnification 4× of the left iliac-obturator lymph node. (**H**) H&E original magnification 40x of the overt FL on the left iliac-obturator lymph node. (**I**) BCL2-. (**J**) CD10+. (**K**) Ki67. (**L**) CD23 immunostains.

3.2. Case n. 5

Dr. Granai submitted and recently published [36] the case of a 72-year-old woman without significant medical history that underwent colonoscopy for enduring complaints and constipation; a 5-mm sessile polypoid lesion in the sigmoid colon was noted. Microscopically, the polypoid lesion displayed a submucosal lymphoid infiltrate with a follicular growth pattern and predominant centroblasts, along with very few centrocytes. The lymphoid population showed immunoreactivity for CD20, CD10, BCL6, BCL2, and MYC, in the context of expanded and disrupted follicular dendritic meshworks. FISH studies identified both *IGH/BCL2* and *IGH/MYC* gene rearrangements, allowing the diagnosis of an extranodal FL grade 3A, with *BCL2* and *MYC* rearrangements (DH-FL). Staging did not show additional sites of disease, and the patient is currently in good health and has never progressed. This case raises several questions related to patient's management, since it is not clear whether to consider DH-FL an indolent lymphoma based on its morphologic aspects or an aggressive lymphoma given its cytogenetic features [37–41]. This dilemma related to the outcome is further enhanced when DH-FL displays partial involvement or is limited to a single site. More studies are needed to clarify this issue.

4. Submitted Cases of Early Lymphoproliferative Lesions Arising in the Setting of Monocytoid Hyperplasia

Case n. 6

Dr. Di Stefano presented the case of a 61-year-old woman with a prior history of invasive breast carcinoma treated with surgical resection, chemotherapy, and radiotherapy, who during follow up developed left supraclavicular lymphadenopathy. The excised lymph node showed follicular hyperplasia with polarized germinal centers; in the perifollicular areas, aggregates of MBC were admixed with rare, scattered large mononucleated or binucleated cells equipped with eosinophilic nucleolus and basophilic cytoplasm (Figure 4). The large cells were immunoreactive for CD30, CD15, PAX5 weak (Figure 5), and MUM1 and negative for CD20, CD3, and CD45. EBV was negative by EBER in situ hybridization. The molecular analysis performed on microdissected atypical, perifollicular areas detected a polyclonal IGH rearrangement, supporting the diagnosis of partial involvement by cHL. Since the radiologic and clinical evidence showed a localized disease, a "watch and wait" approach was chosen, and in the following years, subsequent nodal biopsies of the supraclavicular lymph nodes displayed the same morphological picture. Five years after the first diagnosis, the patient exhibited left inguinal lymphadenopathy and underwent an incisional biopsy. The morphologic examination revealed a subverted architecture by small T lymphocytes, eosinophils, and histiocytes intermingled with classical Reed–Sternberg (RS) and Hodgkin cells (Figure 6). The morpho–phenotypical profile was consistent with cHL, mixed cellularity. After the diagnosis, the patient received appropriate chemotherapy but had frequent hospitalizations due to recurrent nosocomial infections. The following case demonstrated an overt cHL after a history of partial involvement of cHL developing within the context of MBC hyperplasia.

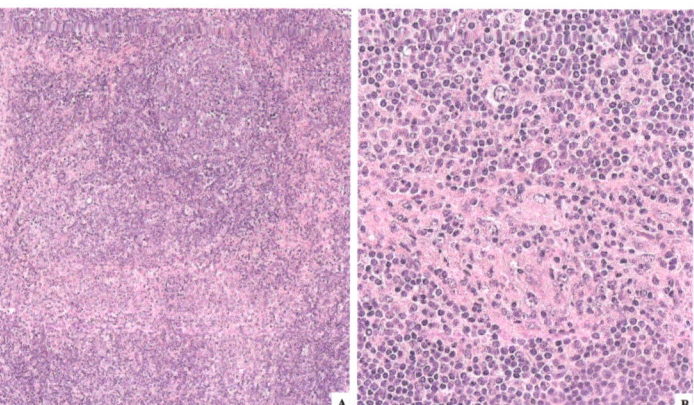

Figure 4. (**A**) H&E original magnification 10× displaying follicular hyperplasia with polarized germinal centers and, in the perifollicular areas, aggregates of MBC. (**B**) H&E original magnification 20× showing, in the perifollicular areas, MBC mixed with rare large mononucleated or binucleated cells containing an eosinophilic nucleolus and basophilic cytoplasm.

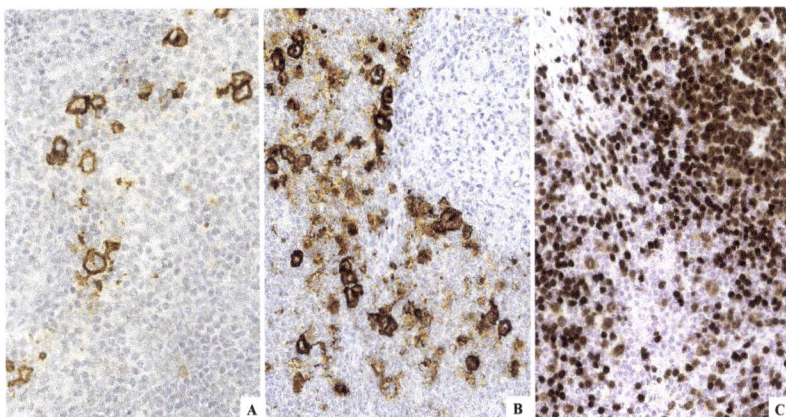

Figure 5. (**A**) CD30+. (**B**) CD15+. (**C**) PAX5+ weak.

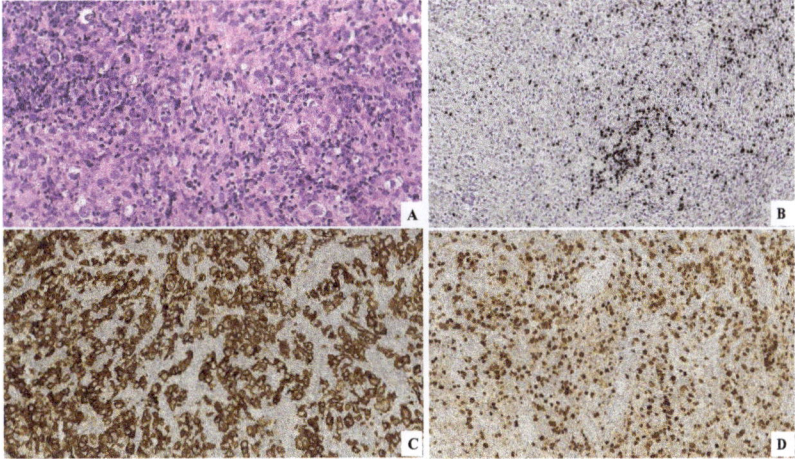

Figure 6. (**A**) H&E original magnification 20× that displays small T lymphocytes, eosinophils, histiocytes, classical Reed–Sternberg cells, and Hodgkin cells. (**B**) PAX5-. (**C**) CD30+. (**D**) MUM1+.

5. Submitted Cases of Early Lymphoproliferative Lesions Associated with Infectious Diseases and Chronic Inflammation

5.1. Case n. 7

Dr. Vittone presented the case of a 76-year-old man with weight loss and low-grade persisting fever for many months. The PET-CT scan revealed multiple lymphoadenomegaly on both sides of the diaphragm with high spleen, bone, and left colon uptake. Histological examination of an axillary lymph node showed an area with well-formed granulomas composed of epithelioid histiocytes and occasional Langhans-type giant cells with central eosinophilic necrosis (Figure 7A). A PCR analysis performed on the paraffin-embedded tissue confirmed the presence of *Mycobacterium tuberculosis* DNA. The residual portion of the lymph node showed predominant follicular hyperplasia; herein, immunohistochemical investigations highlighted two follicles with strong staining for CD10, BCL2 (Figure 7C,D) with a low proliferation index suggestive of ISFN. Therefore, a diagnosis of necrotizing granulomatous lymphadenitis due to *Mycobacterium tuberculosis* infection associated with ISFN was made.

5.2. Case n. 8

Dr. Santi presented a case of a 77-year-old male with a prior history of prostatic adenocarcinoma. During follow-up, left hydroureteronephrosis due to a retroperitoneal mass of 6.5 cm in the maximum diameter developed. The histological examination of left subtotal ureterectomy displayed follicular hyperplasia and predominant mature IgG4+ interfollicular plasma cells with a high IgG4/IgG ratio within the background of septal, storiform fibrosis (Figures 8 and 9). Within this background, a single atypical follicle unusually constituted by monomorphous centrocytes, few centroblasts, and attenuated mantle zones was noticed with a strong positivity for BCL2 and CD10 (Figure 10). A PCR analysis showed a monoclonal IgH rearrangement. The final diagnosis was IgG4-RD with ISFN. A few months after the diagnosis, the patient died of complications due to sepsis.

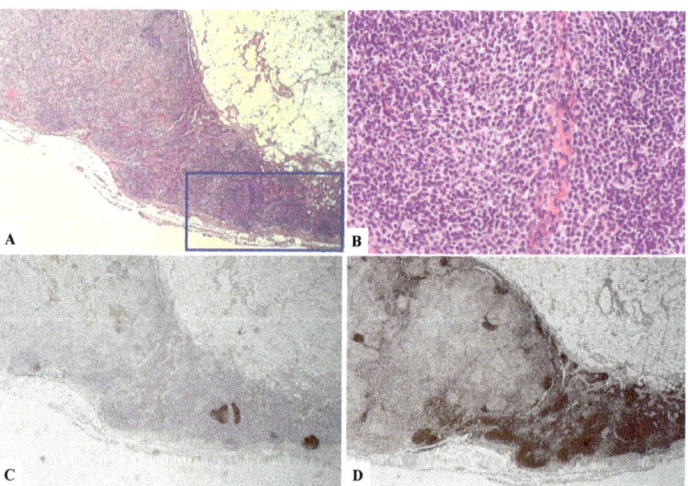

Figure 7. (**A**) H&E original magnification 2.5× of the axillary lymph node displaying an area with well-formed granulomas, and in the remaining part of the lymphoid tissue, follicular hyperplasia was observed with two atypical follicles (blue rectangle). (**B**) H&E original magnification 40× of one of the atypical follicles suggestive of ISFN. (**C**) CD10+. (**D**) BCL2+.

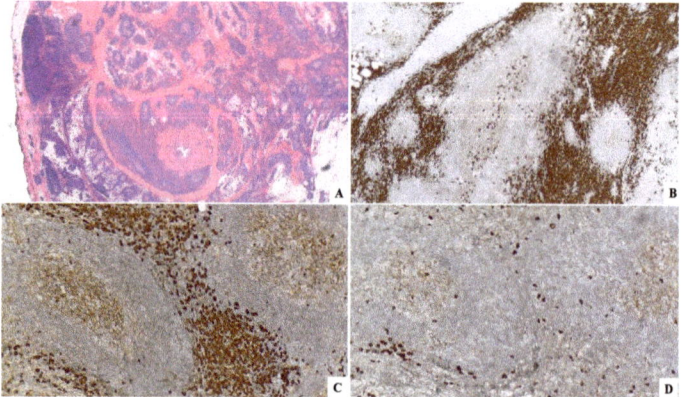

Figure 8. (**A**) H&E original magnification 2× displaying a lymphoproliferative lesion in the background of septal, a storiform fibrosis. (**B**) CD138+. (**C**, **D**) A Kappa light chain restriction.

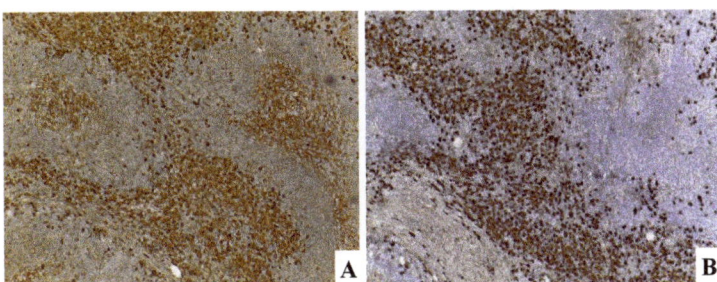

Figure 9. (A) IgG. (B) IgG4.

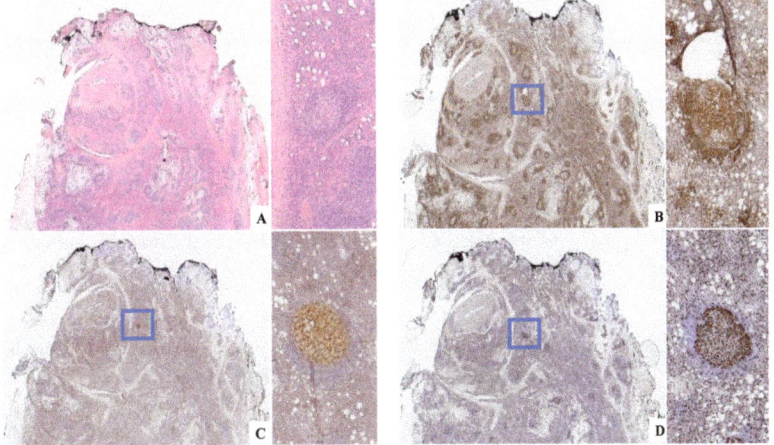

Figure 10. (A) H&E original magnification 4× ISFN highlighted in the blue rectangle. (B) BCL2+. (C) CD10+; (D) Ki-67.

6. Conclusions

Early/in situ lymphoproliferative disorders are still an unclear subject since the evolution of these diseases at the time of the diagnosis is unpredictable on morpho-phenotypical-molecular-cytogenetic grounds. The sequence precancer–cancer in epithelial malignancies does not necessary overlap with the relationship between early lymphoproliferative lesions and overt lymphoma. In fact, most early lymphoid lesions do not progress to an overt lymphoma and may be concomitant with these latter. In the cases presented during the Workshop, the entities ISFN and ISMCN, already recognized by the 4th edition of the WHO classification, were associated with other overt lymphoproliferative processes, and therefore considered a composite lymphoma (Table 2).

Table 2. Clinical cases presented during the Workshop.

Case	Gender	Age	Diagnosis	Presence of Overt Lymphoma	Type of Overt Lymphoma
Case n. 1	F	75 y	FL and ISMCN	Yes	FL
Case n. 2	M	45 y	ISMCN and SLL	Yes	MCL in previous biopsy
Case n. 3	M	45 y	CLL with atypical phenotype and ISFN	Yes	CLL on bone marrow
Case n. 4	M	77 y	FL, 3A with focal localization on the contralateral lymph node	Yes	FL, 3A
Case n. 5	F	72 y	Extranodal FL with *BCL2* and *c-MYC* rearrangement	No	
Case n. 6	F	61 y	Early cHL in monocytoid hyperplasia	Yes	cHL, mixed cellularity
Case n. 7	M	76 y	Necrotizing granulomatous lymphadenitis associated with ISFN	No	
Case n. 8	M	77 y	IgG4-RD with ISFN	No	

The current view of the progression in lymphoproliferative lesion postulates that this process relies on a multistep sequence rather than only on a single event. This concept is exemplified by case #1, confirming that the development of a complex karyotype is the primary cause of the disease's evolution [32], while case #2 highlights the importance of recognizing these early lesions to inform the clinician and carefully look for a possible overt and different lymphoma in another site. In case #3, the association of CLL with an atypical phenotype and ISFN was reported demonstrating that these early lesions concurrent with other lymphoproliferative processes may also be incidental findings discovered by immunohistochemistry. Nevertheless, the observation of such cases, which are usually unrelated to malignant overt counterparts, raises the question of whether there could be an underlying susceptibility for developing B lymphoproliferative processes in certain subjects [42]. The germinal centers are a fragile environment where neoplastic processes can develop. Notwithstanding the overexpression of antiapoptotic molecules such as BCL2 as a result of t(14;18) has been recognized to spy on the occurrence of FL, and case #4 displays that the histopathological examination can be sometimes the only key feature to unravel a lymphoproliferative process. In this case, the lymphoproliferative lesion was suspected on morpho-phenotypic features in two germinal centers, although there was a lack of BCL2 positivity. In this context, the finding of the overt FL on the contralateral lymph node aided the diagnosis of FL t(14;18)-negative that has been proven to be a genetically heterogeneous entity [43], and the NGS analysis performed on the case documented the presence of frequent mutations that have been detected in FL t(14;18)-negative, namely *TNFAIP3* and *NOTCH2* [43]. Therefore, we point out that occasional atypical follicles BCL2-negative in the context of a reactive lymph node should suggest the exclusion of an FL t(14; 18)-negative in other sites. A close correlation between molecular data and morphology is always required, since several studies have detected clonal populations in the context of classical reactive germinal centers or hyperplastic marginal zones [44,45].

In the "early" extra nodal DH-FL (case #5) [36], additional genetic hits are considered necessary for the full transformation of these 'aggressive' in situ neoplasms to a clinically overt disease [12,13]. Furthermore, once these lesions are recognized, clinical characteristics drive treatment decisions, and a close follow-up is mandatory to rule out overt lesions in another site.

Moving outside the germinal center, more specifically in the context of MBC hyperplasia, we notice a possible role of MBC in controlling the neoplastic disease [15,19,20]. In fact, in case #6, all the subsequent biopsies displayed RS cells closely associated with clusters of MBCs, and two previous studies have documented this aspect in overt cHL [19,20]. It has been established that the HL/RS cells originate from the germinal centers [46], and when they migrate to the perifollicular areas, they probably trigger a reaction like MBC hyperplasia. Therefore, even in cHL, MBC hyperplasia may be a physiologic antitumor mechanism of the host that counteracts the development of the full-blown disease [15,19,20].

In the presence of infectious diseases and chronic inflammation syndromes, an underlying lymphoproliferative process, may occur and should be considered. Rarely, non-Hodgkin lymphoma (NHL) and Hodgkin lymphoma were concurrent with chronic infection by *Mycobacterium tuberculosis* and the *Mycobacterium avium* complex [47–55]. Setting aside patients with congenital and cell-mediated immunity defects, it has been hypothesized that *Mycobacterium tuberculosis*, similarly to *Helicobacter pylori*, might induce rearrangements more readily than other infectious agents, since they are both intracellular pathogens [53]. Much caution must be applied in the event of an IgG4-positive lymphoma or plasma cell neoplasm when numerous IgG4+ plasma cells are noticed in the context of a lymphoplasmacytic proliferation [56], and a clinical correlation might be necessary. To our knowledge, a case of necrotizing granulomatous lymphadenitis due to *Mycobacterium tuberculosis* infection and IgG4-RD concomitant to an early lesion have not been reported. Moreover, during the Workshop, it was suggested that the chronic inflammatory process, either created by an infectious agent or by an inflammatory disorder, could be the trigger determining an early lymphoproliferative form. However, to be added to the following hypothesis, we should also consider the well-known role of immunosurveillance of the microenvironment in B-cell lymphomas [15]; therefore, further studies could highlight the control mechanisms and the events determining the onset and progression to an overt disease.

In conclusion, pathologists should emphasize that the above-described early/in situ lesions retain an uncertain potential of malignant progression and require a strong integration with the clinical and imaging findings. Given that, presently, the therapeutic strategy relies on the diagnosis of an overt lymphoma, a conservative management accomplished by an active follow-up must be considered in these early/in situ lymphoproliferations.

Funding: This research received no external funding.

Institutional Review Board Statement: Not applicable.

Informed Consent Statement: Not applicable.

Data Availability Statement: Not applicable.

Conflicts of Interest: The authors declare no conflict of interest.

References

1. Kyle, R.A.; Therneau, T.M.; Rajkumar, S.V.; Larson, D.R.; Plevak, M.F.; Offord, J.R.; Dispenzieri, A.; Katzmann, J.A.; Melton, L.J., 3rd. Prevalence of monoclonal gammopathy of undetermined significance. *N. Engl. J. Med.* **2006**, *354*, 1362–1369. [CrossRef] [PubMed]
2. Swerdlow, S.H.; Campo, E.; Harris, N.L.; Jaffe, E.S.; Pileri, S.A.; Stein, H.; Thiele, J. (Eds.) *WHO Classification of Tumors of Hematopoietic and Lymphoid Tissues*, 4th ed.; IARC: Lyon, France, 2017.
3. Cong, P.; Raffeld, M.; Teruya-Feldstein, J.; Sorbara, L.; Pittaluga, S.; Jaffe, E.S. In situ localization of follicular lymphoma: Description and analysis by laser capture microdissection. *Blood* **2002**, *99*, 3376–3382. [CrossRef] [PubMed]
4. Carbone, A.; Santoro, A. How I treat: Diagnosing and managing "in situ" lymphoma. *Blood* **2011**, *117*, 3954–3960. [CrossRef] [PubMed]
5. Jegalian, A.G.; Eberle, F.C.; Pack, S.D.; Mirvis, M.; Raffeld, M.; Pittaluga, S.; Jaffe, E.S. Follicular lymphoma in situ: Clinical implications and comparisons with partial involvement by follicular lymphoma. *Blood* **2011**, *118*, 2976–3064. [CrossRef]
6. Pillai, R.K.; Surti, U.; Swerdlow, S.H. Follicular lymphoma-like B cells of uncertain significance (in situ follicular lymphoma) may infrequently progress, but precedes follicular lymphoma, is associated with other overt lymphomas and mimics follicular lymphoma in flow cytometric studies. *Haematologica* **2013**, *98*, 1571–1580. [CrossRef]

7. Carvajal-Cuenca, A.; Sua, L.F.; Silva, N.M.; Pittaluga, S.; Royo, C.; Song, J.Y.; Sargent, R.L.; Espinet, B.; Climent, F.; Jacobs, S.A.; et al. In situ mantle cell lymphoma: Clinical implications of an incidental finding with indolent clinical behavior. *Haematologica* **2012**, *97*, 270–278. [CrossRef]
8. Nodit, L.; Bahler, D.W.; Jacobs, S.A.; Locker, J.; Swerdlow, S.H. Indolent mantle cell lymphoma with nodal involvement and mutated immunoglobulin heavy chain genes. *Hum. Pathol.* **2003**, *34*, 1030–1034. [CrossRef]
9. Adam, P.; Schiefer, A.I.; Prill, S.; Henopp, T.; Quintanilla-Martínez, L.; Bösmüller, H.C.; Chott, A.; Fend, F. Incidence of preclinical manifestations of mantle cell lymphoma and mantle cell lymphoma in situ in reactive lymphoid tissues. *Mod. Pathol.* **2012**, *25*, 1629–1636. [CrossRef]
10. Nybakken, G.E.; Bala, R.; Gratzinger, D.; Jones, C.D.; Zehnder, J.L.; Bangs, C.D.; Cherry, A.; Warnke, R.A.; Natkunam, Y. Isolated follicles enriched for centroblasts and lacking t(14;18)/BCL2 in lymphoid tissue: Diagnostic and clinical implications. *PLoS ONE* **2016**, *11*, e0151735. [CrossRef]
11. Granai, M.; Lazzi, S. Early pattern of large B-cell lymphoma with IRF4 rearrangement. *Blood* **2020**, *136*, 769. [CrossRef]
12. Kumar, J.; Butzmann, A.; Wu, S.; Easly, S.; Zehnder, J.L.; Warnke, R.A.; Bangs, C.D.; Jangam, D.; Cherry, A.; Lau, J.; et al. Indolent in situ B-Cell neoplasms with MYC rearrangements show somatic mutations in MYC and TNFRSF14 by Next-generation Sequencing. *Am. J. Surg. Pathol.* **2019**, *43*, 1720–1725. [CrossRef] [PubMed]
13. Knudson, A.G., Jr.; Meadows, A.T.; Nichols, W.W.; Hill, R. Chromosomal deletion and retinoblastoma. *N. Engl. J. Med.* **1976**, *295*, 1120–1123. [CrossRef] [PubMed]
14. Park, D.; Ozkaya, N.; Hariharan, A. Novel insights into the early histopathogenesis of immunodeficiency-associated Burkitt lymphoma: A case report of Burkitt microlymphoma arising within HIV lymphadenitis. *Histopathology* **2016**, *69*, 516–521. [CrossRef] [PubMed]
15. Granai, M.; Lazzi, S.; Mancini, V.; Akarca, A.; Santi, R.; Vergoni, F.; Sorrentino, E.; Guazzo, R.; Mundo, L.; Cevenini, G.; et al. Burkitt lymphoma with a granulomatous reaction: An M1/Th1-polarised microenvironment is associated with controlled growth and spontaneous regression. *Histopathology* **2021**, *80*, 430–442. [CrossRef] [PubMed]
16. Camacho, F.I.; Algara, P.; Mollejo, M.; Garcìa, J.F.; Montalba, C.; Martìnez, N.; Sánchez-Beato, M.; Piris, M.A. Nodal marginal zone B-cell lymphoma: A heterogenous tumor. A comprehensive analysis of a series of 27 cases. *Am. J. Surg. Pathol.* **2003**, *27*, 762–771. [CrossRef]
17. Poppema, S.; Gilchrist, M. Monocytoid B cells and bcl-2 protein negative in contrast to marginal zone cells and monocytoid B-cell lymphoma. *Int. J. Surg. Pathol.* **1995**, *2*, 277.
18. Kojima, M.; Nakamura, S.; Itoh, H.; Yoshida, K.; Shimizu, K.; Motoori, T.; Yamane, N.; Joshita, T.; Suchi, T. Occurrence of monocytoid B-cells in reactive lymph node lesions. *Pathol. Res. Pract.* **1998**, *194*, 559–565. [CrossRef]
19. Mohrmann, R.L.; Nathwani, B.N.; Brynes, R.K.; Sheibani, K. Hodgkin's disease occurring in monocytoid B-cell clusters. *Am. J. Clin. Pathol.* **1991**, *95*, 802–808. [CrossRef]
20. Plank, L.; Hansmann, M.L.; Fischer, R. Monocytoid B-cells occurring in Hodgkin's disease. *Virchows Arch.* **1994**, *424*, 321–326. [CrossRef] [PubMed]
21. Deshpande, V.; Zen, Y.; Chan, J.K.; Yi, E.E.; Sato, Y.; Yoshino, T.; Klöppel, G.; Heathcote, J.G.; Khosroshahi, A.; Ferry, J.A.; et al. Consensus statement on the pathology of IgG4-related disease. *Mod. Pathol.* **2012**, *25*, 1181–1192. [CrossRef]
22. Cheuk, W.; Yuen, H.K.L.; Chan, A.C.L.; Shih, L.Y.; Kuo, T.T.; Ma, M.W.; Lo, Y.F.; Chan, W.K.; Chan, J.K. Ocular adnexal lymphoma associated with IgG4+ chronic sclerosing dacryoadenitis: A previously undescribed complication of IgG4-related sclerosing disease. *Am. J. Surg. Pathol.* **2008**, *32*, 1159–1167. [CrossRef] [PubMed]
23. Sato, Y.; Ohshima, K.; Ichimura, K.; Sato, M.; Yamadori, I.; Tanaka, T.; Takata, K.; Morito, T.; Kondo, E.; Yoshino, T. Ocular adnexal IgG4-related disease has uniform clinicopathology. *Pathol. Int.* **2008**, *58*, 465–470. [CrossRef] [PubMed]
24. Ferry, J.A. IgG4-related lymphadenopathy and IgG4-related lymphoma: Moving targets. *Diagn. Histopathol.* **2013**, *19*, 128–139. [CrossRef]
25. Kanda, G.; Ryu, T.; Shirai, T.; Ijichi, M.; Hishima, T.; Kitamura, S.; Bandai, Y. Peripheral T-cell lymphoma that developed during the follow-up of IgG4-related disease. *Intern. Med.* **2011**, *50*, 155–160. [CrossRef] [PubMed]
26. Ishida, M.; Hodohara, K.; Yoshida, K.; Kagotani, A.; Iwai, M.; Yoshii, M.; Okuno, H.; Horinouchi, A.; Nakanishi, R.; Harada, A.; et al. Occurrence of anaplastic large cell lymphoma following IgG4-related autoimmune pancreatitis and cholecystitis and diffuse large B-cell lymphoma. *Int. J. Clin. Exp. Pathol.* **2013**, *6*, 2560–2568.
27. Uehara, T.; Ikeda, S.; Hamano, H.; Kawa, S.; Moteki, H.; Matsuda, K.; Kaneko, Y.; Hara, E. A case of Mikulicz's disease complicated by malignant lymphoma: A postmortem histopathological finding. *Intern. Med.* **2012**, *51*, 419–423. [CrossRef]
28. Takahashi, N.; Ghazale, A.H.; Smyrk, T.C.; Mandrekar, J.N.; Chari, S.T. Possible association between IgG4-associated systemic disease with or without autoimmune pancreatitis and non-Hodgkin lymphoma. *Pancreas* **2009**, *38*, 523–526. [CrossRef] [PubMed]
29. Yamamoto, M.; Takahashi, H.; Tabeya, T.; Suzuki, C.; Naishiro, Y.; Ishigami, K.; Yajima, H.; Shimizu, Y.; Obara, M.; Yamamoto, H.; et al. Risk of malignancies in IgG4- related disease. *Mod. Rheumatol.* **2012**, *22*, 414–418. [CrossRef]
30. Gupta, R.; Khosroshahi, A.; Shinagare, S.; Fernandez, C.; Ferrone, C.; Lauwers, G.Y.; Stone, J.H.; Deshpande, V. Does autoimmune pancreatitis increase the risk of pancreatic carcinoma? a retrospective analysis of pancreatic resections. *Pancreas* **2013**, *42*, 506–510. [CrossRef]

31. Kussick, S.J.; Kalnoski, M.; Braziel, R.M.; Wood, B.L. Prominent clonal B-cell populations identified by flow cytometry in histologically reactive lymphoid proliferations. *Am. J. Clin. Pathol.* **2004**, *121*, 464–472. [CrossRef]
32. Vivian, L.F.; Magnoli, F.; Campiotti, L.; Chini, C.; Calabrese, G.; Sessa, F.; Tibiletti, M.G.; Uccella, S. Composite follicular lymphoma and "early" (in situ and mantle zone growth pattern) mantle cell neoplasia: A rare entity with peculiar cytogenetic and clinical features. *Pathol. Res. Pract.* **2020**, *216*, 153067. [CrossRef] [PubMed]
33. Fend, F.; Quintanilla-Martinez, L.; Kumar, S.; Beaty, M.W.; Blum, L.; Sorbara, L.; Jaffe, E.S.; Raffeld, M. Composite low grade B-cell lymphomas with two immunophenotypically distinct cell populations are true biclonal lymphomas. A molecular analysis using laser capture microdissection. *Am. J. Pathol.* **1999**, *154*, 1857–1866. [CrossRef]
34. Criel, A.; Michaux, L.; de Wolf-Peeters, C. The concept of typical and atypical chronic lymphocytic leukaemia. *Leuk. Lymphoma* **1999**, *33*, 33–45. [CrossRef] [PubMed]
35. Matutes, E.; Oscier, D.; Garcia-Marco, J.; Ellis, J.; Copplestone, A.; Gillingham, R.; Hamblin, T.; Lens, D.; Swansbury, G.J.; Catovsky, D. Trisomy 12 defines a group of CLL with atypical morphology: Correlation between cytogenetic, clinical and laboratory features in 544 patients. *Br. J. Haematol.* **1996**, *92*, 382–388. [CrossRef]
36. Lazzi, S.; Granai, M.; Capanni, M.; Fend, F. Unusual presentation of extra-nodal double-hit follicular lymphoma: A case report. *BMC Gastroenterol.* **2022**, *22*, 254. [CrossRef]
37. Katsushima, H.; Fukuhara, N.; Konosu-Fukaya, S.; Himuro, M.; Kitawaki, Y.; Ichikawa, S.; Ishizawa, K.; Sasano, H.; Harigae, H.; Ichinohasama, R. Does double-hit follicular lymphoma with translocations of MYC and BCL2 change the definition of transformation? *Leuk. Lymphoma* **2018**, *59*, 758–762. [CrossRef]
38. Miyaoka, M.; Kikuti, Y.Y.; Carreras, J.; Ikoma, H.; Hiraiwa, S.; Ichiki, A.; Kojima, M.; Ando, K.; Yokose, T.; Sakai, R.; et al. Clinicopathological and genomic analysis of double-hit follicular lymphoma: Comparison with high-grade B-cell lymphoma with MYC and BCL2 and/or BCL6 rearrangements. *Mod. Pathol.* **2018**, *31*, 313–326. [CrossRef]
39. Miao, Y.; Hu, S.; Lu, X.; Li, S.; Wang, W.; Medeiros, L.J.; Lin, P. Double-hit follicular lymphoma with MYC and BCL2 translocations: A study of 7 cases with a review of literature. *Hum. Pathol.* **2016**, *58*, 72–77. [CrossRef]
40. Tomita, N.; Tokunaka, M.; Nakamura, N.; Takeuchi, K.; Koike, J.; Motomura, S.; Miyamoto, K.; Kikuchi, A.; Hyo, R.; Yakushijin, Y.; et al. Clinicopathological features of lymphoma/leukemia patients carrying both BCL2 and MYC translocations. *Haematologica* **2009**, *94*, 935–943. [CrossRef]
41. Christie, L.; Kernohan, N.; Levison, D.; Sales, M.; Cunningham, J.; Gillespie, K.; Batstone, P.; Meiklejohn, D.; Goodlad, J. C-MYC translocation in t(14;18) positive follicular lymphoma at presentation: An adverse prognostic indicator? *Leuk. Lymphoma* **2008**, *49*, 470–476. [CrossRef]
42. Landgren, O.; Albitar, M.; Ma, W.; Abbasi, F.; Hayes, R.B.; Ghia, P.; Marti, G.E.; Caporaso, N. B-cell clones as early markers for chronic lymphocytic leukemia. *N. Engl. J. Med.* **2009**, *360*, 659–667. [CrossRef] [PubMed]
43. Nann, D.; Ramis-Zaldivar, J.E.; Müller, I.; Gonzalez-Farre, B.; Schmidt, J.; Egan, C.; Salmeron-Villalobos, J.; Clot, G.; Mattern, S.; Otto, F.; et al. Follicular lymphoma t(14;18)-negative is genetically a heterogeneous disease. *Blood Adv.* **2020**, *4*, 5652–5665. [CrossRef] [PubMed]
44. Nam-Cha, S.H.; San-Millan, B.; Mollejo, M.; Garcia-Cosio, M.; Garijo, G.; Gomez, M.; Warnke, R.A.; Jaffe, E.S.; Piris, M.A. Light-chain-restricted germinal centres in reactive lymphadenitis: Report of eight cases. *Histopathology* **2008**, *52*, 436–444. [CrossRef]
45. Attygalle, A.D.; Liu, H.; Shirali, S.; Diss, T.C.; Loddenkemper, C.; Stein, H.; Dogan, A.; Du, M.Q.; Isaacson, P.G. Atypical marginal zone hyperplasia of mucosa-associated lymphoid tissue: A reactive condition of childhood showing immunoglobulin lambda light-chain restriction. *Blood* **2004**, *104*, 3343–3348. [CrossRef]
46. Weniger, M.A.; Küppers, R. Molecular biology of Hodgkin lymphoma. *Leukemia* **2021**, *35*, 968–981. [CrossRef] [PubMed]
47. Gilroy, D.; Sherigar, J. Concurrent small bowel lymphoma and mycobacterial infection: The use of adesonosine deaminase activity and polymerase chain reaction to facilitated rapid diagnosis and treatment. *Eur. J. Gastroenterol. Hepatol.* **2006**, *18*, 305–307. [CrossRef] [PubMed]
48. Ouedraogo, M.; Ouedraogo, S.M.; Cisse, R.; Lougue, C.; Badoum, G.; Sigani, A.; Drabo, Y.J. Active tuberculosis in a patient with Hodgkin's disease. A case report. *Rev. Pneumol. Clin.* **2000**, *56*, 33–35. [PubMed]
49. Audebert, F.; Schneidewind, A.; Hartmann, P.; Kullmann, F.; Schölmerich, J. Lymph node tuberculosis as primary manifestation of Hodgkin's disease. *Med. Klin.* **2006**, *101*, 500–504. [CrossRef] [PubMed]
50. Klein, T.O.; Soll, B.A.; Issel, B.F.; Fraser, C. Bronchus-associated lymphoid tissue lymphoma and mycobacterium tuberculosis infection: An unusual case and a review of the literature. *Respir. Care* **2007**, *52*, 755–758.
51. Inadome, Y.; Ikezawa, T.; Oyasu, R.; Noguchi, M. Malignant lymphoma of bronchus-associated lymphoid tissue (BALT) coexistent with pulmonary tuberculosis. *Pathol. Int.* **2001**, *51*, 807–811. [CrossRef]
52. Centkowski, P.; Sawczuk-Chabin, J.; Prochorec, M.; Warzocha, K. Hodgkin's lymphoma and tuberculosis coexistence in cervical lymph nodes. *Leuk. Lymphoma* **2005**, *46*, 471–475. [CrossRef] [PubMed]
53. Bellido, M.C.; Martino, R.; Martínez, C.; Sureda, A.; Brunet, S. Extrapulmonary tuberculosis and non-Hodgkin's lymphoma: Coexistence in an abdominal lymph node. *Haematologica* **1995**, *80*, 482–483. [PubMed]

54. Fanourgiakis, P.; Mylona, E.; Androulakis, I.I.; Eftychiou, C.; Vryonis, E.; Georgala, A.; Skoutelis, A.; Aoun, M. Non-Hodgkin's lymphoma and tuberculosis coexistence in the same organs: A report of two cases. *Postgrad. Med. J.* **2008**, *84*, 276–277. [CrossRef]
55. Gaur, S.; Trayner, E.; Aish, L.; Weinstein, R. Bronchus-associated lymphoid tissue lymphoma arising in a patient with bronchiectasis and chronic Mycobacterium avium infection. *Am. J. Hematol.* **2004**, *77*, 22–25. [CrossRef]
56. Geyer, J.T.; Niesvizky, R.; Jayabalan, D.S.; Mathew, S.; Subramaniyam, S.; Geyer, A.I.; Orazi, A.; Ely, S.A. IgG4 plasma cell myeloma: New insights into the pathogenesis of IgG4-related disease. *Mod. Pathol.* **2014**, *27*, 375–381. [CrossRef] [PubMed]

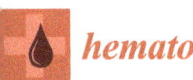 *hemato*

Review

The Clinical Impact of Precisely Defining Mantle Cell Lymphoma: Contributions of Elaine Jaffe

Mark Roschewski [1,*] and Dan L. Longo [2]

1. Lymphoid Malignancies Branch, Center for Cancer Research, National Cancer Institute, National Institutes of Health, Bethesda, MD 20892, USA
2. Hematology Division, Department of Medicine, Brigham and Women's Hospital, Boston, MA 02115, USA
* Correspondence: mark.roschewski@nih.gov

Abstract: Mantle cell lymphoma (MCL) is an aggressive yet incurable B-cell lymphoma that was only first recognized as a distinct subtype in 1992, with early reports suggesting a poor median survival. Elaine Jaffe is a renowned hematopathologist and scientist from the National Cancer Institute who was instrumental in many of the early descriptions of MCL that distinguished it from other B-cell lymphomas. Further, she has led multiple international collaborations that have harmonized the lymphoma classification systems that are currently in use today. The early morphologic descriptions of MCL along with the contributions of immunologic and genetic techniques have confirmed MCL as a distinct entity with unique biology and clinical behavior. Importantly, these scientific discoveries laid the foundation for unprecedented therapeutic breakthroughs that have led to significant improvements in overall survival.

Keywords: centrocytic lymphoma; intermediate lymphocytic lymphoma; Jaffe; mantle cell lymphoma; mantle zone lymphoma; cyclin D1

1. Introduction

Non-Hodgkin lymphoma (NHL) is a generic term applied to a broad range of malignant lymphoid neoplasms with striking underlying clinical and biologic heterogeneity. Lymphomas represent malignant transformation of lymphocytes at various stages of differentiation and have acquired hallmark cancer capabilities, including the ability to proliferate, resist cellular apoptosis, and evade the host immune response. Yet, important biologic differences exist across NHL subtypes that manifest as differences in disease behavior and therapeutic vulnerabilities.

Over the last 7 decades, the classification of lymphoid malignancies has been a complex and iterative process that evolved with the emergence of novel biologic insights and advances in analytic methods. New subtypes are often first introduced as provisional entities and subsequently validated to be sufficiently distinct to merit a unique therapeutic approach. The National Cancer Institute (NCI) has contributed substantially to the body of knowledge on lymphoma biology, classification, and management through the years. The bedrock upon which its lymphoma studies have been built is accurate and reproducible diagnosis, initially based entirely on histologic examination under a microscope and, over time, with a remarkably sophisticated battery of assays for the expression of specific genes and proteins. Indeed, the lymphoma classification systems purport to make scientifically and clinically meaningful distinctions between lymphoma subtypes by defining relatively homogeneous entities from a clinical, morphologic, immunologic, and genetic perspective with the goal of improving clinical outcomes.

For the past nearly 50 years, the precision of the diagnosis of lymphoma at the NCI has been established and maintained by Elaine Jaffe, where she currently serves as the head of the Hematopathology Section of the Laboratory of Pathology. At NCI, the pathologists have participated as full partners in the clinical studies and used their scientific expertise

Citation: Roschewski, M.; Longo, D.L. The Clinical Impact of Precisely Defining Mantle Cell Lymphoma: Contributions of Elaine Jaffe. *Hemato* **2022**, *3*, 508–517. https://doi.org/10.3390/hemato3030035

Academic Editors: Alina Nicolae and Antonino Carbone

Received: 18 July 2022
Accepted: 12 August 2022
Published: 16 August 2022

Publisher's Note: MDPI stays neutral with regard to jurisdictional claims in published maps and institutional affiliations.

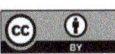

Copyright: © 2022 by the authors. Licensee MDPI, Basel, Switzerland. This article is an open access article distributed under the terms and conditions of the Creative Commons Attribution (CC BY) license (https://creativecommons.org/licenses/by/4.0/).

to establish new insights into lymphoma biology that have direct influence on patient management. The function of a clinical research team requires expertise in several domains: diagnostic imaging, patient care, surgery, pharmacology, and knowledge of the disease being treated. Excellence in each area is critical to obtaining the best outcomes, while variability in a domain can undermine the results. The work at the NCI has been able to rely on the accuracy of lymphoma diagnosis because of the excellence of Dr. Jaffe and her team. If Dr. Jaffe says it, you can count on it. And everyone knows it. A comprehensive recounting of the insights emerging from her work would take volumes to cover. Beyond her role within the NCI, she is a renowned physician scientist who has made numerous seminal contributions to our understanding of the biology and classification of lymphoma subtypes over her illustrious career. In her career, Dr. Jaffe has championed the critical importance of accurate diagnosis in making therapeutic progress. Early on, Dr. Jaffe and her NCI colleagues described important biologic differences between lymphomas arising from B-cell origin compared with those with T-cell or monocytic origin. Indeed, she was the first to demonstrate that nodular lymphomas originated from follicular B lymphocytes [1]. She and her colleagues had the foresight to understand the importance of incorporating the immunologic aspects of lymphoma, including the nature and function of the malignant cell along with the surrounding immune cell infiltrates [2,3]. Throughout her career, she has pioneered scientific discoveries within and across lymphoma subtypes, and she has led international collaborations that modernize lymphoma classification by integrating traditional pathology with the emergence of novel immunologic and genomic approaches. No more illustrative example exists than her scientific contribution to our understanding of the entity mantle cell lymphoma (MCL). She originally described key morphologic and immunologic features of "intermediate lymphocytic lymphoma (ILL)" that suggested it was a distinct B-cell lymphoma and first proposed the term "mantle cell lymphoma" in 1991 [4]. In this article, we highlight the seminal contributions of Dr. Jaffe along a discovery timeline that led to our modern conceptualization of MCL as a B-cell lymphoma with at least two distinct clinical subtypes with divergent clinical behavior (Figure 1). What is striking about this timeline is that numerous therapeutic advances followed from seminal observations in pathobiology and the prognosis has improved. The clinical impact of having a universally recognized set of diagnostic criteria establishing a defined and reproducible clinical entity has allowed clinical research to focus on developing new therapeutic approaches. The Nebraska Lymphoma Study Group has documented therapeutic progress through the last 30 years made possible by defining MCL as a distinct disease entity [5]. Indeed, one can make a cogent argument that the improved clinical outcomes in MCL have outpaced improvements in any other lymphoma subtype and the contributions of Dr. Jaffe and other pioneering scientists enabled that success [5].

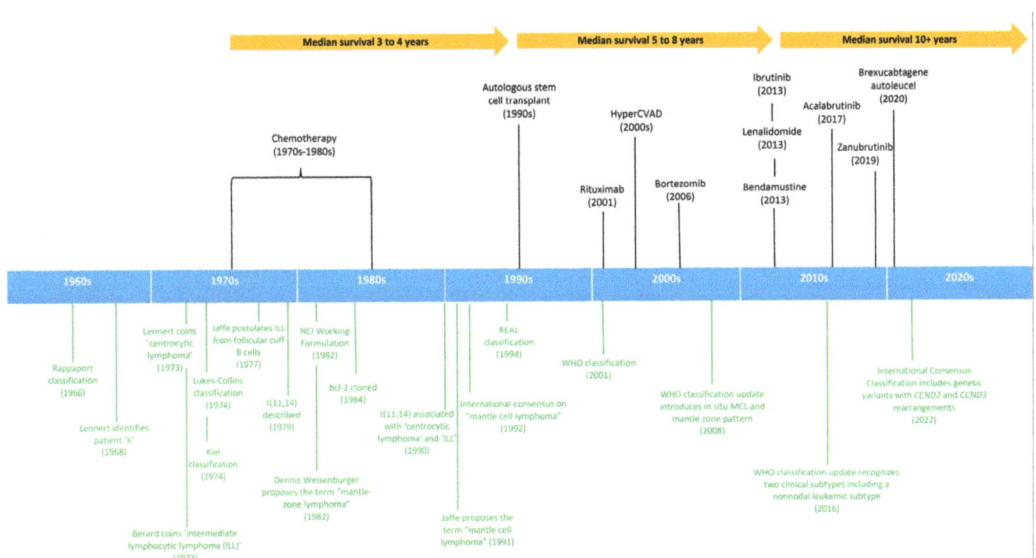

Figure 1. The timeline from the 1960s to the modern day depicting the scientific discoveries that ultimately led to recognition of mantle cell lymphoma (MCL) as a distinct biologic entity and therapeutic advances. Below the timeline are the classification systems of lymphoma and early pathologic descriptions of entities now classified as MCL. Above the timeline are the standard therapies for the period and the corresponding median survival for patients with MCL.

2. History and Evolution of Lymphoid Malignancies Classification

In 1966, Henry Rappaport of the United States Armed Forces Institute of Pathology proposed a simple and reproducible lymphoma classification system that relied exclusively on morphologic criteria [6]. Lymphomas were subdivided based on their underlying growth pattern as either nodular or diffuse. Further, the appearance of the malignant cell and its differentiation state was used to classify tumors as either well-differentiated, poorly differentiated, undifferentiated, or histiocytic [7]. In the Rappaport system, nodular lymphomas were typically composed of small lymphocytes and were comprised mostly of indolent disorders, while the "histiocytic" and poorly differentiated lymphomas were more aggressive and required chemotherapy. Notably, this system predated our modern understanding of cellular immunology and did not classify tumors based on B-cell or T-cell lineage.

In the 1970s, both the German pathologist Karl Lennert and the American pathologists L.J. Lukes and R.D. Collins proposed functional approaches to lymphoma classification that incorporated lymphocytic lineage based on cell surface immune markers and enzyme histochemical features along with morphology [8,9]. During this time period, separate classification schemes were used in different parts of the world and, since no broad international consensus existed, it was difficult to compare pathological and clinical results. Further, all systems lacked extensive clinical correlations and did not consider clinical features when classifying tumors.

In this context, the National Cancer Institute sponsored a panel of expert hematopathologists known as the international Working Formulation (WF) with a goal of providing a reproducible method to translate the various classification systems into clinical trial results and reports of clinical outcomes [10]. The WF system applied many concepts of preceding systems and incorporated clinical data. It defined subtypes based on their general clinical prognosis, and entities were grouped as low-grade, intermediate-grade, or high-grade. Notably, the IWF did not include the immunologic orientation to subclassify, rendering it less reproducible and limiting the discovery of new entities. Indeed, the panel of expert hematopathologists asked to review and classify the cases in the study disagreed with one another and with their own initial reading a substantial and alarming fraction of the time.

In 1994, the International Lymphoma Study Group (ILSG) convened a panel of 19 international expert hematopathologists to develop a consensus list of distinct clinical entities called the Revised European–American Classification of Lymphoid Neoplasms (REAL) classification [11]. The concept behind the REAL classification was to describe disease entities according to all available information (morphology, immunophenotype, genetic, and clinical features), with varying degrees of relative importance for each entity. To further validate the REAL classification, the ILSG conducted a study in which five expert pathologists reviewed over 1300 cases of NHL at various international centers [12,13]. This effort confirmed that the REAL classification was easily used by expert hematopathologists and had greater inter-observer reproducibility than other classification systems [14]. The REAL classification laid the foundation for the World Health Organization (WHO) classification system that was the first true international consensus on the classification of lymphoid malignancies in 2001 [15]. A cardinal feature of the WHO classification system was to periodically review new data and periodically incorporate them into updated classification systems that occurred in both 2008 [16] and 2016 [17].

3. Mantle Cell Lymphoma as a Distinct Entity

A primary objective of all lymphoma classification systems is to build upon previous iterations by describing novel entities that were previously difficult to classify; they are often predicated on the emergence of new technology. For example, in 1968 Karl Lennert described a lymph node biopsy from "patient K" that was comprised of small lymphocytes with a diffuse growth pattern that had completely effaced the lymph node architecture [18]. Lennert recognized that this lymphoma was unclassifiable with existing systems and he labeled this and other similar cases as 'type K'. After analyzing subsequent biopsies from the same patient, he coined the term "centrocytic lymphoma" (CC) to describe lymphomas with a diffuse growth pattern of small cells that resembled cleaved follicular center cells [8,19]. Similarly, the American pathologist Costan Berard had recognized that some lymphomas were not easily classified as either well-differentiated or poorly differentiated by the Rappaport classification system and he proposed the term "malignant lymphoma, lymphocytic type intermediate grade of differentiation" or "intermediate lymphocytic lymphoma" (ILL) [20]. Both CC and ILL shared pathologic features between nodular lymphomas (i.e., follicular lymphoma) and well-differentiated lymphocytic lymphoma (i.e., chronic lymphocytic leukemia). They exhibited a mostly diffuse growth pattern but could also have areas with a vaguely nodular pattern. The cells were small and monotonous with clumped chromatin and scant cytoplasm with nuclei that varied in shape, including round, slightly clefted, and irregular [3]. Immunologically, these tumors also exhibited features intermediate between well-differentiated and poorly differentiated tumors and expressed surface immunoglobulin. In 1977, Dr. Jaffe postulated on the possible cell of origin based on these morphologic and immunologic criteria:

> "The cells of nodular lymphomas are neoplastic counterparts of follicular B lymphocytes whereas well-differentiated lymphocytic lymphoma (WDL) cells are more closely related to medullary-cord B cells. Lymphoma of intermediate differentiation type may derive from B cells of the lymphoid cuff at the margins of follicles and thus exhibit features at the interface between nodular lymphomas and WDL". Jaffe et al., Cancer Treat Rep. 1977;61(6):953–962.

The American pathologist Dennis Weisenburger recognized that there was a distinctive B-cell lymphoma that appeared to originate from the mantle zones of secondary lymphoid follicles [21]. He described 12 cases of lymphoma that morphologically resembled ILL, but with a growth pattern of atypical lymphocytes proliferating as wide mantles around normal appearing germinal centers and proposed the term "mantle-zone lymphoma". Importantly, he reported that the clinical course was often aggressive, which further solidified the need to distinguish them from well-differentiated lymphomas [22]. In 1987, Jaffe and colleagues reviewed the histologic, immunologic, and clinical features of ILL that supported its consideration as a distinct clinicopathologic entity that was virtually identical to CC. The authors concluded that this entity was a tumor derived from lymphocytes of the mantle cuff based on the growth pattern and the expression of alkaline phosphatase on the neoplastic cells, which resembled that seen in mantle cuffs [23,24].

The emergence of molecular biology provided additional methods to sub-classify lymphomas. In 1979, the recurrent rearrangement t(11;14) (q14;q32) was first described in four cases of lymphoid neoplasms [25] and it was soon appreciated that recurrent translocations were often characteristic of specific lymphoma subtypes and this could be a powerful new technology to advance our understanding of distinct pathobiology of specific lymphomas [26]. In 1984, NCI researchers determined that the breakpoint of t(11;14) was within the joining segment of immunoglobulin heavy chain (*IGH*) typically located on chromosome 14 band q32 and characterized a new gene, named *bcl-1* (B-cell lymphoma/leukemia 1), located on chromosome 11 band q13 [27]. It was shortly after that studies linked this recurrent translocation with specific lymphoma subtypes. Rearrangements involving *bcl-1* were enriched in cases of ILL [28], but virtually never observed in follicular lymphoma, Burkitt lymphoma, or diffuse large B-cell lymphomas [29]. In 1990, Mike Williams and colleagues used Southern blotting and probes for immunoglobulin heavy and light chains, *bcl-1*, *bcl-2*, and *c-myc* in 14 patients [30]. They described rearrangements of *bcl-1* in four (29%) cases and none had *bcl-2* rearrangements. At the same time, NCI researchers used a genomic probe of the major breakpoint region in *bcl-1* and showed that 10 (53%) ILL cases were associated with rearrangements [31]. When using multiple probes in 12 cases of CC, Williams and colleagues described that 11 (92%) were associated with *bcl-1* rearrangements [32]. In 1991, it was discovered that the candidate oncogene *PRAD1* located on chromosome 11q13 encoded a protein structurally similar to the cyclins (named cyclin D1) [33–36]. Taken together, we now know that the *bcl-1* rearrangement involves the *PRAD1/CCND1* gene located downstream of its major breakpoint region that encodes cyclin D1 and places it under the transcriptional control of *IGH*. The cyclin D1 translocation leads to unregulated cell cycle control underpinning MCL biology.

In 1991, Raffeld and Jaffe reviewed the morphologic, immunophenotypic, and genetic data supporting the notion that ILL, CC, and mantle zone lymphoma were identical neoplasms that should be unified as a distinct lymphoma subtype [4]. These entities were comprised of small to medium sized lymphocytes with scant neoplasm that expressed pan B-cell markers including CD20, CD19, and CD22 along with the pan T-cell marker CD5 and exhibited characteristically strong surface immunoglobulin expression while lacking CD10, Bcl-6, and CD23. Further, frequent expression of alkaline phosphatase suggested that these tumors were derived from follicular mantle zone cells [4]. They proposed that these entities be unified under the term "mantle cell lymphoma" (MCL) and recognized that diffuse, vaguely nodular, and expanded mantle zone growth patterns could be observed. In 1992, the term MCL was universally accepted to describe ILL, CC, and mantle zone lymphoma based on characteristic clinical features, immunophenotype, and a hallmark translocation [37].

Importantly, the recognition of MCL as a unique B-cell lymphoma did not signify the end of scientific discovery within this entity but represented the beginning. Since the original descriptions, important scientific discoveries have been made in MCL that distinguish it from related B-cell lymphomas that highlight the clinical and biologic heterogeneity within this entity. It is appreciated that tumor proliferation can vary widely in MCL and proliferation signatures by gene expression profiling are closely associated with response to chemotherapy and survival [38]. Further, it is now recognized that not all cases of MCL have demonstrable cyclin D1 expression, and cases of cyclin D1-negative MCL exhibit the classic morphologic and immunologic features of MCL but are often associated with rearrangements involving *CCND2* or *CCND3* [39]. Lastly, it has been noted that select cases of MCL exhibit very indolent behavior and that cyclin D1 positive B cells can occasionally be identified within the inner mantle zones of follicles, a process first described as in situ MCL and later updated to in situ mantle cell neoplasia (ISMN) [16,17,40]. Current classification systems recognize two distinct clinical variants of MCL, including a classical variant that typically expresses SOX11, often involving lymph nodes along with frequent extra-nodal involvement, and can behave aggressively [41,42]. An indolent form of MCL also exists that is frequently SOX11 negative and presents with non-nodal disease involving the spleen, peripheral blood, and bone marrow [17].

4. Therapeutic Advances in Mantle Cell Lymphoma

This article is primarily focused on the contribution of pathologic observations that led to the recognition of MCL as a distinct biologic entity, but it is notable that, since 1991, the prognosis for patients with MCL has improved significantly (Figure 1). Indeed, since the time of original description, research has focused on identifying pathogenetic mechanisms and oncogenic signaling pathways that drive MCL and the translation of these observations into novel therapies. It is beyond the scope of this article to comprehensively review the evolution of therapy for MCL, but we choose to highlight specific therapeutic advances and their effect on outcomes.

A feature of MCL that was initially quite puzzling was the wide range of natural histories associated with the diagnosis. Some patients had a very indolent course and did not require therapeutic intervention for years. Others had an extremely aggressive disease that spread rapidly and killed them in a few months. The initial reports of survival for MCL patients treated with standard lymphoma combination regimens such as cyclophosphamide, vincristine, prednisone (CVP) or cyclophosphamide, doxorubicin, vincristine, and prednisone CHOP showed a very poor outcome compared with other B-cell lymphomas with a median survival of only 3 to 4 years [13,43]. Further, in distinction to aggressive B-cell lymphomas, durable remission was rare and MCL is considered largely incurable with combination chemotherapy. For this reason, the standard approach starting in the 1990s and early 2000s was to intensify chemotherapy to include either autologous stem cell transplantation (ASCT) as part of frontline therapy [44,45] or to treat with highly dose-intensive regimens developed from acute lymphocytic leukemia (ALL) such as fractionated cyclophosphamide, vincristine, doxorubicin, and dexamethasone (hyper-CVAD), often followed by ASCT as consolidation [46]. Although this intensification of therapy was only applicable to patients able to tolerate the myelosuppressive nature of these approaches, the rates of complete response and durable remissions appeared to improve.

In the early 2000s, the monoclonal anti-CD20 antibody rituximab emerged and was tested in combination chemotherapy regimens for NHL, including MCL. Early studies of rituximab added to CHOP demonstrated improvement in rates of complete response, but these data did not translate into a significant improvement in progression-free or overall survival [47,48]. Nonetheless, rituximab was incorporated into virtually all frontline regimens for MCL [49–51] and improved rates of complete response and overall survival when delivered as maintenance therapy after ASCT [52]. Further, for older patients who are not deemed suitable candidates for consolidation with ASCT, rituximab maintenance improved overall survival [53]. Although multiple regimens remain in use for MCL and the approach varies considerably based on practice setting and the age of the patient, both epidemiologic and long term data from clinical trials suggest that rituximab has improved survival in all patients with MCL when added to chemotherapy, including older patients [54–57]. Overall, rituximab along with intensification of chemotherapy in younger patients has improved the median survival of MCL to 5 to 8 years, although this approach is associated with a continuous incidence of relapse and does not cure most patients [56].

In the 2010s, targeted agents emerged that appeared to have unique activity in MCL, including proteasome inhibitors, immunomodulatory agents, and inhibitors of the Bruton tyrosine kinase (BTK) pathway [58–61]. At the same time, bendamustine with rituximab (BR) emerged as a safe and effective induction regimen for MCL that was tolerable for patients of all ages [62]. Indeed, induction therapy with BR is as effective as more intensive induction regimens prior to ASCT and has become the most commonly used chemotherapy regimen in community practice [57,63].

Most recently, combination regimens are being tested in MCL that do not use traditional chemotherapy at all, with the hope of more broad tolerability. Lenalidomide with rituximab has been shown to be safe and highly effective as a frontline regimen with frequent durable remissions [60,64]. The BTK inhibitor ibrutinib has been studied with rituximab in patients with indolent forms of MCL as well as prior to intensive chemotherapy and has shown to induce very high rates of complete response [65]. Ibrutinib also improved the complete response rate and progression free survival when added to BR in a recent randomized study [66]. Finally, the emergence of chimeric antigen receptor T-cell therapy is associated with very high rates of complete response in MCL and is associated with durable remissions [67,68]. Taken together, these data suggest that future studies in MCL will test combinations of targeted agents with and without chemotherapy or immunotherapy. Current estimates suggest that following these therapeutic advances, the overall survival for MCL treated in the modern era may be longer than a decade and should continue to improve [69].

5. Trainees and Mentees

Beyond personal accomplishments as a scientist and researcher, Elaine Jaffe also impacted the field of hematopathology by her mentorship and teaching of close colleagues and trainings for nearly 4 decades. Nearly 75 pathologists have trained under her direct or indirect mentorship since the late 1970s, many of whom also made seminal contributions to our understanding of lymphoma biology and classification. Notable former mentees and/or close collaborators during their formative years include Stefania Pittaluga, Mark Raffeld, Elias Campo, Leticia Quintanilla-Martinez, and Falko Fend. In this way, her approach of identifying novel and biologically relevant associations between pathologic observations and clinical outcomes has been handed down and continues to impact the field.

6. Conclusions

Lymphoma treatment relies on accurate and reproducible diagnosis, while the lymphoma classification systems aim to make scientifically and clinically meaningful distinctions between lymphoma subtypes by defining relatively homogeneous entities from a clinical, morphologic, immunologic, and genetic perspective with the goal of improving clinical outcomes. Throughout her illustrious career, Dr. Elaine Jaffe has made important contributions to the management of individual patients at the NCI and has been instrumental in identifying new lymphoma subtypes, such as MCL. She has championed international efforts to harmonize the classification of lymphoma and these efforts have formed the foundation for therapeutic success.

Funding: This research was funded by the Intramural Research Program of the National Institutes of Health.

Institutional Review Board Statement: Not applicable.

Informed Consent Statement: Not applicable.

Data Availability Statement: Not applicable.

Conflicts of Interest: The authors report no financial conflict of interest.

References

1. Jaffe, E.S.; Shevach, E.M.; Frank, M.M.; Berard, C.W.; Green, I. Nodular lymphoma—Evidence for origin from follicular B lymphocytes. *N. Engl. J. Med.* **1974**, *290*, 813–819. [CrossRef] [PubMed]
2. Jaffe, E.S.; Braylan, R.C.; Nanba, K.; Frank, M.M.; Berard, C.W. Functional markers: A new perspective on malignant lymphomas. *Cancer Treat. Rep.* **1977**, *61*, 953–962. [PubMed]
3. Berard, C.W.; Jaffe, E.S.; Braylan, R.C.; Mann, R.B.; Nanba, K. Immunologic aspects and pathology of the malignant lymphomas. *Cancer* **1978**, *42*, 911–921. [CrossRef]

4. Raffeld, M.; Jaffe, E.S. bcl-1, t(11;14), and mantle cell-derived lymphomas. *Blood* **1991**, *78*, 259–263. [CrossRef] [PubMed]
5. Armitage, J.O.; Longo, D.L. Mantle-Cell Lymphoma. *N. Engl. J. Med.* **2022**, *386*, 2495–2506. [CrossRef] [PubMed]
6. Rappaport, H. *Tumors of the Hematopoietic System*; Armed Forces Institute of Pathology: Washington, DC, USA, 1966.
7. Hicks, E.B.; Rappaport, H.; Winter, W.J. Follicular lymphoma; A re-evaluation of its position in the scheme of malignant lymphoma, based on a survey of 253 cases. *Cancer* **1956**, *9*, 792–821.
8. Lennert, K. *Malignant Lymphomas Other than Hodgkin's Disease: Histology, Cytology, Ultrastructure, Immunology*; Springer: Berlin/Heidelberg, Germany, 1978.
9. Lukes, R.J.; Collins, R.D. Immunologic characterization of human malignant lymphomas. *Cancer* **1974**, *34* (Suppl. 4), 1488–1503. [CrossRef]
10. National Cancer Institute sponsored study of classifications of non-Hodgkin's lymphomas: Summary and description of a working formulation for clinical usage. The Non-Hodgkin's Lymphoma Pathologic Classification Project. *Cancer* **1982**, *49*, 2112–2135. [CrossRef]
11. Harris, N.L.; Jaffe, E.S.; Stein, H.; Banks, P.M.; Chan, J.K.; Cleary, M.L.; Delsol, G.; De Wolf-Peeters, C.; Falini, B.; Gatter, K.C.; et al. A revised European-American classification of lymphoid neoplasms: A proposal from the International Lymphoma Study Group. *Blood* **1994**, *84*, 1361–1392. [CrossRef]
12. A clinical evaluation of the International Lymphoma Study Group classification of non-Hodgkin's lymphoma. The Non-Hodgkin's Lymphoma Classification Project. *Blood* **1997**, *89*, 3909–3918. [CrossRef]
13. Armitage, J.O.; Weisenburger, D.D. New approach to classifying non-Hodgkin's lymphomas: Clinical features of the major histologic subtypes. Non-Hodgkin's Lymphoma Classification Project. *J. Clin. Oncol.* **1998**, *16*, 2780–2795. [CrossRef] [PubMed]
14. Harris, N.L.; Jaffe, E.S.; Diebold, J.; Flandrin, G.; Muller-Hermelink, H.K.; Vardiman, J. Lymphoma classification—From controversy to consensus: The R.E.A.L. and WHO Classification of lymphoid neoplasms. *Ann. Oncol.* **2000**, *11*, S3–S10. [CrossRef]
15. Jaffe, E.S.; Harris, N.L.; Stein, H.; Vardiman, J. *Pathology and Genetics of Tumours of Haematopoietic and Lymphoid Tissues*; IARC Press: Lyon, France, 2001; Volume 3.
16. Campo, E.; Swerdlow, S.H.; Harris, N.L.; Pileri, S.; Stein, H.; Jaffe, E.S. The 2008 WHO classification of lymphoid neoplasms and beyond: Evolving concepts and practical applications. *Blood* **2011**, *117*, 5019–5032. [CrossRef] [PubMed]
17. Swerdlow, S.H.; Campo, E.; Pileri, S.A.; Harris, N.L.; Stein, H.; Advani, R.; Ghielmini, M.; Salles, G.A.; Zelenetz, A.D.; Jaffe, E.S. The 2016 revision of the World Health Organization classification of lymphoid neoplasms. *Blood* **2016**, *127*, 2375–2390. [CrossRef]
18. Klapper, W.; Koch, K.; Mechler, U.; Borck, C.; Fuhry, E.; Siebert, R. Lymphoma 'type K.'-in memory of Karl Lennert (1921–2012). *Leukemia* **2013**, *27*, 519–521. [CrossRef] [PubMed]
19. Tolksdorf, G.; Stein, H.; Lennert, K. Morphological and immunological definition of a malignant lymphoma derived from germinal-centre cells with cleaved nuclei (centrocytes). *Br. J. Cancer* **1980**, *41*, 168–182. [CrossRef]
20. Berard, C.W.; Dorfman, R.F. Histopathology of malignant lymphomas. *Clin. Haematol.* **1974**, *3*, 39–76. [CrossRef]
21. Weisenburger, D.D.; Kim, H.; Rappaport, H. Mantle-zone lymphoma: A follicular variant of intermediate lymphocytic lymphoma. *Cancer* **1982**, *49*, 1429–1438. [CrossRef]
22. Weisenburger, D.D.; Nathwani, B.N.; Diamond, L.W.; Winberg, C.D.; Rappaport, H. Malignant lymphoma, intermediate lymphocytic type: A clinicopathologic study of 42 cases. *Cancer* **1981**, *48*, 1415–1425. [CrossRef]
23. Jaffe, E.S.; Bookman, M.A.; Longo, D.L. Lymphocytic lymphoma of intermediate differentiation–mantle zone lymphoma: A distinct subtype of B-cell lymphoma. *Hum. Pathol.* **1987**, *18*, 877–880. [CrossRef]
24. Nanba, K.; Jaffe, E.S.; Braylan, R.C.; Soban, E.J.; Berard, C.W. Alkaline phosphatase-positive malignant lymphoma. A subtype of B-cell lymphomas. *Am. J. Clin. Pathol.* **1977**, *68*, 535–542. [CrossRef] [PubMed]
25. Van Den Berghe, H.; Parloir, C.; David, G.; Michaux, J.L.; Sokal, G. A new characteristic karyotypic anomaly in lymphoproliferative disorders. *Cancer* **1979**, *44*, 188–195. [CrossRef]
26. Yunis, J.J.; Oken, M.M.; Kaplan, M.E.; Ensrud, K.M.; Howe, R.R.; Theologides, A. Distinctive chromosomal abnormalities in histologic subtypes of non-Hodgkin's lymphoma. *N. Engl. J. Med.* **1982**, *307*, 1231–1236. [CrossRef] [PubMed]
27. Tsujimoto, Y.; Yunis, J.; Onorato-Showe, L.; Erikson, J.; Nowell, P.C.; Croce, C.M. Molecular cloning of the chromosomal breakpoint of B-cell lymphomas and leukemias with the t(11;14) chromosome translocation. *Science* **1984**, *224*, 1403–1406. [CrossRef]
28. Weisenburger, D.D.; Sanger, W.G.; Armitage, J.O.; Purtilo, D.T. Intermediate lymphocytic lymphoma: Immunophenotypic and cytogenetic findings. *Blood* **1987**, *69*, 1617–1621. [CrossRef]
29. Rimokh, R.; Berger, F.; Cornillet, P.; Wahbi, K.; Rouault, J.P.; Ffrench, M.; Bryon, P.A.; Gadoux, M.; Gentilhomme, O.; Germain, D.; et al. Break in the BCL1 locus is closely associated with intermediate lymphocytic lymphoma subtype. *Genes Chromosomes Cancer* **1990**, *2*, 223–226. [CrossRef]
30. Williams, M.E.; Westermann, C.D.; Swerdlow, S.H. Genotypic characterization of centrocytic lymphoma: Frequent rearrangement of the chromosome 11 bcl-1 locus. *Blood* **1990**, *76*, 1387–1391. [CrossRef]
31. Medeiros, L.J.; Van Krieken, J.H.; Jaffe, E.S.; Raffeld, M. Association of bcl-1 rearrangements with lymphocytic lymphoma of intermediate differentiation. *Blood* **1990**, *76*, 2086–2090. [CrossRef]
32. Williams, M.E.; Meeker, T.C.; Swerdlow, S.H. Rearrangement of the chromosome 11 bcl-1 locus in centrocytic lymphoma: Analysis with multiple breakpoint probes. *Blood* **1991**, *78*, 493–498. [CrossRef]
33. Motokura, T.; Bloom, T.; Kim, H.G.; Juppner, H.; Ruderman, J.V.; Kronenberg, H.M.; Arnold, A. A novel cyclin encoded by a bcl1-linked candidate oncogene. *Nature* **1991**, *350*, 512–515. [CrossRef]

34. Bosch, F.; Jares, P.; Campo, E.; Lopez-Guillermo, A.; Piris, M.A.; Villamor, N.; Tassies, D.; Jaffe, E.S.; Monteserrat, E.; Rozman, C.; et al. PRAD-1/cyclin D1 gene overexpression in chronic lymphoproliferative disorders: A highly specific marker of mantle cell lymphoma. *Blood* **1994**, *84*, 2726–2732. [CrossRef] [PubMed]
35. Rosenberg, C.L.; Wong, E.; Petty, E.M.; Bale, A.; Tsujimoto, Y.; Harris, N.L.; Arnold, A. PRAD1, a candidate BCL1 oncogene: Mapping and expression in centrocytic lymphoma. *Proc. Natl. Acad. Sci. USA* **1991**, *88*, 9638–9642. [CrossRef] [PubMed]
36. Rimokh, R.; Berger, F.; Delsol, G.; Charrin, C.; Bertheas, M.F.; Ffrench, M.; Garoscio, M.; Felman, P.; Coiffier, B.; Bryon, P.A.; et al. Rearrangement and overexpression of the BCL-1/PRAD-1 gene in intermediate lymphocytic lymphomas and in t(11q13)-bearing leukemias. *Blood* **1993**, *81*, 3063–3067. [CrossRef] [PubMed]
37. Banks, P.M.; Chan, J.; Cleary, M.L.; Delsol, G.; De Wolf-Peeters, C.; Gatter, K.; Grogan, T.M.; Harris, N.L.; Isaacson, P.G.; Jaffe, E.S.; et al. Mantle cell lymphoma. A proposal for unification of morphologic, immunologic, and molecular data. *Am. J. Surg. Pathol.* **1992**, *16*, 637–640. [CrossRef]
38. Rosenwald, A.; Wright, G.; Wiestner, A.; Chan, W.C.; Connors, J.M.; Campo, E.; Gascoyne, R.D.; Grogan, T.M.; Muller-Hermelink, H.K.; Smeland, E.B.; et al. The proliferation gene expression signature is a quantitative integrator of oncogenic events that predicts survival in mantle cell lymphoma. *Cancer Cell.* **2003**, *3*, 185–197. [CrossRef]
39. Fu, K.; Weisenburger, D.D.; Greiner, T.C.; Dave, S.; Wright, G.; Rosenwald, A.; Chiorazzi, M.; Iqbal, J.; Gesk, S.; Siebert, R.; et al. Cyclin D1-negative mantle cell lymphoma: A clinicopathologic study based on gene expression profiling. *Blood* **2005**, *106*, 4315–4321. [CrossRef]
40. Carvajal-Cuenca, A.; Sua, L.F.; Silva, N.M.; Pittaluga, S.; Royo, C.; Song, J.Y.; Sargent, R.L.; Espinet, B.; Climent, F.; Jacobs, S.A.; et al. In situ mantle cell lymphoma: Clinical implications of an incidental finding with indolent clinical behavior. *Haematologica* **2012**, *97*, 270–278. [CrossRef]
41. Navarro, A.; Clot, G.; Royo, C.; Jares, P.; Hadzidimitriou, A.; Agathangelidis, A.; Bikos, V.; Darzentas, N.; Papadaki, T.; Salaverria, I.; et al. Molecular subsets of mantle cell lymphoma defined by the IGHV mutational status and SOX11 expression have distinct biologic and clinical features. *Cancer Res.* **2012**, *72*, 5307–5316. [CrossRef]
42. Fernandez, V.; Salamero, O.; Espinet, B.; Sole, F.; Royo, C.; Navarro, A.; Carnacho, F.; Bea, S.; Hartmann, E.; Amador, V.; et al. Genomic and gene expression profiling defines indolent forms of mantle cell lymphoma. *Cancer Res.* **2010**, *70*, 1408–1418. [CrossRef]
43. Bosch, F.; Lopez-Guillermo, A.; Campo, E.; Ribera, J.M.; Conde, E.; Piris, M.A.; Vallespi, T.; Woessner, S.; Montserrat, E. Mantle cell lymphoma: Presenting features, response to therapy, and prognostic factors. *Cancer* **1998**, *82*, 567–575. [CrossRef]
44. Vose, J.M.; Bierman, P.J.; Weisenburger, D.D.; Lynch, J.C.; Bociek, Y.; Chan, W.C.; Greiner, T.C.; Armitage, J.O. Autologous hematopoietic stem cell transplantation for mantle cell lymphoma. *Biol. Blood Marrow Transpl.* **2000**, *6*, 640–645. [CrossRef]
45. Vandenberghe, E.; Ruiz de Elvira, C.; Loberiza, F.R.; Conde, E.; Lopez-Guillermo, A.; Gisselbrecht, C.; Guihot, F.; Vose, J.M.; van Biesen, K.; Rizzo, J.D.; et al. Outcome of autologous transplantation for mantle cell lymphoma: A study by the European Blood and Bone Marrow Transplant and Autologous Blood and Marrow Transplant Registries. *Br. J. Haematol.* **2003**, *120*, 793–800. [CrossRef] [PubMed]
46. Khouri, I.F.; Romaguera, J.; Kantarjian, H.; Palmer, J.L.; Pugh, W.C.; Korbling, M.; Hagemeister, F.; Samuels, B.; Rodrigeuz, A.; Giralt, S.; et al. Hyper-CVAD and high-dose methotrexate/cytarabine followed by stem-cell transplantation: An active regimen for aggressive mantle-cell lymphoma. *J. Clin. Oncol.* **1998**, *16*, 3803–3809. [CrossRef] [PubMed]
47. Howard, O.M.; Gribben, J.G.; Neuberg, D.S.; Grossbard, M.; Poor, C.; Janicek, M.J.; Shipp, M.A. Rituximab and CHOP induction therapy for newly diagnosed mantle-cell lymphoma: Molecular complete responses are not predictive of progression-free survival. *J. Clin. Oncol.* **2002**, *20*, 1288–1294. [CrossRef] [PubMed]
48. LaCasce, A.S.; Vandergrift, J.L.; Rodriguez, M.A.; Abel, G.A.; Crosby, A.L.; Czuczman, M.S.; Nademanee, A.P.; Blayney, D.W.; Gordon, L.I.; Millenson, M.; et al. Comparative outcome of initial therapy for younger patients with mantle cell lymphoma: An analysis from the NCCN NHL Database. *Blood* **2012**, *119*, 2093–2099. [CrossRef] [PubMed]
49. Geisler, C.H.; Kolstad, A.; Laurell, A.; Anderson, N.S.; Pederson, L.B.; Jerkeman, M.; Eriksson, M.; Nordstrom, M.; Kimby, E.; Boesen, A.M.; et al. Long-term progression-free survival of mantle cell lymphoma after intensive front-line immunochemotherapy with in vivo-purged stem cell rescue: A nonrandomized phase 2 multicenter study by the Nordic Lymphoma Group. *Blood* **2008**, *112*, 2687–2693. [CrossRef]
50. Romaguera, J.E.; Fayad, L.; Rodriguez, M.A.; Broglio, K.R.; Hagermeister, F.B.; Pro, B.; McLaughlin, P.; Younes, A.; Samaniego, F.; Goy, A.; et al. High rate of durable remissions after treatment of newly diagnosed aggressive mantle-cell lymphoma with rituximab plus hyper-CVAD alternating with rituximab plus high-dose methotrexate and cytarabine. *J. Clin. Oncol.* **2005**, *23*, 7013–7023. [CrossRef]
51. Hermine, O.; Hoster, E.; Walewski, J.; Bosly, A.; Stilgenbauer, S.; Thieblemont, C.; Szymczyk, M.; Bouabdallah, R.; Kneba, M.; Hallek, M.; et al. Addition of high-dose cytarabine to immunochemotherapy before autologous stem-cell transplantation in patients aged 65 years or younger with mantle cell lymphoma (MCL Younger): A randomised, open-label, phase 3 trial of the European Mantle Cell Lymphoma Network. *Lancet* **2016**, *388*, 565–575.
52. Le Gouill, S.; Thieblemont, C.; Oberic, L.; Moreau, A.; Bouabdallah, K.; Dartigeas, C.; Damaj, G.; Gastinne, T.; Ribrag, V.; Feugier, P.; et al. Rituximab after Autologous Stem-Cell Transplantation in Mantle-Cell Lymphoma. *N. Engl. J. Med.* **2017**, *377*, 1250–1260. [CrossRef]

53. Kluin-Nelemans, H.C.; Hoster, E.; Hermine, O.; Walewski, J.; Trney, M.; Geisler, C.H.; Stilgenbauer, S.; Thieblemont, C.; Vehling-Kaiser, U.; Doorduijn, J.K.; et al. Treatment of older patients with mantle-cell lymphoma. *N. Engl. J. Med.* **2012**, *367*, 520–531. [CrossRef]
54. Romaguera, J.E.; Fayad, L.E.; Feng, L.; Hartig, K.; Weaver, P.; Rodriguez, M.A.; Hagemeister, F.B.; Pro, B.; McLaughlin, P.; Younes, A.; et al. Ten-year follow-up after intense chemoimmunotherapy with Rituximab-HyperCVAD alternating with Rituximab-high dose methotrexate/cytarabine (R-MA) and without stem cell transplantation in patients with untreated aggressive mantle cell lymphoma. *Br. J. Haematol.* **2010**, *150*, 200–208. [CrossRef]
55. Griffiths, R.; Mikhael, J.; Gleeson, M.; Danese, M.; Dreyling, M. Addition of rituximab to chemotherapy alone as first-line therapy improves overall survival in elderly patients with mantle cell lymphoma. *Blood* **2011**, *118*, 4808–4816. [CrossRef]
56. Eskelund, C.W.; Kolstad, A.; Jerkeman, M.; Raty, R.; Laurell, A.; Eloranta, S.; Smedby, K.E.; Husby, S.; Pedersen, L.B.; Andersen, N.S.; et al. 15-year follow-up of the Second Nordic Mantle Cell Lymphoma trial (MCL2): Prolonged remissions without survival plateau. *Br. J. Haematol.* **2016**, *175*, 410–418. [CrossRef] [PubMed]
57. Martin, P.; Cohen, J.B.; Wang, M.; Kumar, A.; Hill, B.; Villa, D.; Switchenko, J.M.; Kahl, B.; Maddocks, K.; Grover, N.S.; et al. Treatment Outcomes and Roles of Transplantation and Maintenance Rituximab in Patients With Previously Untreated Mantle Cell Lymphoma: Results From Large Real-World Cohorts. *J. Clin. Oncol.* **2022**, JCO2102698. [CrossRef] [PubMed]
58. Goy, A.; Younes, A.; McLaughlin, P.; Pro, B.; Romaguera, J.E.; Hagermeister, F.; Fayad, L.; Dang, N.H.; Samaniego, F.; Wang, M.; et al. Phase II study of proteasome inhibitor bortezomib in relapsed or refractory B-cell non-Hodgkin's lymphoma. *J. Clin. Oncol.* **2005**, *23*, 667–675. [CrossRef] [PubMed]
59. Robak, T.; Huang, H.; Jin, J.; Zhu, J.; Liu, T.; Samoilova, O.; Pylypenko, H.; Verhoef, G.; Siritanaratkul, N.; Osmanov, E.; et al. Bortezomib-based therapy for newly diagnosed mantle-cell lymphoma. *N. Engl. J. Med.* **2015**, *372*, 944–953. [CrossRef]
60. Ruan, J.; Martin, P.; Shah, B.; Schuster, S.J.; Smith, S.M.; Furman, R.R.; Christos, P.; Rodriguez, A.; Svoboda, J.; Lewis, J.; et al. Lenalidomide plus Rituximab as Initial Treatment for Mantle-Cell Lymphoma. *N. Engl. J. Med.* **2015**, *373*, 1835–1844. [CrossRef]
61. Ladetto, M.; Cortelazzo, S.; Ferrero, S.; Evangelista, A.; Mian, M.; Tavarozzi, R.; Zanni, M.; Cavallo, F.; Di Rocco, A.; Stefoni, V.; et al. Lenalidomide maintenance after autologous haematopoietic stem-cell transplantation in mantle cell lymphoma: Results of a Fondazione Italiana Linfomi (FIL) multicentre, randomised, phase 3 trial. *Lancet Haematol.* **2021**, *8*, e34–e44. [CrossRef]
62. Rummel, M.J.; Niederle, N.; Maschmeyer, G.; Banat, G.A.; von Grunhagen, U.; Losem, C.; Kofahl-Krause, D.; Heil, G.; Welslau, M.; Balser, C.; et al. Bendamustine plus rituximab versus CHOP plus rituximab as first-line treatment for patients with indolent and mantle-cell lymphomas: An open-label, multicentre, randomised, phase 3 non-inferiority trial. *Lancet* **2013**, *381*, 1203–1210. [CrossRef]
63. Chen, R.W.; Li, H.; Bernstein, S.H.; Kahwash, S.; Rimsza, L.M.; Forman, S.J.; Constine, L.; Shea, T.C.; Cashen, A.F.; Blum, K.A.; et al. RB but not R-HCVAD is a feasible induction regimen prior to auto-HCT in frontline MCL: Results of SWOG Study S1106. *Br. J. Haematol.* **2017**, *176*, 759–769. [CrossRef]
64. Ruan, J.; Martin, P.; Christos, P.; Cerchietti, L.; Tam, W.; Shah, B.; Schuster, S.J.; Rodriguez, A.; Hyman, D.; Calvo-Vidal, M.N.; et al. Five-year follow-up of lenalidomide plus rituximab as initial treatment for mantle cell lymphoma. *Blood* **2018**, *132*, 2016–2025. [CrossRef] [PubMed]
65. Gine, E.; de la Cruz, F.; Jimenez Ubieto, A.; Lopez Jimenez, J.; Martin Garcia-Sancho, A.; Terol, M.J.; Gonzalez Barca, E.; Casanova, M.; de la Fuente, A.; Marin-Niebla, A.; et al. Ibrutinib in Combination With Rituximab for Indolent Clinical Forms of Mantle Cell Lymphoma (IMCL-2015): A Multicenter, Open-Label, Single-Arm, Phase II Trial. *J. Clin. Oncol.* **2022**, *40*, 1196–1205. [CrossRef] [PubMed]
66. Wang, M.L.; Jurczak, W.; Jerkeman, M.; Trotman, J.; Zinzani, P.; Belada, D.; Boccomini, C.; Flinn, I.W.; Giri, P.; Goy, A.; et al. Ibrutinib plus Bendamustine and Rituximab in Untreated Mantle-Cell Lymphoma. *N. Engl. J. Med.* **2022**, *386*, 2482–2494. [CrossRef]
67. Wang, M.; Munoz, J.; Goy, A.; Locke, F.L.; Jacobson, C.A.; Hill, B.T.; Timmerman, J.M.; Holmes, H.; Jaglowski, S.; Flinn, I.W.; et al. KTE-X19 CAR T-Cell Therapy in Relapsed or Refractory Mantle-Cell Lymphoma. *N. Engl. J. Med.* **2020**, *382*, 1331–1342. [CrossRef] [PubMed]
68. Wang, M.; Munoz, J.; Goy, A.; Locke, F.L.; Jacobson, C.A.; Hill, B.T.; Timmerman, J.M.; Holmes, H.; Jaglowski, S.; Flinn, I.W.; et al. Three-Year Follow-Up of KTE-X19 in Patients With Relapsed/Refractory Mantle Cell Lymphoma, Including High-Risk Subgroups, in the ZUMA-2 Study. *J. Clin. Oncol.* **2022**, JCO2102370. [CrossRef]
69. Castellino, A.; Wang, Y.; Larson, M.C.; Maurer, M.J.; Link, B.K.; Farooq, U.; Feldman, A.L.; Syrbu, S.I.; Habermann, T.M.; Paludo, J.; et al. Evolving frontline immunochemotherapy for mantle cell lymphoma and the impact on survival outcomes. *Blood Adv.* **2022**, *6*, 1350–1360. [CrossRef]

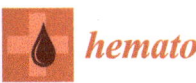

Review

Molecular Pathogenesis of Follicular Lymphoma: From Genetics to Clinical Practice

Cristina López [1,2,3,*,†], Pablo Mozas [1,4,†], Armando López-Guillermo [1,2,3,4] and Sílvia Beà [1,2,3,5]

1. Institut d'Investigacions Biomèdiques August Pi i Sunyer (IDIBAPS), 08036 Barcelona, Spain
2. Centro de Investigación Biomédica en Red de Cáncer (CIBERONC), 28040 Madrid, Spain
3. Universitat de Barcelona, 08036 Barcelona, Spain
4. Department of Hematology, Hospital Clínic, 08036 Barcelona, Spain
5. Hematopathology Section, Department of Pathology, Hospital Clínic, 08036 Barcelona, Spain
* Correspondence: clopez2@recerca.clinic.cat
† These authors contributed equally to this work.

Abstract: Follicular lymphoma (FL), a generally indolent disease that derives from germinal center (GC) B cells, represents around 20–25% of all new lymphomas diagnosed in Western countries. The characteristic t(14;18)(q32;q21) translocation that places the *BCL2* oncogene under control of the immunoglobulin heavy-chain enhancer occurs in pro- or pre-B cells. However, additional secondary alterations are required for the development of overt FL, which mainly affects genes involved in epigenetic and transcriptional regulation, signaling and B cell differentiation, the BCR/NF-κB pathway, and proliferation/apoptosis. On the other hand, new insights into the FL pathogenesis suggest that FL lacking the *BCL2* translocation might be a distinct biological entity with genomic features different from the classical FL. Although FL is considered an indolent disease, around 10–20% of cases eventually transform to an aggressive lymphoma, usually a diffuse large B cell lymphoma, generally by a divergent evolution process from a common altered precursor cell acquiring genomic alterations involved in the cell cycle and DNA damage responses. Importantly, FL tumor cells require interaction with the microenvironment, which sustains cell survival and proliferation. Although the use of rituximab has improved the outlook of most FL patients, further genomic studies are needed to identify those of high risk who can benefit from innovative therapies. This review provides an updated synopsis of FL, including the molecular and cellular pathogenesis, key events of transformation, and targeted treatments.

Keywords: follicular lymphoma; *BCL2* rearrangement; genetic alterations; histological transformation; tumor microenvironment; targeted therapies

1. Introduction

Follicular lymphoma (FL), the most common indolent B cell lymphoma, is histologically characterized by a follicular or nodular pattern of tumor cell growth [1,2]. Its molecular and cellular features make FL the paradigm of a germinal center (GC)-derived neoplasm, with expression of BCL6, CD10, and activation-induced cytidine deaminase (AID), which is critical for immunoglobulin somatic hypermutation. More than 85% of FL cases harbor the characteristic t(14;18)(q32;q21), which occurs in pro- or pre-B cells of the bone marrow [3,4].

The disease generally presents with lymphadenopathy, with eventual dissemination to the bone marrow or other organs [5]. For diagnosis, a tissue biopsy showing the typical histological and immunohistochemical pattern is required, which will also allow histological grading (proportion of centrocytes and centroblasts). FL is characterized by a pattern of continuous relapses, with a progressively shorter duration of response [6]. For this reason, most patients with low tumor burden, non-localized disease are amenable to a watchful waiting strategy without active therapy [5]. In turn, high tumor burden patients require treatment, in the form of immunochemotherapy (ICT) or immunotherapy alone (rituximab). In the event of a relapse, although no standard exists, high-dose therapy and autologous stem cell transplantation (ASCT) are still considered appropriate for a subset of patients, while newer drugs such as bispecific T cell engagers and CAR-T cells will soon be the cornerstone of management for non-transplant-eligible patients and in the event of subsequent relapses.

Although the median overall survival (OS) for FL patients now approaches 20 years [7], specific subsets of patients exhibit a markedly worse prognosis, namely those experiencing an early relapse (progression of disease within 24 months of frontline ICT, POD24) [8] or developing histological transformation (HT) to an aggressive lymphoma [9]. A myriad of prognostic scores have been developed with the aim of identifying individuals with poor outcomes, and eventually tailoring therapy accordingly [10]. However, their success has been limited and most patients receive similar regimens irrespective of prognostic scores, with the exception of obinutuzumab instead of rituximab as part of ICT for high-risk patients in some countries [11].

In the past years, molecular analyses have expanded our knowledge on the mutational landscape of FL, highlighting the importance of epigenetic modifiers, survival pathways, and the tumor microenvironment. However, elucidating the biological mechanisms that underlie the clinical heterogeneity remains a research priority. This review describes the current knowledge regarding the role of the BCL2 rearrangement in FL, the genomic landscape of these tumors, clonal dynamics of transformation, as well as the contribution of the microenvironment. Finally, available and upcoming targeted therapies are summarized.

2. BCL2 Rearrangement in FL

The genetic hallmark of FL is the t(14;18)(q32;q21) translocation, present in 80–85% of patients, which occurs in pro- or pre-B cells in the bone marrow as an error of V(D)J recombination mediated by RAG1 and 2 enzymes [3,4,12]. As a consequence, the BCL2 oncogene is placed under control of the immunoglobulin heavy-chain enhancer, leading to the overexpression of the BCL2 protein, which confers a survival advantage to B cells. The 18q21 breakpoints are mainly clustered within a 2.8 kb major breakpoint region (MBR) located in the 3'UTR of the BCL2 gene [3,12–14] (Figure 1). Breakpoints located within the intermediate cluster region (ICR) and the minor cluster region (MCR), just downstream and far downstream of BCL2, respectively, are less common. The breakpoint in the IGH locus (14q32) occurs in the J and D segments, close to the recombination sequence signal (RSS) site of a J_H gene segment or the 5'RSS of a $D_H J_H$ joint, suggesting that the translocation took place as the cell attempted a D_H to J_H or V_H to $D_H J_H$ rearrangement [4,13–15] (Figure 1). Variant translocations t(2;18)(p12;q21) and t(18;22)(q21;q11) are less frequent and juxtapose the BCL2 gene to the IGK and IGL loci, respectively. In these variants, the breakpoints are located in the 5' end of BCL2 locus [14]. Remarkably, breakpoints in the 5' end of the BCL2 gene have also been described in t(14;18), leading to a higher BCL2 expression compared to that of t(14;18)-positive cells affecting the 3'UTR region of BCL2 [16].

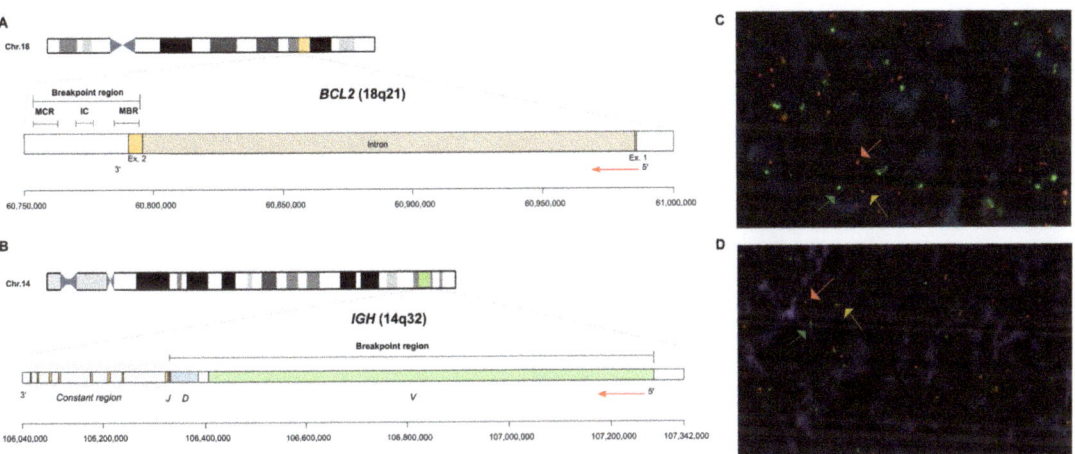

Figure 1. Schematic representation of the *IGH*::*BCL2* translocation breakpoints in follicular lymphoma. (**A**) The figure shows the *BCL2* locus, containing two exons and one intron located in 18q21 and annotated based on ENST00000398117.1 (hg19). The arrow indicates the direction of BCL2 transcription. The breakpoints cluster in three main regions located at 3′ of *BCL2*, namely major breakpoint region (MBR), intermediate cluster region (ICR), and minor cluster region (MCR). Breakpoints located at 5′ of *BCL2* locus have also been described, mainly when BCL2 is rearranged with the light chain loci on 2p12 and 22q11. (**B**) The panel illustrates the IGH locus, representing the constant region (yellow color and highlighted in light gray), the V (green), D (blue), and J (red) regions. The arrow shows the direction of IGH transcription. The distribution of the various breakpoints regions is displayed in the upper part, involving V(D)J region. (**C,D**) Fluorescence in situ hybridization of paraffin-embedded tumor sections using the dual color, dual fusion *IGH*::*BCL2* (**C**) and dual color, break-apart *BCL2* (**D**) probes. (**C**) FISH analysis shows two yellow signals (yellow arrow), indicating an *IGH*::*BCL2* fusion and one green (green arrow) and one red signal (red arrow) corresponding to unrearranged *IGH* and *BCL2*, respectively. Normal cells display two green signals and two red signals. (**D**) Signal constellation shows a break in the *BCL2* locus indicated by a split of the yellow signal into one green and one red and unrearranged *BCL2* labeled with a yellow signal. Normal cells have two yellow signals.

Using sensitive techniques, the t(14;18) may be detected in B cells from peripheral blood and/or lymphoid tissues of a large proportion (up to 70%) of healthy individuals [17–19], although the vast majority of them will never develop FL, indicating that *BCL2* deregulation alone is insufficient for tumorigenesis. Follow-up studies of epidemiological cohorts of healthy individuals have identified t(14;18)+ B cells in the blood for many years [20], with a frequency that increases with age [18,19], and change in the body's immune system due to certain infectious conditions (such as hepatitis C virus) [21]. t(14;18)+ cells, defined as "FL-like cells" (FLLCs), are a clonal population of atypical memory B cells displaying a GC-experienced phenotype that is characteristic of FL [22] and usually display more than one *IGH*::*BCL2* breakpoint, with a similar molecular structure to that seen in follicular lymphoma [23].

3. Genetic and Epigenetic Landscape of FL

In addition to t(14;18), FL has a characteristic genomic profile, with frequent losses of 1p (15–20%), 6q (20–30%), 10q (20%), and 13q (15%), and gains of 1q (25%), 2p (25%), 8q (10%), 12q (20%), and 18q (30%), and trisomies 7 (20%), 18 (20–30%), and chromosome X (20%) [24–26]. Furthermore, recurrent copy-neutral losses of heterozygosity (CN-LOH) involving 1p (30%), 6p (20%), and 16p (20–25%) have been identified [24–26].

Next generation sequencing (NGS) studies have unraveled secondary genomic alterations in FL mainly affecting genes involved in epigenetic and transcriptional regulation, signaling and B cell differentiation, the BCR/NF-κB pathway, and proliferation/apoptosis (Figure 2).

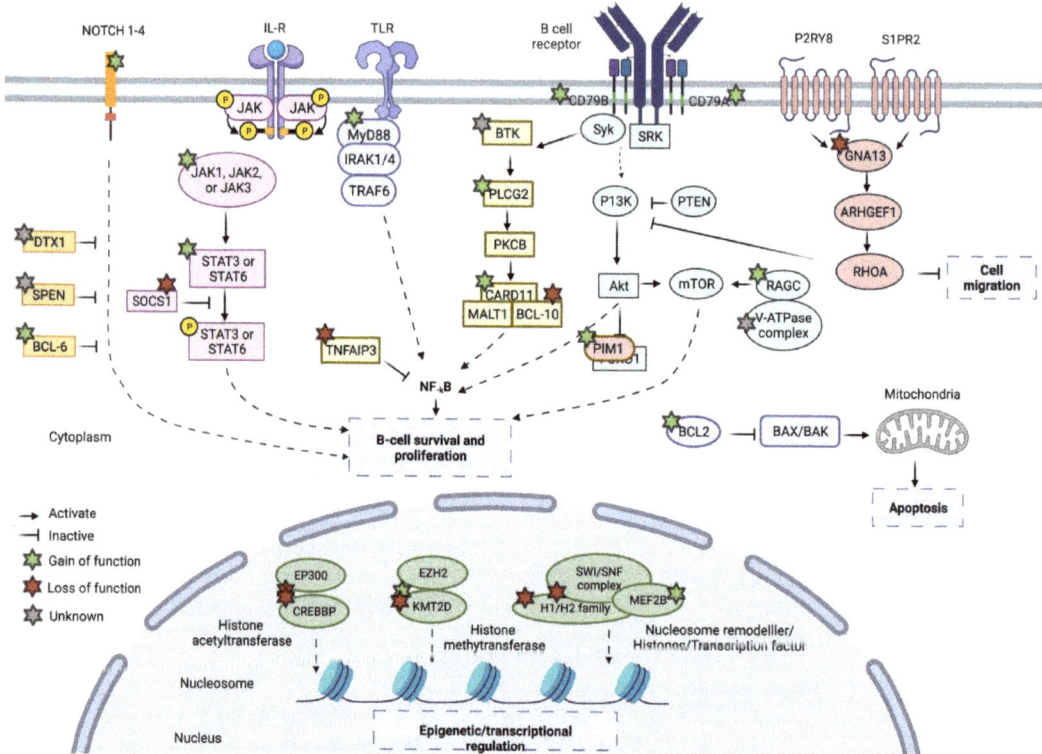

Figure 2. Molecular pathways involved in follicular lymphoma. The figure shows the several pathways dysregulated in follicular lymphoma. Gain-of-function alterations are labeled with a green star, loss-of-function with a red star, and unknown functions with a grey star. BCL2 overexpression leads to apoptosis inhibition. Genomic alterations affecting Janus Kinase (JAK) signal, B cell receptor (BCR) pathways, MYD88, and NOTCH pathway directly stimulate B cell survival and proliferation. Alterations in sphingosine 1-phosphatase receptor 2 (S1PR2) and guanine nucleotide binding protein subunit (GNA13) enhance dissemination outside the germinal centers. Figure created with BioRender.com (accessed on 13 July 2022).

3.1. Epigenetic and Transcriptional Regulation

Genomic alterations in histone-modifying enzymes, including *KMT2D*, *CREBBP*, *EP300*, and *EZH2*, are detected in virtually all FL patients [27–31]. The *KMT2D* gene encodes a H3K4 methyltransferase and is the most frequently altered gene in FL (70–80% of cases) [32–34]. The majority of these alterations are nonsense or frameshift somatic mutations leading to a loss of function and, consequently, a loss of active transcription marks (H3 lysine 4 methylation, H3K4me) [35]. Studies using mouse models have shown that the ablation of Kmt2d in B cells leads to GC expansion and impaired terminal differentiation promoting lymphomagenesis [35,36]. The *CREBBP* gene encodes a lysine acetyltransferase that acetylates histone 3 at lysines 18 (H3K18Ac) and 27 (H3K27Ac) [37] and is altered in 70% of FL cases [29,31,33,35,38]. Around 80% of somatic mutations cluster within the KAT domain, reducing its acetyltransferase activity [29,30,38,39]. Murine studies reported that loss of Crebbp promotes B cell lymphoma, especially in cooperation with BCL2 overexpression [38], and that the regions of decreased histone acetylation were primarily located at distal enhancer elements, including MHC class II genes [38,40–42]. Moreover, *CREBBP* mutations have been previously associated with a reduction of acetylation of nonhistone proteins such as TP53 and BCL6, highlighting the crucial role of alterations in this gene in lymphomagenesis [30]. In addition, the alteration of *EP300*, also encoding for a histone acetyltransferase, occurs in 15% of FL cases [29,31,33]. EP300 regulates different GC transcriptional programs and cooperates with CREBBP in the GC reaction [43]. The *EZH2* gene encodes a lysine methyltransferase that catalyzes the trimethylation of H3K27 (H3K27me3) as part of the polycomb repressive complex 2 (PRC2). *EZH2* mutations, present in 25–30% of FL cases, were the first recurrent chromatin modifying gene mutations described [27,44–46]. The majority of the mutations are located in the catalytic SET domain, mostly involving tyrosine 646 (Y646). These mutations result in a gain of function, increasing the transcriptional repressive H3K27me3 mark [47,48]. Altered EZH2 regulates the GC phenotype by repressing specific cell cycle genes (e.g., *CDKN1A* and *CDKN1B*) and abrogates GC formation [44]. In addition, mutations in linker histones (*HIST1H1B-E*) [28,49] and core histone genes and in genes encoding members of SWI/SNF (e.g., *ARID1A, ARID1B, BCL7A*, and *SMARCA4*) are also frequently found in FL [29,31,33,35,50].

The transcriptional regulator BCL6 is altered by somatic mutations or translocation in 5–10% of FL cases [50–53]. Rearrangements involving *BCL6*, mainly t(3;14)(q27;q32), leading to the *IGH::BCL6* fusion, are commonly found in grade 3B cases [54]. On the other hand, mutations in the transcriptional activator *MEF2B* involved in the recruitment of demethylases and deacetylases to promoters and enhancers, are present in 12–15% of FL patients [32,55]. *MEF2B* mutations modify the ability of MEF2B to bind to DNA or to the co-repressor CABIN1, leading to increased transcriptional activity [55,56].

3.2. BCR/NF-κB Pathway

Genomic alterations in genes encoding proteins in the BCR/NF-κB signaling pathway (*CARD11, TNFAIP3, CD79A, CD79B*, and *MYD88*) are present in approximately 30% of FL patients [28,57]. *CARD11* gain of function mutations occur in 10% of the cases and affect mainly the coiled-coil domain [58]. Less prevalent are *TNFAIP3* somatic mutations, occurring in 5% of patients [29,59,60], although *TNFAIP3* deletions have a prevalence of 20% [25,26]. On the other hand, mutations in other components such as *CD79A*, *CD79B*, and *MYD88* are less frequent in FL as compared to other germinal center-derived B cell lymphomas [57]. The molecular consequence of the genomic alterations described above is the activation of the NF-κB signaling pathway via tonic BCR (e.g., CD79A and CD79B), chronic BCR (e.g., CARD11), and toll receptor and interleukin-1 receptor signaling (e.g., MYD88) [61]. *BTK* and *FOXO1* somatic mutations are found in about 5–10% of FL cases [29,33,62]. FOXO1 is a transcription factor activated downstream of BCR and the molecular consequence of the mutations described in FL is a gain of function [50]. Nonetheless, the functional consequences of *BTK* mutations warrant further investigations. Somatic mutations in the variable regions of the immunoglobulin heavy and light chain loci, which promote N-glycosylation, occur in up to 80% of FL cases [59,63,64].

3.3. Signaling Pathways

Genes involved in JAK-STAT (*SOCS1, STAT6, STAT3*) and NOTCH signaling (*NOTCH1, NOTCH2, NOTCH3, NOTCH4, DTX1*, and *SPEN*) are frequently altered in FL, promoting proliferation and survival of tumor cells [26,29,63,65,66]. *SOCS1* or *STAT6* mutations are found in around 10% of FL cases [60,67]. Somatic mutations involving the C-terminal PEST domain of the NOTCH1 and NOTCH2 proteins are similar to those observed in other B cell lymphomas [57,62], as well as alterations in the *NOTCH3* and *NOTCH4* loci and signaling regulators such as *DTX1* and *SPEN* [57,62]. Overall, the NOTCH pathway is altered in 18% of FL patients.

Recurrent mutations in genes encoding components of the mTOR complex 1 (mTORC1) pathway have been identified in FL. mTORC1 promotes protein synthesis in response to growth factors and nutrient signals. Intracellular amino acid levels are detected via a supercomplex that includes Rag GTPases, the Regulator complex, the v-ATPase complex, and SLC38A9 that cooperate to activate mTORC1 signaling in the presence of sufficient amino acids [68–70]. In the context of an acid-rich medium, active RAG GTPase heterodimers recruit mTORC1 to the lysosomal membrane [65,66,71]. Activating mutations in *RRAGC* enhance mTORC1 even after amino acid depletion and are found in 17% of FL patients. In addition, mutations in components of the V-ATPase complex have also been observed in FL [65,66]. Finally, inactivating mutations of the *S1PR2*-guanine nucleotide-binding protein subunit (Gα13) pathway, responsible for retaining B cells into the GC niche, are present in around 10% of FL patients, promoting both dissemination and survival of FL cells [35,62,72].

3.4. Immune Regulation/Evasion

The *TNFRSF14* gene encodes the herpes virus entry mediator A (HVEM) which is the most recurrently altered gene via inactivating mutations, deletions, and CN-LOH [27,29,73], besides the epigenetic family members. HVEM induces activation or inactivation of B and T cells depending on its interaction with different ligands, including B and T-lymphocyte (BTLA) and LIGHT [74,75]. In BCL2 mouse models, HVEM or BTLA knockdown promoted the development of FL [76]. Remarkably, B cells lacking HVEM produce increased tumor necrosis factor (TNF)-associated cytokines, promoting an abnormal stroma activation, which induces a supportive tumor microenvironment and recruitment of T follicular helper cells which, in turn, support the survival of tumor cells.

3.5. Apoptosis and Proliferation

BCL2 mutations have been described together with the *BCL2* rearrangement in around half of FL cases [77]. Furthermore, *PIM1* mutations have been reported in around 10% of FL patients [57]. PIM1 is a kinase which promotes NF-κB signaling [78].

3.6. DNA Damage Response

Although *TP53* mutations are identified in a low proportion of FL patients at diagnosis (6%), they are enriched in subgroups of patients with an older age, higher-risk scores, and a shorter progression-free survival [79].

4. Follicular Lymphoma Lacking BCL2 Rearrangement: A Different Entity?

FL lacking the *BCL2* translocation (*BCL2* − FL) comprises 10–15% of all FL patients [1,72]. Several studies have investigated whether this subset of patients is biologically and clinically different to classical FL with *BCL2* rearrangement (*BCL2* + FL). Katzenberger and colleagues [73] identified that *BCL2* − FL were characterized by a diffuse growth pattern, frequent inguinal presentation, and 1p36 deletions. Subsequent studies trying to define the molecular profile of *BCL2* − FL cases revealed: (i) somatic hypermutation, aberrant somatic hypermutation and expression of activation-induced cytidine deaminase at similar levels compared to the *BCL2* + FL cases [72,80]; (ii) frequent gains of 2p16 involving *REL* [72]; (iii) absence of molecular features resembling marginal zone lymphoma [72]; and (iv) enrichment in late GC B cell and NF-κB and proliferation signatures and significant downregulation of miR16 expression [72,81]. Intriguingly, the vast majority of *BCL2* − FL cases express BCL2, suggesting an alternative molecular mechanism to induce BCL2 expression in this subset of cases [51].

Similar clinical features have been identified in *BCL2* + and *BCL2* − FL [51]. However, diffuse and pediatric forms of FL, which often lack *BCL2* translocation, exhibit a better clinical prognosis compared to *BCL2* + FL cases [73,82]. On the other hand, some studies have compared the clinical features of *BCL2* − FL with and without *BCL6* rearrangements and, although most studies point towards a similar clinical presentation, some differences have been identified, e.g., advanced clinical stages, higher histological grades, and less frequent expression of the CD10 marker in *BCL2* − FL cases with *BCL6* rearrangement [54,83,84].

Katzenberger and colleagues [73] were the first authors to delineate a subgroup of FL patients with a diffuse growth pattern, characterized by CD23 expression, lack of *BCL2* rearrangement, and 1p36 deletion. Later on, Siddiqi confirmed these findings in 2016 [85], proposed the *TNFRSF14* locus as the candidate gene of 1p36 deletion, and identified recurrent mutations in the *STAT6* and *TNFRSF14* loci. In addition, current NGS studies of *BCL2* − FL cases have identified recurrent mutations in *CREBBP* [85–89], an enrichment in immune response and N-glycosylation signatures and less frequent N-glycosylation sites [88].

A recent comprehensive study conducted in the largest cohort of *BCL2* − FL cases identified that this subtype is genetically heterogeneous. Patients were more commonly women, presented in early clinical stages at diagnosis, and had a favorable clinical behavior [86]. Two molecular clusters were identified: cluster A, characterized by *TNFRSF14* alterations and frequent mutations in epigenetic regulators, with recurrent losses of 6q21-q24, resembling *BCL2* + FL cases; and cluster B, showing few genetic alterations, namely *STAT6* mutations concurrent with *CREBBP* alterations, lacking *TNFRSF14* and *EZH2* mutations [86]. Furthermore, an association between *STAT6* mutations and CD23 expression, an uncommon marker in *BCL2* + FL, was identified, especially in cases with a diffuse growth pattern. Importantly, the study concludes that *BCL2* − FL cases are mainly characterized by a follicular growth pattern and only a few cases have a diffuse component [86].

Recently, the International Consensus Classification (ICC) proposed the BCL2-R-negative (here described as *BCL2* − FL), CD23-positive follicle center lymphoma subtype as a new provisional entity [2]. Besides, pediatric-type and testicular FL are also proposed as distinct entities [2]. Pediatric-type FL is characterized by recurrent mutations in the MAPK pathway, lack of *BCL2* rearrangement, and an excellent prognosis FL [90–92], and has also been included as a new subtype in the 5th edition of the WHO Classification [83]. Furthermore, testicular FL, identified as a new FL entity in young boys, which confers good prognosis, is also characterized by the lack of *BCL2* translocations [84,93].

5. Molecular Mechanisms of Transformation

Histological transformation of FL (tFL) into an aggressive lymphoma (mainly diffuse large B cell lymphoma—DLBCL) [94–98] can occur during the course of the disease and affects approximately 10–20% of patients [9,99–101]. Several studies have been conducted to describe the genetic landscape of tFL and compare it to baseline biopsy samples. The studies of paired diagnostic and tFL cases identified that tFL arises mainly through a divergent or branching evolution from a common altered precursor cell (CPC) [29,73,102,103] (Figure 3). Remarkably, none of these studies identified a single genetic event driving transformation.

Initial studies described an increased number of copy-number alterations (CNA), including gains of oncogenes *REL/BCL11A* (2p16), *BCL6* (3q27), and *MYC* (8q24), and losses of tumor suppressor genes like *TP53* (17p13) and *CDKN2A/B* (9p21) in transformed compared to diagnostic samples [104–107]. Somatic mutations enriched at transformation involve signaling pathways (e.g., *PIM1*, *SOCS1*, *STAT6*, *MYD88*, *TNFAIP3*, and *ITPKB*), the cell cycle (e.g., *CCND3*), sphingosine-1-phosphate signaling (*GNA13*, *S1PR2*, and *P2RY8*), B cell development (*EBF1*), and immune evasion (*B2M* and *CD58*) [29,73,102]. The majority of tFL cases fall into the germinal center B (GCB) molecular subtype of DLBCL, although 20% of cases are of the activated B cell (ABC) subtype. The genomic profile differs between the GCB and ABC subtypes of tFL, indicating that the different biological backgrounds modulate the transformation process, mainly concerning the activation of the BCR and NF-κB pathways associated with the ABC subtype [25,108].

Transcriptomic analysis of tFL suggests the implication of an embryonic stem cell signature maintained by MYC activation, or the role of the NF-κB pathway in the transformation event [99,109]. On the other hand, transformation in FL is also modulated by the interaction of tumor cells with the immune system. Consequently, the composition and distribution of the immune cells infiltrating the tumor, such as CD4+ T helper cells, have been identified as a predictor of transformation [100].

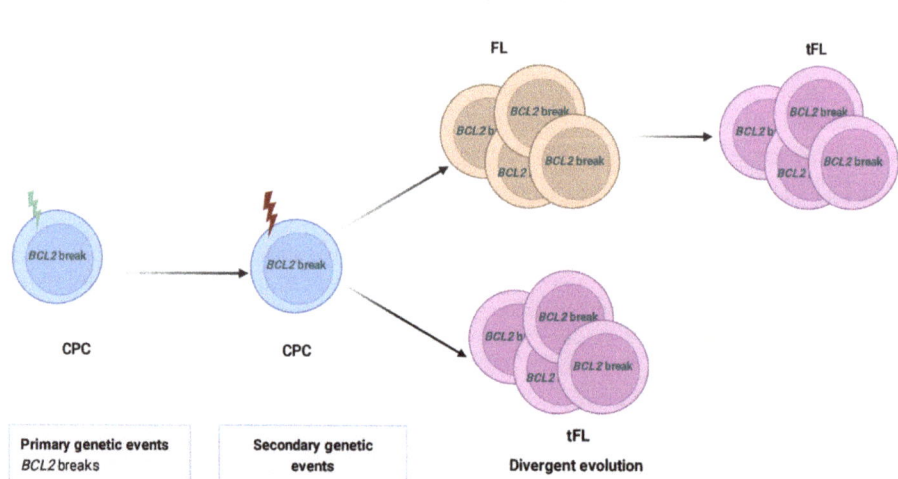

Figure 3. Clonal dynamics of transformed follicular lymphoma. Models of clonal evolution during FL transformation. FL tumors derived from a common progenitor cell (CPC), that has acquired the primary genetic events, e.g., *BCL2* rearrangements (green thunderbolt). The CPC subsequently harbors additional secondary alterations leading to the neoplasm (red thunderbolt). The transformed FL (tFL) clone might originate from the FL clone after the acquisition of additional alterations corresponding to a linear evolution, or derive from a CPC through an independent acquisition of distinct mutations suggesting a divergent evolution. Figure created with BioRender.com (accessed on 13 July 2022).

6. Role of the Tumor Microenvironment (TME)

Despite the crucial role of genomic alterations of lymphoma cells in the development, progression, and relapse of FL, their crosstalk with non-malignant tumor-infiltrating cells might be even more relevant [101,102] (Figure 4). While some other lymphomas, such as Burkitt's, are dependent on an intense proliferation of tumor cells, and others (Hodgkin's) recruit reactive cells, FL recapitulates the GC organization and uses the support of follicular dendritic cells and T follicular helper (T$_{FH}$) cells to build three-dimensional structures.

The tumor-promoting activity of the TME has been explained by the development of an ecosystem that sustains the growth and survival of lymphoma cells and by the induction of mechanisms of evasion of the host antitumor immunity. These effects are exerted by means of genetic modifications (e.g., mutations in epigenetic modifiers), a modulation of immune cell subsets (dampening of antitumor populations, stimulation of immune suppressive cells), and an induction of T cell exhaustion mechanisms. For the sake of practicality, cells of the TME can be categorized into T cells, tumor-associated macrophages (TAM), and stromal cells.

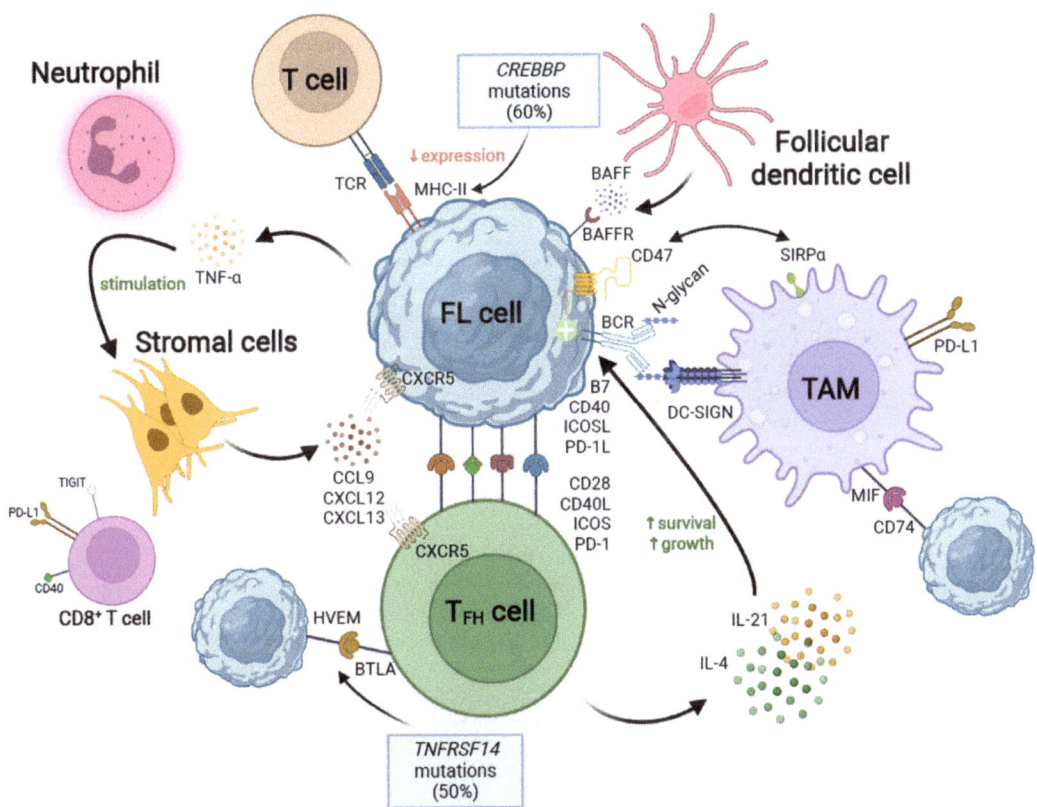

Figure 4. Schematic representation of the crosstalk between follicular lymphoma (FL) cells and the tumor microenvironment. From the upper right corner, clockwise: follicular dendritic cells secrete BAFF, which is sensed by BAFFR on FL cells. The "don't eat me" signal CD47 expressed by FL cells interacts with SIRPα in tumor-associated macrophages (TAM), which induces immune tolerance towards tumor growth. N-glycan-modified residues of the B cell receptor (BCR) are recognized by DC-SIGN on the TAM. T_{FH} cells secrete IL-4 and IL-21, which promote survival and growth of the FL cell. The immunological synapse is established, among others, between B7, CD40, ICOS, and PD-1L (FL cell) and CD28, CD40L, ICOS, and PD-1 (T_{FH} cell). TNFRSF14 mutations affect the HVEM–BTLA interaction between FL and T_{FH} cells. Stromal cells secrete chemokines, which are sensed by CXCR5 on FL cells. In turn, tumor cells release TNF-α, which stimulates stromal cells. Mutations in CREBBP induce a decreased MHC-II expression on FL cells, which reduce the interaction with the T cell receptor (TCR), thus hampering the detection of tumor cells by the immune system. Figure created with BioRender.com (accessed on 13 July 2022).

6.1. T Cells

$CD4^+$ cells: FL follicles show a higher proportion of some types of T cells compared to healthy germinal centers [103,110]. First, T_{FH} cells are a subgroup of $CD4^+$ T lymphocytes implicated in normal GC biology and antibody production. However, T_{FH} cells of FL patients are not superimposable to those of healthy individuals [111,112]: they overexpress IL-2 and IL-4 and have activated STAT6 signaling, which increases proliferation and prevents apoptosis. Tumor immune evasion is also facilitated by T cell exhaustion and tolerance: dysfunctional $CD4^+$ and $CD8^+$ and functional T_{FH} cells express PD-1, and some of them secrete IL-4, IL-21, and TNF-α, sustaining malignant development [113].

Second, regulatory T cells (T_{reg}), a CD4$^+$ immunosuppressive subset expressing CD25 and FOXP3, are crucial guarantors of peripheral immune tolerance [114]. However, their frequency is higher than in normal lymph nodes. By means of an increased number of immune checkpoint molecules (GITR, TIGIT, ICOS), they have a stronger suppressive capacity [115–117]. It has even been suggested that the T_{reg} population is oligoclonal [118], a fact that would explain their role in sustaining tumor growth. Finally, a recently described type of infiltrating lymphocytes are T_{FR} (follicular regulatory T cells) [110,119], which express FOXP3 and CXCR5. Indeed, the T_{FH}/T_{FR} ratio could be important for the biology of FL.

CD8$^+$ (cytotoxic) cells: This cell subset is key to antitumor immunity. Some studies have established that a higher proportion of CD8$^+$ cells is an independent favorable prognostic factor [120,121]. These cells build synaptic relationships with tumor cells and exert direct cytotoxicity by means of lytic granules containing granzyme B. However, their effector function can be lost with time, due to persistent antigen stimulation and the expression of inhibitory receptors (PD-1, LAG3, TIM3, TIGIT) [122,123]. A deeper understanding of these exhaustion mechanisms will be crucial for the development of novel immunotherapeutic strategies [102].

6.2. Tumor-Associated Macrophages (TAM)

Besides being part of the innate immune system, macrophages are professional antigen-presenting cells. Classically, two macrophage phenotypes were described: M1 (receiving activating signals in the form of lipopolysaccharide or IFN-γ) and M2 or activated (sensitive to IL-4 and IL-13) [124]. However, this dichotomic classification is now considered too simplistic and unable to grasp the plasticity of these cells [125].

Concerning the prognostic impact of macrophages, Dave and colleagues [126] demonstrated that FL cases with high expression of genes mainly related to macrophages and follicular dendritic cells ("immune response 2") had shorter survival, while those of patients with high expression of T cell-related genes ("immune response 1") were longer. The real importance of TAM in FL is yet to be determined, especially when evaluated using immunohistochemistry (CD68 and CD163). Although a higher proportion of CD68$^+$ cells was associated with a poorer prognosis in chemotherapy-treated FL patients, this effect was lost when rituximab was incorporated [127,128]. These apparently contradicting findings suggest that therapeutic strategies modulate the composition of the TME.

Macrophages are important players in antibody-dependent cellular phagocytosis and rituximab-induced cytotoxicity [129] and express SIRPα, which is part of the "don't eat me" signaling pathway. A higher proportion of macrophages expressing this protein has been linked to poorer outcomes [130]. Furthermore, M2 macrophages enhance a dendritic cell-specific intercellular adhesion molecule-3-grabbing nonintegrin (DC-SIGN)-dependent adhesion via N-glycan-modified residues of the BCR and generate BCR-associated kinase activation [131].

6.3. Stromal Cells

Although initially viewed as not immunologically active, non-immune elements of the TME (endothelial cells, fibroblasts, mesenchymal stromal cells) are considered increasingly important in the pathogenesis of FL. Ongoing interesting studies are attempting to characterize the composition and cell organization of the lymph nodes, blood, and bone marrow. In this sense, the role of the crosstalk between the tumor and stromal cells needs to be highlighted [132]. Cancer-associated fibroblasts, emerging from the reprogramming of lymph node lymphoid stromal cells, directly support malignant B cell growth and orchestrate a permissive FL cell niche by recruiting and polarizing immune TME subsets.

7. Clinical Implications

7.1. Molecular Prognostic Scores

With the advent of NGS, attempts at incorporating molecular data to refine prognosis have been made. The first of such efforts was the m7-FLIPI, a clinicogenetic risk model encompassing clinical (FLIPI and ECOG performance status) and genetic data [133]. After applying a 74-gene deep sequencing panel to 151 lymph nodes from FL patients in need of treatment, the authors found that mutations in *EP300*, *FOXO1*, *CREBBP*, and *CARD11* (conferring poor prognosis), and in *MEF2B*, *ARID1A*, and *EZH2* (conferring good prognosis), enhanced the prognostic ability of the clinical parameters. The primary endpoint of the study was failure-free survival, but the score was similarly predictive of OS. Subsequent applications of the score to patients treated with different regimens have yielded diverse results, which, together with its unavailability in common practice, has limited its widespread use.

The same German and Canadian cohorts from the m7-FLIPI gave rise to the POD24 prognostic index (POD24-PI) [8], which was specifically designed to predict early treatment failure. Selecting only mutations in *EP300*, *EZH2*, and *FOXO1*, the sensitivity to predict POD24 was higher, at a cost of lower accuracy and specificity. Likewise, it has not reached clinical practice.

Finally, with the intention of capturing the complexity of FL biology and the crosstalk between tumor and accompanying cells, a gene expression profile score was devised, the 23-GEP [134]. After genes independently associated with PFS were selected, 23 of them were shown to have a strong correlation between the experimental platform and the standard Nanostring® technology. Those genes were finally included in a score that was predictive of PFS. The incorporation of a risk score using GEP is even more challenging than that of NGS-based indexes.

It must not be forgotten that molecular prognostic scores calculated using lymphoid tissue samples will always face the limitation of sampling bias: the mutational spectrum, akin to histological grading, might change according to the site of biopsy [135]. This drawback may be overcome by the incorporation of the circulating tumor DNA (ctDNA) technology [136], which could integrate/recapitulate the overall genomic landscape of a neoplasm.

7.2. Therapies Targeting the Molecular Pathogenesis of FL

Considering the importance of the t(14;18) and the *BCL2* oncogene in the pathogenesis of FL, its selective inhibitor, venetoclax, would be expected to have notable efficacy, akin to that seen in chronic lymphocytic leukemia. Results have been, however, underwhelming [137,138]. The phase 2 CONTRALTO study [138] compared venetoclax (V), bendamustine (B), and rituximab (R) with BR alone in the relapsed/refractory (RR) setting, with similar efficacy but higher toxicity in the VBR arm, leading to a high discontinuation rate of venetoclax. A chemotherapy-free arm with VR was also tested, with only 17% of complete responses. Several mechanisms explaining this insensitivity to BCL2 inhibitors have been postulated [102]: (i) the expression of BCL2 might be heterogeneous, (ii) other components of the anti-apoptotic BCL2 family might be active (MCL-1, BCL-XL), and (iii) a plethora of genetic and microenvironmental stimuli might make overt FL tumors less dependent on BCL2 expression.

One of the few genetically-targeted therapies available in this disease is tazemetostat, an oral selective inhibitor of the epigenetic regulator *EZH2*, which has been recently approved by the Food and Drug Administration (FDA) for RR FL. A phase 2 study [139] tested tazemetostat in 99 RR FL patients (45 $EZH2^{mut}$ and 54 $EZH2^{wt}$), and the overall response rate (ORR) was 69% and 35% in $EZH2^{mut}$ and $EZH2^{wt}$ patients, respectively. Median progression-free survival (PFS) was around one year, and toxicity was acceptable, mainly in the form of cytopenias. This makes tazemetostat an excellent candidate for drug combinations.

In contrast to *EZH2*, which is predominantly affected by activating mutations, the function of most epigenetic regulators, such as *CREBBP* and *KMT2D*, is disrupted by loss-of-function mutations, which are less easily amenable to pharmacological targeting. Acetyltransferase inactivating mutations are frequent in FL, which is why vorinostat, an oral histone deacetylase (HDAC) inhibitor, has been tested in this disease. By targeting HDAC, this drug would restore the epigenetic homeostasis of the tumor. In the phase 2 study including 39 FL patients [140], the ORR was 49% and median PFS was 20 months, with cytopenias as main adverse events. Vorinostat has later been combined with rituximab, with comparable results [141]. The pan-HDAC inhibitor panobinostat [142] has also been studied in FL, as well as newer-generation inhibitors, such as mocetinostat [143], albeit with limited efficacy. It remains to be seen whether genetically-targeted drugs and their combinations become relevant tools in the management of this neoplasm, in which epigenetic dysregulation is a hallmark.

Several immunomodulatory drugs targeting the TME have been tested, and some of them approved for both frontline and RR FL: lenalidomide [144,145] (a molecule unleashing pleiotropic antitumor effects), the anti-CD47 antibody Hu5F9-G4 [146] (inhibiting the "don't eat me" signal on FL cells), as well as various CD20 × CD3 bispecific antibodies, such as mosunetuzumab [147]. Moreover, with the incorporation of CAR-T cells in earlier lines of therapy, prognosis for FL patients is likely to change significantly in the coming years.

8. Discussion

The t(14;18) is considered the primary genetic event in FL, juxtaposing the *BCL2* oncogene to the immunoglobulin heavy-chain enhancer, which promotes BCL2 overexpression [3,4,12]. Important progress has been made to identify the additional genomic alterations cooperating with BCL2 deregulation [28–31,33,35,77], although how these alterations interact with each other, and which specific alterations are maintained or emerge during the course of the disease remain unclear. Studies using more sensitive techniques (e.g., single cell whole genome sequencing/RNAseq) will be needed to understand the chronological evolution of single aberrations throughout the course of the disease. By comparison with other germinal center-derived B cell lymphomas, FL is addicted to epigenetic alterations [148], as over 90% of patients have mutations in genes encoding epigenetic modifiers [29,31,73,102], suggesting its potential as an attractive therapeutic target in this disease. Moreover, genomic alterations in signaling and B cell differentiation, the BCR/NF-κB pathway, and proliferation/apoptosis have been identified in FL, cooperating in tumorigenesis [29,31,33,38,73,77,102].

Although the *BCL2* rearrangement is the hallmark of FL, 10–15% of patients lack this translocation [1,72]. Several studies have suggested that this subset of patients is different to the classical *BCL2* + FL and consequently emerge as a new provisional entity in the ICC classification [51,72,73,80–82,85,86,88,149].

The identification of high-risk patient groups at diagnosis in FL is still challenging. New molecular prognostic scores have been developed during the last years, combining mutational (m7-FLIPI and POD24-PI) [8,133] or gene expression data (23-GEP) [134]. Nevertheless, their use in the clinical setting is limited, and the vast majority of patients are treated independently of prognostic scores.

The rate of transformation to a more aggressive lymphoma is estimated between 10% and 20% of all patients [101,150]. Studies conducted in paired diagnostic and tFL cases showed a divergent or branching evolution from a CPC, which is responsible for generating each new event (e.g., progression, transformation) of FL [29,73,102,103]. Genomic alterations in genes involving the cell cycle (*CDKN2A/B*), apoptosis (*TP53*), and signaling pathways and immune evasion (*B2M, CD58*) are more prevalent at transformation [73,110,111,113]. However, further studies using high resolution genomic techniques are needed to understand the evolution pattern and to identify whether these genomic alterations are acquired or present at low frequency at diagnosis. On the other hand, the composition of the TME is crucial for the development, progression, and relapse of FL [101,102]. A better understanding of the TME could help develop novel targeted therapies.

Reflecting the clinical and molecular heterogeneity of FL, not all high-risk patients (e.g., early relapse or primary refractory) are equal, and their clinical outcomes will differ based on the genetic tumor profile, patterns of clonal evolution, composition and interaction of tumor cells with the TME, and the timing and location of the relapse. Furthermore, a deeper knowledge of specific high-risk groups will be essential to understand the wide clinical spectrum of the disease.

Several therapies targeting key alterations in the pathogenesis of FL have been approved, highlighting the importance to expand our knowledge on the mutational profile of FL. Although the efficacy of venetoclax, targeting BCL2, is insufficient [137,138], tazemetostat, an EZH2 inhibitor, seems to be a good candidate for drug combinations [145]. Moreover, drugs targeting the TME, such as lenalidomide, have been investigated as new alternatives to modulate the interactions between tumor and non-tumor cells in FL [144,145].

9. Conclusions

FL, one of the most common lymphomas, is a heterogeneous disease, both genetically and clinically. Although the *IGH::BCL2* rearrangement and mutations in epigenetic modifiers are very common, the potential prognostic role of other genetic abnormalities remains to be consolidated. Since a majority of patients will have prolonged survival, tools to identify those at higher risk of early relapse, multiple relapses, or HT are eagerly sought. In this sense, refined molecular prognostic scores and ctDNA will most likely be of help. With the integration of those data, the practicing clinician will face the challenge of selecting the most appropriate management strategy for each patient, including watchful waiting, single-agent monoclonal antibodies, ICT, ASCT, immunomodulatory drugs, epigenetic therapies, bispecifics, and CAR-T cells

Author Contributions: C.L. and P.M. drafting of the manuscript. A.L.-G. and S.B. supervision the manuscript. C.L. conception and supervision of the manuscript. All authors have read and agreed to the published version of the manuscript.

Funding: This study was supported by Fundación AECC/CIBER: PROYE1820BEA (S.B.), Fondo de Investigaciones Sanitarias, Instituto de Salud Carlos III and European Regional Development Fund "Una manera de hacer Europa" [Grant Number: PI17/01061 (S.B.), PI19/00887 (A.L.-G). Generalitat de Catalunya Suport Grups de Recerca AGAUR 2017-SGR-709 (S.B.). C.L. is supported by postdoctoral Beatriu de Pinós grant from Secretaria d'Universitats i Recerca del Departament d'Empresa I Coneixement de la Generalitat de Catalunya and by Marie Sklodowska-Curie COFUND program from H2020 (2018-BP-00055).

Institutional Review Board Statement: Not applicable.

Informed Consent Statement: Not applicable.

Data Availability Statement: Not applicable.

Conflicts of Interest: The authors declare no conflict of interest.

References

1. Swerdlow, S.H.; Campo, E.; Harris, N.L.; Jaffe, E.S.; Pileri, S.A.; Stein, H.; Thiele, J. *WHO Classification of Tumours of Haematopoietic and Lymphoid Tissues*, 4th ed.; IARC: Lyon, France, 2017.
2. Campo, E.; Jaffe, E.S.; Cook, J.R.; Quintanilla-Martinez, L.; Swerdlow, S.H.; Anderson, K.C.; Brousset, P.; Cerroni, L.; de Leval, L.; Dirnhofer, S.; et al. The International Consensus Classification of Mature Lymphoid Neoplasms: A Report from the Clinical Advisory Committee. *Blood* **2022**, *140*, 1229–1253. [CrossRef] [PubMed]
3. Tsujimoto, Y.; Cossman, J.; Jaffe, E.; Croce, C.M. Involvement of the bcl-2 gene in human follicular lymphoma. *Science* **1985**, *228*, 1440–1443. [CrossRef] [PubMed]
4. Küppers, R.; Dalla-Favera, R. Mechanisms of chromosomal translocations in B cell lymphomas. *Oncogene* **2001**, *20*, 5580–5594. [CrossRef]

5. Dreyling, M.; Ghielmini, M.; Rule, S.; Salles, G.; Ladetto, M.; Tonino, S.H.; Herfarth, K.; Seymour, J.F.; Jerkeman, M. Newly diagnosed and relapsed follicular lymphoma: ESMO Clinical Practice Guidelines for diagnosis, treatment and follow-up. *Ann. Oncol.* **2021**, *32*, 298–308. [CrossRef]
6. Rivas-Delgado, A.; Magnano, L.; Moreno-Velázquez, M.; García, O.; Nadeu, F.; Mozas, P.; Dlouhy, I.; Baumann, T.; Rovira, J.; González-Farre, B.; et al. Response duration and survival shorten after each relapse in patients with follicular lymphoma treated in the rituximab era. *Br. J. Haematol.* **2019**, *184*, 753–759. [CrossRef] [PubMed]
7. Bachy, E.; Seymour, J.F.; Feugier, P.; Offner, F.; López-Guillermo, A.; Belada, D.; Xerri, L.; Catalano, J.V.; Brice, P.; Lemonnier, F.; et al. Sustained Progression-Free Survival Benefit of Rituximab Maintenance in Patients With Follicular Lymphoma: Long-Term Results of the PRIMA Study. *J. Clin. Oncol.* **2019**, *37*, 2815–2824. [CrossRef] [PubMed]
8. Casulo, C.; Byrtek, M.; Dawson, K.L.; Zhou, X.; Farber, C.M.; Flowers, C.R.; Hainsworth, J.D.; Maurer, M.J.; Cerhan, J.R.; Link, B.K.; et al. Early Relapse of Follicular Lymphoma After Rituximab Plus Cyclophosphamide, Doxorubicin, Vincristine, and Prednisone Defines Patients at High Risk for Death: An Analysis From the National LymphoCare Study. *J. Clin. Oncol.* **2015**, *33*, 2516–2522. [CrossRef] [PubMed]
9. Alonso-Álvarez, S.; Magnano, L.; Alcoceba, M.; Andrade-Campos, M.; Espinosa-Lara, N.; Rodríguez, G.; Mercadal, S.; Carro, I.; Sancho, J.M.; Moreno, M.; et al. Risk of, and survival following, histological transformation in follicular lymphoma in the rituximab era. A retrospective multicentre study by the Spanish GELTAMO group. *Br. J. Haematol.* **2017**, *178*, 699–708. [CrossRef] [PubMed]
10. Mozas, P.; Rivero, A.; López-Guillermo, A. Past, present and future of prognostic scores in follicular lymphoma. *Blood Rev.* **2021**, *50*, 100865. [CrossRef] [PubMed]
11. McNamara, C.; Montoto, S.; Eyre, T.A.; Ardeshna, K.; Burton, C.; Illidge, T.; Linton, K.; Rule, S.; Townsend, W.; Wong, W.L.; et al. The investigation and management of follicular lymphoma. *Br. J. Haematol.* **2020**, *191*, 363–381. [CrossRef] [PubMed]
12. Szankasi, P.; Bolia, A.; Liew, M.; Schumacher, J.A.; Gee, E.P.S.; Matynia, A.P.; Li, K.D.; Patel, J.L.; Xu, X.; Salama, M.E.; et al. Comprehensive detection of chromosomal translocations in lymphoproliferative disorders by massively parallel sequencing. *J. Hematop.* **2019**, *12*, 121–133. [CrossRef]
13. Akasaka, T.; Akasaka, H.; Yonetani, N.; Ohno, H.; Yamabe, H.; Fukuhara, S.; Okuma, M. Refinement of the BCL2/immunoglobulin heavy chain fusion gene in t(14;18)(q32;q21) by polymerase chain reaction amplification for long targets. *Genes Chromosom. Cancer* **1998**, *21*, 17–29. [CrossRef]
14. Chong, L.C.; Ben-Neriah, S.; Slack, G.W.; Freeman, C.; Ennishi, D.; Mottok, A.; Collinge, B.; Abrisqueta, P.; Farinha, P.; Boyle, M.; et al. High-resolution architecture and partner genes of MYC rearrangements in lymphoma with DLBCL morphology. *Blood Adv.* **2018**, *2*, 2755–2765. [CrossRef] [PubMed]
15. Dyer, M.J.S.; Akasaka, T.; Capasso, M.; Dusanjh, P.; Lee, Y.F.; Karran, E.L.; Nagel, I.; Vater, I.; Cario, G.; Siebert, R. Immunoglobulin heavy chain locus chromosomal translocations in B cell precursor acute lymphoblastic leukemia: Rare clinical curios or potent genetic drivers? *Blood* **2010**, *115*, 1490–1499. [CrossRef] [PubMed]
16. Yonetani, N.; Ueda, C.; Akasaka, T.; Nishikori, M.; Uchiyama, T.; Ohno, H. Heterogeneous breakpoints on the immunoglobulin genes are involved in fusion with the 5' region of BCL2 in B-cell tumors. *Jpn. J. Cancer Res.* **2001**, *92*, 933–940. [CrossRef] [PubMed]
17. Liu, Y.; Hernandez, A.M.; Shibata, D.; Cortopassi, G.A. BCL2 translocation frequency rises with age in humans. *Proc. Natl. Acad. Sci. USA* **1994**, *91*, 8910–8914. [CrossRef] [PubMed]
18. Roulland, S.; Lebailly, P.; Roussel, G.; Briand, M.; Cappellen, D.; Pottier, D.; Hardouin, A.; Troussard, X.; Bastard, C.; Henry-Amar, M.; et al. BCL-2/JH translocation in peripheral blood lymphocytes of unexposed individuals: Lack of seasonal variations in frequency and molecular features. *Int. J. Cancer* **2003**, *104*, 695–698. [CrossRef] [PubMed]
19. Schüler, F.; Dölken, L.; Hirt, C.; Kiefer, T.; Berg, T.; Fusch, G.; Weitmann, K.; Hoffmann, W.; Fusch, C.; Janz, S.; et al. Prevalence and frequency of circulating t(14;18)-MBR translocation carrying cells in healthy individuals. *Int. J. Cancer* **2009**, *124*, 958–963. [CrossRef] [PubMed]
20. Roulland, S.; Lebailly, P.; Lecluse, Y.; Heutte, N.; Nadel, B.; Gauduchon, P. Long-term clonal persistence and evolution of t(14;18)-bearing B cells in healthy individuals. *Leukemia* **2006**, *20*, 158–162. [CrossRef] [PubMed]
21. Giannelli, F.; Moscarella, S.; Giannini, C.; Caini, P.; Monti, M.; Gragnani, L.; Romanelli, R.G.; Solazzo, V.; Laffi, G.; La Villa, G.; et al. Effect of antiviral treatment in patients with chronic HCV infection and t(14;18) translocation. *Blood* **2003**, *102*, 1196–1201. [CrossRef] [PubMed]
22. Roulland, S.; Navarro, J.M.; Grenot, P.; Milili, M.; Agopian, J.; Montpellier, B.; Gauduchon, P.; Lebailly, P.; Schiff, C.; Nadel, B. Follicular lymphoma-like B cells in healthy individuals: A novel intermediate step in early lymphomagenesis. *J. Exp. Med.* **2006**, *203*, 2425–2431. [CrossRef] [PubMed]
23. Limpens, J.; Stad, R.; Vos, C.; De Vlaam, C.; De Jong, D.; Van Ommen, G.J.B.; Schuuring, E.; Kluin, P.M. Lymphoma-associated translocation t(14;18) in blood B cells of normal individuals. *Blood* **1995**, *85*, 2528–2536. [CrossRef] [PubMed]
24. Qu, X.; Li, H.; Braziel, R.M.; Passerini, V.; Rimsza, L.M.; His, E.D.; Leonard, J.P.; Smith, S.M.; Kridel, R.; Press, O.; et al. Genomic alterations important for the prognosis in patients with follicular lymphoma treated in SWOG study S0016. *Blood* **2019**, *133*, 81–93. [CrossRef] [PubMed]
25. Bouska, A.; McKeithan, T.W.; Deffenbacher, K.E.; Lachel, C.; Wright, G.W.; Iqbal, J.; Smith, L.M.; Zhang, W.; Kucuk, C.; Rinaldi, A.; et al. Genome-wide copy-number analyses reveal genomic abnormalities involved in transformation of follicular lymphoma. *Blood* **2014**, *123*, 1681–1690. [CrossRef] [PubMed]

26. Cheung, K.J.J.; Shah, S.P.; Steidl, C.; Johnson, N.; Relander, T.; Telenius, A.; Lai, B.; Murphy, K.P.; Lam, W.; Al-Tourah, A.J.; et al. Genome-wide profiling of follicular lymphoma by array comparative genomic hybridization reveals prognostically significant DNA copy number imbalances. *Blood* **2009**, *113*, 137–148. [CrossRef] [PubMed]
27. Morin, R.D.; Johnson, N.A.; Severson, T.M.; Mungall, A.J.; An, J.; Goya, R.; Paul, J.E.; Boyle, M.; Woolcock, B.W.; Kuchenbauer, F.; et al. Somatic mutations altering EZH2 (Tyr641) in follicular and diffuse large B-cell lymphomas of germinal-center origin. *Nat. Genet.* **2010**, *42*, 181–185. [CrossRef]
28. Okosun, J.; Bödör, C.; Wang, J.; Araf, S.; Yang, C.Y.; Pan, C.; Boller, S.; Cittaro, D.; Bozek, M.; Iqbal, S.; et al. Integrated genomic analysis identifies recurrent mutations and evolution patterns driving the initiation and progression of follicular lymphoma. *Nat. Genet.* **2014**, *46*, 176–181. [CrossRef] [PubMed]
29. Green, M.R.; Kihira, S.; Liu, C.L.; Nair, R.V.; Salari, R.; Gentles, A.J.; Irish, J.; Stehr, H.; Vicente-Dueñas, C.; Romero-Camarero, I.; et al. Mutations in early follicular lymphoma progenitors are associated with suppressed antigen presentation. *Proc. Natl. Acad. Sci. USA* **2015**, *112*, E1116–E1125. [CrossRef]
30. Pasqualucci, L.; Dominguez-Sola, D.; Chiarenza, A.; Fabbri, G.; Grunn, A.; Trifonov, V.; Kasper, L.H.; Lerach, S.; Tang, H.; Ma, J.; et al. Inactivating mutations of acetyltransferase genes in B-cell lymphoma. *Nature* **2011**, *471*, 189–196. [CrossRef] [PubMed]
31. Bödör, C.; Grossmann, V.; Popov, N.; Okosun, J.; O'Riain, C.; Tan, K.; Marzec, J.; Araf, S.; Wang, J.; Lee, A.M.; et al. EZH2 mutations are frequent and represent an early event in follicular lymphoma. *Blood* **2013**, *122*, 3165–3168. [CrossRef] [PubMed]
32. Morin, R.D.; Mendez-Lago, M.; Mungall, A.J.; Goya, R.; Mungall, K.L.; Corbett, R.D.; Johnson, N.A.; Severson, T.M.; Chiu, R.; Field, M.; et al. Frequent mutation of histone-modifying genes in non-Hodgkin lymphoma. *Nature* **2011**, *476*, 298–303. [CrossRef] [PubMed]
33. Hübschmann, D.; Kleinheinz, K.; Wagener, R.; Bernhart, S.H.; López, C.; Toprak, U.H.; Sungalee, S.; Ishaque, N.; Kretzmer, H.; Kreuz, M.; et al. Mutational mechanisms shaping the coding and noncoding genome of germinal center derived B-cell lymphomas. *Leukemia* **2021**, *35*, 2002–2016. [CrossRef] [PubMed]
34. Green, M.R.; Gentles, A.J.; Nair, R.V.; Irish, J.M.; Kihira, S.; Liu, C.L.; Kela, I.; Hopmans, E.S.; Myklebust, J.H.; Ji, H.; et al. Hierarchy in somatic mutations arising during genomic evolution and progression of follicular lymphoma. *Blood* **2013**, *121*, 1604–1611. [CrossRef] [PubMed]
35. Zhang, J.; Dominguez-Sola, D.; Hussein, S.; Lee, J.E.; Holmes, A.B.; Bansal, M.; Vlasevska, S.; Mo, T.; Tang, H.; Basso, K.; et al. Disruption of KMT2D perturbs germinal center B cell development and promotes lymphomagenesis. *Nat. Med.* **2015**, *21*, 1190–1198. [CrossRef] [PubMed]
36. Ortega-Molina, A.; Boss, I.W.; Canela, A.; Pan, H.; Jiang, Y.; Zhao, C.; Jiang, M.; Hu, D.; Agirre, X.; Niesvizky, I.; et al. The histone lysine methyltransferase KMT2D sustains a gene expression program that represses B cell lymphoma development. *Nat. Med.* **2015**, *21*, 1199–1208. [CrossRef] [PubMed]
37. Calo, E.; Wysocka, J. Modification of enhancer chromatin: What, how, and why? *Mol. Cell* **2013**, *49*, 825–837. [CrossRef]
38. García-Ramírez, I.; Tadros, S.; González-Herrero, I.; Martín-Lorenzo, A.; Rodríguez-Hernández, G.; Moore, D.; Ruiz-Roca, L.; Blanco, O.; Alonso-López, D.; De Las Rivas, J.; et al. Crebbp loss cooperates with Bcl2 overexpression to promote lymphoma in mice. *Blood* **2017**, *129*, 2645–2656. [CrossRef]
39. Mullighan, C.G.; Zhang, J.; Kasper, L.H.; Lerach, S.; Payne-Turner, D.; Phillips, L.A.; Heatley, S.L.; Holmfeldt, L.; Collins-Underwood, J.R.; Ma, J.; et al. CREBBP mutations in relapsed acute lymphoblastic leukaemia. *Nature* **2011**, *471*, 235–241. [CrossRef]
40. Horton, S.J.; Giotopoulos, G.; Yun, H.; Vohra, S.; Sheppard, O.; Bashford-Rogers, R.; Rashid, M.; Clipson, A.; Chan, W.I.; Sasca, D.; et al. Early loss of Crebbp confers malignant stem cell properties on lymphoid progenitors. *Nat. Cell Biol.* **2017**, *19*, 1093–1104. [CrossRef]
41. Jiang, Y.; Ortega-Molina, A.; Geng, H.; Ying, H.Y.; Hatzi, K.; Parsa, S.; McNally, D.; Wang, L.; Doane, A.S.; Agirre, X.; et al. CREBBP Inactivation Promotes the Development of HDAC3-Dependent Lymphomas. *Cancer Discov.* **2017**, *7*, 38–53. [CrossRef]
42. Zhang, J.; Vlasevska, S.; Wells, V.A.; Nataraj, S.; Holmes, A.B.; Duval, R.; Meyer, S.N.; Mo, T.; Basso, K.; Brindle, P.K.; et al. The CREBBP Acetyltransferase Is a Haploinsufficient Tumor Suppressor in B-cell Lymphoma. *Cancer Discov.* **2017**, *7*, 323–337. [CrossRef] [PubMed]
43. Meyer, S.N.; Scuoppo, C.; Vlasevska, S.; Bal, E.; Holmes, A.B.; Holloman, M.; Garcia-Ibanez, L.; Nataraj, S.; Duval, R.; Vantrimpont, T.; et al. Unique and Shared Epigenetic Programs of the CREBBP and EP300 Acetyltransferases in Germinal Center B Cells Reveal Targetable Dependencies in Lymphoma. *Immunity* **2019**, *51*, 535–547.e9. [CrossRef] [PubMed]
44. Béguelin, W.; Popovic, R.; Teater, M.; Jiang, Y.; Bunting, K.L.; Rosen, M.; Shen, H.; Yang, S.N.; Wang, L.; Ezponda, T.; et al. EZH2 is required for germinal center formation and somatic EZH2 mutations promote lymphoid transformation. *Cancer Cell* **2013**, *23*, 677–692. [CrossRef]
45. Béguelin, W.; Teater, M.; Gearhart, M.D.; Calvo Fernández, M.T.; Goldstein, R.L.; Cárdenas, M.G.; Hatzi, K.; Rosen, M.; Shen, H.; Corcoran, C.M.; et al. EZH2 and BCL6 Cooperate to Assemble CBX8-BCOR Complex to Repress Bivalent Promoters, Mediate Germinal Center Formation and Lymphomagenesis. *Cancer Cell* **2016**, *30*, 197–213. [CrossRef]
46. Souroullas, G.P.; Jeck, W.R.; Parker, J.S.; Simon, J.M.; Liu, J.Y.; Paulk, J.; Xiong, J.; Clark, K.S.; Fedoriw, Y.; Qi, J.; et al. An oncogenic Ezh2 mutation induces tumors through global redistribution of histone 3 lysine 27 trimethylation. *Nat. Med.* **2016**, *22*, 632–640. [CrossRef]

47. Sneeringer, C.J.; Scott, M.P.; Kuntz, K.W.; Knutson, S.K.; Pollock, R.M.; Richon, V.M.; Copeland, R.A. Coordinated activities of wild-type plus mutant EZH2 drive tumor-associated hypertrimethylation of lysine 27 on histone H3 (H3K27) in human B-cell lymphomas. *Proc. Natl. Acad. Sci. USA* **2010**, *107*, 20980–20985. [CrossRef] [PubMed]
48. Yap, D.B.; Chu, J.; Berg, T.; Schapira, M.; Cheng, S.W.G.; Moradian, A.; Morin, R.D.; Mungall, A.J.; Meissner, B.; Boyle, M.; et al. Somatic mutations at EZH2 Y641 act dominantly through a mechanism of selectively altered PRC2 catalytic activity, to increase H3K27 trimethylation. *Blood* **2011**, *117*, 2451–2459. [CrossRef]
49. Li, H.; Kaminski, M.S.; Li, Y.; Yildiz, M.; Ouillette, P.; Jones, S.; Fox, H.; Jacobi, K.; Saiya-Cork, K.; Bixby, D.; et al. Mutations in linker histone genes HIST1H1 B, C, D, and E; OCT2 (POU2F2); IRF8; and ARID1A underlying the pathogenesis of follicular lymphoma. *Blood* **2014**, *123*, 1487–1498. [CrossRef]
50. Schmitz, R.; Wright, G.W.; Huang, D.W.; Johnson, C.A.; Phelan, J.D.; Wang, J.Q.; Roulland, S.; Kasbekar, M.; Young, R.M.; Shaffer, A.L.; et al. Genetics and Pathogenesis of Diffuse Large B-Cell Lymphoma. *N. Engl. J. Med.* **2018**, *378*, 1396–1407. [CrossRef]
51. Leich, E.; Hoster, E.; Wartenberg, M.; Unterhalt, M.; Siebert, R.; Koch, K.; Klapper, W.; Engelhard, M.; Puppe, B.; Horn, H.; et al. Similar clinical features in follicular lymphomas with and without breaks in the BCL2 locus. *Leukemia* **2016**, *30*, 854–860. [CrossRef]
52. Jardin, F.; Gaulard, P.; Buchonnet, G.; Contentin, N.; Leprêtre, S.; Lenain, P.; Stamatoullas, A.; Picquenot, J.M.; Duval, C.; Parmentier, F.; et al. Follicular lymphoma without t(14;18) and with BCL-6 rearrangement: A lymphoma subtype with distinct pathological, molecular and clinical characteristics. *Leukemia* **2002**, *16*, 2309–2317. [CrossRef] [PubMed]
53. Jardin, F.; Sahota, S.S. Targeted somatic mutation of the BCL6 proto-oncogene and its impact on lymphomagenesis. *Hematology* **2005**, *10*, 115–129. [CrossRef] [PubMed]
54. Bosga-Bouwer, A.G.; Van Imhoff, G.W.; Boonstra, R.; Van der Veen, A.; Haralambieva, E.; Van den Berg, A.; De Jong, B.; Krause, V.; Palmer, M.C.; Coupland, R.; et al. Follicular lymphoma grade 3B includes 3 cytogenetically defined subgroups with primary t(14;18), 3q27, or other translocations: T(14;18) and 3q27 are mutually exclusive. *Blood* **2003**, *101*, 1149–1154. [CrossRef] [PubMed]
55. Ying, C.Y.; Dominguez-Sola, D.; Fabi, M.; Lorenz, I.C.; Hussein, S.; Bansal, M.; Califano, A.; Pasqualucci, L.; Basso, K.; Dalla-Favera, R. MEF2B mutations lead to deregulated expression of the oncogene BCL6 in diffuse large B cell lymphoma. *Nat. Immunol.* **2013**, *14*, 1084–1092. [CrossRef]
56. Pon, J.R.; Wong, J.; Saberi, S.; Alder, O.; Moksa, M.; Cheng, S.-W.G.; Morin, G.B.; Hoodless, P.A.; Hirst, M.; Marra, M.A. MEF2B mutations in non-Hodgkin lymphoma dysregulate cell migration by decreasing MEF2B target gene activation. *Nat. Commun.* **2015**, *6*, 7953. [CrossRef]
57. Krysiak, K.; Gomez, F.; White, B.S.; Matlock, M.; Miller, C.A.; Trani, L.; Fronick, C.C.; Fulton, R.S.; Kreisel, F.; Cashen, A.F.; et al. Recurrent somatic mutations affecting B-cell receptor signaling pathway genes in follicular lymphoma. *Blood* **2017**, *129*, 473–483. [CrossRef]
58. Jeelall, Y.S.; Wang, J.Q.; Law, H.-D.; Domaschenz, H.; Fung, H.K.H.; Kallies, A.; Nutt, S.L.; Goodnow, C.C.; Horikawa, K. Human lymphoma mutations reveal CARD11 as the switch between self-antigen-induced B cell death or proliferation and autoantibody production. *J. Exp. Med.* **2012**, *209*, 1907–1917. [CrossRef]
59. Zhu, D.; McCarthy, H.; Ottensmeier, C.H.; Johnson, P.; Hamblin, T.J.; Stevenson, F.K. Acquisition of potential N-glycosylation sites in the immunoglobulin variable region by somatic mutation is a distinctive feature of follicular lymphoma. *Blood* **2002**, *99*, 2562–2568. [CrossRef]
60. Yildiz, M.; Li, H.; Bernard, D.; Amin, N.A.; Ouillette, P.; Jones, S.; Saiya-Cork, K.; Parkin, B.; Jacobi, K.; Shedden, K.; et al. Activating STAT6 mutations in follicular lymphoma. *Blood* **2015**, *125*, 668–679. [CrossRef]
61. Young, R.M.; Staudt, L.M. Targeting pathological B cell receptor signalling in lymphoid malignancies. *Nat. Rev. Drug Discov.* **2013**, *12*, 229–243. [CrossRef]
62. Karube, K.; Martínez, D.; Royo, C.; Navarro, A.; Pinyol, M.; Cazorla, M.; Castillo, P.; Valera, A.; Carrió, A.; Costa, D.; et al. Recurrent mutations of NOTCH genes in follicular lymphoma identify a distinctive subset of tumours. *J. Pathol.* **2014**, *234*, 423–430. [CrossRef] [PubMed]
63. Radcliffe, C.M.; Arnold, J.N.; Suter, D.M.; Wormald, M.R.; Harvey, D.J.; Royle, L.; Mimura, Y.; Kimura, Y.; Sim, R.B.; Inogès, S.; et al. Human follicular lymphoma cells contain oligomannose glycans in the antigen-binding site of the B-cell receptor. *J. Biol. Chem.* **2007**, *282*, 7405–7415. [CrossRef] [PubMed]
64. McCann, K.J.; Ottensmeier, C.H.; Callard, A.; Radcliffe, C.M.; Harvey, D.J.; Dwek, R.A.; Rudd, P.M.; Sutton, B.J.; Hobby, P.; Stevenson, F.K. Remarkable selective glycosylation of the immunoglobulin variable region in follicular lymphoma. *Mol. Immunol.* **2008**, *45*, 1567–1572. [CrossRef] [PubMed]
65. Okosun, J.; Wolfson, R.L.; Wang, J.; Araf, S.; Wilkins, L.; Castellano, B.M.; Escudero-Ibarz, L.; Al Seraihi, A.F.; Richter, J.; Bernhart, S.H.; et al. Recurrent mTORC1-activating RRAGC mutations in follicular lymphoma. *Nat. Genet.* **2016**, *48*, 183–188. [CrossRef]
66. Ying, Z.X.; Jin, M.; Peterson, L.F.; Bernard, D.; Saiya-Cork, K.; Yildiz, M.; Wang, S.; Kaminski, M.S.; Chang, A.E.; Klionsky, D.J.; et al. Recurrent Mutations in the MTOR Regulator RRAGC in Follicular Lymphoma. *Clin. Cancer Res.* **2016**, *22*, 5383–5393. [CrossRef]
67. Mottok, A.; Renné, C.; Seifert, M.; Oppermann, E.; Bechstein, W.; Hansmann, M.L.; Küppers, R.; Bräuninger, A. Inactivating SOCS1 mutations are caused by aberrant somatic hypermutation and restricted to a subset of B-cell lymphoma entities. *Blood* **2009**, *114*, 4503–4506. [CrossRef]

68. Kim, E.; Goraksha-Hicks, P.; Li, L.; Neufeld, T.P.; Guan, K.L. Regulation of TORC1 by Rag GTPases in nutrient response. *Nat. Cell Biol.* **2008**, *10*, 935–945. [CrossRef]
69. Sancak, Y.; Bar-Peled, L.; Zoncu, R.; Markhard, A.L.; Nada, S.; Sabatini, D.M. Ragulator-Rag complex targets mTORC1 to the lysosomal surface and is necessary for its activation by amino acids. *Cell* **2010**, *141*, 290–303. [CrossRef]
70. Zoncu, R.; Bar-Peled, L.; Efeyan, A.; Wang, S.; Sancak, Y.; Sabatini, D.M. mTORC1 senses lysosomal amino acids through an inside-out mechanism that requires the vacuolar H(+)-ATPase. *Science* **2011**, *334*, 678–683. [CrossRef]
71. Lawrence, R.E.; Cho, K.F.; Rappold, R.; Thrun, A.; Tofaute, M.; Kim, D.J.; Moldavski, O.; Hurley, J.H.; Zoncu, R. A nutrient-induced affinity switch controls mTORC1 activation by its Rag GTPase-Ragulator lysosomal scaffold. *Nat. Cell Biol.* **2018**, *20*, 1052–1063. [CrossRef]
72. Leich, E.; Salaverria, I.; Bea, S.; Zettl, A.; Wright, G.; Moreno, V.; Gascoyne, R.D.; Chan, W.C.; Braziel, R.M.; Rimsza, L.M.; et al. Follicular lymphomas with and without translocation t(14;18) differ in gene expression profiles and genetic alterations. *Blood* **2009**, *114*, 826–834. [CrossRef] [PubMed]
73. Katzenberger, T.; Kalla, J.; Leich, E.; Stöcklein, H.; Hartmann, E.; Barnickel, S.; Wessendorf, S.; Ott, M.M.; Hans Konrad, M.H.; Rosenwald, A.; et al. A distinctive subtype of t(14;18)-negative nodal follicular non-Hodgkin lymphoma characterized by a predominantly diffuse growth pattern and deletions in the chromosomal region 1p36. *Blood* **2009**, *113*, 1053–1061. [CrossRef] [PubMed]
74. Cai, G.; Freeman, G.J. The CD160, BTLA, LIGHT/HVEM pathway: A bidirectional switch regulating T-cell activation. *Immunol. Rev.* **2009**, *229*, 244–258. [CrossRef] [PubMed]
75. Murphy, K.M.; Nelson, C.A.; Šedý, J.R. Balancing co-stimulation and inhibition with BTLA and HVEM. *Nat. Rev. Immunol.* **2006**, *6*, 671–681. [CrossRef] [PubMed]
76. Boice, M.; Salloum, D.; Mourcin, F.; Sanghvi, V.; Amin, R.; Oricchio, E.; Jiang, M.; Mottok, A.; Denis-Lagache, N.; Ciriello, G.; et al. Loss of the HVEM Tumor Suppressor in Lymphoma and Restoration by Modified CAR-T Cells. *Cell* **2016**, *167*, 405–418.e13. [CrossRef] [PubMed]
77. Huet, S.; Szafer-Glusman, E.; Tesson, B.; Xerri, L.; Fairbrother, W.J.; Mukhyala, K.; Bolen, C.; Punnoose, E.; Tonon, L.; Chassagne-Clément, C.; et al. BCL2 mutations do not confer adverse prognosis in follicular lymphoma patients treated with rituximab. *Am. J. Hematol.* **2017**, *92*, 515–519. [CrossRef] [PubMed]
78. Wang, J.; Anderson, P.D.; Luo, W.; Gius, D.; Roh, M.; Abdulkadir, S.A. Pim1 kinase is required to maintain tumorigenicity in MYC-expressing prostate cancer cells. *Oncogene* **2012**, *31*, 1794–1803. [CrossRef]
79. O'Shea, D.; O'Riain, C.; Taylor, C.; Waters, R.; Carlotti, E.; MacDougall, F.; Gribben, J.; Rosenwald, A.; Ott, G.; Rimsza, L.M.; et al. The presence of TP53 mutation at diagnosis of Follicular Lymphoma identifies a high-risk group of patients with shortened time to disease progression and poorer overall survival. *Blood* **2008**, *112*, 3126–3129. [CrossRef]
80. Gagyi, É.; Balogh, Z.; Bödör, C.; Timár, B.; Reiniger, L.; Deák, L.; Csomor, J.; Csernus, B.; Szepesi, Á.; Matolcsy, A. Somatic hypermutation of IGVH genes and aberrant somatic hypermutation in follicular lymphoma without BCL-2 gene rearrangement and expression. *Haematologica* **2008**, *93*, 1822–1828. [CrossRef]
81. Leich, E.; Zamo, A.; Horn, H.; Haralambieva, E.; Puppe, B.; Gascoyne, R.D.; Chan, W.C.; Braziel, R.M.; Rimsza, L.M.; Weisenburger, D.D.; et al. MicroRNA profiles of t(14;18)-negative follicular lymphoma support a late germinal center B-cell phenotype. *Blood* **2011**, *118*, 5550–5558. [CrossRef]
82. Martin-Guerrero, I.; Salaverria, I.; Burkhardt, B.; Szczepanowski, M.; Baudis, M.; Bens, S.; de Leval, L.; Garcia-Orad, A.; Horn, H.; Lisfeld, J.; et al. Recurrent loss of heterozygosity in 1p36 associated with TNFRSF14 mutations in IRF4 translocation negative pediatric follicular lymphomas. *Haematologica* **2013**, *98*, 1237–1241. [CrossRef]
83. Khoury, J.D.; Solary, E.; Abla, O.; Akkari, Y.; Alaggio, R.; Apperley, J.F.; Bejar, R.; Berti, E.; Busque, L.; Chan, J.K.C.; et al. The 5th edition of the World Health Organization Classification of Haematolymphoid Tumours: Myeloid and Histiocytic/Dendritic Neoplasms. *Leukemia* **2022**, *36*, 1703–1719. [CrossRef] [PubMed]
84. Lones, M.A.; Raphael, M.; McCarthy, K.; Wotherspoon, A.; Terrier-Lacombe, M.J.; Ramsay, A.D.; MacLennan, K.; Cairo, M.S.; Gerrard, M.; Michon, J.; et al. Primary follicular lymphoma of the testis in children and adolescents. *J. Pediatr. Hematol. Oncol.* **2012**, *34*, 68–71. [CrossRef]
85. Siddiqi, I.N.; Friedman, J.; Barry-Holson, K.Q.; Ma, C.; Thodima, V.; Kang, I.; Padmanabhan, R.; Dias, L.M.; Kelly, K.R.; Brynes, R.K.; et al. Characterization of a variant of t(14;18) negative nodal diffuse follicular lymphoma with CD23 expression, 1p36/TNFRSF14 abnormalities, and STAT6 mutations. *Mod. Pathol.* **2016**, *29*, 570–581. [CrossRef] [PubMed]
86. Nann, D.; Ramis-Zaldivar, J.E.; Müller, I.; Gonzalez-Farre, B.; Schmidt, J.; Egan, C.; Salmeron-Villalobos, J.; Clot, G.; Mattern, S.; Otto, F.; et al. Follicular lymphoma t(14;18)-negative is genetically a heterogeneous disease. *Blood Adv.* **2020**, *4*, 5652–5665. [CrossRef] [PubMed]
87. Zamò, A.; Pischimarov, J.; Horn, H.; Ott, G.; Rosenwald, A.; Leich, E. The exomic landscape of t(14;18)-negative diffuse follicular lymphoma with 1p36 deletion. *Br. J. Haematol.* **2018**, *180*, 391–394. [CrossRef] [PubMed]
88. Zamò, A.; Pischimarov, J.; Schlesner, M.; Rosenstiel, P.; Bomben, R.; Horn, H.; Grieb, T.; Nedeva, T.; López, C.; Haake, A.; et al. Differences between BCL2-break positive and negative follicular lymphoma unraveled by whole-exome sequencing. *Leukemia* **2018**, *32*, 685–693. [CrossRef]

89. Xian, R.R.; Xie, Y.; Haley, L.M.; Yonescu, R.; Pallavajjala, A.; Pittaluga, S.; Jaffe, E.S.; Duffield, A.S.; McCall, C.M.; Gheith, S.M.F.; et al. CREBBP and STAT6 co-mutation and 16p13 and 1p36 loss define the t(14;18)-negative diffuse variant of follicular lymphoma. *Blood Cancer J.* **2020**, *10*, 69. [CrossRef] [PubMed]
90. Louissaint, A.; Schafernak, K.T.; Geyer, J.T.; Kovach, A.E.; Ghandi, M.; Gratzinger, D.; Roth, C.G.; Paxton, C.N.; Kim, S.; Namgyal, C.; et al. Pediatric-type nodal follicular lymphoma: A biologically distinct lymphoma with frequent MAPK pathway mutations. *Blood* **2016**, *128*, 1093–1100. [CrossRef]
91. Schmidt, J.; Gong, S.; Marafioti, T.; Mankel, B.; Gonzalez-Farre, B.; Balagué, O.; Mozos, A.; Cabeçadas, J.; Van Der Walt, J.; Hoehn, D.; et al. Genome-wide analysis of pediatric-type follicular lymphoma reveals low genetic complexity and recurrent alterations of TNFRSF14 gene. *Blood* **2016**, *128*, 1101–1111. [CrossRef] [PubMed]
92. Liu, Q.; Salaverria, I.; Pittaluga, S.; Jegalian, A.G.; Xi, L.; Siebert, R.; Raffeld, M.; Hewitt, S.M.; Jaffe, E.S. Follicular lymphomas in children and young adults: A comparison of the pediatric variant with usual follicular lymphoma. *Am. J. Surg. Pathol.* **2013**, *37*, 333–343. [CrossRef] [PubMed]
93. Finn, L.S.; Viswanatha, D.S.; Belasco, J.B.; Snyder, H.; Huebner, D.; Sorbara, L.; Raffeld, M.; Jaffe, E.S.; Salhany, K.E. Primary follicular lymphoma of the testis in childhood. *Cancer* **1999**, *85*, 1626–1635. [CrossRef]
94. Gascoyne, R.D. XIV. The pathology of transformation of indolent B cell lymphomas. *Hematol. Oncol.* **2015**, *33*, 75–79. [CrossRef] [PubMed]
95. Fischer, T.; Zing, N.P.C.; Chiattone, C.S.; Federico, M.; Luminari, S. Transformed follicular lymphoma. *Ann. Hematol.* **2018**, *97*, 17–29. [CrossRef] [PubMed]
96. Federico, M.; Caballero Barrigón, M.D.; Marcheselli, L.; Tarantino, V.; Manni, M.; Sarkozy, C.; Alonso-Álvarez, S.; Wondergem, M.; Cartron, G.; Lopez-Guillermo, A.; et al. Rituximab and the risk of transformation of follicular lymphoma: A retrospective pooled analysis. *Lancet Haematol.* **2018**, *5*, e359–e367. [CrossRef]
97. Wagner-Johnston, N.D.; Link, B.K.; Byrtek, M.; Dawson, K.L.; Hainsworth, J.; Flowers, C.R.; Friedberg, J.W.; Bartlett, N.L. Outcomes of transformed follicular lymphoma in the modern era: A report from the National LymphoCare Study (NLCS). *Blood* **2015**, *126*, 851–857. [CrossRef]
98. Sarkozy, C.; Maurer, M.J.; Link, B.K.; Ghesquieres, H.; Nicolas, E.; Thompson, C.A.; Traverse-Glehen, A.; Feldman, A.L.; Allmer, C.; Slager, S.L.; et al. Cause of death in follicular lymphoma in the first decade of the rituximab era: A pooled analysis of French and US cohorts. *J. Clin. Oncol.* **2019**, *37*, 144–152. [CrossRef] [PubMed]
99. Gentles, A.J.; Alizadeh, A.A.; Lee, S.I.; Myklebust, J.H.; Shachaf, C.M.; Shahbaba, B.; Levy, R.; Koller, D.; Plevritis, S.K. A pluripotency signature predicts histologic transformation and influences survival in follicular lymphoma patients. *Blood* **2009**, *114*, 3158–3166. [CrossRef]
100. Glas, A.M.; Knoops, L.; Delahaye, L.; Kersten, M.J.; Kibbelaar, R.E.; Wessels, L.A.; Van Laar, R.; Van Krieken, J.H.J.M.; Baars, J.W.; Raemaekers, J.; et al. Gene-expression and immunohistochemical study of specific T-cell subsets and accessory cell types in the transformation and prognosis of follicular lymphoma. *J. Clin. Oncol.* **2007**, *25*, 390–398. [CrossRef] [PubMed]
101. Huet, S.; Sujobert, P.; Salles, G. From genetics to the clinic: A translational perspective on follicular lymphoma. *Nat. Rev. Cancer* **2018**, *18*, 224–239. [CrossRef] [PubMed]
102. Kumar, E.; Pickard, L.; Okosun, J. Pathogenesis of follicular lymphoma: Genetics to the microenvironment to clinical translation. *Br. J. Haematol.* **2021**, *194*, 810–821. [CrossRef] [PubMed]
103. Hilchey, S.P.; De, A.; Rimsza, L.M.; Bankert, R.B.; Bernstein, S.H. Follicular lymphoma intratumoral CD4$^+$CD25$^+$GITR$^+$ regulatory T cells potently suppress CD3/CD28-costimulated autologous and allogeneic CD8$^+$CD25$^-$ and CD4$^+$CD25$^-$ T cells. *J. Immunol.* **2007**, *178*, 4051–4061. [CrossRef] [PubMed]
104. Martinez-Climent, J.A.; Alizadeh, A.A.; Segraves, R.; Blesa, D.; Rubio-Moscardo, F.; Albertson, D.G.; Garcia-Conde, J.; Dyer, M.J.S.; Levy, R.; Pinkel, D.; et al. Transformation of follicular lymphoma to diffuse large cell lymphoma is associated with a heterogeneous set of DNA copy number and gene expression alterations. *Blood* **2003**, *101*, 3109–3117. [CrossRef] [PubMed]
105. Sander, C.A.; Yano, T.; Clark, H.M.; Harris, C.; Longo, D.L.; Jaffe, E.S.; Raffeld, M. p53 mutation is associated with progression in follicular lymphomas. *Blood* **1993**, *82*, 1994–2004. [CrossRef] [PubMed]
106. Pinyol, M.; Cobo, F.; Bea, S.; Jares, P.; Nayach, I.; Fernandez, P.L.; Montserrat, E.; Cardesa, A.; Campo, E. p16^{INK4a} gene inactivation by deletions, mutations, and hypermethylation is associated with transformed and aggressive variants of non-Hodgkin's lymphomas. *Blood* **1998**, *91*, 2977–2984. [CrossRef] [PubMed]
107. Akasaka, T.; Lossos, I.S.; Levy, R. BCL6 gene translocation in follicular lymphoma: A harbinger of eventual transformation to diffuse aggressive lymphoma. *Blood* **2003**, *102*, 1443–1448. [CrossRef] [PubMed]
108. Kridel, R.; Mottok, A.; Farinha, P.; Ben-Neriah, S.; Ennishi, D.; Zheng, Y.; Chavez, E.A.; Shulha, H.P.; Tan, K.; Chan, F.C.; et al. Cell of origin of transformed follicular lymphoma. *Blood* **2015**, *126*, 2118–2127. [CrossRef] [PubMed]
109. Brodtkorb, M.; Lingjærde, O.C.; Huse, K.; Trøen, G.; Hystad, M.; Hilden, V.I.; Myklebust, J.H.; Leich, E.; Rosenwald, A.; Delabie, J.; et al. Whole-genome integrative analysis reveals expression signatures predicting transformation in follicular lymphoma. *Blood* **2014**, *123*, 1051–1054. [CrossRef]
110. Yang, Z.Z.; Kim, H.J.; Villasboas, J.C.; Price-Troska, T.; Jalali, S.; Wu, H.; Luchtel, R.A.; Polley, M.Y.C.; Novak, A.J.; Ansell, S.M. Mass Cytometry Analysis Reveals that Specific Intratumoral CD4$^+$ T Cell Subsets Correlate with Patient Survival in Follicular Lymphoma. *Cell Rep.* **2019**, *26*, 2178–2193.e3. [CrossRef] [PubMed]

111. Pangault, C.; Amé-Thomas, P.; Ruminy, P.; Rossille, D.; Caron, G.; Baia, M.; De Vos, J.; Roussel, M.; Monvoisin, C.; Lamy, T.; et al. Follicular lymphoma cell niche: Identification of a preeminent IL-4-dependent T(FH)-B cell axis. *Leukemia* **2010**, *24*, 2080–2089. [CrossRef] [PubMed]
112. Amé-Thomas, P.; Le Priol, J.; Yssel, H.; Caron, G.; Pangault, C.; Jean, R.; Martin, N.; Marafioti, T.; Gaulard, P.; Lamy, T.; et al. Characterization of intratumoral follicular helper T cells in follicular lymphoma: Role in the survival of malignant B cells. *Leukemia* **2012**, *26*, 1053–1063. [CrossRef] [PubMed]
113. Amé-Thomas, P.; Hoeller, S.; Artchounin, C.; Misiak, J.; Braza, M.S.; Jean, R.; Le Priol, J.; Monvoisin, C.; Martin, N.; Gaulard, P.; et al. CD10 delineates a subset of human IL-4 producing follicular helper T cells involved in the survival of follicular lymphoma B cells. *Blood* **2015**, *125*, 2381–2385. [CrossRef] [PubMed]
114. Hori, S.; Nomura, T.; Sakaguchi, S. Control of regulatory T cell development by the transcription factor Foxp3. *Science* **2003**, *299*, 981–985. [CrossRef] [PubMed]
115. Fuhrman, C.A.; Yeh, W.-I.; Seay, H.R.; Saikumar Lakshmi, P.; Chopra, G.; Zhang, L.; Perry, D.J.; McClymont, S.A.; Yadav, M.; Lopez, M.-C.; et al. Divergent Phenotypes of Human Regulatory T Cells Expressing the Receptors TIGIT and CD226. *J. Immunol.* **2015**, *195*, 145–155. [CrossRef]
116. Nedelkovska, H.; Rosenberg, A.F.; Hilchey, S.P.; Hyrien, O.; Burack, W.R.; Quataert, S.A.; Baker, C.M.; Azadniv, M.; Welle, S.L.; Ansell, S.M.; et al. Follicular Lymphoma Tregs Have a Distinct Transcription Profile Impacting Their Migration and Retention in the Malignant Lymph Node. *PLoS ONE* **2016**, *11*, e0155347. [CrossRef] [PubMed]
117. Le, K.S.; Thibult, M.L.; Just-Landi, S.; Pastor, S.; Gondois-Rey, F.; Granjeaud, S.; Broussais, F.; Bouabdallah, R.; Colisson, R.; Caux, C.; et al. Follicular B Lymphomas Generate Regulatory T Cells via the ICOS/ICOSL Pathway and Are Susceptible to Treatment by Anti-ICOS/ICOSL Therapy. *Cancer Res.* **2016**, *76*, 4648–4660. [CrossRef] [PubMed]
118. Liu, X.; Venkataraman, G.; Lin, J.; Kiyotani, K.; Smith, S.; Montoya, M.; Nakamura, Y.; Kline, J. Highly clonal regulatory T-cell population in follicular lymphoma—Inverse correlation with the diversity of $CD8^+$ T cells. *Oncoimmunology* **2015**, *4*, e1002728. [CrossRef]
119. Linterman, M.A.; Pierson, W.; Lee, S.K.; Kallies, A.; Kawamoto, S.; Rayner, T.F.; Srivastava, M.; Divekar, D.P.; Beaton, L.; Hogan, J.J.; et al. $Foxp3^+$ follicular regulatory T cells control the germinal center response. *Nat. Med.* **2011**, *17*, 975–982. [CrossRef] [PubMed]
120. Álvaro-Naranjo, T.; Lejeune, M.; Salvadó, M.T.; Lopez, C.; Jaén, J.; Bosch, R.; Pons, L.E. Immunohistochemical patterns of reactive microenvironment are associated with clinicobiologic behavior in follicular lymphoma patients. *J. Clin. Oncol.* **2006**, *24*, 5350–5357. [CrossRef] [PubMed]
121. Laurent, C.; Müller, S.; Do, C.; Al-Saati, T.; Allart, S.; Larocca, L.M.; Hohaus, S.; Duchez, S.; Quillet-Mary, A.; Laurent, G.; et al. Distribution, function, and prognostic value of cytotoxic T lymphocytes in follicular lymphoma: A 3-D tissue-imaging study. *Blood* **2011**, *118*, 5371–5379. [CrossRef] [PubMed]
122. Yang, Z.Z.; Kim, H.J.; Villasboas, J.C.; Chen, Y.P.; Price-Troska, T.P.; Jalali, S.; Wilson, M.; Novak, A.J.; Ansell, S.M. Expression of LAG-3 defines exhaustion of intratumoral $PD-1^+$ T cells and correlates with poor outcome in follicular lymphoma. *Oncotarget* **2017**, *8*, 61425–61439. [CrossRef] [PubMed]
123. Gravelle, P.; Do, C.; Franchet, C.; Mueller, S.; Oberic, L.; Ysebaert, L.; Larocca, L.M.; Hohaus, S.; Calmels, M.N.; Frenois, F.X.; et al. Impaired functional responses in follicular lymphoma $CD8^+$ $TIM-3^+$ T lymphocytes following TCR engagement. *Oncoimmunology* **2016**, *5*, e1224044. [CrossRef]
124. Schmieder, A.; Michel, J.; Schönhaar, K.; Goerdt, S.; Schledzewski, K. Differentiation and gene expression profile of tumor-associated macrophages. *Semin. Cancer Biol.* **2012**, *22*, 289–297. [CrossRef] [PubMed]
125. Guilliams, M.; Mildner, A.; Yona, S. Developmental and Functional Heterogeneity of Monocytes. *Immunity* **2018**, *49*, 595–613. [CrossRef] [PubMed]
126. Dave, S.S.; Wright, G.; Tan, B.; Rosenwald, A.; Gascoyne, R.D.; Chan, W.C.; Fisher, R.I.; Braziel, R.M.; Rimsza, L.M.; Grogan, T.M.; et al. Prediction of survival in follicular lymphoma based on molecular features of tumor-infiltrating immune cells. *N. Engl. J. Med.* **2004**, *351*, 2159–2169. [CrossRef] [PubMed]
127. Kridel, R.; Xerri, L.; Gelas-Dore, B.; Tan, K.; Feugier, P.; Vawda, A.; Canioni, D.; Farinha, P.; Boussetta, S.; Moccia, A.A.; et al. The Prognostic Impact of CD163-Positive Macrophages in Follicular Lymphoma: A Study from the BC Cancer Agency and the Lymphoma Study Association. *Clin. Cancer Res.* **2015**, *21*, 3428–3435. [CrossRef]
128. Stevens, W.B.C.; Mendeville, M.; Redd, R.; Clear, A.J.; Bladergroen, R.; Calaminici, M.; Rosenwald, A.; Hoster, E.; Hiddemann, W.; Gaulard, P.; et al. Prognostic relevance of CD163 and CD8 combined with EZH2 and gain of chromosome 18 in follicular lymphoma: A study by the Lunenburg Lymphoma Biomarker Consortium. *Haematologica* **2017**, *102*, 1413–1423. [CrossRef] [PubMed]
129. Manches, O.; Lui, G.; Chaperot, L.; Gressin, R.; Molens, J.P.; Jacob, M.C.; Sotto, J.J.; Leroux, D.; Bensa, J.C.; Plumas, J. In vitro mechanisms of action of rituximab on primary non-Hodgkin lymphomas. *Blood* **2003**, *101*, 949–954. [CrossRef] [PubMed]
130. Chen, Y.P.; Kim, H.J.; Wu, H.; Price-Troska, T.; Villasboas, J.C.; Jalali, S.; Feldman, A.L.; Novak, A.J.; Yang, Z.Z.; Ansell, S.M. SIRPα expression delineates subsets of intratumoral monocyte/macrophages with different functional and prognostic impact in follicular lymphoma. *Blood Cancer J.* **2019**, *9*, 84. [CrossRef] [PubMed]

131. Amin, R.; Mourcin, F.; Uhel, F.; Pangault, C.; Ruminy, P.; Dupré, L.; Guirriec, M.; Marchand, T.; Fest, T.; Lamy, T.; et al. DC-SIGN-expressing macrophages trigger activation of mannosylated IgM B-cell receptor in follicular lymphoma. *Blood* **2015**, *126*, 1911–1920. [CrossRef]
132. Lamaison, C.; Tarte, K. B cell/stromal cell crosstalk in health, disease, and treatment: Follicular lymphoma as a paradigm. *Immunol. Rev.* **2021**, *302*, 273–285. [CrossRef] [PubMed]
133. Pastore, A.; Jurinovic, V.; Kridel, R.; Hoster, E.; Staiger, A.M.; Szczepanowski, M.; Pott, C.; Kopp, N.; Murakami, M.; Horn, H.; et al. Integration of gene mutations in risk prognostication for patients receiving first-line immunochemotherapy for follicular lymphoma: A retrospective analysis of a prospective clinical trial and validation in a population-based registry. *Lancet Oncol.* **2015**, *16*, 1111–1122. [CrossRef]
134. Huet, S.; Tesson, B.; Jais, J.P.; Feldman, A.L.; Magnano, L.; Thomas, E.; Traverse-Glehen, A.; Albaud, B.; Carrère, M.; Xerri, L.; et al. A gene-expression profiling score for prediction of outcome in patients with follicular lymphoma: A retrospective training and validation analysis in three international cohorts. *Lancet. Oncol.* **2018**, *19*, 549–561. [CrossRef]
135. Sorigue, M.; Sancho, J.M. Current prognostic and predictive factors in follicular lymphoma. *Ann. Hematol.* **2018**, *97*, 209–227. [CrossRef]
136. Lauer, E.M.; Mutter, J.; Scherer, F. Circulating tumor DNA in B-cell lymphoma: Technical advances, clinical applications, and perspectives for translational research. *Leukemia* **2022**, *36*, 2151–2164. [CrossRef]
137. Davids, M.S.; Roberts, A.W.; Seymour, J.F.; Pagel, J.M.; Kahl, B.S.; Wierda, W.G.; Puvvada, S.; Kipps, T.J.; Anderson, M.A.; Salem, A.H.; et al. Phase I First-in-Human Study of Venetoclax in Patients With Relapsed or Refractory Non-Hodgkin Lymphoma. *J. Clin. Oncol.* **2017**, *35*, 826–833. [CrossRef]
138. Zinzani, P.L.; Flinn, I.W.; Yuen, S.L.S.; Topp, M.S.; Rusconi, C.; Fleury, I.; Le Dû, K.; Arthur, C.; Pro, B.; Gritti, G.; et al. Venetoclax-rituximab with or without bendamustine vs bendamustine-rituximab in relapsed/refractory follicular lymphoma. *Blood* **2020**, *136*, 2628–2637. [CrossRef]
139. Morschhauser, F.; Tilly, H.; Chaidos, A.; McKay, P.; Phillips, T.; Assouline, S.; Batlevi, C.L.; Campbell, P.; Ribrag, V.; Damaj, G.L.; et al. Tazemetostat for patients with relapsed or refractory follicular lymphoma: An open-label, single-arm, multicentre, phase 2 trial. *Lancet Oncol.* **2020**, *21*, 1433–1442. [CrossRef]
140. Ogura, M.; Ando, K.; Suzuki, T.; Ishizawa, K.; Oh, S.Y.; Itoh, K.; Yamamoto, K.; Au, W.Y.; Tien, H.F.; Matsuno, Y.; et al. A multicentre phase II study of vorinostat in patients with relapsed or refractory indolent B-cell non-Hodgkin lymphoma and mantle cell lymphoma. *Br. J. Haematol.* **2014**, *165*, 768–776. [CrossRef]
141. Chen, R.; Frankel, P.; Popplewell, L.; Siddiqi, T.; Ruel, N.; Rotter, A.; Thomas, S.H.; Mott, M.; Nathwani, N.; Htut, M.; et al. A phase II study of vorinostat and rituximab for treatment of newly diagnosed and relapsed/refractory indolent non-Hodgkin lymphoma. *Haematologica* **2015**, *100*, 357–362. [CrossRef]
142. Oki, Y.; Buglio, D.; Fanale, M.; Fayad, L.; Copeland, A.; Romaguera, J.; Kwak, L.W.; Pro, B.; De Castro Faria, S.; Neelapu, S.; et al. Phase I study of panobinostat plus everolimus in patients with relapsed or refractory lymphoma. *Clin. Cancer Res.* **2013**, *19*, 6882–6890. [CrossRef] [PubMed]
143. Batlevi, C.L.; Crump, M.; Andreadis, C.; Rizzieri, D.; Assouline, S.E.; Fox, S.; van der Jagt, R.H.C.; Copeland, A.; Potvin, D.; Chao, R.; et al. A phase 2 study of mocetinostat, a histone deacetylase inhibitor, in relapsed or refractory lymphoma. *Br. J. Haematol.* **2017**, *178*, 434–441. [CrossRef] [PubMed]
144. Leonard, J.P.; Trneny, M.; Izutsu, K.; Fowler, N.H.; Hong, X.; Zhu, J.; Zhang, H.; Offner, F.; Scheliga, A.; Nowakowski, G.S.; et al. AUGMENT: A Phase III study of lenalidomide plus rituximab versus placebo plus rituximab in relapsed or refractory indolent lymphoma. *J. Clin. Oncol.* **2019**, *37*, 1188–1199. [CrossRef] [PubMed]
145. Morschhauser, F.; Fowler, N.H.; Feugier, P.; Bouabdallah, R.; Tilly, H.; Palomba, M.L.; Fruchart, C.; Libby, E.N.; Casasnovas, R.-O.; Flinn, I.W.; et al. Rituximab plus Lenalidomide in Advanced Untreated Follicular Lymphoma. *N. Engl. J. Med.* **2018**, *379*, 934–947. [CrossRef]
146. Advani, R.; Flinn, I.; Popplewell, L.; Forero, A.; Bartlett, N.L.; Ghosh, N.; Kline, J.; Roschewski, M.; LaCasce, A.; Collins, G.P.; et al. CD47 Blockade by Hu5F9-G4 and Rituximab in Non-Hodgkin's Lymphoma. *N. Engl. J. Med.* **2018**, *379*, 1711–1721. [CrossRef]
147. Budde, L.E.; Sehn, L.H.; Matasar, M.J.; Schuster, S.J.; Assouline, S.; Giri, P.; Kuruvilla, J.; Canales, M.; Dietrich, S.; Fay, K.; et al. Mosunetuzumab Monotherapy Is an Effective and Well-Tolerated Treatment Option for Patients with Relapsed/Refractory (R/R) Follicular Lymphoma (FL) Who Have Received ≥2 Prior Lines of Therapy: Pivotal Results from a Phase I/II Study. *Blood* **2021**, *138*, 127. [CrossRef]
148. Korfi, K.; Ali, S.; Heward, J.A.; Fitzgibbon, J. Follicular lymphoma, a B cell malignancy addicted to epigenetic mutations. *Epigenetics* **2017**, *12*, 370–377. [CrossRef]
149. Horsman, D.E.; Okamoto, I.; Ludkovski, O.; Le, N.; Harder, L.; Gesk, S.; Siebert, R.; Chhanabhai, M.; Sehn, L.; Connors, J.M.; et al. Follicular lymphoma lacking the t(14;18)(q32;q21): Identification of two disease subtypes. *Br. J. Haematol.* **2003**, *120*, 424–433. [CrossRef]
150. Carbone, A.; Roulland, S.; Gloghini, A.; Younes, A.; von Keudell, G.; López-Guillermo, A.; Fitzgibbon, J. Follicular lymphoma. *Nat. Rev. Dis. Prim.* **2019**, *5*, 83. [CrossRef]

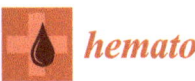

Review

Genetics of Transformed Follicular Lymphoma

Miguel Alcoceba [1,†], María García-Álvarez [1,†], Jessica Okosun [2], Simone Ferrero [3], Marco Ladetto [4,5], Jude Fitzgibbon [2] and Ramón García-Sanz [1,*]

1. Department of Haematology, University Hospital of Salamanca (HUS/IBSAL), CIBERONC, Cancer Research Centre–IBMCC (USAL-CSIC), 37007 Salamanca, Spain
2. Centre for Haemato-Oncology, Barts Cancer Institute, Queen Mary University of London, London EC1M 5PZ, UK
3. Department of Molecular Biotechnologies and Health Sciences–Hematology Division, University of Torino, 10126 Torino, Italy
4. Department of Translational Medicine, University of Eastern Piedmont, 28100 Novara, Italy
5. Division of Hematology, Azienda Ospedaliera SS Antonio e Biagio e Cesare Arrigo, 15121 Alessandria, Italy
* Correspondence: rgarcias@usal.es
† These authors contributed equally to this work.

Abstract: Histological transformation (HT) to a more aggressive disease–mostly diffuse large B-cell lymphoma–is considered one of the most dismal events in the clinical course of follicular lymphoma (FL). Current knowledge has not found a single biological event specific for HT, although different studies have highlighted common genetic alterations, such as *TP53* and *CDKN2A/B* loss, and *MYC* translocations, among others. Together, they increase genomic complexity and mutational burden at HT. A better knowledge of HT pathogenesis would presumably help to find diagnostic biomarkers allowing the identification of patients at high-risk of transformation, as well as the discrimination from patients with FL recurrence, and those who remain in remission. This would also help to identify new drug targets and the design of clinical trials for the treatment of transformation. In the present review we provide a comprehensive overview of the genetic events frequently identified in transformed FL contributing to the switch towards aggressive behaviour, and we will discuss current open questions in the field of HT.

Keywords: transformed follicular lymphoma; genetics; histological transformation

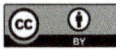

1. Introduction

Follicular lymphoma (FL) is a B-cell lymphoid neoplasm whose origin is the germinal centre cells present in the lymphoid follicle of the lymph nodes. It constitutes the second most frequent non-Hodgkin's lymphoma (NHL), with an estimated incidence of 20–30% of all lymphomas in western countries, and approximately 2.2 new cases per 100,000 inhabitants per year [1–4]. In a prospective epidemiological registry of lymphoid neoplasms (RELINF) initiated in 2014 by the Spanish GELTAMO group (Grupo Español de Linfoma y Trasplante de Médula Ósea), 23.1% (*n* = 2099) of B-cell lymphomas were FL [5]. The median age of presentation is ~60 years, being infrequent in young patients.

The number of centroblasts (enlarged activated B-cells) visualised by light microscopy distinguishes the histological grades of FL: grade 1 (0–5 centroblasts per high-power–40×magnification, 0.159 mm^2–microscopic field–HPF), grade 2 (6–15 centroblasts per HPF), and grade 3, further differentiated into 3A (>15 centroblasts per HPF, with centrocytes -B-cells with irregular or cleaved nucleus-still present) and 3B (extensive and diffuse infiltration by centroblasts or immunoblasts). In the clinical practice, grade 3B FL management is similar to that of diffuse large B-cell lymphoma (DLBCL), due to its more aggressive clinical behaviour. In the recent updates of the classification of lymphoid neoplasms [6,7], in addition to classical nodal FL, there are other types of FL recognised, including the in situ follicular B-cell neoplasm, duodenal type FL, paediatric FL, as well as the provisional entity BCL2-rearrangement negative, CD23-positive follicle centre lymphoma, which will not be the subject of the present review.

The prognosis of patients with nodal FL is relatively favourable, reflecting their generally indolent behaviour, with median survival over 15 years, thanks in part to the introduction of immunotherapy both at induction and relapse [8–10]. However, continuous relapses, decreases in the response duration, and the gradual acquisition of drug resistance defines the clinical pattern of this lymphoma, often leading to the death of the patients [2,11]. Additionally ~20% of patients progress within 24 months of treatment and half of them die within five years [12,13]; on the other hand, those who remain in complete remission within 24 months of treatment have a similar overall survival (OS) as the general population [14].

Historically, approximately 3% of FL patients per year transform into an aggressive lymphoma, commonly DLBCL, as a first or a later event, even in the absence of treatment. More recently, the cumulative incidence of histological transformation (HT) is lower since the incorporation of rituximab. In a European series with more than 5000 patients studied, the cumulative incidence of HT as a first event at five years was 7% in patients who had not received rituximab, while it was 5% in those who had received rituximab only at induction, and 3% in patients who received rituximab not only at induction but also at maintenance [15]. HT has been considered one of the most unfavourable events in FL's natural history, with a five-year survival from transformation (SFT) of ~20–30% both prior to and in the rituximab era [16–22], although this survival increases up to 40–50% when considering only transformation as a first event [15]. Those cases experiencing early histological transformation show a reduced five-year SFT compared to late histological transformation, although the time point to define early/late HT has to be validated [15,19,23]. Therefore, the prediction of histological transformation at diagnosis remains a challenge [24].

In the present work we will review the most frequent genetic events described in transformed FL and discuss current open questions in this field.

2. Definition of FL Transformation

The gold standard for determining FL transformation is based on the histologically confirmed progression of grade 1, 2, or 3A FL to a high-grade lymphoma, consisting of a predominance of large cells and the loss of the follicular architecture [23,25]. Most of the transformed cases have a DLBCL histology (>80% of the cases) according to the current WHO classification, although other histologies have been described, such as high-grade B-cell lymphoma, FL grade 3B, Burkitt lymphoma, B lymphoblastic leukemia/lymphoma, and plasmablastic lymphoma [25–28]. There are other atypical forms suggestive of histological transformation, such as the presence at diagnosis of both FL and DLBCL cells, at the same site, referred to as composite lymphoma, or at different sites such as DLBCL in the lymph node and FL in bone marrow, as well as DLBCL cases that undergo a process of reverse transformation, relapsing as a lower grade lymphoma. These forms are not addressed in the present review.

Since lymphoma lesions are not isolated, other tumour areas might have a FL component at the same time in addition to the transformation area [23,29,30]. Positron emission tomography and computerized tomography (PET/CT) could help by selecting the biopsy site according to the highest standardized uptake value (SUV) of 18[F] fluorodeoxyglucose, since a high value (generally > 14) is correlated with more aggressive histology [31]. However, only ~50% of patients are biopsied, with inaccessibility of the tumour, the patient's clinical situation or refusal among the main reasons [32]. Based on the clinical behaviour of transformed patients, several clinical criteria of transformation suspicion could be of utility in these cases, including an increase in lactate dehydrogenase (LDH) levels or hypercalcemia, rapid lymphadenopathy growth or the appearance of lymphoma masses or conglomerates, and the novel involvement of extranodal sites and new B symptoms. However, these criteria vary between studies and are not standardised [16,18,19]. Moreover, these clinical criteria are also present in patients who progress without transformation [32].

3. Clonal Evolution

Clonality analysis to test the relationship between the transformation and diagnosis samples is essential to distinguish true transformed cases from a secondary de novo DLBCL, and is especially recommended when the transformation occurs years later after the FL biopsy [25,33]. It is well known in transformation from chronic lymphocytic leukaemia (CLL), namely Richter syndrome (RS), that clonally unrelated cases can represent up to 20% of all histological transformations in this setting. This fact can have clinical implications, because clonally unrelated cases have a superior survival rate compared to clonally related cases [3,34]. Studies in FL suggest that up to 5% of the transformed cases are clonally unrelated to their FL counterpart at diagnosis [35,36]. Due to the lack of clonality testing in several studies, the availability of paired low-grade and transformed samples and the relatively low incidence of clonally unrelated cases, it is currently unknown whether these cases could have a different clinical outcome compared to clonally related cases.

The pattern of clonal evolution in transformed FLs follows two main models: (i) the linear model, a direct evolution of the transformed clone from the indolent lymphoma by the acquisition of new lesions, and therefore retaining the genetic aberrations of the indolent phase; (ii) the divergent/branching model, in which both the FL and the clonal related transformed samples presumably derived from a common progenitor clone (CPC), which independently acquired some genetic events at each phase. Both indolent and aggressive clones will share the genetic events present in the CPC, such as t(14;18), and mutations in *KMT2D*, and *CREBBP*, which drives lymphomagenesis (Figure 1).

Few studies have analysed paired clonally related FL and transformed FL samples with next-generation sequencing (NGS), mainly due to the difficulties in case recruitment, or in obtaining DNA with good quality and quantity at both events. Previous work using karyotype, SNP-arrays or custom NGS panels to analyse a limited set of mutations have observed a slightly higher incidence of the divergent evolution model (>50%) [37–40]. However, accurate classification of transformed cases on each model highly depends on the number of genetic alterations studied and the inclusion of other samples of the FL evolution. Indeed, up to 70% of transformations were classified as divergent when FL relapse samples were added to the analysis [39,41]. In addition, when we consider studies using whole-genome (WGS) or whole-exome sequencing (WES), most cases (~90%) present a divergent evolution [28,41,42]. This predominance of the divergent model contrasts with other transformed B-cell lymphoproliferative disorders, such as in RS-CLL, in which the evolution usually follows a linear model [43]. In addition, two patterns of evolution from the CPC have been identified. The most frequent (~80%) is the 'rich' CPC pattern, in which there is high similarity of genetic events shared in FL and transformed samples. The other one is the 'sparse' CPC pattern, in which only a few genetic alterations are shared between both samples [41].

Despite the use of different treatments, the CPC is difficult to eradicate and can persist over time. The development of a donor-derived FL several years after an allogeneic stem-cell transplantation (allo-SCT), sharing identical t(14;18) breakpoint, immunoglobulin heavy chain (IGHV) usage, and different genetic events between recipient and donor, further support the existence of this CPC and its persistence over time [44,45].

In FL progression, the responsible progression-contributing clones are already present at diagnosis. In contrast, the dominant clone(s) at transformation were very rarely detected (<1%) or absent at diagnosis even after analyses with ultra-sensitive variant detection methods [28]. Several possibilities can explain why the responsible clone at transformation was not seen at diagnosis: (1) very low numbers, which would have required even more sensitive detection methods to identify the original clone at diagnosis; (2) the presence of the responsible subclone at a different site compared to the primary site, perhaps requiring the analyses of several lymphoma biopsies or liquid biopsy [46]; or (3) the emergence of new clones being responsible for the transformation after the diagnosis.

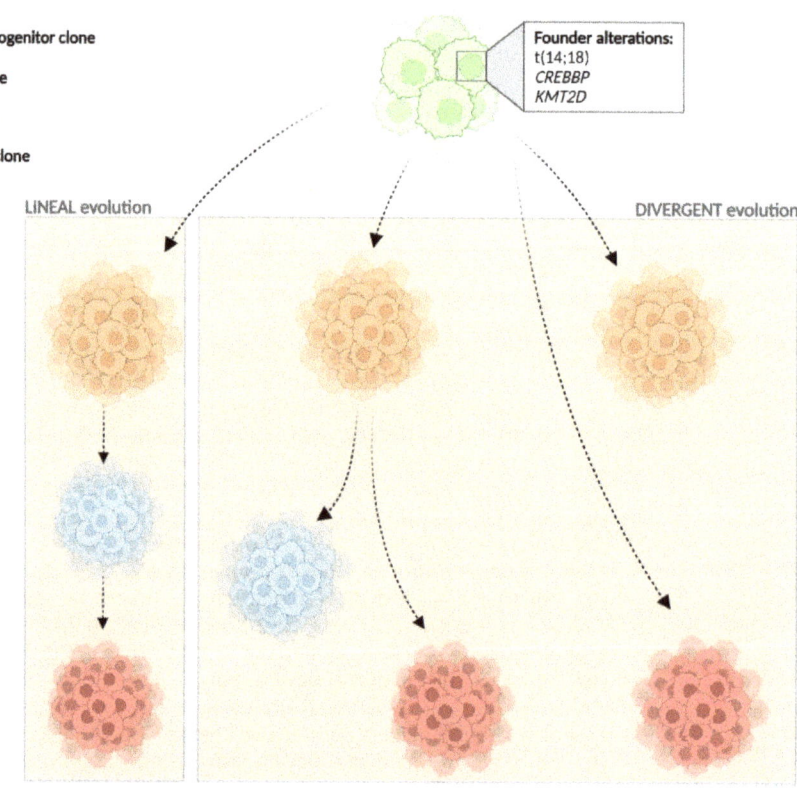

Figure 1. Models of clonal evolution in histological transformation.

Similarly, three evolution models have been proposed by analysing the somatic hypermutation of IGHV. In one, CPCs could coexist in FL and HT in the same lymph node. In the second, CPCs could be present only in the pre-lymphoma germinal centre, with the FL and HT arising independently of these CPCs. The third model proposes that the CPCs are maintained in bone marrow niches before acquiring new lesions and migrating to cause HT [44]; the last model is also supported by the development of FL in healthy individuals in whom a t(14;18) was detectable years before the diagnosis, as well as by the two transformed FL cases of donor origin after an allo-SCT [44,45,47]. It is plausible that the three models occur in different patients or even coexist in some cases.

These data, together with the predominance of the divergent model, implies that the predominant tumour clone at FL diagnosis is not the direct precursor of the transformed clone in most of the cases, and therefore the genetic events identified at diagnosis probably would not help to predict transformation.

4. Cell of Origin and Pathogenesis of FL Transformation

Transformed cases may have changes in their immunophenotype, with an antigenic drift including CD10 loss or positivity of MUM1/IRF4. Although most transformed FLs are of germinal B-cell DLBCL subtype (GCB), up to 15–20% of the cases change to an activated B-cell (ABC) without differences in survival between both subtypes [27,48,49]. This contrasts with transformation in other B-cell lymphoproliferative disorders, such as CLL, Waldenström macroglobulinemia or marginal zone lymphoma, in which transformed cases are mostly ABC/non-GCB [50–52].

Recurrent rearranged genes in DLBCL include *BCL2*, *BCL6* and *MYC*. There are no major changes in the frequency of *BCL2* or *BCL6* translocations in transformed samples compared to FL diagnosis, however, *MYC* translocations are commonly acquired and are present in 25% of transformed cases [27,42]. The acquisition of *MYC* translocations implies an increase in the proportion of double-hit lymphomas (presence of both *BCL2* and *MYC* translocations) in transformed patients, which is associated with a shorter SFT [27], although differences were not statistically significant likely due to the low number of cases analysed.

High-resolution genome wide analysis using SNP-array, WGS or WES, and targeted next-generation sequencing studies in transformed FL identify increased genomic complexity and mutational burden at transformation in comparison to FL [28,39,41,42,53–56]. The most recurrent genetic lesions acquired in transformed FL cases are summarized in Table 1 and Figure 2, and include alterations (mainly mutations and/or deletions) in *TP53* in approximately 15–30% transformed cases, *CDKN2A/B* deletions in 20–30% of cases, and *B2M* mutations and/or deletions in 20–25% of cases, together with the previously mentioned *MYC* translocations [28,39,41,42,54,55,57]. Of note, although these lesions are commonly acquired in transformation, they are not specific, as they could also be present at diagnosis or acquired during disease recurrence, representing markers of more aggressive disease [25,28,39,41,42,54,55,58]. In fact, these are also common acquired lesions in refractoriness and/or transformation in other haematological disorders [43,59].

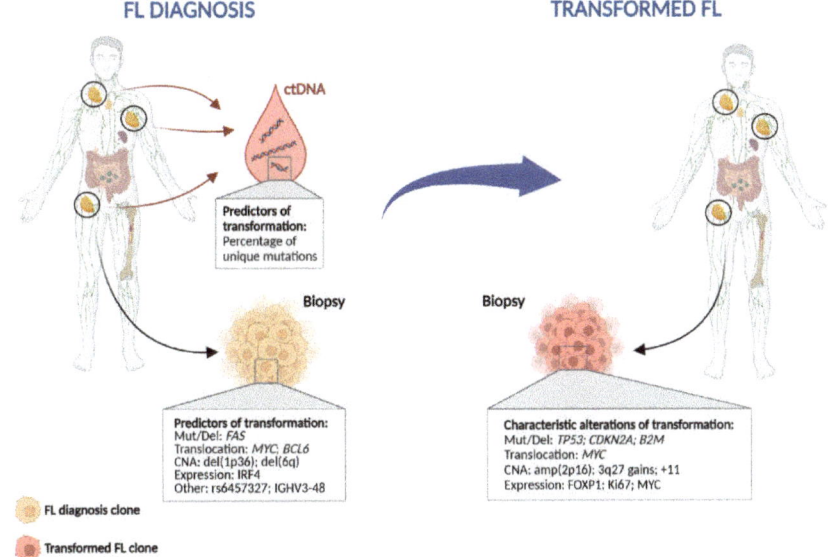

Figure 2. Characteristic genetic events in follicular lymphoma histological transformation. Left: Potential predictors of transformation; Right: Genetic alterations commonly found at histological transformation. CNA: copy number alteration; ctDNA: circulating tumour DNA; Mut/Del: mutation and/or deletion.

Other commonly acquired events include mutations in *MYC*, *CCND3*, *CD58*, *EBF1*, *GNA13*, *P2RY8*, and *S1PR2*, as well as gains of 3q27.3-q28 (*BCL6*), amplification of 2p16 (*REL*), and gains in chromosomes 2, 5, and 11 [28,35,41,42,54,55,60,61]. All of these alterations together indicate that different pathways may be involved in transformation, including both cell cycle and DNA damage dysregulation, immune escape, JAK-STAT or NF-κB pathways, increased proliferation, and lymphoma cell migration.

When transformed cases are classified according to their cell-of-origin, different patterns of mutations are observed in each group. *MYD88*, *CD79B*, and *BCL10* mutations are more frequently (~15–25%) identified in ABC transformed cases, while amplification of 2p16 (*REL*) are more common in GCB, consistent with what is observed in DLBCL [28,54,55,61]. This suggests that there could be at least two different subgroups of transformed FLs. Moreover, recent studies have classified de novo DLBCL into different molecular clusters according to their mutation, copy-number and structural variation profile, and these clusters are associated with different outcomes [62,63]. There is no information regarding the distribution of these clusters in transformed FL, although some of the most common alterations in HT such as *TP53* mutations/deletions, *CDKN2A/B* deletions and *REL* amplification are present in cluster C2, while C5 and MCD comprised mostly ABC-DLBCL, with mutations in *CD79B* and *MYD88* [62,63]. This suggests that different clusters of transformed FL could be present, possibly with different pathways leading to transformation, and perhaps a distinct outcome. In line with this, a previous study showed an increased proliferation rate by gene expression analysis at transformation in a subgroup of HT, which was enriched with aberrations in *TP53*, *CDKN2A/B*, and *REL* in contrast to other HT, suggesting different mechanisms of transformation [48]. Similarly, previous studies in CLL have suggested three groups of RS, one of them with alterations in *TP53* and deletions in *CDKN2A/B* with poorer prognosis than other RS [64]

Table 1. Biological and genetic factors enriched at follicular lymphoma histological transformation in the literature.

Category	Variable	Biological Effect	Effect on Transformation
IHQ and microenvironment	IRF4 expression	-	Increased at HT [27]
	MYC expression	-	Increased at HT [65]
	FOXP1 expression	-	Increased at HT [66]
	TP53 mutation and deletion	Cell cycle	Increased at HT [28,39,41,42,55]
	B2microglobulin mutation and deletion	Immune surveillance	Increased at HT [28,42]
	FAS mutation and deletion	Apoptosis	Enriched in transformed cases [42]
	MYC mutation and translocation	Cell cycle	Increased at HT [27,42]
	CCND3 mutation	Cell cycle, JAK-STAT signalling	Increased at HT [28,39]
	EBF1 mutation	B-cell development	Increased at HT [28,41]
	GNA13 mutation	NF-kB/BCR signalling	Increased at HT [28]
	P2RY8 mutation	B-cell migration	Increased at HT [28]
	S1PR2 mutation	Proliferation	Increased at HT [28]
	CD58 mutation	Immune surveillance	Increased at HT [42]
	MYD88 mutation	NF-kB/BCR signalling	Increased at HT, ABC-HT related [28,39,41,55]
Genomic variants	CD79B mutation	NF-kB/BCR signalling	Increased at HT, ABC-HT related [28,39,55]
	BCL10 mutation	NF-kB/BCR signalling	Increased at HT, ABC-HT related [28,55]
	CDKN2A/B deletion	Cell cycle	Increased at HT [28,41,42,54,57,61]
	BCL6 translocation	B-cell differentiation	Increased at HT [27,67]
	2p16 (REL) amplification	NF-kB/BCR signalling	Increased at HT, GCB-HT related [35,42,54,60,61]
	3q27.3-q28 (BCL6) gains	B-cell differentiation	Increased at HT [35,42,54,60]
	Chromosomes 2, 5 and 11 gains	-	Increased at HT [35,54]
	Genomic complexity -copy-number changes-	-	Increased at HT [28,41,42,53–56]
	Genetic complexity -mutations-	-	Increased at HT [28,39,41,42,55,68]

HT: Histological transformation.

5. Can We Predict Transformation at Diagnosis?

5.1. Clinical, Biological and Immunohistochemical Factors

Several retrospective and prospective studies analysing clinical variables in the rituximab era have suggested that a higher Follicular Lymphoma International Prognostic Index (FLIPI) at diagnosis as well as some of their individual factors (elevated serum LDH, advanced stage or low haemoglobin) associates with a higher risk of transformation [18–22,32]. Other clinical indexes evaluated, including FLIPI-2 and PRIMA-PI, are of limited value in predicting HT [69]. Moreover, an association with higher risk of transformation is also observed in patients experiencing a poor response to first-line treatment, especially in those cases which are refractory [22,70]. The FLIPI index is prognostic of OS and therefore it could be a poor tool to specifically predict transformation. Overall, lymphoma-related death is the main cause of mortality in FL [71]. However, lymphoma-related death is prominent in patients who experience transformation in contrast to patients who do not, thus indicating that transformation in FL is the major cause of lymphoma-related death. In line with this, a higher cumulative incidence of lymphoma-related death has also been observed in patients with a higher FLIPI, as well as those who do not achieve event-free survival at 24 months [71]. Thus, FLIPI will potentially play a role in predicting transformation, probably as part of an integrated clinical and biological score.

According to the histological grade, FL grade 3A patients have a higher risk of transformation according to some studies [27,32] but not in others [19–22]. MUM1/IRF4 expression is significantly higher in FL grade 3A than in FL grades 1–2 [72,73], and the positive MUM1/IRF4 expression at diagnosis has been associated with transformation [27], as well as lower progression-free (PFS) survival and OS in FL [74,75].

Different individual protein expressions have been associated with unfavourable outcomes in FL. For example, FOXP1 protein levels have been previously associated with failure-free survival and shorter OS in immunochemotherapy-treated patients [66,76], although no impact on progression of disease within 24 months (POD24) was observed in clinical trials [77]. FOXP1 regulates germinal centre differentiation and promotes B cell survival [78–80]. FOXP1 protein levels were higher in non-GCB DLBCL, and have also been associated with shorter PFS and OS in DLBCL [81]. Although higher FOXP1 protein levels at transformation were observed [66], their role at diagnosis in transformation prediction have not been assessed. Similarly, higher MYC expression has been identified in HT as compared to diagnosis [65], although its role at diagnosis is unknown.

5.2. Genetic Aberrations

All FL cells harbour a clonal rearrangement of the immunoglobulin heavy chain gene (*IGH*). Previous reports showed a biased repertoire in FL in comparison with normal CD5 negative lymphocytes, with *IGHV3-23*, and *IGHV3-48* genes the commonest in FLs [36,82,83]. We have recently reported that patients carrying the *IGHV3-48* gene have a higher risk of transformation (Figure 2) [36]. IGHV gene usage was previously associated with higher risk of transformation in CLL bearing the *IGHV4-39* gene [84]. These findings require further validation in prospective series.

At diagnosis, the role in transformation of the frequent individual genetic alterations is controversial. Although *TP53* alterations (mutations or deletions) are rare at diagnosis (~5%), they have been associated with high POD24, shorter PFS and shorter OS, but not with risk of transformation [56,68,85–88]. *MYC* translocations at diagnosis are also an infrequent event (<3%), and most of these cases would therefore be double-hit lymphomas with *BCL2* and *MYC* translocations [89,90]. These cases usually have a shorter PFS, OS and SFT [91], although the very low number of *MYC* translocated cases precludes drawing definitive conclusions. *CDKN2A/B* deletions (<10%) have also been correlated with inferior PFS and OS [56,58]. Interestingly, methylation of *CDKN2A* is a more frequent event (~20%) and is also correlated with shorter OS [58]. Together, these genetic alterations are rare events at diagnosis (<5%), but they have not been generally studied in large cohorts, especially analysing their role in transformation.

Other genetic events are present at similar frequency at diagnosis and at transformation, however a potential role in transformation has been suggested. *FAS* mutations (~5–10%) and deletions (~20%) are predominant in patients who will transform, suggesting that *FAS* alterations could be an early biomarker in transformation, although these findings require further validation [42]. *FAS* mutations have also been observed in GCB-DLBCL associated with an inferior outcome [92]. *BCL6* translocations at diagnosis are associated with a high risk of transformation [27,67], with a slightly increased frequency at transformation (25% at HT and 10% at diagnosis). *BCL6* translocations were similarly found in GCB or ABC HT [27], in contrast to DLBCL, in which they are more frequent in ABC cases [93].

At diagnosis, chromosomal imbalances have been recurrently identified in FL, including gains of 1q, 2p, +7, 12, 18, X, and losses in 1p36, 6q, 10q, and a copy-neutral loss of heterozygosity (CNN-LOH) in 1p, 6p and 16p, some of them correlated with a worse prognosis [53,54,56,94–98]. Losses in 1p36, 6q and CNN-LOH in 16p were also associated with high risk of transformation (Figure 2 and Table 2) [53,94,97]. although most of these studies included patients treated prior to the rituximab era and require validation.

Some genetic mutations alter FL B-cell interaction with the microenvironment. HVEM, encoded by the *TNFRSF14* gene, regulates T-cell response, delivering costimulatory or coinhibitory signals, depending on the ligand [99,100]. The BTLA ligand is expressed by B-cells and its interaction with HVEM inhibits T-cell response [99]. The *TNFRSF14* gene is disrupted by mutations (~30–40%), deletions, (~20–30%) and/or CNN-LOHs (~10%) in FL patients [41,53,54,68,97]. This would lead to reduced HVEM expression [101,102] and higher BTLA signalling [102]. Therefore, the inhibitory signalling of the HVEM-BTLA axis is disrupted by *TNFRSF14* aberrations modifying the microenvironment and inducing B-cell expansion, activated lymphoid stroma and increased number of follicular T helper cells [102]. Other genetic mutations altering the microenvironment include *CREBBP* mutations, which are involved in FL immune evasion by both decreasing the proliferation of T-cells and antigen presentation via downregulating the major histocompatibility complex (MHC) class II [103], and mutations in *CTSS* or *RRAGC*, which alter CD4+ T-cell interactions [104,105].

Table 2. Biological, genetic and clinical risk factors at follicular lymphoma diagnosis associated with histological transformation in the literature.

Category	Variable	Effect on Transformation
Clinical	High FLIPI (≥ 3)	Higher risk of HT [18–22,32]
	FL Grade 3A	Higher risk of HT (controversial) [27,32]
	High IRF4 expression	Higher risk of HT [27]
IHQ and microenvironment	High levels of lymphoma-associated macrophages	Shorter time to HT [106]
	High density of CD21 Follicular dendritic cells	Shorter time to HT, absent at HT [106]
	High levels of CD4+, CD8+, CD57+, PD1+, and FOXP3+	Higher risk of HT [106]
	Follicular pattern of FOXP3+ T-cells	Higher risk of HT [107]
	Low tumour distance to blood vessels	Higher risk of HT [108]
Genomic variants	1p36, 6q deletions	Higher risk of HT [94,97]
	BCL6, MYC translocations	Higher risk of HT [27,42,67]
	16p CNN-LOH	Higher risk of HT [53]
	IGHV3-48 gene usage	Higher risk of HT [36]
	SNP rs6457327 (6p region)	Higher risk of HT [109]
	Circulating tumour DNA mutations	Higher risk of HT [46]

CNN-LOH: copy number neutral loss of heterozygosity; HT: Histological transformation; SNP: single nucleotide polymorphism.

In summary, no single factor has been shown to accurately predict transformation, but the combination of several genomic aberrations could be a good predictor of transformation. The m7-FLIPI index, which integrates the FLIPI clinical variables and performance status with the mutational status of 7 genes—*ARID1A, CARD11, CREBBP, EP300, EZH2, FOXO1,* and *MEF2B*—better classified patients with treatment failure, POD24 and OS than FLIPI [86,87]. The POD24-PI, which includes FLIPI and the mutational status of 3 genes—*EZH2, EP300,* and *FOXO1,* demonstrated superiority to identify POD24 patients in comparison with FLIPI and m7-FLIPI [87]. However, none of these scores has been used to assess the risk of transformation. The same can be said for genomic (copy-number aberrations -CNAs- or CNN-LOH) or genetic (mutations) complexity, which is associated with POD24, and inferior PFS, and OS when they are present at diagnosis [56,68]. Although their frequencies are increased at transformation, their role in prediction is still unknown.

In addition, several genetic expression signatures have been associated with higher risk of transformation in FL in the pre-rituximab era, which includes a pluripotency signature composed of embryonic stem cell genes [110], and a six NF-kβ target signature scores [111], being the BTK score later validated in a series of patients receiving immunotherapy [112].

5.3. Tumour Microenvironment

Several components of the tumour microenvironment, including lymphoma-associated macrophages (LAMs), follicular dendritic cells (FDCs), and different T-cell subsets, may play a key role in FL outcome [113–116].

A higher level of LAMs has been associated with a worse PFS and OS in the pre-rituximab era [113,114,117], although the unfavourable prognosis of LAMs has been reversed in the rituximab era [74,115,116], possibly due to the binding of the macrophages to the rituximab-opsonized lymphoma cells and its phagocytosis [118]. The number of LAMs at diagnosis is not related to a higher risk of transformation, although this cohort was heterogeneously treated including pre-rituximab and rituximab patients [106]. However, within FL patients who transform, the number of LAMs at diagnosis is associated with shorter time to transformation [106].

Similarly, the high density of CD21+ FDCs at diagnosis have been correlated with inferior PFS, OS and, in those who transform, shorter time to transformation [106,119,120], although not with higher risk of transformation at diagnosis [106]. At transformation, most cases showed the absence of CD21+ FDCs [106].

CD8+ tumour-infiltrating T-cells (TIL) have been correlated with better outcomes in FLs, presumably due to their cytotoxic effect, and this association was stronger when high expression of granzyme B is present [121–123]. Conversely, CD4+ cells are associated with poor outcome, presumably due to B-cell stimulation [122].

Some studies have identified a higher risk of transformation in patients with high levels of CD4+, CD8+, CD57+, PD1+, and FOXP3+ T-cells at diagnosis, as well as a FOXP3+ follicular pattern, a low tumour distance to blood vessels (TDV) or the high expression of vimentin [106–108,124]. Interestingly, both the FOXP3 pattern and TDV are correlated with the higher number of LAMs, although these studies included patients not treated with an anti-CD20 monoclonal antibody [107,108].

All of these observations could be related to the therapy [119,125,126] and the presence of other cell populations such as mast cells [127,128]. Moreover, the differences between studies could also be due to small cohorts of patients, different cut-offs, and variability in the interpretation by distinct pathologists. Therefore, the role of the microenvironment immune cells in predicting FL transformation in the current scenario requires further research, without forgetting the treatment and the balance between immune cell subsets, to create a score/model for both prognosis and transformation with rituximab [117,121,122].

MHC (HLA in humans) is located in the 6p21.3 region, which is frequently disrupted by loss or CNN-LOH in FL as previously mentioned [53,54,97]. Genome-wide studies identify the 6p21.3 region as a susceptibility region for FL [129,130]. Previous studies have reported an association between certain HLA polymorphisms and the higher susceptibility of B-cell lymphoproliferative disorders, including FL [131–134]. Studies analysing the role of HLA specificities in FL prognosis are scarce, and no studies have focused on the risk of HT [132]. Interestingly, the single-nucleotide polymorphism rs6457327, located in this region, has been associated with poor outcome and higher risk of transformation [109,135].

5.4. Liquid Biopsy

Liquid biopsy has emerged as a non-invasive method that allows the detection of tumour-associated alterations in circulating tumour DNA (ctDNA) in plasma, and has shown clinical utility in different lymphoproliferative disorders [136–139]. Since tumour ctDNA may arise from different clones, the ctDNA may better reflect the spatial and/or intra-tumour heterogeneity, a feature that is especially relevant in FL [30]. Focused on FL, the detection of high levels of ctDNA has been correlated with shorter PFS [137,140]. Interestingly, in one FL patient who transformed into DLBCL, mutations specific to the transformed clone were detected in the ctDNA at diagnosis but were not present in the FL lymph node biopsy, thus suggesting that the clone responsible for the transformation could be detected in the ctDNA at diagnosis at least in some cases [46]. The authors of this work described a predictive model only based on the mutations identified in plasma, which could be a promising biomarker for transformation prediction [46].

6. Discussion and Concluding Remarks

Histological transformation is an unfavourable event of FL course which clearly affects patient survival. In the last years, several works have increased the genetic knowledge of FL transformation, helping to dissect different possible mechanisms of transformation.

The predominance of the divergent model in transformed FL suggests the existence of an ancestral CPC driving FL recurrence and transformation. Whether this CPC (or the subclone responsible for transformation) was already present at diagnosis still remains unknown, and this could preclude prediction, at least in some transformed cases. The driver events that trigger HT from the CPC are still unknown. There is most probably not a single mechanism, but several distinct pathways driving HT from the CPC, as suggested by gene-expression analysis and the differences in genetic alterations between HT groups, for instance, according to the cell-of-origin of the HT, and these pathways could be different according to the CPC niche [27,28,54,61]. Moreover, the variable histologies observed at transformation also suggest different mechanisms, and this is highlighted by the different incidence of some alterations such as *TP53* mutations in DLBCL-HT compared to composite-HT [28].

There is still not an accurate predictor of transformation. This may in part result from the lack of biomarker validation, which, in turn, could be due to the heterogeneity of the series included in the different studies, for other reasons. Much research has focused on genetic aberrations, although some studies do not include FL relapse samples, or even do not distinguish FL samples at diagnosis or FL relapse, which could lead to missing or confounding information. The tumour microenvironment may play a key role in FL outcome and probably in transformation. As mentioned, this microenvironment is affected by the treatment and the presence of certain genetic alterations. Few studies have analysed the role of immune cell crosstalk together with genetic events, and this was performed in short and/or heterogeneous series. This emphasizes the need to perform comprehensive biological and clinical analysis in large-scale series of clonally related FL-HT, including at least genetic aberrations together with gene expression and microenvironment composition, in homogeneous cohorts, to better identify the different pathways triggering transformation. Moreover, emerging treatments, including EZH2 inhibitors, HDAC inhibitors, bispecific antibodies and CAR T-cells, would probably improve the survival of FL transformed patients, thus highlighting the need to perform these studies to help identify targets to personalize treatment approaches [141–143].

However, there are several challenges to address these studies in transformed FLs. First, not all cases can be biopsied at suspicion of transformation. There are limited available biopsies, and these are stored in formalin-fixed paraffin-embedded which fragments and partially degrades DNA, limiting the availability of quality samples for the experiments. Therefore, it is difficult to have paired samples both at diagnosis and at transformation, and even more so when samples from different events, such as FL or transformation relapses, are included.

In summary, collaborative efforts are required to obtain high and robust FL-HT collections, to generate and collect genetic data of large-scale series of HT, and to identify the CPCs that if eradicated could potentially prevent both FL recurrence and transformation. We hope the increasing biological knowledge on FL transformation will enable personalized treatment strategies avoiding transformation.

Author Contributions: Conception and design: All authors; Manuscript writing: All authors; Final approval of manuscript: All authors. All authors have read and agreed to the published version of the manuscript.

Funding: This work was supported in part by grants from the Health Research Program of the Institute of Health Carlos III (ISCIII), the Spanish Ministry of Economy and Competitiveness, PI15/01393, PI18/00410, CIBERONC (CB16/12/00233), the Cancer Research UK [C355/A26819], FC AECC and AIRC under the "Accelerator Award Program" [EDITOR], AECC (PROYE18020BEA), the Education and Health Counselings of Castilla y León (CAS102P17, GRS 1180/A/15), Gilead Sciences (GLD17/00334), and the European Regional Development Fund (ERDF) 'Una manera de hacer Europa' (Innocampus; CEI-2010-1-0010). All Spanish funding was co-sponsored by the European Union FEDER program. Figures were created by BioRender.com accessed on 1 September 2022.

Conflicts of Interest: The authors declare no conflict of interest.

References

1. Sant, M.; Allemani, C.; Tereanu, C.; De, A.R.; Capocaccia, R.; Visser, O.; Marcos-Gragera, R.; Maynadié, M.; Simonetti, A.; Lutz, J.M.; et al. Incidence of hematologic malignancies in Europe by morphologic subtype: Results of the HAEMACARE project. *Blood* **2010**, *116*, 3724–3734. [CrossRef] [PubMed]
2. Kridel, R.; Sehn, L.H.; Gascoyne, R.D. Pathogenesis of follicular lymphoma. *J. Clin. Investig.* **2012**, *122*, 3424–3431. [CrossRef] [PubMed]
3. Swerdlow, S.H.; Campo, E.; Pileri, S.A.; Harris, N.L.; Stein, H.; Siebert, R.; Advani, R.; Ghielmini, M.; Salles, G.A.; Zelenetz, A.D.; et al. The 2016 revision of the World Health Organization classification of lymphoid neoplasms. *Blood* **2016**, *127*, 2375–2390. [CrossRef] [PubMed]
4. Carbone, A.; Roulland, S.; Gloghini, A.; Younes, A.; von Keudell, G.; López-Guillermo, A.; Fitzgibbon, J. Follicular lymphoma. *Nat. Rev. Dis. Primers* **2019**, *5*, 83. [CrossRef]
5. Bastos-Oreiro, M.; Muntañola, A.; Panizo, C.; Gonzalez-Barca, E.; de Villambrosia, S.G.; Córdoba, R.; López, J.L.B.; González-Sierra, P.; Terol, M.J.; Gutierrez, A.; et al. RELINF: Prospective epidemiological registry of lymphoid neoplasms in Spain. A project from the GELTAMO group. *Ann. Hematol.* **2020**, *99*, 799–808. [CrossRef]
6. Campo, E.; Jaffe, E.S.; Cook, J.R.; Quintanilla-Martinez, L.; Swerdlow, S.H.; Anderson, K.C.; Brousset, P.; Cerroni, L.; de Leval, L.; Dirnhofer, S.; et al. The International Consensus Classification of Mature Lymphoid Neoplasms: A Report from the Clinical Advisory Committee. *Blood* **2022**, *140*, 1229–1253. [CrossRef]
7. Alaggio, R.; Amador, C.; Anagnostopoulos, I.; Attygalle, A.D.; Araujo, I.B.O.; Berti, E.; Bhagat, G.; Borges, A.M.; Boyer, D.; Calaminici, M.; et al. The 5th edition of the World Health Organization Classification of Haematolymphoid Tumours: Lymphoid Neoplasms. *Leukemia* **2022**, *36*, 1720–1748. [CrossRef]
8. Hiddemann, W.; Kneba, M.; Dreyling, M.; Schmitz, N.; Lengfelder, E.; Schmits, R.; Reiser, M.; Metzner, B.; Harder, H.; Hegewisch-Becker, S.; et al. Frontline therapy with rituximab added to the combination of cyclophosphamide, doxorubicin, vincristine, and prednisone (CHOP) significantly improves the outcome for patients with advanced-stage follicular lymphoma compared with therapy with CHOP alone: Results of a prospective randomized study of the German Low-Grade Lymphoma Study Group. *Blood* **2005**, *106*, 3725–3732.
9. Marcus, R.; Imrie, K.; Solal-Celigny, P.; Catalano, J.V.; Dmoszynska, A.; Raposo, J.C.; Offner, F.C.; Gomez-Codina, J.; Belch, A.; Cunningham, D.; et al. Phase III study of R-CVP compared with cyclophosphamide, vincristine, and prednisone alone in patients with previously untreated advanced follicular lymphoma. *J. Clin. Oncol.* **2008**, *26*, 4579–4586. [CrossRef]
10. Salles, G.; Seymour, J.F.; Offner, F.; Lopez-Guillermo, A.; Belada, D.; Xerri, L.; Feugier, P.; Bouabdallah, R.; Catalano, J.V.; Brice, P.; et al. Rituximab maintenance for 2 years in patients with high tumour burden follicular lymphoma responding to rituximab plus chemotherapy (PRIMA): A phase 3, randomised controlled trial. *Lancet* **2011**, *377*, 42–51. [CrossRef]
11. Swerdlow, S.H.; Campo, E.; Harris, N.L.; Jaffe, E.S.; Pileri, S.A.; Stein, H.; Thiele, J.; Vardiman, J.W. *WHO Classification of Tumours of Haematopoietic and Lymphoid Tissues*; IARC Press: Lyon, France, 2008.

12. Casulo, C.; Byrtek, M.; Dawson, K.L.; Zhou, X.; Farber, C.M.; Flowers, C.R.; Hainsworth, J.D.; Maurer, M.J.; Cerhan, J.R.; Link, B.K.; et al. Early Relapse of Follicular Lymphoma After Rituximab Plus Cyclophosphamide, Doxorubicin, Vincristine, and Prednisone Defines Patients at High Risk for Death: An Analysis From the National LymphoCare Study. *J. Clin. Oncol.* **2015**, *33*, 2516–2522. [CrossRef] [PubMed]
13. Sorigue, M.; Mercadal, S.; Alonso, S.; Fernández-Álvarez, R.; García, O.; Moreno, M.; Pomares, H.; Alcoceba, M.; González-García, E.; Motlló, C.; et al. Refractoriness to immunochemotherapy in follicular lymphoma: Predictive factors and outcome. *Hematol. Oncol.* **2017**, *35*, 520–527. [CrossRef] [PubMed]
14. Magnano, L.; Alonso-Alvarez, S.; Alcoceba, M.; Rivas-Delgado, A.; Muntañola, A.; Nadeu, F.; Setoain, X.; Rodríguez, S.; Andrade-Campos, M.; Espinosa-Lara, N.; et al. Life expectancy of follicular lymphoma patients in complete response at 30 months is similar to that of the Spanish general population. *Br. J. Haematol.* **2019**, *185*, 480–491. [CrossRef] [PubMed]
15. Federico, M.; Caballero, B.; Marcheselli, L.; Tarantino, V.; Manni, M.; Sarkozy, C.; Alonso-Álvarez, S.; Wondergem, M.; Cartron, G.; Lopez-Guillermo, A.; et al. Rituximab and the risk of transformation of follicular lymphoma: A retrospective pooled analysis. *Lancet Haematol.* **2018**, *5*, e359–e367. [CrossRef]
16. Bastion, Y.; Sebban, C.; Berger, F.; Felman, P.; Salles, G.; Dumontet, C.; Bryon, P.A.; Coiffier, B. Incidence, predictive factors, and outcome of lymphoma transformation in follicular lymphoma patients. *J. Clin. Oncol.* **1997**, *15*, 1587–1594. [CrossRef]
17. Montoto, S.; Davies, A.J.; Matthews, J.; Calaminici, M.; Norton, A.J.; Amess, J.; Vinnicombe, S.; Waters, R.; Rohatiner, A.Z.; Lister, T.A. Risk and clinical implications of transformation of follicular lymphoma to diffuse large B-cell lymphoma. *J. Clin. Oncol.* **2007**, *25*, 2426–2433. [CrossRef]
18. Al-Tourah, A.J.; Gill, K.K.; Chhanabhai, M.; Hoskins, P.J.; Klasa, R.J.; Savage, K.J.; Sehn, L.H.; Shenkier, T.N.; Gascoyne, R.D.; Connors, J.M. Population-based analysis of incidence and outcome of transformed non-Hodgkin's lymphoma. *J. Clin. Oncol.* **2008**, *26*, 5165–5169. [CrossRef]
19. Link, B.K.; Maurer, M.J.; Nowakowski, G.S.; Ansell, S.M.; Macon, W.R.; Syrbu, S.I.; Slager, S.L.; Thompson, C.A.; Inwards, D.J.; Johnston, P.B.; et al. Rates and outcomes of follicular lymphoma transformation in the immunochemotherapy era: A report from the University of Iowa/MayoClinic Specialized Program of Research Excellence Molecular Epidemiology Resource. *J. Clin. Oncol.* **2013**, *31*, 3272–3278. [CrossRef]
20. Wagner-Johnston, N.D.; Link, B.K.; Byrtek, M.; Dawson, K.L.; Hainsworth, J.; Flowers, C.R.; Friedberg, J.W.; Bartlett, N.L. Outcomes of transformed follicular lymphoma in the modern era: A report from the National LymphoCare Study (NLCS). *Blood* **2015**, *126*, 851–857. [CrossRef]
21. Sarkozy, C.; Trneny, M.; Xerri, L.; Wickham, N.; Feugier, P.; Leppa, S.; Brice, P.; Soubeyran, P.; Gomes Da Silva, M.; Mounier, C.; et al. Risk Factors and Outcomes for Patients With Follicular Lymphoma Who Had Histologic Transformation After Response to First-Line Immunochemotherapy in the PRIMA Trial. *J. Clin. Oncol.* **2016**, *34*, 2575–2582. [CrossRef]
22. Alonso-Álvarez, S.; Magnano, L.; Alcoceba, M.; Andrade-Campos, M.; Espinosa-Lara, N.; Rodríguez, G.; Mercadal, S.; Carro, I.; Sancho, J.M.; Moreno, M.; et al. Risk of, and survival following, histological transformation in follicular lymphoma in the rituximab era. A retrospective multicentre study by the Spanish GELTAMO group. *Br. J. Haematol.* **2017**, *178*, 699–708. [CrossRef] [PubMed]
23. Casulo, C.; Burack, W.R.; Friedberg, J.W. Transformed follicular non-Hodgkin lymphoma. *Blood* **2015**, *125*, 40–47. [CrossRef] [PubMed]
24. Kridel, R.; Sehn, L.H.; Gascoyne, R.D. Can histologic transformation of follicular lymphoma be predicted and prevented? *Blood* **2017**, *130*, 258–266. [CrossRef] [PubMed]
25. Lossos, I.S.; Gascoyne, R.D. Transformation of follicular lymphoma. *Best Pract. Res. Clin. Haematol.* **2011**, *24*, 147–163. [CrossRef]
26. Ouansafi, I.; He, B.; Fraser, C.; Nie, K.; Mathew, S.; Bhanji, R.; Hoda, R.; Arabadjief, M.; Knowles, D.; Cerutti, A.; et al. Transformation of follicular lymphoma to plasmablastic lymphoma with c-myc gene rearrangement. *Am. J. Clin. Pathol.* **2010**, *134*, 972–981. [CrossRef]
27. Kridel, R.; Mottok, A.; Farinha, P.; Ben-Neriah, S.; Ennishi, D.; Zheng, Y.; Chavez, E.A.; Shulha, H.P.; Tan, K.; Chan, F.C.; et al. Cell of origin of transformed follicular lymphoma. *Blood* **2015**, *126*, 2118–2127. [CrossRef]
28. Kridel, R.; Chan, F.C.; Mottok, A.; Boyle, M.; Farinha, P.; Tan, K.; Meissner, B.; Bashashati, A.; McPherson, A.; Roth, A.; et al. Histological Transformation and Progression in Follicular Lymphoma: A Clonal Evolution Study. *PLoS Med.* **2016**, *13*, e1002197. [CrossRef]
29. Salles, G.; Coiffier, B. Histologic transformation in follicular lymphoma. *Ann. Oncol.* **1998**, *9*, 803–805. [CrossRef]
30. Araf, S.; Wang, J.; Korfi, K.; Pangault, C.; Kotsiou, E.; Rio-Machin, A.; Rahim, T.; Heward, J.; Clear, A.; Iqbal, S.; et al. Genomic profiling reveals spatial intra-tumor heterogeneity in follicular lymphoma. *Leukemia* **2018**, *32*, 1261–1265. [CrossRef]
31. Bodet-Milin, C.; Kraeber-Bodere, F.; Moreau, P.; Campion, L.; Dupas, B.; Le, G.S. Investigation of FDG-PET/CT imaging to guide biopsies in the detection of histological transformation of indolent lymphoma. *Haematologica* **2008**, *93*, 471–472. [CrossRef]
32. Gine, E.; Montoto, S.; Bosch, F.; Arenillas, L.; Mercadal, S.; Villamor, N.; Martinez, A.; Colomo, L.; Campo, E.; Montserrat, E.; et al. The Follicular Lymphoma International Prognostic Index (FLIPI) and the histological subtype are the most important factors to predict histological transformation in follicular lymphoma. *Ann. Oncol.* **2006**, *17*, 1539–1545. [CrossRef] [PubMed]
33. Gascoyne, R.D. The pathology of transformation of indolent B cell lymphomas. *Hematol. Oncol.* **2015**, *33* (Suppl. 1), 75–79. [CrossRef] [PubMed]

34. Rossi, D.; Spina, V.; Deambrogi, C.; Rasi, S.; Laurenti, L.; Stamatopoulos, K.; Arcaini, L.; Lucioni, M.; Rocque, G.B.; Xu-Monette, Z.Y.; et al. The genetics of Richter syndrome reveals disease heterogeneity and predicts survival after transformation. *Blood* **2011**, *117*, 3391–3401. [CrossRef]
35. Eide, M.B.; Liestol, K.; Lingjaerde, O.C.; Hystad, M.E.; Kresse, S.H.; Meza-Zepeda, L.; Myklebost, O.; Troen, G.; Aamot, H.V.; Holte, H.; et al. Genomic alterations reveal potential for higher grade transformation in follicular lymphoma and confirm parallel evolution of tumor cell clones. *Blood* **2010**, *116*, 1489–1497. [CrossRef]
36. García-Álvarez, M.; Alonso-Álvarez, S.; Prieto-Conde, I.; Jiménez, C.; Sarasquete, M.E.; Chillón, M.C.; Medina, A.; Balanzategui, A.; Maldonado, R.; Antón, A.; et al. Immunoglobulin gene rearrangement IGHV3–48 is a predictive marker of histological transformation into aggressive lymphoma in follicular lymphomas. *Blood Cancer J.* **2019**, *9*, 52. [CrossRef] [PubMed]
37. Fitzgibbon, J.; Iqbal, S.; Davies, A.; O'Shea, D.; Carlotti, E.; Chaplin, T.; Matthews, J.; Raghavan, M.; Norton, A.; Lister, T.A.; et al. Genome-wide detection of recurring sites of uniparental disomy in follicular and transformed follicular lymphoma. *Leukemia* **2007**, *21*, 514–1520. [CrossRef]
38. Johnson, N.A.; Al-Tourah, A.; Brown, C.J.; Connors, J.M.; Gascoyne, R.D.; Horsman, D.E. Prognostic significance of secondary cytogenetic alterations in follicular lymphomas. *Genes Chromosom. Cancer* **2008**, *47*, 1038–1048. [CrossRef] [PubMed]
39. García-Álvarez, M.; Alonso-Álvarez, S.; Prieto-Conde, M.I.; Jiménez, C.; Sarasquete, M.E.; Chillón, M.C.; Medina, A.; Balanzategui, A.; Antón, A.; Maldonado, R.; et al. Molecular study of the clonal evolution of follicular lymphoma to aggressive lymphoma. A single center experience. *Haematologica* **2018**, *103*, 15.
40. González-Rincón, J.; Méndez, M.; Gómez, S.; García, J.F.; Martín, P.; Bellas, C.; Pedrosa, L.; Rodríguez-Pinilla, S.M.; Camacho, F.I.; Quero, C.; et al. Unraveling transformation of follicular lymphoma to diffuse large B-cell lymphoma. *PLoS ONE* **2019**, *14*, e0212813. [CrossRef]
41. Okosun, J.; Bodor, C.; Wang, J.; Araf, S.; Yang, C.Y.; Pan, C.; Boller, S.; Cittaro, D.; Bozek, M.; Iqbal, S.; et al. Integrated genomic analysis identifies recurrent mutations and evolution patterns driving the initiation and progression of follicular lymphoma. *Nat. Genet.* **2014**, *46*, 176–181. [CrossRef]
42. Pasqualucci, L.; Khiabanian, H.; Fangazio, M.; Vasishtha, M.; Messina, M.; Holmes, A.B.; Ouillette, P.; Trifonov, V.; Rossi, D.; Tabbo, F.; et al. Genetics of follicular lymphoma transformation. *Cell Rep.* **2014**, *6*, 130–140. [CrossRef] [PubMed]
43. Fabbri, G.; Khiabanian, H.; Holmes, A.B.; Wang, J.; Messina, M.; Mullighan, C.G.; Pasqualucci, L.; Rabadan, R.; Dalla-Favera, R. Genetic lesions associated with chronic lymphocytic leukemia transformation to Richter syndrome. *J. Exp. Med.* **2013**, *210*, 2273–2288. [CrossRef] [PubMed]
44. Carlotti, E.; Wrench, D.; Matthews, J.; Iqbal, S.; Davies, A.; Norton, A.; Hart, J.; Lai, R.; Montoto, S.; Gribben, J.G.; et al. Transformation of follicular lymphoma to diffuse large B-cell lymphoma may occur by divergent evolution from a common progenitor cell or by direct evolution from the follicular lymphoma clone. *Blood* **2009**, *113*, 3553–3557. [CrossRef]
45. Weigert, O.; Kopp, N.; Lane, A.A.; Yoda, A.; Dahlberg, S.E.; Neuberg, D.; Bahar, A.Y.; Chapuy, B.; Kutok, J.L.; Longtine, J.A.; et al. Molecular ontogeny of donor-derived follicular lymphomas occurring after hematopoietic cell transplantation. *Cancer Discov.* **2012**, *2*, 47–55. [CrossRef] [PubMed]
46. Scherer, F.; Kurtz, D.M.; Newman, A.M.; Stehr, H.; Craig, A.F.; Esfahani, M.S.; Lovejoy, A.F.; Chabon, J.J.; Klass, D.M.; Liu, C.L.; et al. Distinct biological subtypes and patterns of genome evolution in lymphoma revealed by circulating tumor DNA. *Sci. Transl. Med.* **2016**, *8*, 364ra155. [CrossRef]
47. Roulland, S.; Kelly, R.S.; Morgado, E.; Sungalee, S.; Solal-Celigny, P.; Colombat, P.; Jouve, N.; Palli, D.; Pala, V.; Tumino, R.; et al. t(14;18) Translocation: A predictive blood biomarker for follicular lymphoma. *J. Clin. Oncol.* **2014**, *32*, 1347–1355. [CrossRef]
48. Davies, A.J.; Rosenwald, A.; Wright, G.; Lee, A.; Last, K.W.; Weisenburger, D.D.; Chan, W.C.; Delabie, J.; Braziel, R.M.; Campo, E.; et al. Transformation of follicular lymphoma to diffuse large B-cell lymphoma proceeds by distinct oncogenic mechanisms. *Br. J. Haematol.* **2007**, *136*, 286–293. [CrossRef]
49. Maeshima, A.M.; Taniguchi, H.; Toyoda, K.; Yamauchi, N.; Makita, S.; Fukuhara, S.; Munakata, W.; Maruyama, D.; Kobayashi, Y.; Tobinai, K. Clinicopathological features of histological transformation from extranodal marginal zone B-cell lymphoma of mucosa-associated lymphoid tissue to diffuse large B-cell lymphoma: An analysis of 467 patients. *Br. J. Haematol.* **2016**, *174*, 923–931. [CrossRef]
50. Zanwar, S.; Abeykoon, J.P.; Durot, E.; King, R.; Perez Burbano, G.E.; Kumar, S.; Gertz, M.A.; Quinquenel, A.; Delmer, A.; Gonsalves, W.; et al. Impact of MYD88(L265P) mutation status on histological transformation of Waldenström Macroglobulinemia. *Am. J. Hematol.* **2020**, *95*, 274–281. [CrossRef]
51. Abrisqueta, P.; Delgado, J.; Alcoceba, M.; Oliveira, A.C.; Loscertales, J.; Hernández-Rivas, J.A.; Ferrà, C.; Cordoba, R.; Yáñez, L.; Medina, A.; et al. Clinical outcome and prognostic factors of patients with Richter syndrome: Real-world study of the Spanish Chronic Lymphocytic Leukemia Study Group (GELLC). *Br. J. Haematol.* **2020**, *190*, 854–863. [CrossRef]
52. Bastidas-Mora, G.; Beà, S.; Navarro, A.; Gine, E.; Costa, D.; Delgado, J.; Baumann, T.; Magnano, L.; Rivas-Delgado, A.; Villamor, N.; et al. Clinico-biological features and outcome of patients with splenic marginal zone lymphoma with histological transformation. *Br. J. Haematol.* **2022**, *196*, 146–155. [CrossRef] [PubMed]
53. O'Shea, D.; O'Riain, C.; Gupta, M.; Waters, R.; Yang, Y.; Wrench, D.; Gribben, J.; Rosenwald, A.; Ott, G.; Rimsza, L.M.; et al. Regions of acquired uniparental disomy at diagnosis of follicular lymphoma are associated with both overall survival and risk of transformation. *Blood* **2009**, *113*, 2298–2301. [CrossRef] [PubMed]

54. Bouska, A.; McKeithan, T.W.; Deffenbacher, K.E.; Lachel, C.; Wright, G.W.; Iqbal, J.; Smith, L.M.; Zhang, W.; Kucuk, C.; Rinaldi, A.; et al. Genome-wide copy-number analyses reveal genomic abnormalities involved in transformation of follicular lymphoma. *Blood* **2014**, *123*, 1681–1690. [CrossRef] [PubMed]
55. Bouska, A.; Zhang, W.; Gong, Q.; Iqbal, J.; Scuto, A.; Vose, J.; Ludvigsen, M.; Fu, K.; Weisenburger, D.D.; Greiner, T.C.; et al. Combined copy number and mutation analysis identifies oncogenic pathways associated with transformation of follicular lymphoma. *Leukemia* **2017**, *31*, 83–91. [CrossRef] [PubMed]
56. Qu, X.; Li, H.; Braziel, R.M.; Passerini, V.; Rimsza, L.M.; Hsi, E.D.; Leonard, J.P.; Smith, S.M.; Kridel, R.; Press, O.; et al. Genomic alterations important for the prognosis in patients with follicular lymphoma treated in SWOG study S0016. *Blood* **2019**, *133*, 81–93. [CrossRef]
57. Elenitoba-Johnson, K.S.; Gascoyne, R.D.; Lim, M.S.; Chhanabai, M.; Jaffe, E.S.; Raffeld, M. Homozygous deletions at chromosome 9p21 involving p16 and p15 are associated with histologic progression in follicle center lymphoma. *Blood* **1998**, *91*, 4677–4685. [CrossRef]
58. Alhejaily, A.; Day, A.G.; Feilotter, H.E.; Baetz, T.; Lebrun, D.P. Inactivation of the CDKN2A tumor-suppressor gene by deletion or methylation is common at diagnosis in follicular lymphoma and associated with poor clinical outcome. *Clin. Cancer Res.* **2014**, *20*, 1676–1686. [CrossRef]
59. Martello, M.; Poletti, A.; Borsi, E.; Solli, V.; Dozza, L.; Barbato, S.; Zamagni, E.; Tacchetti, P.; Pantani, L.; Mancuso, K.; et al. Clonal and subclonal TP53 molecular impairment is associated with prognosis and progression in multiple myeloma. *Blood Cancer J.* **2022**, *12*, 15. [CrossRef]
60. Martinez-Climent, J.A.; Alizadeh, A.A.; Segraves, R.; Blesa, D.; Rubio-Moscardo, F.; Albertson, D.G.; Garcia-Conde, J.; Dyer, M.J.; Levy, R.; Pinkel, D.; et al. Transformation of follicular lymphoma to diffuse large cell lymphoma is associated with a heterogeneous set of DNA copy number and gene expression alterations. *Blood* **2003**, *101*, 3109–3117. [CrossRef]
61. Kwiecinska, A.; Ichimura, K.; Berglund, M.; Dinets, A.; Sulaiman, L.; Collins, V.P.; Larsson, C.; Porwit, A.; Lagercrantz, S.B. Amplification of 2p as a genomic marker for transformation in lymphoma. *Genes Chromosom. Cancer* **2014**, *53*, 750–768. [CrossRef]
62. Chapuy, B.; Stewart, C.; Dunford, A.J.; Kim, J.; Kamburov, A.; Redd, R.A.; Lawrence, M.S.; Roemer, M.G.M.; Li, A.J.; Ziepert, M.; et al. Molecular subtypes of diffuse large B cell lymphoma are associated with distinct pathogenic mechanisms and outcomes. *Nat. Med.* **2018**, *24*, 679–690. [CrossRef] [PubMed]
63. Schmitz, R.; Wright, G.W.; Huang, D.W.; Johnson, C.A.; Phelan, J.D.; Wang, J.Q.; Roulland, S.; Kasbekar, M.; Young, R.M.; Shaffer, A.L.; et al. Genetics and Pathogenesis of Diffuse Large B-Cell Lymphoma. *N. Engl. J. Med.* **2018**, *378*, 1396–1407. [CrossRef] [PubMed]
64. Chigrinova, E.; Rinaldi, A.; Kwee, I.; Rossi, D.; Rancoita, P.M.; Strefford, J.C.; Oscier, D.; Stamatopoulos, K.; Papadaki, T.; Berger, F.; et al. Two main genetic pathways lead to the transformation of chronic lymphocytic leukemia to Richter syndrome. *Blood* **2013**, *122*, 2673–2682. [CrossRef]
65. Aukema, S.M.; van Pel, R.; Nagel, I.; Bens, S.; Siebert, R.; Rosati, S.; van den Berg, E.; Bosga-Bouwer, A.G.; Kibbelaar, R.E.; Hoogendoorn, M.; et al. MYC expression and translocation analyses in low-grade and transformed follicular lymphoma. *Histopathology* **2017**, *71*, 960–971. [CrossRef]
66. Musilova, K.; Devan, J.; Cerna, K.; Seda, V.; Pavlasova, G.; Sharma, S.; Oppelt, J.; Pytlik, R.; Prochazka, V.; Prouzova, Z.; et al. miR-150 downregulation contributes to the high-grade transformation of follicular lymphoma by upregulating FOXP1 levels. *Blood* **2018**, *132*, 2389–2400. [CrossRef]
67. Akasaka, T.; Lossos, I.S.; Levy, R. BCL6 gene translocation in follicular lymphoma: A harbinger of eventual transformation to diffuse aggressive lymphoma. *Blood* **2003**, *102*, 1443–1448. [CrossRef]
68. García Álvarez, M.; Alonso-Álvarez, S.; Prieto-Conde, I.; Jiménez, C.; Sarasquete, M.E.; Chillón, M.C.; Medina, A.; Balanzategui, A.; Maldonado, R.; Antón, A.; et al. Genetic complexity impacts the clinical outcome of follicular lymphoma patients. *Blood Cancer J.* **2021**, *11*, 11. [CrossRef]
69. Mozas, P.; Rivero, A.; Rivas-Delgado, A.; Correa, J.G.; Condom, M.; Nadeu, F.; Giné, E.; Delgado, J.; Villamor, N.; Campo, E.; et al. Prognostic ability of five clinical risk scores in follicular lymphoma: A single-center evaluation. *Hematol. Oncol.* **2021**, *39*, 639–649. [CrossRef]
70. Alonso-Álvarez, S.; Manni, M.; Montoto, S.; Sarkozy, C.; Morschhauser, F.; Wondergem, M.J.; Guarini, A.; Magnano, L.; Alcoceba, M.; Chamuleau, M.; et al. Primary refractory follicular lymphoma: A poor outcome entity with high risk of transformation to aggressive B cell lymphoma. *Eur. J. Cancer* **2021**, *157*, 132–139. [CrossRef]
71. Sarkozy, C.; Maurer, M.J.; Link, B.K.; Ghesquieres, H.; Nicolas, E.; Thompson, C.A.; Traverse-Glehen, A.; Feldman, A.L.; Allmer, C.; Slager, S.L.; et al. Cause of Death in Follicular Lymphoma in the First Decade of the Rituximab Era: A Pooled Analysis of French and US Cohorts. *J. Clin. Oncol.* **2019**, *37*, 144–152. [CrossRef]
72. Naresh, K.N. MUM1 expression dichotomises follicular lymphoma into predominantly, MUM1-negative low-grade and MUM1-positive high-grade subtypes. *Haematologica* **2007**, *92*, 267–268. [CrossRef] [PubMed]
73. Koch, K.; Hoster, E.; Ziepert, M.; Unterhalt, M.; Ott, G.; Rosenwald, A.; Hansmann, M.L.; Bernd, W.; Stein, H.; Pöschel, V.; et al. Clinical, pathological and genetic features of follicular lymphoma grade 3A: A joint analysis of the German low-grade and high-grade lymphoma study groups GLSG and DSHNHL. *Ann. Oncol.* **2016**, *27*, 1323–1329. [CrossRef] [PubMed]

74. Sweetenham, J.W.; Goldman, B.; LeBlanc, M.L.; Cook, J.R.; Tubbs, R.R.; Press, O.W.; Maloney, D.G.; Fisher, R.I.; Rimsza, L.M.; Braziel, R.M.; et al. Prognostic value of regulatory T cells, lymphoma-associated macrophages, and MUM-1 expression in follicular lymphoma treated before and after the introduction of monoclonal antibody therapy: A Southwest Oncology Group Study. *Ann. Oncol.* **2010**, *21*, 1196–1202. [CrossRef] [PubMed]
75. Xerri, L.; Bachy, E.; Fabiani, B.; Canioni, D.; Chassagne-Clement, C.; Dartigues-Cuilleres, P.; Charlotte, F.; Brousse, N.; Rousselet, M.C.; Foussard, C.; et al. Identification of MUM1 as a prognostic immunohistochemical marker in follicular lymphoma using computerized image analysis. *Hum. Pathol.* **2014**, *45*, 2085–2093. [CrossRef]
76. Mottok, A.; Jurinovic, V.; Farinha, P.; Rosenwald, A.; Leich, E.; Ott, G.; Horn, H.; Klapper, W.; Boesl, M.; Hiddemann, W.; et al. FOXP1 expression is a prognostic biomarker in follicular lymphoma treated with rituximab and chemotherapy. *Blood* **2018**, *131*, 226–235. [CrossRef]
77. Sohani, A.R.; Maurer, M.J.; Giri, S.; Pitcher, B.; Chadburn, A.; Said, J.W.; Bartlett, N.L.; Czuczman, M.S.; Martin, P.; Rosenbaum, C.A.; et al. Biomarkers for Risk Stratification in Patients With Previously Untreated Follicular Lymphoma Receiving Anti-CD20-based Biological Therapy. *Am. J. Surg. Pathol.* **2021**, *45*, 384–393. [CrossRef]
78. Sagardoy, A.; Martinez-Ferrandis, J.I.; Roa, S.; Bunting, K.L.; Aznar, M.A.; Elemento, O.; Shaknovich, R.; Fontán, L.; Fresquet, V.; Perez-Roger, I.; et al. Downregulation of FOXP1 is required during germinal center B-cell function. *Blood* **2013**, *121*, 4311–4320. [CrossRef]
79. Gascoyne, D.M.; Banham, A.H. The significance of FOXP1 in diffuse large B-cell lymphoma. *Leuk. Lymphoma* **2017**, *58*, 1037–1051. [CrossRef]
80. Patzelt, T.; Keppler, S.J.; Gorka, O.; Thoene, S.; Wartewig, T.; Reth, M.; Förster, I.; Lang, R.; Buchner, M.; Ruland, J. Foxp1 controls mature B cell survival and the development of follicular and B-1 B cells. *Proc. Natl. Acad. Sci. USA* **2018**, *115*, 3120–3125. [CrossRef]
81. Barrans, S.L.; Fenton, J.A.; Banham, A.; Owen, R.G.; Jack, A.S. Strong expression of FOXP1 identifies a distinct subset of diffuse large B-cell lymphoma (DLBCL) patients with poor outcome. *Blood* **2004**, *104*, 2933–2935. [CrossRef]
82. Noppe, S.M.; Heirman, C.; Bakkus, M.H.; Brissinck, J.; Schots, R.; Thielemans, K. The genetic variability of the VH genes in follicular lymphoma: The impact of the hypermutation mechanism. *Br. J. Haematol.* **1999**, *107*, 625–640. [CrossRef] [PubMed]
83. Berget, E.; Molven, A.; Lokeland, T.; Helgeland, L.; Vintermyr, O.K. IGHV gene usage and mutational status in follicular lymphoma: Correlations with prognosis and patient age. *Leuk. Res.* **2015**, *39*, 702–708. [CrossRef] [PubMed]
84. Rossi, D.; Cerri, M.; Capello, D.; Deambrogi, C.; Rossi, F.M.; Zucchetto, A.; De, P.L.; Cresta, S.; Rasi, S.; Spina, V.; et al. Biological and clinical risk factors of chronic lymphocytic leukaemia transformation to Richter syndrome. *Br. J. Haematol.* **2008**, *142*, 202–215. [CrossRef]
85. O'Shea, D.; O'Riain, C.; Taylor, C.; Waters, R.; Carlotti, E.; Macdougall, F.; Gribben, J.; Rosenwald, A.; Ott, G.; Rimsza, L.M.; et al. The presence of TP53 mutation at diagnosis of follicular lymphoma identifies a high-risk group of patients with shortened time to disease progression and poorer overall survival. *Blood* **2008**, *112*, 3126–3129. [CrossRef] [PubMed]
86. Pastore, A.; Jurinovic, V.; Kridel, R.; Hoster, E.; Staiger, A.M.; Szczepanowski, M.; Pott, C.; Kopp, N.; Murakami, M.; Horn, H.; et al. Integration of gene mutations in risk prognostication for patients receiving first-line immunochemotherapy for follicular lymphoma: A retrospective analysis of a prospective clinical trial and validation in a population-based registry. *Lancet Oncol.* **2015**, *16*, 1111–1122. [CrossRef]
87. Jurinovic, V.; Kridel, R.; Staiger, A.M.; Szczepanowski, M.; Horn, H.; Dreyling, M.H.; Rosenwald, A.; Ott, G.; Klapper, W.; Zelenetz, A.D.; et al. Clinicogenetic risk models predict early progression of follicular lymphoma after first-line immunochemotherapy. *Blood* **2016**, *128*, 1112–1120. [CrossRef]
88. Krysiak, K.; Gomez, F.; White, B.S.; Matlock, M.; Miller, C.A.; Trani, L.; Fronick, C.C.; Fulton, R.S.; Kreisel, F.; Cashen, A.F.; et al. Recurrent somatic mutations affecting B-cell receptor signaling pathway genes in follicular lymphoma. *Blood* **2017**, *129*, 473–483. [CrossRef]
89. Miao, Y.; Hu, S.; Lu, X.; Li, S.; Wang, W.; Medeiros, L.J.; Lin, P. Double-hit follicular lymphoma with MYC and BCL2 translocations: A study of 7 cases with a review of literature. *Hum. Pathol.* **2016**, *58*, 72–77. [CrossRef]
90. Chaudhary, S.; Brown, N.; Song, J.Y.; Yang, L.; Skrabek, P.; Nasr, M.R.; Wong, J.T.; Bedell, V.; Murata-Collins, J.; Kochan, L.; et al. Relative frequency and clinicopathologic characteristics of MYC-rearranged follicular lymphoma. *Hum. Pathol.* **2021**, *114*, 19–27. [CrossRef]
91. Bussot, L.; Chevalier, S.; Cristante, J.; Grange, B.; Tesson, B.; Deteix-Santana, C.; Orsini-Piocelle, F.; Leyronnas, C.; Dupire, S.; Gressin, R.; et al. Adverse outcome in follicular lymphoma is associated with MYC rearrangements but not MYC extra copies. *Br. J. Haematol.* **2021**, *194*, 382–392. [CrossRef]
92. Razzaghi, R.; Agarwal, S.; Kotlov, N.; Plotnikova, O.; Nomie, K.; Huang, D.W.; Wright, G.W.; Smith, G.A.; Li, M.; Takata, K.; et al. Compromised counterselection by FAS creates an aggressive subtype of germinal center lymphoma. *J. Exp. Med.* **2021**, *218*, e20201173. [CrossRef] [PubMed]
93. Iqbal, J.; Greiner, T.C.; Patel, K.; Dave, B.J.; Smith, L.; Ji, J.; Wright, G.; Sanger, W.G.; Pickering, D.L.; Jain, S.; et al. Distinctive patterns of BCL6 molecular alterations and their functional consequences in different subgroups of diffuse large B-cell lymphoma. *Leukemia* **2007**, *21*, 2332–2343. [CrossRef] [PubMed]
94. Tilly, H.; Rossi, A.; Stamatoullas, A.; Lenormand, B.; Bigorgne, C.; Kunlin, A.; Monconduit, M.; Bastard, C. Prognostic value of chromosomal abnormalities in follicular lymphoma. *Blood* **1994**, *84*, 1043–1049. [CrossRef] [PubMed]

95. Viardot, A.; Möller, P.; Högel, J.; Werner, K.; Mechtersheimer, G.; Ho, A.D.; Ott, G.; Barth, T.F.; Siebert, R.; Gesk, S.; et al. Clinicopathologic correlations of genomic gains and losses in follicular lymphoma. *J. Clin. Oncol.* **2002**, *20*, 4523–4530. [CrossRef]
96. Schwaenen, C.; Viardot, A.; Berger, H.; Barth, T.F.; Bentink, S.; Döhner, H.; Enz, M.; Feller, A.C.; Hansmann, M.L.; Hummel, M.; et al. Microarray-based genomic profiling reveals novel genomic aberrations in follicular lymphoma which associate with patient survival and gene expression status. *Genes Chromosom. Cancer* **2009**, *48*, 39–54. [CrossRef]
97. Cheung, K.J.; Shah, S.P.; Steidl, C.; Johnson, N.; Relander, T.; Telenius, A.; Lai, B.; Murphy, K.P.; Lam, W.; Al-Tourah, A.J.; et al. Genome-wide profiling of follicular lymphoma by array comparative genomic hybridization reveals prognostically significant DNA copy number imbalances. *Blood* **2009**, *113*, 137–148. [CrossRef]
98. Cheung, K.J.; Johnson, N.A.; Affleck, J.G.; Severson, T.; Steidl, C.; Ben-Neriah, S.; Schein, J.; Morin, R.D.; Moore, R.; Shah, S.P.; et al. Acquired TNFRSF14 mutations in follicular lymphoma are associated with worse prognosis. *Cancer Res.* **2010**, *70*, 9166–9174. [CrossRef]
99. Murphy, K.M.; Nelson, C.A.; Sedý, J.R. Balancing co-stimulation and inhibition with BTLA and HVEM. *Nat. Rev. Immunol.* **2006**, *6*, 671–681. [CrossRef]
100. Cai, G.; Freeman, G.J. The CD160, BTLA, LIGHT/HVEM pathway: A bidirectional switch regulating T-cell activation. *Immunol. Rev.* **2009**, *229*, 244–258. [CrossRef]
101. Kotsiou, E.; Okosun, J.; Besley, C.; Iqbal, S.; Matthews, J.; Fitzgibbon, J.; Gribben, J.G.; Davies, J.K. TNFRSF14 aberrations in follicular lymphoma increase clinically significant allogeneic T-cell responses. *Blood* **2016**, *128*, 72–81. [CrossRef]
102. Boice, M.; Salloum, D.; Mourcin, F.; Sanghvi, V.; Amin, R.; Oricchio, E.; Jiang, M.; Mottok, A.; Denis-Lagache, N.; Ciriello, G.; et al. Loss of the HVEM Tumor Suppressor in Lymphoma and Restoration by Modified CAR-T Cells. *Cell* **2016**, *167*, 405–418. [CrossRef] [PubMed]
103. Green, M.R.; Kihira, S.; Liu, C.L.; Nair, R.V.; Salari, R.; Gentles, A.J.; Irish, J.; Stehr, H.; Vicente-Dueñas, C.; Romero-Camarero, I.; et al. Mutations in early follicular lymphoma progenitors are associated with suppressed antigen presentation. *Proc. Natl. Acad. Sci. USA* **2015**, *112*, E1116–E1125. [CrossRef] [PubMed]
104. Okosun, J.; Wolfson, R.L.; Wang, J.; Araf, S.; Wilkins, L.; Castellano, B.M.; Escudero-Ibarz, L.; Al Seraihi, A.F.; Richter, J.; Bernhart, S.H.; et al. Recurrent mTORC1-activating RRAGC mutations in follicular lymphoma. *Nat. Genet.* **2016**, *48*, 183–188. [CrossRef] [PubMed]
105. Bararia, D.; Hildebrand, J.A.; Stolz, S.; Haebe, S.; Alig, S.; Trevisani, C.P.; Osorio-Barrios, F.; Bartoschek, M.D.; Mentz, M.; Pastore, A.; et al. Cathepsin S Alterations Induce a Tumor-Promoting Immune Microenvironment in Follicular Lymphoma. *Cell Rep.* **2020**, *31*, 107522. [CrossRef] [PubMed]
106. Blaker, Y.N.; Spetalen, S.; Brodtkorb, M.; Lingjaerde, O.C.; Beiske, K.; Ostenstad, B.; Sander, B.; Wahlin, B.E.; Melen, C.M.; Myklebust, J.H.; et al. The tumour microenvironment influences survival and time to transformation in follicular lymphoma in the rituximab era. *Br. J. Haematol.* **2016**, *175*, 102–114. [CrossRef]
107. Farinha, P.; Al-Tourah, A.; Gill, K.; Klasa, R.; Connors, J.M.; Gascoyne, R.D. The architectural pattern of FOXP3-positive T cells in follicular lymphoma is an independent predictor of survival and histologic transformation. *Blood* **2010**, *115*, 289–295. [CrossRef]
108. Farinha, P.; Kyle, A.H.; Minchinton, A.I.; Connors, J.M.; Karsan, A.; Gascoyne, R.D. Vascularization predicts overall survival and risk of transformation in follicular lymphoma. *Haematologica* **2010**, *95*, 2157–2160. [CrossRef]
109. Berglund, M.; Enblad, G.; Thunberg, U. SNP rs6457327 is a predictor for overall survival in follicular lymphoma as well as survival after transformation. *Blood* **2011**, *118*, 4489. [CrossRef]
110. Gentles, A.J.; Alizadeh, A.A.; Lee, S.I.; Myklebust, J.H.; Shachaf, C.M.; Shahbaba, B.; Levy, R.; Koller, D.; Plevritis, S.K. A pluripotency signature predicts histologic transformation and influences survival in follicular lymphoma patients. *Blood* **2009**, *114*, 3158–3166. [CrossRef]
111. Brodtkorb, M.; Lingjaerde, O.C.; Huse, K.; Troen, G.; Hystad, M.; Hilden, V.I.; Myklebust, J.H.; Leich, E.; Rosenwald, A.; Delabie, J.; et al. Whole-genome integrative analysis reveals expression signatures predicting transformation in follicular lymphoma. *Blood* **2014**, *123*, 1051–1054. [CrossRef]
112. Steen, C.B.; Leich, E.; Myklebust, J.H.; Lockmer, S.; Wise, J.F.; Wahlin, B.E.; Østenstad, B.; Liestøl, K.; Kimby, E.; Rosenwald, A.; et al. A clinico-molecular predictor identifies follicular lymphoma patients at risk of early transformation after first-line immunotherapy. *Haematologica* **2019**, *104*, e460–e464. [CrossRef] [PubMed]
113. Farinha, P.; Masoudi, H.; Skinnider, B.F.; Shumansky, K.; Spinelli, J.J.; Gill, K.; Klasa, R.; Voss, N.; Connors, J.M.; Gascoyne, R.D. Analysis of multiple biomarkers shows that lymphoma-associated macrophage (LAM) content is an independent predictor of survival in follicular lymphoma (FL). *Blood* **2005**, *106*, 2169–2174. [CrossRef] [PubMed]
114. Alvaro, T.; Lejeune, M.; Camacho, F.I.; Salvado, M.T.; Sanchez, L.; Garcia, J.F.; Lopez, C.; Jaen, J.; Bosch, R.; Pons, L.E.; et al. The presence of STAT1-positive tumor-associated macrophages and their relation to outcome in patients with follicular lymphoma. *Haematologica* **2006**, *91*, 1605–1612. [PubMed]
115. Taskinen, M.; Karjalainen-Lindsberg, M.L.; Nyman, H.; Eerola, L.M.; Leppa, S. A high tumor-associated macrophage content predicts favorable outcome in follicular lymphoma patients treated with rituximab and cyclophosphamide-doxorubicin-vincristine-prednisone. *Clin. Cancer Res.* **2007**, *13*, 5784–5789. [CrossRef]

116. Canioni, D.; Salles, G.; Mounier, N.; Brousse, N.; Keuppens, M.; Morchhauser, F.; Lamy, T.; Sonet, A.; Rousselet, M.C.; Foussard, C.; et al. High numbers of tumor-associated macrophages have an adverse prognostic value that can be circumvented by rituximab in patients with follicular lymphoma enrolled onto the GELA-GOELAMS FL-2000 trial. *J. Clin. Oncol.* **2008**, *26*, 440–446. [CrossRef]
117. Richendollar, B.G.; Pohlman, B.; Elson, P.; Hsi, E.D. Follicular programmed death 1-positive lymphocytes in the tumor microenvironment are an independent prognostic factor in follicular lymphoma. *Hum. Pathol.* **2011**, *42*, 552–557. [CrossRef]
118. Leidi, M.; Gotti, E.; Bologna, L.; Miranda, E.; Rimoldi, M.; Sica, A.; Roncalli, M.; Palumbo, G.A.; Introna, M.; Golay, J. M2 macrophages phagocytose rituximab-opsonized leukemic targets more efficiently than m1 cells in vitro. *J. Immunol.* **2009**, *182*, 4415–4422. [CrossRef]
119. de Jong, D.; Koster, A.; Hagenbeek, A.; Raemaekers, J.; Veldhuizen, D.; Heisterkamp, S.; de Boer, J.P.; van Glabbeke, M. Impact of the tumor microenvironment on prognosis in follicular lymphoma is dependent on specific treatment protocols. *Haematologica* **2009**, *94*, 70–77. [CrossRef]
120. Smeltzer, J.P.; Jones, J.M.; Ziesmer, S.C.; Grote, D.M.; Xiu, B.; Ristow, K.M.; Yang, Z.Z.; Nowakowski, G.S.; Feldman, A.L.; Cerhan, J.R.; et al. Pattern of CD14+ follicular dendritic cells and PD1+ T cells independently predicts time to transformation in follicular lymphoma. *Clin. Cancer Res.* **2014**, *20*, 2862–2872. [CrossRef]
121. Alvaro, T.; Lejeune, M.; Salvadó, M.T.; Lopez, C.; Jaén, J.; Bosch, R.; Pons, L.E. Immunohistochemical patterns of reactive microenvironment are associated with clinicobiologic behavior in follicular lymphoma patients. *J. Clin. Oncol.* **2006**, *24*, 5350–5357. [CrossRef]
122. Wahlin, B.E.; Aggarwal, M.; Montes-Moreno, S.; Gonzalez, L.F.; Roncador, G.; Sanchez-Verde, L.; Christensson, B.; Sander, B.; Kimby, E. A unifying microenvironment model in follicular lymphoma: Outcome is predicted by programmed death-1–positive, regulatory, cytotoxic, and helper T cells and macrophages. *Clin. Cancer Res.* **2010**, *16*, 637–650. [CrossRef] [PubMed]
123. Laurent, C.; Müller, S.; Do, C.; Al-Saati, T.; Allart, S.; Larocca, L.M.; Hohaus, S.; Duchez, S.; Quillet-Mary, A.; Laurent, G.; et al. Distribution, function, and prognostic value of cytotoxic T lymphocytes in follicular lymphoma: A 3-D tissue-imaging study. *Blood* **2011**, *118*, 5371–5379. [CrossRef] [PubMed]
124. Madsen, C.; Lauridsen, K.L.; Plesner, T.L.; Monrad, I.; Honoré, B.; Hamilton-Dutoit, S.; D'Amore, F.; Ludvigsen, M. High intratumoral expression of vimentin predicts histological transformation in patients with follicular lymphoma. *Blood Cancer J.* **2019**, *9*, 35. [CrossRef] [PubMed]
125. Kridel, R.; Xerri, L.; Gelas-Dore, B.; Tan, K.; Feugier, P.; Vawda, A.; Canioni, D.; Farinha, P.; Boussetta, S.; Moccia, A.A.; et al. The Prognostic Impact of CD163-Positive Macrophages in Follicular Lymphoma: A Study from the BC Cancer Agency and the Lymphoma Study Association. *Clin. Cancer Res.* **2015**, *21*, 3428–3435. [CrossRef]
126. Menter, T.; Tzankov, A.; Zucca, E.; Kimby, E.; Hultdin, M.; Sundström, C.; Beiske, K.; Cogliatti, S.; Banz, Y.; Cathomas, G.; et al. Prognostic implications of the microenvironment for follicular lymphoma under immunomodulation therapy. *Br. J. Haematol.* **2020**, *189*, 707–717. [CrossRef] [PubMed]
127. Taskinen, M.; Karjalainen-Lindsberg, M.L.; Leppa, S. Prognostic influence of tumor-infiltrating mast cells in patients with follicular lymphoma treated with rituximab and CHOP. *Blood* **2008**, *111*, 4664–4667. [CrossRef] [PubMed]
128. Chu, F.; Neelapu, S.S. Anti-PD-1 antibodies for the treatment of B-cell lymphoma: Importance of PD-1(+) T-cell subsets. *Oncoimmunology* **2014**, *3*, e28101. [CrossRef]
129. Skibola, C.F.; Bracci, P.M.; Halperin, E.; Conde, L.; Craig, D.W.; Agana, L.; Iyadurai, K.; Becker, N.; Brooks-Wilson, A.; Curry, J.D.; et al. Genetic variants at 6p21.33 are associated with susceptibility to follicular lymphoma. *Nat. Genet.* **2009**, *41*, 873–875. [CrossRef]
130. Conde, L.; Halperin, E.; Akers, N.K.; Brown, K.M.; Smedby, K.E.; Rothman, N.; Nieters, A.; Slager, S.L.; Brooks-Wilson, A.; Agana, L.; et al. Genome-wide association study of follicular lymphoma identifies a risk locus at 6p21.32. *Nat. Genet.* **2010**, *42*, 661–664. [CrossRef]
131. Wang, S.S.; Abdou, A.M.; Morton, L.M.; Thomas, R.; Cerhan, J.R.; Gao, X.; Cozen, W.; Rothman, N.; Davis, S.; Severson, R.K.; et al. Human leukocyte antigen class I and II alleles in non-Hodgkin lymphoma etiology. *Blood* **2010**, *115*, 4820–4823. [CrossRef]
132. Lu, Y.; Abdou, A.M.; Cerhan, J.R.; Morton, L.M.; Severson, R.K.; Davis, S.; Cozen, W.; Rothman, N.; Bernstein, L.; Chanock, S.; et al. Human leukocyte antigen class I and II alleles and overall survival in diffuse large B-cell lymphoma and follicular lymphoma. *ScientificWorldJournal* **2011**, *11*, 2062–2070. [CrossRef] [PubMed]
133. Alcoceba, M.; Sebastian, E.; Marin, L.; Balanzategui, A.; Sarasquete, M.E.; Chillón, M.C.; Jiménez, C.; Puig, N.; Corral, R.; Pardal, E.; et al. HLA specificities are related to development and prognosis of diffuse large B-cell lymphoma. *Blood* **2013**, *122*, 1448–1454. [CrossRef] [PubMed]
134. García-, M.; Alcoceba, M.; López-Parra, M.; Puig, N.; Antón, A.; Balanzategui, A.; Prieto-Conde, I.; Jiménez, C.; Sarasquete, M.E.; Chillón, M.C.; et al. HLA specificities are associated with prognosis in IGHV-mutated CLL-like high-count monoclonal B cell lymphocytosis. *PLoS ONE* **2017**, *12*, e0172978.
135. Wrench, D.; Leighton, P.; Skibola, C.F.; Conde, L.; Cazier, J.B.; Matthews, J.; Iqbal, S.; Carlotti, E.; Bodor, C.; Montoto, S.; et al. SNP rs6457327 in the HLA region on chromosome 6p is predictive of the transformation of follicular lymphoma. *Blood* **2011**, *117*, 3147–3150. [CrossRef] [PubMed]

136. Roschewski, M.; Dunleavy, K.; Pittaluga, S.; Moorhead, M.; Pepin, F.; Kong, K.; Shovlin, M.; Jaffe, E.S.; Staudt, L.M.; Lai, C.; et al. Circulating tumour DNA and CT monitoring in patients with untreated diffuse large B-cell lymphoma: A correlative biomarker study. *Lancet Oncol.* **2015**, *16*, 541–549. [CrossRef]
137. Sarkozy, C.; Huet, S.; Carlton, V.E.; Fabiani, B.; Delmer, A.; Jardin, F.; Delfau-Larue, M.H.; Hacini, M.; Ribrag, V.; Guidez, S.; et al. The prognostic value of clonal heterogeneity and quantitative assessment of plasma circulating clonal IG-VDJ sequences at diagnosis in patients with follicular lymphoma. *Oncotarget* **2017**, *8*, 8765–8774. [CrossRef]
138. Alcoceba, M.; García-Álvarez, M.; Chillón, M.C.; Jiménez, C.; Medina, A.; Antón, A.; Blanco, O.; Díaz, L.G.; Tamayo, P.; González-Calle, V.; et al. Liquid biopsy: A non-invasive approach for Hodgkin lymphoma genotyping. *Br. J. Haematol.* **2021**, *195*, 542–551. [CrossRef]
139. Lakhotia, R.; Melani, C.; Dunleavy, K.; Pittaluga, S.; Saba, N.S.; Lindenberg, L.; Mena, E.; Bergvall, E.; Lucas, A.N.; Jacob, A.P.; et al. Circulating Tumor DNA Predicts Therapeutic Outcome in Mantle Cell Lymphoma. *Blood Adv.* **2022**, *6*, 2667–2680. [CrossRef]
140. Delfau-Larue, M.H.; van der Gucht, A.; Dupuis, J.; Jais, J.P.; Nel, I.; Beldi-Ferchiou, A.; Hamdane, S.; Benmaad, I.; Laboure, G.; Verret, B.; et al. Total metabolic tumor volume, circulating tumor cells, cell-free DNA: Distinct prognostic value in follicular lymphoma. *Blood Adv.* **2018**, *2*, 807–816. [CrossRef]
141. Höpken, U.E. Targeting HDAC3 in CREBBP-Mutant Lymphomas Counterstrikes Unopposed Enhancer Deacetylation of B-cell Signaling and Immune Response Genes. *Cancer Discov.* **2017**, *7*, 14–16. [CrossRef]
142. Morschhauser, F.; Tilly, H.; Chaidos, A.; McKay, P.; Phillips, T.; Assouline, S.; Batlevi, C.L.; Campbell, P.; Ribrag, V.; Damaj, G.L.; et al. Tazemetostat for patients with relapsed or refractory follicular lymphoma: An open-label, single-arm, multicentre, phase 2 trial. *Lancet Oncol.* **2020**, *21*, 1433–1442. [CrossRef]
143. Patel, A.; Oluwole, O.; Savani, B.; Dholaria, B. Taking a BiTE out of the CAR T space race. *Br. J. Haematol.* **2021**, *195*, 689–697. [CrossRef] [PubMed]

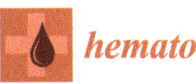

Review

Primary Cutaneous B-Cell Lymphoma: An Update on Pathologic and Molecular Features

Marco Lucioni [1], Sara Fraticelli [2], Giuseppe Neri [1], Monica Feltri [1], Giuseppina Ferrario [1], Roberta Riboni [1] and Marco Paulli [1,2,*]

[1] Anatomic Pathology Unit, Department of Molecular Medicine, University of Pavia, Fondazione IRCCS Policlinico San Matteo, Via Forlanini 14, 27100 Pavia, Italy; marco.lucioni@unipv.it (M.L.); giuseppe.joseph.neri@gmail.com (G.N.); moniechloe@gmail.com (M.F.); g.ferrario@smatteo.pv.it (G.F.); r.riboni@smatteo.pv.it (R.R.)

[2] Anatomic Pathology Unit, Department of Molecular Medicine, University of Pavia, 27100 Pavia, Italy; sara.fraticelli@unipv.it

* Correspondence: marco.paulli@unipv.it; Tel.: +39-0382-501-241; Fax: +39-0382-525-866

Abstract: Primary cutaneous B-cell lymphomas (PCBCLs) account for 25% of all primary cutaneous lymphomas. Three major types are currently recognized by the WHO classification: primary cutaneous marginal zone B-cell lymphoma (PCMZL), primary cutaneous follicle centre lymphoma (PCFCL) (both considered indolent lymphomas) and primary cutaneous diffuse large B-cell lymphoma, leg-type (PCDLBCL-LT), which is, instead, a very aggressive disease. Nowadays, the PCBCL's category also includes some rare entities such as intravascular B-cell lymphoma (IVBL) and the EBV+ mucocutaneous ulcer (EBVMCU). Furthermore, controversies still exist concerning the category of primary cutaneous diffuse large B-cell lymphoma (PCDLBCL), because some cases may present with clinical and histological features between PCFCL and PCDLBCL-LT. Therefore, some authors proposed introducing another category called PCDLBCL, not otherwise specified (NOS). Regardless, PCBCLs exhibit distinct features and differ in prognosis and treatment from their nodal/systemic counterparts. Therefore, clinicopathologic analysis is a key diagnostic element in the work-up of these lymphomas.

Keywords: primary cutaneous B-cell lymphoma; primary cutaneous marginal zone B-cell lymphoma; primary cutaneous follicle centre lymphoma; primary cutaneous diffuse large B-cell lymphoma, leg-type; primary cutaneous diffuse large B-cell lymphoma, not otherwise specified; intravascular B-cell lymphoma; EBV+ mucocutaneous ulcer

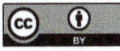

1. Introduction

Primary cutaneous B-cell lymphomas (PCBCLs) are a clinically and pathologically heterogeneous group of extranodal non-Hodgkin's lymphomas (NHLs) that primarily involve the skin, do not have evidence of extracutaneous disease at diagnosis and do not exhibit extracutaneous spread for a long time (or for the entire course of the disease) [1].

PCBCLs make up about 25% of all primary cutaneous lymphomas, but less than 1% of all NHLs [2,3]. PCBCLs exhibit distinct clinical, histological, immunophenotypic and genetic features and differ in prognosis and treatment from their nodal/systemic counterparts [4,5].

PCBCL diagnosis and management is a multidisciplinary task, involving dermatologists, pathologists, haemato-oncologists and radiation oncologists [6]. The diagnosis of PCBCL needs careful histomorphological and immunophenotypical analyses, corroborated by clinical data and, when necessary, by molecular and cytogenetic investigations. The preanalytical phase is crucial, and adequate (in size and quality) lesional samples should be obtained. Whenever possible, excisional biopsies should be recommended [2].

Careful clinical examination and staging at presentation are mandatory to exclude secondary cutaneous localization of systemic B-cell lymphomas—these can be histologically indistinguishable from their primary cutaneous counterparts [7].

Current WHO (2017) classification [8] recognizes three types of PCBCLs as being most frequent: (1) primary cutaneous marginal zone B-cell lymphoma (PCMZL); (2) primary cutaneous follicle centre lymphoma (PCFCL); and (3) primary cutaneous diffuse large B-cell lymphoma, leg-type (PCDLBCL-LT). PCMZL and PCFCL are considered to be indolent lymphomas with a good prognosis and a five-year disease-specific survival rate of >95%. In contrast, PCDLBCL-LT is an aggressive lymphoma, with a five-year survival rate between 40 and 60%. PCBCL also includes some rare entities such as intravascular B-cell lymphoma (IVBL) and the EBV+ mucocutaneous ulcer (EBVMCU), a provisional entity [3].

In spite of these classificational advances, the diagnosis of PCBCL can be challenging and some issues are still a matter of debate. In some cases, a clear-cut distinction between PCMZL and/or PCFCL and reactive cutaneous lymphoid infiltrates (so-called "pseudolymphoma") may be difficult through histology alone [9].

Furthermore, controversies still exist concerning the category of primary cutaneous diffuse large B-cell lymphoma (PCDLBCL) [10]. The border between centroblast-rich PCFCL and PCDLBCL is not clear; similarly, the term "PCDLBCL-LT" sounds inadequate for describing the whole spectrum of PCDLBCLs. Cases of PCDLBCL that are mostly composed of centroblast-like cells may also arise in sites other than the legs and pursue a less aggressive clinical course. Based on such findings, some authors proposed the definition of PCDLBCL, not otherwise specified (NOS) for these cases [11].

2. Primary Cutaneous Marginal Zone B-Cell Lymphoma

PCMZL is a very indolent type of extranodal marginal zone lymphoma (MZL), originating from the skin associated lymphoid tissue (SALT) that presents in the skin with some distinctive features [3,12]. It accounts for about 20–40% of all PCBCLs in western countries (0.4 per 1,000,000 per year in the U.S.A.) [8]. It affects mainly adults and the elderly (median age at diagnosis >50 years with a male predominance) [13] and, exceptionally, children and adolescents. However, the occurrence of primary cutaneous MZL in the paediatric age range is a matter of debate [14,15].

As in other extranodal MZL, a link with chronic antigenic stimulation has also been suggested for PCMZL, including bacterial and viral agents, tattoo pigments, vaccines and iatrogenic agents (fluoxetine). Borrelia burgdorferi infection has been associated with PCBCL, including the PCMZL type, according to studies from some European countries (Scotland and Austria); however, other studies, mostly from Asia and the U.S.A., did not confirm such an association, suggesting geographic variability [16,17]. Other infections possibly associated with the development of PCMZL are herpes simplex virus type 1 and hepatitis virus [18]. Notably, hepatitis C virus (HCV) infections have been found in association with up to 43% of PCMZL, according to one Italian study, and rare cases responding to antiviral therapy have been reported [19–22]. PCMZL may also arise in an autoimmune disease setting, such as Sjögren syndrome or Hashimoto's thyroiditis [23–25].

2.1. Clinical Features

PCMZL usually presents on the arms and trunk, but other sites, including the head and neck, may also be involved. Lesions are often multifocal, in contrast to PCFCL, and consist of red to purple papules, nodules and/or plaques. Ulceration is exceptional [26,27]. In some cases, mostly in the context of autoimmune disorders, the lesion may spontaneously regress, leaving a localized area of flaccid skin (so-called anetoderma) due to loss of dermal elastic tissue [28,29]. One peculiar subset of PCMZL, which is associated with HCV infection and has a female predilection, presents with confined subcutaneous nodular lesions, clinically mimicking lipoma [22].

2.2. Pathology

PCMZL infiltrates initially involve the reticular dermis and may subsequently extend throughout the whole dermis and hypodermis—the epidermis is spared. Periadnexal infiltration around eccrine glands and hair follicles is frequently seen, but lymphoepithelial lesions are uncommon and not critical for diagnosis [24].

The overall architecture is usually nodular, but it may also be diffuse (Figure 1). Lymphoid follicles with reactive germinal centres and preserved mantle zones are frequently seen. In the initial lesion, the neoplastic marginal zone (MZ) circumscribes the reactive follicles. At disease progression, the follicles can be colonized by MZ B cells with partial and/or diffuse effacement of dendritic meshwork [12]. The lymphoma population includes small- to medium-sized centrocyte-like MZ B cells, monocytoid B cells (Figure 1), lymphoplasmacytic cells, scattered centroblasts and/or immunoblast-like cells. A variable degree of plasmacytic differentiation may occur (Figure 1), the plasma cells usually being located at the periphery of the infiltrate. Amyloid deposition can be found in cases with prominent plasmacytic differentiation. Some morphological variants of PCMZL have been described, including small-cell lymphocytic variants, monocytoid variants and variants with diffuse plasmacytic differentiation [30]. A variable amount of inflammatory cells may be admixed with the neoplastic population, including T-cell lymphocytes, histiocytes, mast cells and eosinophils. The reactive inflammatory population may be prominent, obscuring the lymphoma cells [31].

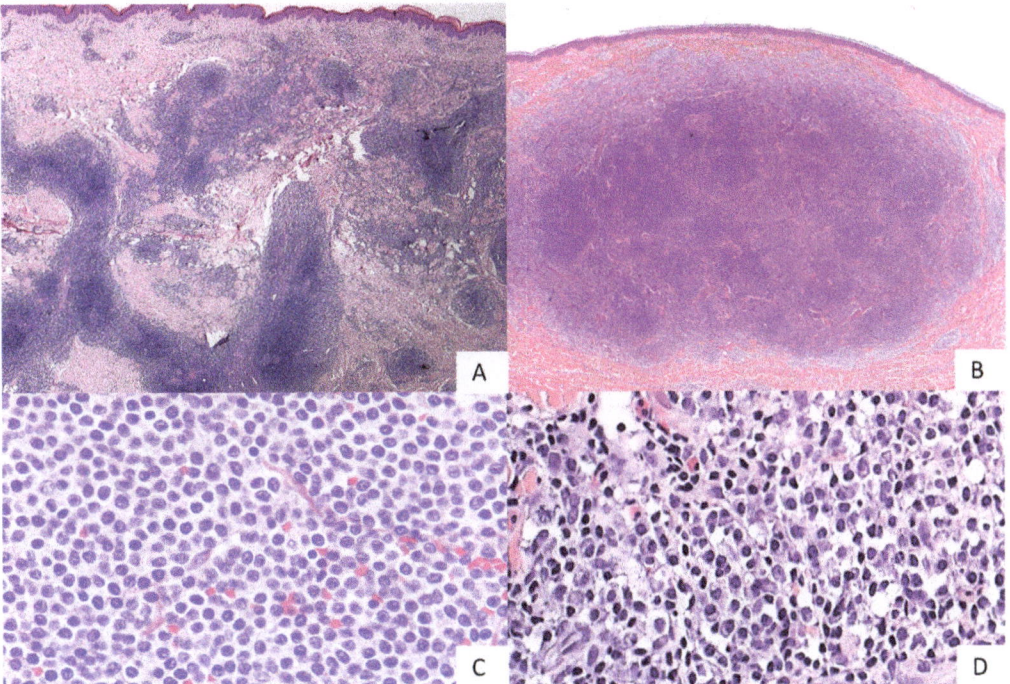

Figure 1. PCMZL. At histological evaluation, this lymphoma shows a nodular ((**A**), HE 2×) or a diffuse growth pattern ((**B**), HE 2×) and is composed of small- to medium-sized B cells, sometimes with a monocytoid appearance ((**C**), HE 40×) or a plasmacytic differentiation ((**D**), HE 40×).

No specific immunophenotype profile exists for MZLs in general, including cutaneous ones. Lymphoma cells express B-cell antigens (CD19, CD20, CD22 and CD79a), and bcl-2 being negative for CD5, CD10, bcl-6 and Cyclin D1. CD23 expression is variable. Plasma cell components express CD38, CD138 and CD79a, but not CD20. Light chain clonal restrictions can be demonstrated with immunohistochemistry, as well as by in situ hybridization. Follicular markers (CD10 and bcl-6), coupled with Ki-67, are helpful in highlighting residual reactive germinal centres, in which CD21 and CD23 immunostainings may evidentiate the disruption of the dendritic meshwork [32].

Increased numbers of plasmacytoid dendritic cells (CD123+) have been reported in PCMZL when compared with very few or absent plasmacytoid dendritic cells in PCFCL and PCLBCL, respectively [33].

Recently, PCMZL has been subdivided into two subtypes, one carrying class-switched immunoglobulins, the other carrying non-class-switched ones [34]. The class-switched form of the disease (90% of cases) contains monotypic plasma cells with expressions of IgG and, to a lesser extent, IgA or IgE, which are mainly localized at the periphery of the infiltrate. It lacks CXCR3, shows a predominant type 2 helper T cell environment and lacks reactive germinal centre colonization [35]. In contrast, the non-class-switched PCMZL (10% of cases) shows CXCR3 and IgM expression and more frequently reveals a diffuse proliferation of large nodules of neoplastic B cells. The class-switched subtype seems to pursue an indolent course, with an extremely low risk of progression to large B-cell lymphoma and/or of extracutaneous spread [36].

On such a basis, it seems reasonable to retain the class-switched subtype as a clonal chronic lymphoproliferative disorder, rather than as a lymphoma. Up to 40% of IgG-positive PCMZL cases express IgG4, but they are unrelated to systemic IgG4-related diseases [37].

2.3. Molecular and Cytogenetic Features

Clonal IGH or IGK gene rearrangements may be detected in up to 80–92% of PCMZLs [24,38]. Cytogenetic abnormalities usually associated with MALT lymphoma have been variably reported in PCMZL: the t(14;18)(q32;q21) (IGH-MALT1) is the most frequent one (in up to 25% of PCMZL), whereas t(11;18)(q21;q21) (BIRC3-MALT1) and t(3;14)(p14.1;q32) (IGH-FOXP1) rearrangements are less common. The t(1;14)(p22;q32) involving IGH and BCL10 has not been identified [39]. Trisomies of chromosomes 3 and 18 have been reported in up to 20% of PCMZLs. BCL6 rearrangements have been sporadically observed, but IGH-BCL2 translocations are absent. Activating MYD88^{L265P} mutations, more commonly associated with lymphoplasmacytic lymphoma and PCDLBCL-LT, have been detected in 6% of PCMZLs, however, exclusively in IgM-positive types (three of six IgM-positive PCMZLs) [40]. The mutational landscape of PCMZL may also include alterations of FAS (24 of 38, 63%), SLAMF1 (9 of 38, 24%), SPEN (7 of 38, 18%) and NCOR2 (5 of 38, 13%) [41].

2.4. Differential Diagnosis

Particularly in the early phase of PCMZL, the lymphoma infiltrate may appear to be not specific. Differential diagnoses include other lymphomas (i.e., lymphoplasmacytic lymphoma, plasma cell myeloma and primary cutaneous follicular helper T-cell lymphoma (PCFHTCL)), as well as inflammatory, non-neoplastic cutaneous lymphoid hyperplasia (CLH) [24]. The distinction between PCMZL lymphoma and CLH may sometimes be very difficult to determine (Table 1) as they often share histopathological features (abundant reactive background and B follicles with germinal centres) [42].

Table 1. Differential diagnosis between PCFCL, PCMZL and CLH.

Characteristics	PCFCL	PCMZL	CLH
Age	50–60	>50	50
Sex	M > F	M > F	F > M
Site	head, trunk, leg	arms, trunk, head, neck	face (nose and cheeks), trunk, extremities
Clinical features	plaque, nodule, tumour	papules, nodules, plaques	nodule, papules
Single/multiple lesions	usually single	often multifocal	usually single
Histology			
Cells morphology	centrocytes (prevalent) and centroblasts	centrocyte-like, monocytoid, lymphoplasmacytic. Plasma cells often present in superficial dermis and at the lymphoma's periphery	small lymphocytes
Pattern	nodular, nodular and diffuse, diffuse	nodular (more often), diffuse	nodular/diffuse
Skin ulceration	absent	absent	absent
Necrosis	no	No	no
Adnexal effacement	usually absent	usually absent	usually absent
Reactive T-cell CD3+ infiltrate	present, abundant	present, abundant	present
Dendritic meshwork	present/absent	present/absent	present
Immunophenotype	CD20+, CD79a+ bcl6+, CD10+, bcl2- (73%)	CD20+, CD79a+, bcl2+, CD10-, bcl6-, CD5-Cyclin-D1-, CD23- (most cases)	mixed infiltrates of B and T cells with reactive germinal centres
Ki67	usually low (up to 30%)	usually low	high in reactive germinal centres
Molecular features	rarely translocation IGH-BCL2 up to 40% BCL2 aberrations	80–92% clonal IGH/IGK gene rearrangements, 25% translocation IGH-MALT1	80–90% polyclonal
Prognosis	indolent	indolent	usually good

The presence of lymphoepithelial lesions has a limited diagnostic value in PCMZL. Ancillary studies may corroborate lymphoma diagnosis, documenting clonal IGH rearrangements by means of molecular analyses and/or light chain restriction by means of immunohistochemistry or ISH technique. However, it is important to stress that clonal rearrangements may also occur in some reactive lymphoid infiltrates. As a consequence, a definitive diagnosis may not always be achieved, even after a judicious integration of pathological and clinical data. In these cases, only clinical "follow-ups" and repeated biopsies may finally confirm the lymphoma diagnosis [12].

Distinction of PCMZL from other PCBCLs requires the careful evaluation of a series of cytological and architectural features combined with a proper immunohistochemical panel. The B-cell follicles in PCMZL typically exhibit reactive germinal centres. The follicles in PCFCL are monomorphic in appearance, with low Ki-67 proliferation, while bcl6+ and CD10+/− B cells are detectable in the interfollicular areas (Table 1). Cases with prominent plasmacytic differentiation must be distinguished from lymphoplasmacytic lymphoma and plasma cell myeloma [43]. PCMZL usually lacks the MYD88^{L265P} mutation typical of lymphoplasmacytic lymphoma; nevertheless, it is important to remember that plasmacytic differentiation may occur in PCMZL [44,45]. In the skin infiltrated by systemic myeloma, the detection of the sheet-like proliferation of monotypic plasma cells and/or plasmablasts (without a CD20+ lymphocytic component) support the myeloma diagnosis.

Cytoarchitectural features and immunostainings for CD5, CD23, SOX11 and cyclin D1 usually allow for the exclusion of cutaneous localizations of mantle cell lymphoma (MCL) and chronic lymphocytic leukaemia [8].

2.5. Prognosis and Treatment

PCMZL prognosis is excellent, with a five-year survival rate of 98%. Complete response to therapy occurs in 93% of patients with solitary lesions and 75% of patients with a multifocal disease [46]. Relapses are common within five years, occurring in 39% of patients with solitary lesions and 77% of patients with multifocal lesions. PCMZL rarely exhibits extracutaneous spread (lymph nodes and MALT sites) or large cell transformations [47,48].

PCMZL with solitary or few contiguous lesions can be treated with radiotherapy or excision with curative intent. Antibiotic treatment is required in Borrelia antibody-positive cases. Lesional regression has also been reported in cases of HCV-related PCMZL, including the so-called "lipoma-like" variant. Topical therapies are sometimes employed, including clobetasol, nitrogen mustard, cryotherapy and imiquimod [49–51].

2.6. Summing Up

PCMZL is an uncommon lymphoma subtype clinically characterized by a very indolent course and a favourable outcome. In addition, spontaneous lesional regression has been reported in various cases. In contrast, some studies have reported high rates of relapse, mostly cutaneous. Particularly in the early stage of the disease, differential diagnosis between PCMZL and CLH may be difficult. Recently, an MZL classification based on IgH switching revealed two disease subsets, one of which (class-switched form) usually shows a better clinical course and outcome. On such a basis, it is reasonable to postulate that at least a part of PCMZL indeed represents atypical lymphoid proliferation rather than true lymphoma. The high relapse rates reported in certain studies might be, at least in part, ascribed to an incomplete lesional surgical excision, thus representing a local disease recurrence rather that a true relapse.

3. Primary Cutaneous Follicle Centre Lymphoma

PCFCL is a low-grade lymphoid malignancy that develops from a mature germinal centre (GC) B cell in the skin. PCFCL accounts for about 50% of PCBCL, and for 10–20% of all cutaneous lymphomas. PCFCL is more frequent in Caucasian males (median age: 55), and its occurrence in the paediatric age range is matter of debate; male-to-female ratio is 1.5:1 [8,52–54]. Borrelia burgdorferi infections have also been reported in a fraction of PCFCL cases from endemic areas [55,56]. Prognosis is very favourable, but relapses may occur. Transformation into diffuse large B-cell lymphoma (DLBCL) has been reported [57].

3.1. Clinical Features

PCFCL usually presents with solitary, localized or (less often) multifocal (15%), painless, non-pruritic, erythematous to violaceous plaques, nodules or tumours that vary in size and are not usually ulcerated. The most frequently involved sites include the head (in particular the forehead and scalp) and trunk [8,58].

PCFCL presenting on the trunk—historically known as "reticulohistiocytoma of the dorsum" or "Crosti lymphoma—is characterized by a central core of plaques and tumours centrifugally surrounded by papules and macules [59]. Localization on the legs occur in about 5% of cases, and it seems to be associated with a less favourable outcome [8].

Without treatment, lesions tend to slowly progress and may assume a pattern of infiltrating and destroying [60]. Recurrences usually occur at the same site or in proximity of initial presentation [8].

3.2. Pathology

In the early stage, PCFCL usually shows a nodular growth pattern with closely spaced, monotonous neoplastic follicular aggregates (Figure 2). Lymphoma follicles have no polarization, have diminished (or absent) mantle zones and lack tingible body macrophages. Typically, a "grenz zone" beneath the epidermis surface is observed. At disease progression, the neoplastic follicles tend to fuse, resulting in a nodular and/or diffuse growth pattern, often with hypodermis involvement (Figure 2). Occasionally, an "inverted nodular pattern" can be encountered, with neoplastic cells located in pale areas at the periphery of follicles and small reactive lymphocytes in dark areas at the centre [61].

PCFCL populations consist of an admixture of centrocytes and centroblasts. Sometimes it may consist predominantly of large, often multilobated, cells or exhibit a spindle-like cytological appearance, mimicking sarcomatoid neoplasms (mostly due to intermingled reactive fibrosis) [62].

In contrast with its nodal counterpart, in PCFCL, the grading (number of large centroblast-like cells) and predominant growth pattern (follicular versus diffuse) retain limited prognostic relevance.

PCFCL may be associated with a variable amount of reactive T cells and histiocytes. Dendritic meshwork (highlighted by CD21/CD23 immunostainings) is usually disrupted and/or effaced. PCFCL cells express B-cell markers (CD20, CD79a, CD19, CD22 and PAX5) and GC markers (bcl6, CD10, MEF2B and HGAL). The CD10 expression on paraffin sections is variable, being influenced by antibody clones and fixation time. Notably, PCFCLs showing a diffuse growth pattern frequently lack CD10. Some studies have reported a lack of bcl-2 in the vast majority of PCFCL cases. In contrast, in our and other researchers' experience, bcl-2 may be expressed in at least 25–27% of PCFCL cases; the evaluation of bcl-2 expression in PCFCL may be difficult in cases with T-cell-rich reactive infiltrates that are uniformly bcl-2+. The proliferation index is variable, from low to up to 30%.

Cases showing a diffuse growth pattern, coupled with an increased number of centroblast-like cells, usually have a higher Ki-67 rate [8].

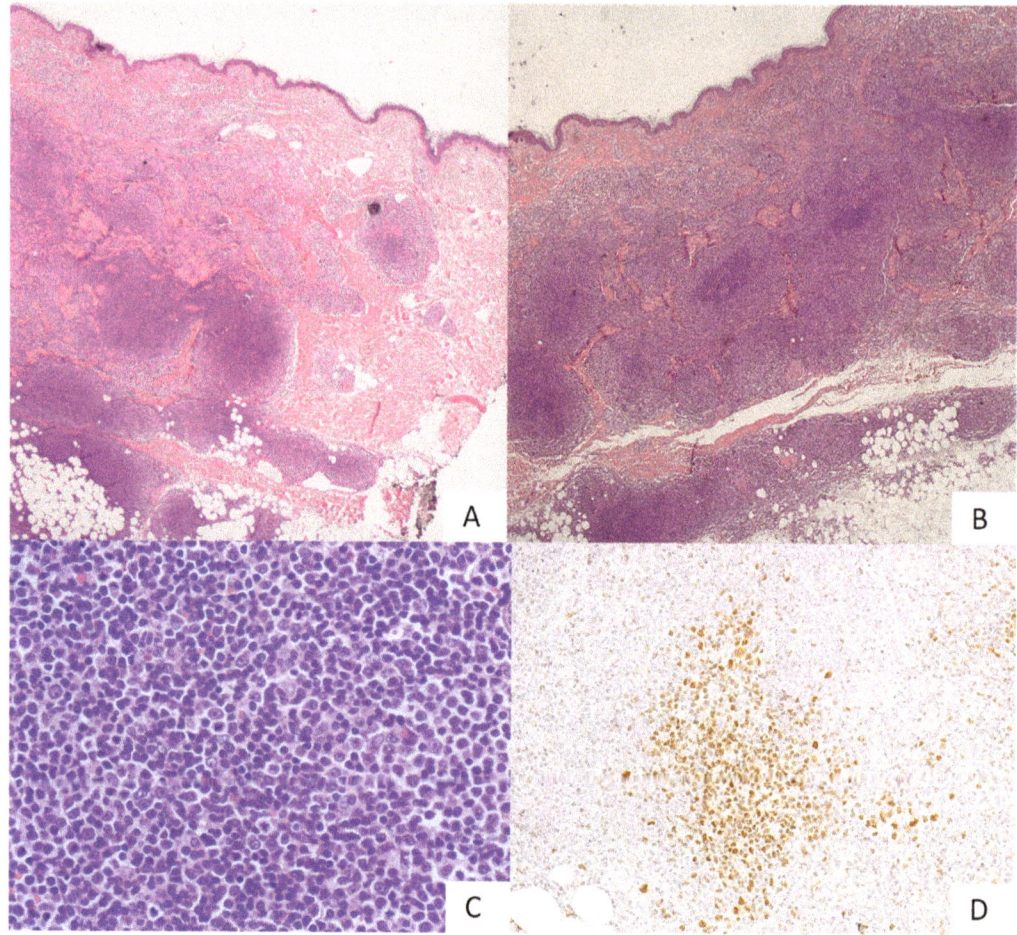

Figure 2. PCFCL. At histological evaluation, this lymphoma shows a nodular growth pattern ((**A**), HE 2×), sometimes nodular and vaguely diffuse ((**B**), 2×), composed of an admixture of centrocytes and centroblasts ((**C**), HE 40×), and is usually bcl6-positive ((**D**), 10×).

3.3. Molecular and Cytogenetic Features

In the past, t(14;18)(q23;q21), the genetic hallmark of nodal follicular lymphoma (FL) involving BCL2 and IGH genes, has been retained as an exceedingly rare occurrence in PCFCLs. This lack was proposed as a way to distinguish secondary skin localizations of nodal FL from PCFCL [63]. In contrast, in the last decade, several groups have documented BCL2 chromosomal aberrations in up to 40% of PCFCL cases [63–71]. Such divergent findings could be partially related to the molecular technique employed, with a higher incidence observed with PCR analysis [69].

In some studies, the presence of BCL2 rearrangements has been more frequently associated with a predominantly centrocytic morphology, a high probability of skin relapse and a higher risk of extracutaneous spread [72,73].

Other reported chromosomal alterations include loss of heterozygosity in chromosomes 6p and 9p, deletion of 1p36, 14q32.33, 2p11.2 (IGKV locus), 9p21.3 (CDKN2A locus) and 14q32.33 (IGH locus), gains involving chromosomes 7 and 18 and high-level amplifications at 2p16.1 (REL gene). Aberrant somatic hypermutations targeting BCL6, PAX5,

RhoH/TTF and/or MYC genes have also been reported. NGS analysis documented somatic mutations on TNFRSF14, CREBBP, TNFAIP3, KMT2D, SOCS1, EP300, STAT6 and FOXO1 genes, as well as nucleotide substitutions (C>T transitions) associated with UV-damage [74]. Concomitant 1p36 deletion and TNFRSF14 mutations in PCFCL seem to be associated with elevated levels of EZH2 protein expression [75,76].

3.4. Differential Diagnosis

PCFCL with a predominant follicular growth pattern must primarily be distinguished from reactive CLH (Table 1). The differential diagnosis between PCFCL and CLH mainly relies on the lack of the typical features that characterize the reactive follicles, such as heterogeneity in shape and size, compartmentalization (polarization) into light and dark zones, detectable mantle and marginal zone areas and the presence of tingible body macrophages. Reactive follicles have also retained the CD21/CD23+ dendritic meshwork and a high Ki-67 proliferation index. PCFCL favours the reduction or disappearance of mantle and marginal zone areas coupled with the absence of tingible body macrophages and a low proliferation index. Similarly, lymphoma favours an expansion of follicular centre B cells (bcl-6+ and CD10+) in the interfollicular areas. Detection of clonal Ig gene rearrangements may support lymphoma diagnosis, but some cases remain doubtful and clinical follow-ups should be recommended [77].

The distinction of PCDLBL from secondary cutaneous localizations of nodal FL is a clinically relevant issue because of divergences in prognosis and therapy. PCFCL and secondary cutaneous involvement by a nodal FL can be indistinguishable in skin biopsies by morphology alone; thus, a complete clinical staging is mandatory. However, the primary cutaneous forms often lack CD10 and bcl-2 immunoreactivity as well as BCL2 rearrangements [63]. In skin localizations of systemic FL, the neoplastic cells usually show strong co-expressions of bcl2 and bcl6 and carry BCL-2 translocation.

Recently, a whole-exome sequencing study on a series of FLs—, including both systemic and primary cutaneous ones—proposed three criteria: BCL2 rearrangement, chromatin-modifying gene mutations (CREBBP, KMT2D, EZH2, and EP300) and proliferation rate to identify PCFCL subsets at different degrees of risk for concurrent or future systemic spread [78]. PCFCLs with diffuse growth patterns and a high content of large, centroblast-like cells, enter the differential diagnosis with PCDLBCL-LT (Table 2).

Table 2. Differential diagnosis between PCFCL, PCDLBCL NOS and PCDLBCL-LT.

Characteristics	PCFCL	PCDLBL NOS	PCDLBCL-LT
Age	50–60	60	70–80
Sex	M>F	M>F	F>M
Site	head, trunk, leg	trunk, head-neck, lower limbs, upper limbs	leg, trunk, head-neck, upper extremities
Clinical features	plaque, nodule, tumour	nodule, plaque	tumour, nodule
Single/multiple lesions	usually single	single	single or multiple
Histology			
Cells morphology	centrocytes (prevalent) and centroblasts	centroblasts with <10% of medium sized cells	centroblast and/or immunoblast
Pattern	nodular, nodular and diffuse, diffuse	diffuse, vaguely nodular	diffuse
Skin ulceration	Absent	present or absent	mostly present
Necrosis	no	rare	yes
Adnexal effacement	usually absent	May be present	mostly present
Reactive T-cell CD3+ infiltrate	present, abundant	present, mild to moderate	few or absent
Dendritic meshwork	present/absent	absent	absent
Immunophenotype	CD20+, CD79a+, Bcl6+, CD10+, Bcl2-(73%)	CD20+, CD79a+, Bcl6+, CD10-/-, MUM1+/-, IgM+/-, c-Myc+/-, bcl2-/+	CD20+, CD79a+, Bcl2+, MUM1+, Bcl6+, c-myc+, IgM+, CD10-
Ki67	usually low (up to 30%)	moderate (40%)	high (>70%)
DE phenotype	no	infrequent	>60% of cases
Molecular features	rarely translocation IGH-BCL2, up to 40% BCL2 aberrations	rearrangements of BCL6 or MYC, rarely BCL2 alterations	IGH clonal rearrangements, translocations involving BCL6, MYC and IGH, MYD88[L265P] mutations
DH/TH status	no	DH status reported in literature (one case)	yes
Prognosis	indolent	less aggressive than PCDLBCL-LT, GC cases more similar to PCFCL, Non-GC cases in between PCFCL and PCDLBCL-LT	aggressive

The presence of large, cohesive sheets of centroblasts and immunoblasts with an activated B-cell-like (ABC) profile usually leads to the diagnosis of DLBCL; the presence of a vaguely residual nodular pattern (at low magnification), a residual dendritic meshwork (although disrupted), an intense, intermingled reactive T cell infiltrate, a weak to absent bcl-2 expression and negativity for IgM and MUM1 favour a PCFCL. Additional molecular analysis can also be useful, as PCDLBCLs variably carry MYC and/or BCL6 translocations, BCL2 and MALT1 region amplifications, CDKN2A loss on chromosome 9p21.3 (more than 50% of cases) and MYD88^{L265P} mutations [79].

Differential diagnosis between PCFCL and PCMZL mainly concerns cases of PCFCL presenting with an inverted nodular pattern, or cases of PCMZL with prominent follicular colonization. The presence of a clonal plasmacytic component, rarely seen in PCFCL, and negativity for GC markers (bcl6 and CD10) in neoplastic cells may be a useful diagnostic clue to recognize PCMZL, along with negativity for STMN1, LMO2, HGAL, MNDA and AID, and the absence of 1p36 deletion [80–82].

PCFHTCL is a follicular centre T-helper CD4+ neoplasm, not yet well characterized, which can mimic, both clinically and histologically, PCFCL. Cases of PCFHTCL misdiagnosed as PCFCL have been recognized only after an ineffective therapy with rituximab [83].

PCFHTCL usually contains a large amount of accompanying reactive B follicles; neoplastic T cells are medium to large in size, have irregular nuclei with small nucleoli and express T-cell markers (including CD2, CD3, CD4), T follicular helper markers (PD1, CXCL13 and ICOS) and GC markers (such as CD10 and bcl6); T-cell clonality can be detected in most cases. PCFCL with prominent spindle-shaped cytology must be distinguished from other spindle-cell tumours, including spindle cell melanoma, spindle squamous cell carcinoma, and spindle cell mesenchymal neoplasms [62,84].

3.5. Prognosis and Treatment

PCFCL is an indolent disease, with a 95% disease-specific five-year survival rate.

After treatment (see below), 99% of patients achieve complete remission; cutaneous relapses occur in about 30% of cases, but only 10% of patients have extracutaneous spread (lymph nodes, bone marrow and/or extralymphoid organs) [52–54].

Progression into large B-cell lymphomas is rare, and usually does not fit with leg-type features. Histology and multifocal diseasedo not influence prognosis. PCFCLs presenting on the legs seem to pursue a less favourable outcome (overall five-year survival rate: 41%). The prognostic significance of BCL-2 translocation in PCFCL is a controversial issue. In our experience and in other studies, the presence of such translocation seems to be associated with less favourable outcomes and an elevated risk of recurrence [73].

Treatment choices include the "watch and wait" approach, excision, radiotherapy and local or systemic therapy based on clinical presentation and disease extension [6].

Cutaneous relapses do not usually require a more aggressive treatment. Low-dose radiation therapy is recommended for localized lesions, allowing a complete response rate of 99%. Intralesional corticosteroids or rituximab and other topical agents (such as mustard, cryotherapy and imiquimod) can also be employed. Skin-disseminated diseases can achieve complete remission after systemic biological therapy with single-agent rituximab, while multiagent chemotherapy (R-CHOP) is reserved for refractory diseases, extracutaneous dissemination and cases arising on the legs [3,6].

3.6. Summing Up

PCFCL is the most frequent subtype of PCBCL, usually with a favourable clinical outcome—other than for cases presenting on the leg. Histologically, PCFCL exhibits, in the early stage, a nodular/follicular pattern. Subsequently, lymphoma follicles tend to merge, resulting in a diffuse pattern extending into subcutis. Lymphoma populations consist of an admixture of centrocyte- and centroblast-like cells. They sometimes present with peculiar cytological features, including polylobated centroblasts and a spindle-like cell appearance. The number of centroblastic cells and the growth pattern are retained as not being prognostically significant. PCFCL has a B cell phenotype with variable expressions of GC markers and bcl-2, the latter often negative. Mainly in PCFCL, CD10 may also be negative, showing a diffuse growth pattern. The presence of BCL-2 rearrangements is still debated, but some studies have reported that cases of PCFCL with BCL-2 translocations are associated with a less favourable outcome.

4. Primary Cutaneous Diffuse Large B Cell Lymphoma, Leg-Type

PCDLBCL-LT is an aggressive DLBCL characterized by sheets of centroblasts and/or immunoblasts with no/few admixed reactive cells, usually arising on the leg and showing an ABC phenotype [8,85]. According to the most recent WHO classification of skin tumours, 4% of all primary cutaneous lymphomas are PCDLBCL-LT and it accounts for the 20% of PCBCLs [8,86]. It typically occurs in the eighth decade of life. Elderly women are more commonly affected, with a male-to-female ratio of 1:3–4 [8,87].

4.1. Clinical Features

PCDLBCL-LT is a rapidly progressive disease which involves mostly the lower legs (one or both), however in 10–15% of cases it may arise at other sites, such as the trunk, the head–neck area, and the upper extremities [88].

Clinically, PCDLBCL-LT presents with one or multiple red to bluish tumours which can be ulcerated, otherwise it may appear as a multicoloured or verrucous nodule. Larger tumours may be surrounded by smaller satellite lesions [8,89]. Moreover, extracutaneous dissemination is frequent [90].

4.2. Pathology

Morphologically, PCDLBCL-LT is characterized by a diffuse, non-epidermotropic, dense infiltrate with a grenz zone, which involves the entire dermis, effaces adnexal structures and often extends to the subcutaneous tissue. Overlying skin is frequently ulcerated. Cytologically, the infiltrate is usually monomorphic, consisting of round centroblastic and/or immunoblastic cells arranged in sheets (Figure 3), with very few reactive T-lymphocytes and minimal stromal reaction; occasionally pleomorphic to anaplastic cells are seen. Numerous mitoses and necrosis are usually found, while follicular structures and CD21+/CD23+ dendritic meshwork are typically lacking [86,90].

The immunophenotype of PCDLBCL-LT resembles that of the non-germinal centre-type of nodal DLBCL [91]. Neoplastic cells are positive for CD20, CD79a, bcl-2, MUM-1/IRF4 and (usually) bcl-6, but negative for CD10. FOXP1, c-MYC and cytoplasmic IgM are positive in most cases (Figure 3), whereas CD30 is usually not expressed [8,86,92]. Since bcl-2 is positive in more than 90% of cases and c-MYC is positive in over 65%, more than 60% of PCDLBCL-LT have a double-expressor (DE) phenotype [12,86]. EBV search is negative [87].

PD-L1 and CD33 may be expressed by tumour cells or by myeloid-derived suppressor cells (MDSCs), therefore, it has been suggested that they may shield the tumour against PD-1+ tumour-infiltrating lymphocytes [93]. A high proliferative index (usually >70%) is seen [8].

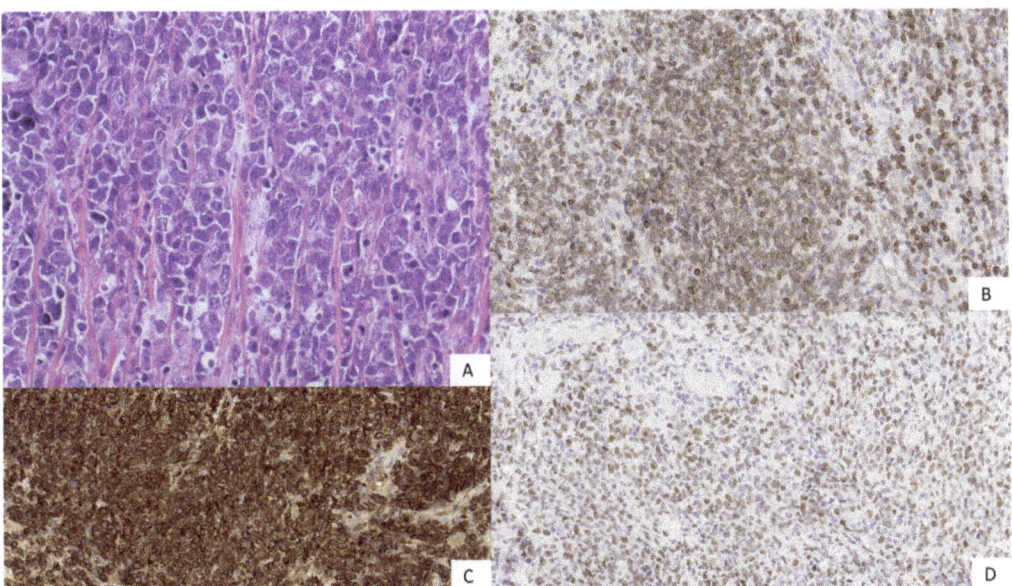

Figure 3. PCDLBCL LT. At histological evaluation, this lymphoma is composed of sheets of large, atypical cells (centroblasts and/or immunoblasts) with numerous mitoses and no/few reactive backgrounds ((**A**), HE 40×). PCDLBCL-LT frequently expresses bcl2 ((**B**), 20×), IgM ((**C**), 20×), and c-MYC ((**D**), 20×).

4.3. Molecular and Cytogenetic Features

Clonal rearrangements of IGH genes are detected in most PCDLBCLs. According to a post-germinal centre derivation, rearranged IGH genes usually carry somatic hypermutation, often with concurrent BCL-6 mutations. However, the precise definition of the cell of origin (COO) of PCDLBCL-LT is incomplete.

A study by Hoefangel et al. [85], based on gene expression analyses techniques, reported that PCDLBCL-LT has a profile similar to that of ABC-like nodal DLBCL.

On the other hand, a more recent study by Schrader et al. [94], based on Lymph2Cx algorithm, documented that the COO classification of PCLBCL-LT is more heterogeneous than expected, with only 18% of cases resulting as ABCs, 39% as germinal centre B cells (GCBs) and 43% as unclassifiable.

FISH analysis reveals translocations involving IGH, MYC, and BCL6 genes [38,92].

Recently, cases of PCDLBCL-LT with a double or triple hit status have been described [11].

In spite of bcl-2 protein overexpression, BCL-2 rearrangements are usually absent, whereas BCL-2 amplification was found in a fraction of cases. Loss of CDKN2A and CDKN2B have also been reported in more than 50% of cases. MYD88^{L265P} mutations are the most common, being found in two thirds of patients, [8,95,96] but mutations in PIM1 and CD79B have also been seen. MYD88^{L265P} mutations and mutations in CARD11, CD79B and TNFAIP3/A20 may indicate a constitutive activation of the NF-kB pathway [12,97,98].

Moreover, Zhou et al. [99] reported that in the MYD-88 wild-type PCDLBCL-LT, there may be a cancer-promoting mutation which activates the NF-kB pathway through different genes or activates other cancer pathways. They also found PDL1/PDL2 translocations in 40% of PCBLBCL-LT cases. Most of these genes' mutations are commonly found in primary DLBCL of the central nervous system and in primary testicular DLBCL. Therefore, even though the mutational profile of PCDLBCL-LT seems to overlap with that of the ABC subtype of DLBCL, it is actually most similar to that of these two entities [12,99–102].

Furthermore, another study about microRNA profiling of PCBCL showed that microRNAs with a higher expression in the ABC-type of nodal DLBCL were not differentially expressed in PCDLBCL-LT, suggesting different pathogenetic mechanisms for PCDLBCL-LT cases than for nodal ones [103].

4.4. Differential Diagnosis

PCDLBCL-LT is relatively easy to diagnose once sheets of large B cells with typical morphology and immunophenotype are seen. The differential diagnosis of PCFCL with a diffuse growth pattern and large-cell cytology is the most challenging issue, which has already been discussed in the paragraph above (Table 2). Secondary skin involvement from systemic DLBCL—histologically and immunophenotypically indistinguishable from primary cutaneous forms—is frequent and can be excluded only based on clinical staging.

Predominantly blastoid or pleomorphic variants of MCL can infiltrate the skin, mimicking the histopathologic features of PCDLBCL-LT. Immunostaining for Cyclin D1 and SOX11 must be performed to exclude secondary skin involvement by MCL. Cases with Cyclin D1 expression should be tested by FISH analysis for CCND1 gene translocation [104,105].

An EBV search is required to exclude EBV+ DLBCL, which typically arises in elderly patients [8].

In cases with plasmablastic and immunoblastic differentiation, molecular and immunohistochemical tests for EBV and HHV8 are recommended. EBV and HHV8 infection associations should also be tested in any immunodeficient patient. The possibility of a precursor lymphoblastic lymphoma must be excluded by performing TdT immunostaining [104]. Some T-cell lymphomas, as mycosis fungoides, tumour stage, might show aberrant expressions of CD20 [106]. Rare, non-haematological neoplasms, such as Merkel cell carcinoma, might express B-cell markers, in particular PAX5 [104,107].

Cases with anaplastic cytology must be differentiated from CD30+/CD30-, anaplastic large T-cell lymphoma [108] and non-lymphoid, large-cell neoplasms, including melanoma, carcinoma and mesenchymal malignancies [109].

4.5. Prognosis and Treatment

PCDLBCL-LT is an aggressive disease with a five-year, disease-specific survival rate of around 50%, and many patients experience relapse despite treatment [88].

Adverse prognostic factors are the presence of multiple skin lesions (on one or both legs), involvement of both legs, inactivation of CDKN2A by gene deletion or promoter methylation, and the presence of the somatic mutation MYD88^{L265P} [38,79,89,90,96,110].

As for the DE profile, there have been discordant observations; while Menguy et al. [91,110] observed impaired survival in cases with a DE phenotype, both Schrader et al. [92] and Lucioni et al. [11] did not correlate a DE status with a significantly worse prognosis.

Similarly, the prognostic impact of MYC rearrangements is not completely understood. While Schrader et al. [92] suggested a poorer prognosis for patients with MYC translocations, this has not been confirmed by the study by Lucioni et al. [11] that documented a poor response to treatment and a more rapid disease progression only in association with a double/triple hit status.

Standard first-line treatment is based on polychemotherapy (CHOP regimen) in combination with rituximab. However, many patients with PCDLBCL-LT are elderly and frail, making them unfit for chemotherapy [87,88,111].

When the disease is confined to the leg, another option is radiation therapy, which can be used in combination with systemic therapies or as a monotherapy for palliative purposes. For single lesions, or for lesions confined in a single area, surgery with debulking intent may also be considered [87]. Although there are no uniform recommendations for second-line treatment in case of relapse, the management of recurrences seems to be comparable to that of relapsed systemic DLBCL with an activated phenotype and, for this reason, the use of lenalidomide has been reported [89,112].

4.6. Summing Up

PCDLBCL-LT is an aggressive disease, usually arising on the leg. It is characterized by sheets of centroblasts and/or immunoblasts, with no/few admixed reactive cells. Neoplastic cells are usually positive for bcl-2, MUM-1/IRF4, bcl-6, c-MYC and IgM, but negative for CD10, and more than 60% of PCDLBCL-LT cases have a DE phenotype.

The precise definition of the COO of this lymphoma is still incomplete and its mutational profile seems to be more similar to those of primary DLBCL of the central nervous system and primary testicular DLBCL.

5. Primary Cutaneous Diffuse Large B Cell Lymphoma, Not Otherwise Specified/Other

The 2005 WHO-EORTC classification of skin tumours included a further subgroup of PCDLBCL that was named primary cutaneous diffuse large B-cell lymphoma, other (PCDL-BCL, other). This group included rare cases not belonging either to the PCDLBCL-LT or to the PCFCL categories. However, since PCDLBCL, other was not a clearly defined entity, the 2018 update of the WHO-EORTC classification decided to delete it to avoid further confusion [12,113].

As of today, the debate about this entity is still ongoing. Recent articles have highlighted the presence of a group of large B-cell lymphomas, primarily arising on the skin, with peculiar morphological features and a slightly different prognosis than PCDLBCL-LT and PCFCL. This group has been called primary cutaneous B-cell lymphoma, not otherwise specified/unclassifiable (PCDLBCL-NOS/PCDLBCL-U) [10,11,73,91,114].

PCDLBCL-NOS seems to affect younger patients than PCDLBCL-LT, with a median age of 60 years at diagnosis and a male prevalence [10,11,115]. It usually develops over a longer period of time [10] and it most commonly arises as a single nodular or plaque lesion on the trunk, followed by the head and neck region, the lower limbs and finally the upper limbs [10,11,90].

Histologically, PCDLBCL-NOS is distinguished from PCDLBCL-LT (Table 2) because it is composed of large centroblastic cells with a minority (<10%) of medium-sized cells and/or a mild to moderate reactive cellular background of small CD3+ T lymphocytes. The infiltrate most commonly presents with a diffuse growth pattern, but (rarely) vaguely nodular areas may also be seen (Figure 4). Usually, necrosis and effacement of cutaneous adnexa, along with the dendritic meshwork, are not found. PCDLBCL-NOS cells display a B cell phenotype with expressions of CD20, CD79a, bcl-6 and variable positivity for bcl2 in a minority of cases (Figure 4). PCDLBCL-NOS can be positive for c-MYC, CD10, IgM and MUM1/IRF4, but the DE status is infrequent. The proliferative index is lower than in the PCDLBCL-LT cases, with a median value of 40%. The histogenetic characterization according to the Hans algorithm showed cases with a GC profile and cases with a non-GC phenotype [10,11,73].

FISH analysis revealed BCL6 as the most frequently translocated gene, followed by MYC rearrangements; rarely, BCL2 alterations, rearrangements or an increase in gene copy number, were found. A single case of PCDLBCL-NOS with a DH status (translocations of MYC and BCL6) has been reported; the patient presented a GC histogenetic profile and bcl2 negativity by means of immunohistochemistry [11,73].

PCDLBCL-NOS seems to be less aggressive than PCDLBCL-LT. The histogenetic profile may be retained as a significant prognostic factor in this disease. In fact, there seems to be differences in survival rates between PCDLBCL-NOS GC-type and PCDLBCL-NOS non-GC-type, with the first group more similar to PCFCL and the latter presenting instead with an intermediate behaviour between PCFCL and PCDLBCL-LT [73].

Interestingly, it has been noted that BCL6 translocations have correlated with inferior survival rates in PCDLBCL-NOS [11]. Since PCDLBCL-NOS is not an entirely recognized entity, no standardized treatment protocol exists. Local radiotherapy, chemotherapy, radiotherapy in association with chemotherapy, or in a few cases, a wait-and-see approach, were used [11,73].

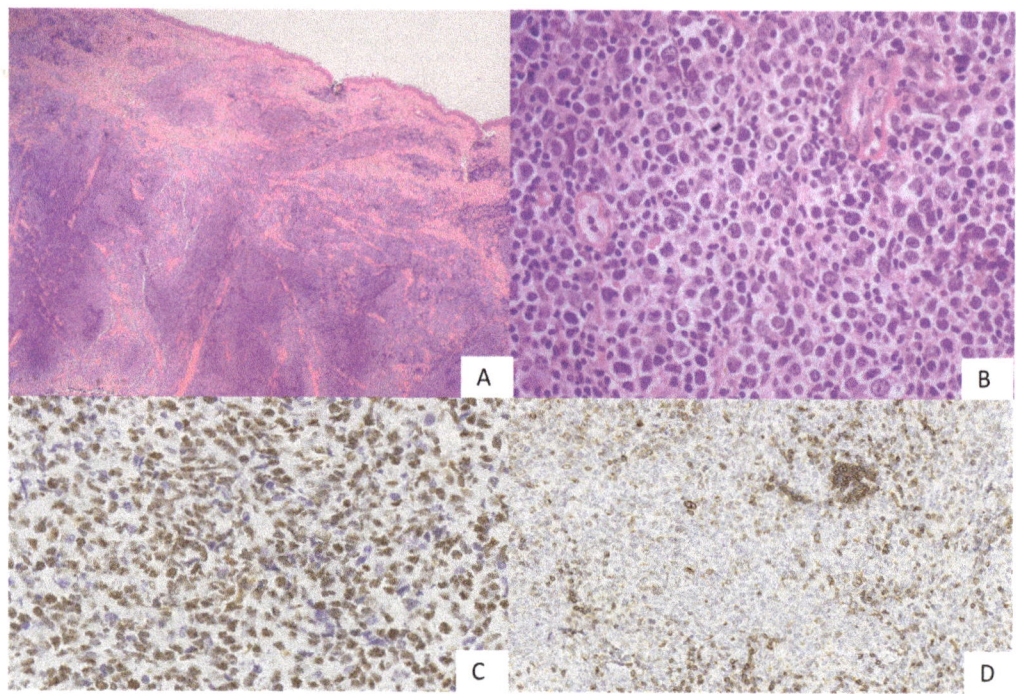

Figure 4. PCDLBCL-NOS. At histological evaluation, this lymphoma shows a diffuse growth pattern, sometimes with vaguely nodular areas ((**A**), HE 2×) and is composed of large centroblasts with a minority of medium-sized cells ((**B**), HE 40×). PCDLBCL-NOS is frequently bcl6-positive ((**C**), 40×) and bcl-2-negative ((**D**), 20×).

5.1. Diffuse Large B-Cell Lymphoma, Rare Subtypes

Primary cutaneous lymphomas with plasmablastic features are exceedingly rare. Most of these cases occur in settings of immunodeficiency (HIV-associated or iatrogenic) [86] or during the course of systemic T-cell lymphoma (such as angioimmunoblastic T-cell lymphoma). Plasmablastic lymphomas are clinically very aggressive. Histologically, they are composed of sheets of cells resembling immunoblasts, with variable degrees of plasmacytic differentiation. The lymphoma cells phenotype is consistent with terminal stages of B-cell differentiation, with negativity for CD20 and PAX5 and variable positivity for CD79a, CD38/CD138 and MUM1. Approximately 75% of cases are EBV-positive, exhibiting a latency I phenotype (EBERs expression and negativity for LMP1 and EBNA2). CD30 is frequently positive, correlating with EBV positivity, whereas, in contrast with plasma cell myeloma, CD56 is usually negative [8,116]. Plasmablastic lymphoma harbours frequent MYC rearrangements, with c-MYC protein expression by immunohistochemistry [86,116].

Intravascular B-cell lymphoma (IVBL) may present in the skin or localize to the skin during the course of the disease. IVBL is characterized by the presence of large lymphoid cells within the lumina of small- to medium-sized blood vessels, particularly capillaries and postcapillary venules [8]. This peculiar intravascular growth pattern has been attributed to a defect in homing receptors and adhesion molecules on the tumour cells (such as the lack of CD29 (b1 integrin) and CD54 (ICAM1)) [108,117]. Lymphoma cells express B-cell-associated antigens and may be positive for CD5 (38%) [8]; the majority of cases are positive for MUM1 and negative for CD10, suggesting an ABC phenotype [116] and show an overexpression of bcl-2 in the absence of BCL2 rearrangements [118].

In keeping with an ABC origin, a subset of IVBLs carry MYD88^{L265P} and CD79B mutations [86,116]. Skin is a common site for presentation of IVBL, although most patients have a widespread, disseminated disease at the time of diagnosis. Dermatologic manifestations include a wide range of skin lesions, including erythematous patches and plaques, panniculitis-like lesions, as well as painful telangiectasias and nodular lesions with a predilection for the trunk and lower extremities [3,108].

Clinical symptoms include fever and, due to the frequent involvement of the central nervous system, focal neurological defects. Lungs, adrenal glands, thyroid, gastrointestinal system, kidneys, genitourinary tract and eyes can also be involved. IVBL is an aggressive disease, requiring systemic immunochemotherapy. However, patients presenting with a cutaneous disease have a better prognosis in most series, probably because of earlier detection and treatment [8,108,119].

5.2. EBV-Positive Mucocutaneous Ulcer

EBVMCU is a provisional entity included in the *WHO Classification of Tumours of Haematopoietic and Lymphoid Tissues* of 2017 [8,120]. It occurs in patients with primary or secondary immunodeficiencies, including age-related or iatrogenic immunosuppression for immune disorders, transplant recipients and HIV infection. The median age is about 66 years [121].

Clinically, EBVMCU presents as a solitary, sharply demarcated ulcer occurring mostly in the oral mucosa; other involved sites may be the skin and the gastrointestinal tract with (rarely) locoregional lymph node involvement and without systemic symptoms [12,122].

Histologically, there is a mucosal/cutaneous ulceration with the underlying presence of EBV-positive, large, atypical cells resembling immunoblasts or Hodgkin/Reed–Sternberg cells in a polymorphic background containing lymphocytes, histiocytes, plasma cells and granulocytes. Angioinvasion, necrosis and apoptotic bodies may occur. An important characteristic is the presence of a rim of CD8+ T cells at the base of the ulcer [123].

The atypical cells show expression of CD30, PAX5, MUM1/IRF4 and OCT2, with variable positivity for CD20, CD79a and BOB1. They have an ABC phenotype with negativity for CD10 and bcl6. Half of these cases express CD15 [3]. EBV positivity may be detected using an LMP1 antibody or in situ hybridization for EBV-encoded RNA (EBER) [123].

Up to 40% of cases show clonal immunoglobulin gene rearrangements and/or T-cell receptor gene (TCR) rearrangements [116,123].

Differential diagnosis includes classic Hodgkin's lymphoma and EBV-positive DLBCL-NOS. Both of these diseases usually form masses and are more widespread (most commonly involving lymph nodes) than EBVMCU. As such, the correlation between clinical and pathological features is crucial to discriminate between these entities [122,123].

Other differential diagnoses include primary cutaneous or primary oropharyngeal anaplastic large-cell lymphoma (negativity for PAX5 and EBV) and lymphomatoid granulomatosis (almost always involving the lungs) [122].

EBVMCU usually has a benign, self-limited course with spontaneous remission or regression upon reduction of immunosuppressive medications. If a therapy is required, the use of rituximab, local radiotherapy or chemotherapy has been reported. Only rare cases experience recurrences or disease progression (mostly local spread) [3,8,12,121,123].

6. Conclusions

PCBCL is a heterogeneous group of lymphoproliferative disorders with distinct clinicopathologic features comparable with their nodal counterparts. In the last decade, we have achieved significant advancements in our understanding of the clinicopathologic features and molecular background of PCBCL with the identification of characteristic molecular alterations in different lymphoma subtypes. In addition, some novel provisional entities have been described, such as EBVMCU, further expanding the spectrum of PCBCLs. However, in spite of such advances, the histopathological diagnosis of PCBCL is still challenging, and a number of issues continue to be a matter of debate. The most compelling topics include the differential diagnosis between PCMZL, PCFCL and reactive cutaneous lymphoid infiltrates, the border between centroblast-rich PCFCL and PCDLBCL and the putative prognostic subcategorization of PCDLBCL. The hope is that, in the future, the identification of new genetic markers will be useful for refining PCBCL categories, opening up new diagnostic and therapeutic perspectives.

Funding: This research received no external funding.

Institutional Review Board Statement: Not applicable. This study is a review of current literature; it is not based on original data from patients series.

Informed Consent Statement: Not applicable.

Data Availability Statement: Not applicable.

Conflicts of Interest: The authors declare no conflict of interest.

References

1. Kempf, W.; Zimmermann, A.-K.; Mitteldorf, C. Cutaneous lymphomas—An update 2019. *Hematol. Oncol.* **2019**, *37* (Suppl. S1), 43–47. [CrossRef] [PubMed]
2. Chen, S.T.; Barnes, J.; Duncan, L. Primary cutaneous B-cell lymphomas—Clinical and histopathologic features, differential diagnosis, and treatment. *Semin. Cutan. Med. Surg.* **2018**, *37*, 49–55. [CrossRef] [PubMed]
3. Vitiello, P.; Sica, A.; Ronchi, A.; Caccavale, S.; Franco, R.; Argenziano, G. Primary Cutaneous B-Cell Lymphomas: An Update. *Front. Oncol.* **2020**, *10*, 651. [CrossRef] [PubMed]
4. Hope, C.B.; Pincus, L.B. Primary Cutaneous B-cell Lymphomas. *Clin. Lab. Med.* **2017**, *37*, 547–574. [CrossRef]
5. Grandi, V.; Violetti, S.A.; La Selva, R.; Cicchelli, S.; Delfino, C.; Fava, P.; Fierro, M.T.; Pileri, A.; Pimpinelli, N.; Quaglino, P.; et al. Primary cutaneous B-cell lymphoma: Narrative review of the literature. *G. Ital. Dermatol. Venereol.* **2019**, *154*, 466–479. [CrossRef]
6. Wilcox, R.A. Cutaneous B-cell lymphomas: 2019 update on diagnosis, risk stratification, and management. *Am. J. Hematol.* **2018**, *93*, 1427–1430. [CrossRef]
7. Goyal, A.; LeBlanc, R.E.; Carter, J.B. Cutaneous B-Cell Lymphoma. *Hematol. Clin. N. Am.* **2019**, *33*, 149–161. [CrossRef]
8. Swerdlow, S.H.; Campo, E.; Harris, N.L.; Jaffe, E.S.; Pileri, S.A.; Stein, H.; Thiele, J. (Eds.) *WHO Classification of Tumours of Haematopoietic and Lymphoid Tissues, Revised*, 4th ed.; IARC: Lyon, France, 2017.
9. Malachowski, S.J.; Sun, J.; Chen, P. L.; Seminario Vidal, L. Diagnosis and Management of Cutaneous B-Cell Lymphomas. *Dermatol. Clin.* **2019**, *37*, 443–454. [CrossRef]
10. Felcht, M.; Klemke, C.-D.; Nicolay, J.P.; Weiss, C.; Assaf, C.; Wobser, M.; Schlaak, M.; Hillen, U.; Moritz, R.; Tantcheva-Poor, I.; et al. Primary cutaneous diffuse large B-cell lymphoma, NOS and leg type: Clinical, morphologic and prognostic differences. *JDDG J. Dtsch. Dermatol. Ges.* **2019**, *17*, 275–285. [CrossRef]
11. Lucioni, M.; Pescia, C.; Bonometti, A.; Fraticelli, S.; Moltrasio, C.; Ramponi, A.; Riboni, R.; Roccio, S.; Ferrario, G.; Arcaini, L.; et al. Double expressor and double/triple hit status among primary cutaneous diffuse large B-cell lymphoma: A comparison between leg type and not otherwise specified subtypes. *Hum. Pathol.* **2021**, *111*, 1–9. [CrossRef]
12. Willemze, R.; Cerroni, L.; Kempf, W.; Berti, E.; Facchetti, F.; Swerdlow, S.H.; Jaffe, E.S. The 2018 update of the WHO-EORTC clas-sification for primary cutaneous lymphomas. *Blood* **2019**, *134*, 1112.
13. Hoefnagel, P.; Vermeer, M.; Jansen, P.; Heule, F.; Vader, P.C.V.V.; Sanders, C.J.G.; Gerritsen, M.J.P.; Geerts, M.L.; Meijer, C.J.L.M.; Noordijk, E.M.; et al. Primary Cutaneous Marginal Zone B-Cell Lymphoma: Clinical and therapeutic features in 50 cases. *Arch. Dermatol.* **2005**, *141*, 1139–1145. [CrossRef] [PubMed]
14. Fink-Puches, R.; Chott, A.; Ardigo, M.; Simonitsch, I.; Ferrara, G.; Kerl, H.; Cerroni, L. The Spectrum of Cutaneous Lymphomas in Patients Less than 20 Years of Age. *Pediatr. Dermatol.* **2004**, *21*, 525–533. [CrossRef] [PubMed]
15. Kempf, W.; Kazakov, D.; Buechner, S.A.; Graf, M.; Zettl, A.; Zimmermann, D.R.; Tinguely, M. Primary Cutaneous Marginal Zone Lymphoma in Children: A report of 3 cases and review of the literature. *Am. J. Dermatopathol.* **2014**, *36*, 661–666. [CrossRef] [PubMed]
16. Goodlad, J.R.; Davidson, M.M.; Hollowood, K.; Ling, C.; MacKenzie, C.; Christie, I.; Batstone, P.J.; Ho-Yen, D.O. Primary Cutaneous B-Cell Lymphoma and Borrelia burgdorferi Infection in Patients from the Highlands of Scotland. *Am. J. Surg. Pathol.* **2000**, *24*, 1279–1285. [CrossRef]
17. Takino, H.; Li, C.; Hu, S.; Kuo, T.-T.; Geissinger, E.; Muller-Hermelink, H.K.; Kim, B.; Swerdlow, S.H.; Inagaki, H. Primary cutaneous marginal zone B-cell lymphoma: A molecular and clinicopathological study of cases from Asia, Germany, and the United States. *Mod. Pathol.* **2008**, *21*, 1517–1526. [CrossRef]
18. Suarez, F.; Lortholary, O.; Hermine, O.; Lecuit, M. Infection-associated lymphomas derived from marginal zone B cells: A model of antigen-driven lymphoproliferation. *Blood* **2006**, *107*, 3034–3044. [CrossRef]
19. Arcaini, L.; Bruno, R. Hepatitis C Virus Infection and Antiviral Treatment in Marginal Zone Lymphomas. *Curr. Clin. Pharmacol.* **2010**, *5*, 74–81. [CrossRef]

20. Arcaini, L.; Burcheri, S.; Rossi, A.; Paulli, M.; Bruno, R.; Passamonti, F.; Brusamolino, E.; Molteni, A.; Pulsoni, A.; Cox, M.; et al. Prevalence of HCV infection in nongastric marginal zone B-cell lymphoma of MALT. *Ann. Oncol.* **2007**, *18*, 346–350. [CrossRef]
21. Arcaini, L.; Merli, M.; Volpetti, S.; Rattotti, S.; Gotti, M.; Zaja, F. Indolent B-Cell Lymphomas Associated with HCV Infection: Clinical and Virological Features and Role of Antiviral Therapy. *Clin. Dev. Immunol.* **2012**, *2012*, 638185. [CrossRef]
22. Paulli, M.; Arcaini, L.; Lucioni, M.; Boveri, E.; Capello, D.; Passamonti, F.; Merli, M.; Rattotti, S.; Rossi, D.; Riboni, R.; et al. Subcutaneous 'lipoma-like' B-cell lymphoma associated with HCV infection: A new presentation of primary extranodal marginal zone B-cell lymphoma of MALT. *Ann. Oncol.* **2009**, *21*, 1189–1195. [CrossRef] [PubMed]
23. Tsuji, K.; Suzuki, D.; Naito, Y.; Sato, Y.; Yoshino, T.; Iwatsuki, K. Primary cutaneous marginal zone B-cell lymphoma. *Eur. J. Dermatol.* **2005**, *15*, 480–483. [PubMed]
24. Gibson, S.E.; Swerdlow, S.H. How I Diagnose Primary Cutaneous Marginal Zone Lymphoma. *Am. J. Clin. Pathol.* **2020**, *154*, 428–449. [CrossRef] [PubMed]
25. Russo, I.; Fagotto, L.; Sernicola, A.; Alaibac, M. Primary Cutaneous B-Cell Lymphomas in Patients with Impaired Immunity. *Front. Oncol.* **2020**, *10*, 1296. [CrossRef] [PubMed]
26. Cicogna, G.T.; Ferranti, M.; Alaibac, M. Diagnostic Workup of Primary Cutaneous B Cell Lymphomas: A Clinician's Approach. *Front. Oncol.* **2020**, *10*, 988. [CrossRef]
27. Ronchi, A.; Sica, A.; Vitiello, P.; Franco, R. Dermatological Considerations in the Diagnosis and Treatment of Marginal Zone Lymphomas. *Clin. Cosmet. Investig. Dermatol.* **2021**, *14*, 231–239. [CrossRef]
28. Cook, J.C.; Puckett, Y. *Anetoderma*; StatPearls Publishing: Treasure Island, FL, USA, 2022.
29. Hodak, E.; Feuerman, H.; Barzilai, A.; David, M.; Cerroni, L.; Feinmesser, M. Anetodermic Primary Cutaneous B-Cell Lymphoma: A unique clinicopathological presentation of lymphoma possibly associated with antiphospholipid antibodies. *Arch. Dermatol.* **2010**, *146*, 175–182. [CrossRef]
30. Dalle, S.; Thomas, L.; Balme, B.; Dumontet, C.; Thieblemont, C. Primary cutaneous marginal zone lymphoma. *Crit. Rev. Oncol.* **2010**, *74*, 156–162. [CrossRef]
31. Farhadian, J.; Terushkin, V.; Meehan, S.A.; Latkowski, J.A. Primary cutaneous marginal-zone lymphoma. *Derm. Online J.* **2016**, *22*, 13030. [CrossRef]
32. Cho-Vega, J.H.; Vega, F.; Rassidakis, G.; Medeiros, L.J. Primary cutaneous marginal zone B-cell lymphoma. *Am. J. Clin. Pathol.* **2006**, *125*, S38–S49. [CrossRef]
33. Kempf, W.; Kerl, H.; Kutzner, H. CD123-Positive Plasmacytoid Dendritic Cells in Primary Cutaneous Marginal Zone B-Cell Lymphoma: A Crucial Role and a New Lymphoma Paradigm. *Am. J. Dermatopathol.* **2010**, *32*, 194–196. [CrossRef]
34. Edinger, J.T.; Kant, J.A.; Swerdlow, S.H. Cutaneous Marginal Zone Lymphomas Have Distinctive Features and Include 2 Subsets. *Am. J. Surg. Pathol.* **2010**, *34*, 1830–1841. [CrossRef]
35. Kogame, T.; Takegami, T.; Sakai, T.; Kataoka, T.; Hirata, M.; Budair, F.M.; Ueshima, C.; Matsui, M.; Nomura, T.; Kabashima, K. Immunohistochemical analysis of class-switched subtype of primary cutaneous marginal zone lymphoma in terms of inducible skin-associated lymphoid tissue. *J. Eur. Acad. Dermatol. Venereol.* **2019**, *33*, e401–e403. [CrossRef]
36. Van Maldegem, F.; van Dijk, R.; Wormhoudt, T.A.M.; Kluin, P.M.; Willemze, R.; Cerroni, L.; van Noesel, C.J.M.; Bende, R.J. The majority of cutaneous marginal zone B-cell lymphomas expresses class-switched immunoglobulins and develops in a T-helper type 2 inflammatory environment. *Blood* **2008**, *112*, 3355–3361. [CrossRef]
37. Sun, J.R.; Nong, L.; Liu, X.Q.; Tu, P.; Wang, Y. Frequent immunoglobulin G4 expression in a common variant of primary cutaneous marginal zone B-cell lymphoma. *Australas. J. Dermatol.* **2017**, *59*, 141–145. [CrossRef]
38. Hallermann, C.; Kaune, K.; Gesk, S.; Martin-Subero, J.; Gunawan, B.; Griesinger, F.; Vermeer, M.; Santucci, M.; Pimpinelli, N.; Willemze, R.; et al. Molecular Cytogenetic Analysis of Chromosomal Breakpoints in the IGH, MYC, BCL6, and MALT1 Gene Loci in Primary Cutaneous B-cell Lymphomas. *J. Investig. Dermatol.* **2004**, *123*, 213–219. [CrossRef]
39. Li, C.; Inagaki, H.; Kuo, T.-T.; Hu, S.; Okabe, M.; Eimoto, T. Primary Cutaneous Marginal Zone B-Cell Lymphoma: A molecular and clinicopathologic study of 24 asian cases. *Am. J. Surg. Pathol.* **2003**, *27*, 1061–1069. [CrossRef]
40. Swerdlow, S.H. Cutaneous marginal zone lymphomas. *Semin. Diagn. Pathol.* **2017**, *34*, 76–84. [CrossRef]
41. Maurus, K.; Appenzeller, S.; Roth, S.; Kuper, J.; Rost, S.; Meierjohann, S.; Arampatzi, P.; Goebeler, M.; Rosenwald, A.; Geissinger, E.; et al. Panel Sequencing Shows Recurrent Genetic FAS Alterations in Primary Cutaneous Marginal Zone Lymphoma. *J. Investig. Dermatol.* **2018**, *138*, 1573–1581. [CrossRef]
42. Baldassano, M.F.; Bailey, E.M.; Ferry, J.A.; Harris, N.L.; Duncan, L.M. Cutaneous Lymphoid Hyperplasia and Cutaneous Marginal Zone Lymphoma: Comparison of morphologic and immunophenotypic features. *Am. J. Surg. Pathol.* **1999**, *23*, 88–96. [CrossRef]
43. Lin, P.; Molina, T.; Cook, J.R.; Swerdlow, S.H. Lymphoplasmacytic Lymphoma and Other Non–Marginal Zone Lymphomas with Plasmacytic Differentiation. *Am. J. Clin. Pathol.* **2011**, *136*, 195–210. [CrossRef]
44. Molina, T.J.; Lin, P.; Swerdlow, S.H.; Cook, J.R. Marginal Zone Lymphomas with Plasmacytic Differentiation and Related Disorders. *Am. J. Clin. Pathol.* **2011**, *136*, 211–225. [CrossRef]
45. Brenner, I.; Roth, S.; Puppe, B.; Wobser, M.; Rosenwald, A.; Geissinger, E. Primary cutaneous marginal zone lymphomas with plasmacytic differentiation show frequent IgG4 expression. *Mod. Pathol.* **2013**, *26*, 1568–1576. [CrossRef]
46. Servitje, O.; Muniesa, C.; Benavente, Y.; Monsálvez, V.; Garcia-Muret, M.P.; Gallardo, F.; Domingo-Domenech, E.; Lucas, A.; Climent, F.; Rodriguez-Peralto, J.L.; et al. Primary cutaneous marginal zone B-cell lymphoma: Response to treatment and disease-free survival in a series of 137 patients. *J. Am. Acad. Dermatol.* **2013**, *69*, 357–365. [CrossRef]

47. Prieto-Torres, L.; Manso, R.; Cieza-Díaz, D.E.; Jo, M.; Pérez, L.K.; Montenegro-Damaso, T.; Eraña, I.; Lorda, M.; Massa, D.S.; Machan, S.; et al. Large Cells with CD30 Expression and Hodgkin-like Features in Primary Cutaneous Marginal Zone B-Cell Lymphoma: A Study of 13 Cases. *Am. J. Surg. Pathol.* **2019**, *43*, 1191–1202. [CrossRef]
48. Palmedo, G.; Hantschke, M.; Rütten, A.; Mentzel, T.; Kempf, W.; Tomasini, D.; Kutzner, H. Primary Cutaneous Marginal Zone B-cell Lymphoma May Exhibit Both the t(14;18)(q32;q21) IGH/BCL2 and the t(14;18)(q32;q21) IGH/MALT1 Translocation: An Indicator for Clonal Transformation Towards Higher-Grade B-cell Lymphoma? *Am. J. Dermatopathol.* **2007**, *29*, 231–236. [CrossRef]
49. Boudreaux, B.W.; Patel, M.H.; Brumfiel, C.M.; Besch-Stokes, J.; DiCaudo, D.J.; Craig, F.; Rosenthal, A.C.; Rule, W.G.; Pittelkow, M.R.; Mangold, A.R. Primary cutaneous epidermotropic marginal zone B-cell lymphoma treated with total skin electron beam therapy. *JAAD Case Rep.* **2021**, *15*, 15–18. [CrossRef]
50. Wobser, M. Therapie indolenter kutaner B-Zell-Lymphome [Treatment of indolent cutaneous B-cell lymphoma]. *Hautarzt* **2017**, *68*, 721–726. [CrossRef]
51. Lang, C.C.V.; Ramelyte, E.; Dummer, R. Innovative Therapeutic Approaches in Primary Cutaneous B Cell Lymphoma. *Front. Oncol.* **2020**, *10*, 1163. [CrossRef]
52. Skala, S.L.; Hristov, B.; Hristov, A.C. Primary Cutaneous Follicle Center Lymphoma. *Arch. Pathol. Lab. Med.* **2018**, *142*, 1313–1321. [CrossRef]
53. Senff, N.J.; Hoefnagel, J.J.; Jansen, P.M.; Vermeer, M.; Van Baarlen, J.; Blokx, W.; Dijk, M.R.C.-V.; Geerts, M.-L.; Hebeda, K.M.; Kluin, P.M.; et al. Reclassification of 300 Primary Cutaneous B-Cell Lymphomas According to the New WHO–EORTC Classification for Cutaneous Lymphomas: Comparison with Previous Classifications and Identification of Prognostic Markers. *J. Clin. Oncol.* **2007**, *25*, 1581–1587. [CrossRef]
54. Zinzani, P.L.; Quaglino, P.; Pimpinelli, N.; Berti, E.; Baliva, G.; Rupoli, S.; Martelli, M.; Alaibac, M.; Borroni, G.; Chimenti, S.; et al. Prognostic Factors in Primary Cutaneous B-Cell Lymphoma: The Italian Study Group for Cutaneous Lymphomas. *J. Clin. Oncol.* **2006**, *24*, 1376–1382. [CrossRef]
55. Travaglino, A.; Varricchio, S.; Pace, M.; Russo, D.; Picardi, M.; Baldo, A.; Staibano, S.; Mascolo, M. Borrelia burgdorferi in primary cutaneous lymphomas: A systematic review and meta-analysis. *JDDG: J. Dtsch. Dermatol. Ges.* **2020**, *18*, 1379–1384. [CrossRef]
56. Slater, D.N. Borrelia burgdorferi-associated primary cutaneous B-cell lymphoma. *Histopathology* **2001**, *38*, 73–77. [CrossRef]
57. Petković, I.Z.; Pejcic, I.; Tiodorović, D.; Krstić, M.; Stojnev, S.; Vrbic, S. Transformation of primary cutaneous follicle centre lymphoma into primary cutaneous diffuse large B-cell lymphoma of other type. *Adv. Dermatol. Allergol.* **2017**, *34*, 625–628. [CrossRef]
58. Uy, M.; Sprowl, G.; Lynch, D.T. *Primary Cutaneous Follicle Center Lymphoma*; StatPearls Publishing: Treasure Island, FL, USA, 2022.
59. Berti, E.; Alessi, E.; Caputo, R.; Gianotti, R.; Delia, D.; Vezzoni, P. Reticulohistiocytoma of the dorsum. *J. Am. Acad. Dermatol.* **1988**, *19*, 259–272. [CrossRef]
60. Fierro, M.T.; Marenco, F.; Novelli, M.; Fava, P.; Quaglino, P.; Bernengo, M.G. Long-Term Evolution of an Untreated Primary Cutaneous Follicle Center Lymphoma of the Scalp. *Am. J. Dermatopathol.* **2010**, *32*, 91–94. [CrossRef]
61. Cerroni, L.; Arzberger, E.; Pütz, B.; Höfler, G.; Metze, D.; Sander, C.A.; Rose, C.; Wolf, P.; Rütten, A.; McNiff, J.M.; et al. Primary cutaneous follicle center cell lymphoma with follicular growth pattern. *Blood* **2000**, *95*, 3922–3928. [CrossRef]
62. Cerroni, L.; El-Shabrawi-Caelen, L.; Fink-Puches, R.; LeBoit, P.E.; Kerl, H. Cutaneous Spindle-Cell B-Cell Lymphoma. *Am. J. Dermatopathol.* **2000**, *22*, 299–304. [CrossRef]
63. Child, F.; Russell-Jones, R.; Woolford, A.; Calonje, E.; Photiou, A.; Orchard, G.; Whittaker, S. Absence of the t(14;18) chromosomal translocation in primary cutaneous B-cell lymphoma. *Br. J. Dermatol.* **2001**, *144*, 735–744. [CrossRef]
64. Abdul-Wahab, A.; Tang, S.-Y.; Robson, A.; Morris, S.; Agar, N.; Wain, E.M.; Child, F.; Scarisbrick, J.; Neat, M.; Whittaker, S. Chromosomal anomalies in primary cutaneous follicle center cell lymphoma do not portend a poor prognosis. *J. Am. Acad. Dermatol.* **2014**, *70*, 1010–1020. [CrossRef]
65. Cerroni, L.; Volkenandt, M.; Rieger, E.; Soyer, H.P.; Kerl, H. bcl-2 Protein Expression and Correlation with the Interchromoso-mal 14;18 Translocation in Cutaneous Lymphomas and Pseudolymphomas. *J. Invest Dermatol.* **1994**, *102*, 231–235. [CrossRef]
66. Geelen, F.A.; Vermeer, M.; Meijer, C.J.; Van Der Putte, S.C.; Kerkhof, E.; Kluin, P.M.; Willemze, R. bcl-2 protein expression in primary cutaneous large B-cell lymphoma is site-related. *J. Clin. Oncol.* **1998**, *16*, 2080–2085. [CrossRef]
67. Goodlad, J.R.; Krajewski, A.S.; Batstone, P.J.; McKay, P.; White, J.M.; Benton, E.C.; Kavanagh, G.M.; Lucraft, H.H. Primary Cutaneous Follicular Lymphoma. *Am. J. Surg. Pathol.* **2002**, *26*, 733–741. [CrossRef]
68. Hallermann, C.; Kaune, K.M.; Siebert, R.; Vermeer, M.H.; Tensen, C.P.; Willemze, R.; Gunawan, B.; Bertsch, H.P.; Neumann, C. Chromosomal Aberration Patterns Differ in Subtypes of Primary Cutaneous B Cell Lymphomas. *J. Investig. Dermatol.* **2004**, *122*, 1495–1502. [CrossRef]
69. Vergier, B.; Belaud-Rotureau, M.-A.; Benassy, M.-N.; Beylot-Barry, M.; Dubus, P.; Delaunay, M.; Garroste, J.-C.; Taine, L.; Merlio, J.-P. Neoplastic Cells Do Not Carry bcl2-JH Rearrangements Detected in a Subset of Primary Cutaneous Follicle Center B-cell Lymphomas. *Am. J. Surg. Pathol.* **2004**, *28*, 748–755. [CrossRef]
70. Aguilera, N.S.I.; Tomaszewski, M.-M.; Moad, J.C.; Bauer, F.A.; Taubenberger, J.K.; Abbondanzo, S.L. Cutaneous Follicle Center Lymphoma: A Clinicopathologic Study of 19 Cases. *Mod. Pathol.* **2001**, *14*, 828–835. [CrossRef]
71. Mirza, I.; Macpherson, N.; Paproski, S.; Gascoyne, R.D.; Yang, B.; Finn, W.G.; Hsi, E.D. Primary Cutaneous Follicular Lymphoma: An Assessment of Clinical, Histopathologic, Immunophenotypic, and Molecular Features. *J. Clin. Oncol.* **2002**, *20*, 647–655. [CrossRef]

72. Pham-Ledard, A.; Cowppli-Bony, A.; Doussau, A.; Prochazkova-Carlotti, M.; Laharanne, E.; Jouary, T.; Belaud-Rotureau, M.-A.; Vergier, B.; Merlio, J.-P.; Beylot-Barry, M. Diagnostic and Prognostic Value of BCL2 Rearrangement in 53 Patients with Follicular Lymphoma Presenting as Primary Skin Lesions. *Am. J. Clin. Pathol.* **2015**, *143*, 362–373. [CrossRef]
73. Lucioni, M.; Berti, E.; Arcaini, L.; Croci, G.A.; Maffi, A.; Klersy, C.; Goteri, G.; Tomasini, C.; Quaglino, P.; Riboni, R.; et al. Primary cutaneous B-cell lymphoma other than marginal zone: Clinicopathologic analysis of 161 cases: Comparison with current classification and definition of prognostic markers. *Cancer Med.* **2016**, *5*, 2740–2755. [CrossRef]
74. Brash, D.E. UV Signature Mutations. *Photochem. Photobiol.* **2015**, *91*, 15–26. [CrossRef]
75. Szablewski, V.; Ingen-Housz-Oro, S.; Baia, M.; Delfau-Larue, M.-H.; Copie-Bergman, C.; Ortonne, N. Primary Cutaneous Follicle Center Lymphomas Expressing BCL2 Protein Frequently Harbor BCL2 Gene Break and May Present 1p36 Deletion. *Am. J. Surg. Pathol.* **2016**, *40*, 127–136. [CrossRef]
76. Gángó, A.; Bátai, B.; Varga, M.; Kapczár, D.; Papp, G.; Marschalkó, M.; Kuroli, E.; Schneider, T.; Csomor, J.; Matolcsy, A.; et al. Concomitant 1p36 deletion and TNFRSF14 mutations in primary cutaneous follicle center lymphoma frequently expressing high levels of EZH2 protein. *Virchows Arch.* **2018**, *473*, 453–462. [CrossRef]
77. Schafernak, K.T.; Variakojis, D.; Goolsby, C.L.; Tucker, R.M.; Martínez-Escala, M.E.; Smith, F.A.; Dittman, D.; Chenn, A.; Guitart, J. Clonality Assessment of Cutaneous B-Cell Lymphoid Proliferations. *Am. J. Dermatopathol.* **2014**, *36*, 781–795. [CrossRef]
78. Zhou, X.A.; Yang, J.; Ringbloom, K.G.; Martinez-Escala, M.E.; Stevenson, K.E.; Wenzel, A.T.; Fantini, D.; Martin, H.K.; Moy, A.P.; Morgan, E.A.; et al. Genomic landscape of cutaneous follicular lymphomas reveals 2 subgroups with clinically predictive molecular features. *Blood Adv.* **2021**, *5*, 649–661. [CrossRef]
79. Menguy, S.; Gros, A.; Pham-Ledard, A.; Battistella, M.; Ortonne, N.; Comoz, F.; Balme, B.; Szablewski, V.; Lamant, L.; Carlotti, A.; et al. MYD88 Somatic Mutation Is a Diagnostic Criterion in Primary Cutaneous Large B-Cell Lymphoma. *J. Investig. Dermatol.* **2016**, *136*, 1741–1744. [CrossRef]
80. Verdanet, E.; Dereure, O.; René, C.; Tempier, A.; Benammar-Hafidi, A.; Gallo, M.; Frouin, E.; Durand, L.; Gazagne, I.; Costes-Martineau, V.; et al. Diagnostic value of STMN1, LMO2, HGAL, AID expression and 1p36 chromosomal abnormalities in primary cutaneous B cell lymphomas. *Histopathology* **2017**, *71*, 648–660. [CrossRef]
81. Metcalf, R.A.; Monabati, A.; Vyas, M.; Roncador, G.; Gualco, G.; Bacchi, C.E.; Younes, S.F.; Natkunam, Y.; Freud, A.G. Myeloid cell nuclear differentiation antigen is expressed in a subset of marginal zone lymphomas and is useful in the differential diagnosis with follicular lymphoma. *Hum. Pathol.* **2014**, *45*, 1730–1736. [CrossRef]
82. Kanellis, G.; Roncador, G.; Arribas, A.; Mollejo, M.; Montes-Moreno, S.; Maestre, L.; Campos-Martin, Y.; Gonzalez, J.L.R.; Martinez-Torrecuadrada, J.L.; Sanchez-Verde, L.; et al. Identification of MNDA as a new marker for nodal marginal zone lymphoma. *Leukemia* **2009**, *23*, 1847–1857. [CrossRef]
83. Battistella, M.; Beylot-Barry, M.; Bachelez, H.; Rivet, J.; Vergier, B.; Bagot, M. Primary Cutaneous Follicular Helper T-cell Lymphoma. *Arch. Dermatol.* **2012**, *148*, 832–839. [CrossRef]
84. Ferrara, G.; Bevilacqua, M.; Argenziano, G. Cutaneous Spindle B-Cell Lymphoma: A Reappraisal. *Am. J. Dermatopathol.* **2002**, *24*, 526–527. [CrossRef]
85. Hoefnagel, J.J.; Dijkman, R.; Basso, K.; Jansen, P.M.; Hallermann, C.; Willemze, R.; Tensen, C.P.; Vermeer, M. Distinct types of primary cutaneous large B-cell lymphoma identified by gene expression profiling. *Blood* **2005**, *105*, 3671–3678. [CrossRef]
86. Sukswai, N.; Lyapichev, K.; Khoury, J.D.; Medeiros, L.J. Diffuse large B-cell lymphoma variants: An update. *Pathology* **2020**, *52*, 53–67. [CrossRef]
87. Nicolay, J.P.; Wobser, M. Cutaneous B-cell lymphomas—pathogenesis, diagnostic workup, and therapy. *JDDG J. Dtsch. Dermatol. Ges.* **2016**, *14*, 1207–1224. [CrossRef]
88. Vermeer, M.; Willemze, R. Recent advances in primary cutaneous B-cell lymphomas. *Curr. Opin. Oncol.* **2014**, *26*, 230–236. [CrossRef]
89. Hristov, A.C.; Tejasvi, T.; Wilcox, R.A. Cutaneous B-cell lymphomas: 2021 update on diagnosis, risk-stratification, and management. *Am. J. Hematol.* **2020**, *95*, 1209–1213. [CrossRef]
90. Kempf, W.; Denisjuk, N.; Kerl, K.; Cozzio, A.; Sander, C. Primary cutaneous B-cell lymphomas. *J. Dtsch Dermatol Ges.* **2012**, *10*, 12–23. [CrossRef]
91. Menguy, S.; Beylot-Barry, M.; Parrens, M.; Ledard, A.; Frison, E.; Comoz, F.; Battistella, M.; Szablewski, V.; Balme, B.; Croue, A.; et al. Primary cutaneous large B-cell lymphomas: Relevance of the 2017 World Health Organization classification: Clinicopathological and molecular analyses of 64 cases. *Histopathology* **2019**, *74*, 1067–1080. [CrossRef]
92. Schrader, A.M.R.; Jansen, P.M.; Vermeer, M.H.; Kleiverda, J.K.; Vermaat, J.S.P.; Willemze, R. High Incidence and Clinical Significance of MYC Rearrangements in Primary Cutaneous Diffuse Large B-Cell Lymphoma, Leg Type. *Am. J. Surg. Pathol.* **2018**, *42*, 1488–1494. [CrossRef]
93. Mitteldorf, C.; Berisha, A.; Pfaltz, M.C.; Broekaert, S.M.C.; Schön, M.P.; Kerl, K.; Kempf, W. Tumor Microenvironment and Check-point Molecules in Primary Cutaneous Diffuse Large B-Cell Lymphoma-New Therapeutic Targets. *Am. J. Surg. Pathol.* **2017**, *41*, 998–1004. [CrossRef]
94. Schrader, A.M.R.; de Groen, R.A.L.; Willemze, R.; Jansen, P.M.; Quint, K.D.; van Wezel, T.; van Eijk, R.; Ruano, D.; Tensen, C.P.; Hauben, E.; et al. Cell-of-origin classification using the Hans and Lymph2Cx algorithms in primary cutaneous large B-cell lymphomas. *Virchows Arch.* **2022**, *480*, 667–675. [CrossRef] [PubMed]

95. Senff, N.J.; Zoutman, W.H.; Vermeer, M.H.; Assaf, C.; Berti, E.; Cerroni, L.; Espinet, B.; Cabrera, R.F.D.M.; Geerts, M.-L.; Kempf, W.; et al. Fine-Mapping Chromosomal Loss at 9p21: Correlation with Prognosis in Primary Cutaneous Diffuse Large B-Cell Lymphoma, Leg Type. *J. Investig. Dermatol.* **2009**, *129*, 1149–1155. [CrossRef] [PubMed]
96. Pham-Ledard, A.; Beylot-Barry, M.; Barbe, C.; LeDuc, M.; Petrella, T.; Vergier, B.; Martinez, F.; Cappellen, D.; Merlio, J.-P.; Grange, F. High Frequency and Clinical Prognostic Value of MYD88 L265P Mutation in Primary Cutaneous Diffuse Large B-Cell Lymphoma, Leg-Type. *JAMA Dermatol.* **2014**, *150*, 1173–1179. [CrossRef] [PubMed]
97. Pham-Ledard, A.; Prochazkova-Carlotti, M.; Andrique, L.; Cappellen, D.; Vergier, B.; Martinez, F.; Grange, F.; Petrella, T.; Beylot-Barry, M.; Merlio, J.-P. Multiple genetic alterations in primary cutaneous large B-cell lymphoma, leg type support a common lymphomagenesis with activated B-cell-like diffuse large B-cell lymphoma. *Mod. Pathol.* **2014**, *27*, 402–411. [CrossRef]
98. Koens, L.; Zoutman, W.H.; Ngarmlertsirichai, P.; Przybylski, G.K.; Grabarczyk, P.; Vermeer, M.H.; Willemze, R.; Jansen, P.M.; Schmidt, C.A.; Tensen, C.P. Nuclear factor-κB pathway-activating gene aberrancies in primary cutaneous large B-cell lympho-ma, leg type. *J. Invest. Dermatol.* **2014**, *134*, 290–292. [CrossRef]
99. Zhou, X.A.; Louissaint, A., Jr.; Wenzel, A.; Yang, J.; Martinez-Escala, M.E.; Moy, A.P.; Morgan, E.A.; Paxton, C.N.; Hong, B.; Andersen, E.F.; et al. Genomic Analyses Identify Recurrent Alterations in Immune Evasion Genes in Diffuse Large B-Cell Lymphoma, Leg Type. *J. Invest. Dermatol.* **2018**, *138*, 2365–2376. [CrossRef]
100. Nayyar, N.; White, M.D.; Gill, C.M.; Lastrapes, M.; Bertalan, M.; Kaplan, A.; D'Andrea, M.R.; Bihun, I.; Kaneb, A.; Dietrich, J.; et al. MYD88 L265P mutation and CDKN2A loss are early mutational events in primary central nervous system diffuse large B-cell lymphomas. *Blood Adv.* **2019**, *3*, 375–383. [CrossRef]
101. Zhou, Y.; Liu, W.; Xu, Z.; Zhu, H.; Xiao, D.; Su, W.; Zeng, R.; Feng, Y.; Duan, Y.; Zhou, J.; et al. Analysis of Genomic Alteration in Primary Central Nervous System Lymphoma and the Expression of Some Related Genes. *Neoplasia* **2018**, *20*, 1059–1069. [CrossRef]
102. Chapuy, B.; Roemer, M.G.M.; Stewart, C.; Tan, Y.; Abo, R.P.; Zhang, L.; Dunford, A.J.; Meredith, D.M.; Thorner, A.R.; Jordanova, E.S.; et al. Targetable genetic features of primary testicular and primary central nervous system lymphomas. *Blood* **2016**, *127*, 869–881. [CrossRef]
103. Koens, L.; Qin, Y.; Leung, W.Y.; Corver, W.; Jansen, P.M.; Willemze, R.; Vermeer, M.; Tensen, C. MicroRNA Profiling of Primary Cutaneous Large B-Cell Lymphomas. *PLoS ONE* **2013**, *8*, e82471. [CrossRef]
104. Oschlies, I.; Wehkamp, U. Cutaneous B cell lymphomas: Standards in diagnostic and clinical work-up. Hints, pitfalls and recent advances. *Histopathology* **2022**, *80*, 184–195. [CrossRef] [PubMed]
105. Wehkamp, U.; Pott, C.; Unterhalt, M.; Koch, K.; Weichenthal, M.; Klapper, W.; Oschlies, I. Skin Involvement of Mantle Cell Lymphoma May Mimic Primary Cutaneous Diffuse Large B-cell Lymphoma, Leg Type. *Am. J. Surg. Pathol.* **2015**, *39*, 1093–1101. [CrossRef] [PubMed]
106. Harms, K.L.; Harms, P.; Anderson, T.; Betz, B.L.; Ross, C.W.; Fullen, D.R.; Hristov, A.C. Mycosis fungoides with CD20 expression: Report of two cases and review of the literature. *J. Cutan. Pathol.* **2014**, *41*, 494–503. [CrossRef]
107. Cm, B.J.; Sahi, H.; Koljonen, V.; Böhling, T. The expression of terminal deoxynucleotidyl transferase and paired box gene 5 in Merkel cell carcinomas and its relation to the presence of Merkel cell polyomavirus DNA. *J. Cutan. Pathol.* **2019**, *46*, 26–32. [CrossRef]
108. Kempf, W.; Kazakov, D.; Mitteldorf, C. Cutaneous Lymphomas. *Am. J. Dermatopathol.* **2014**, *36*, 197–210. [CrossRef] [PubMed]
109. Forcucci, J.; Ralston, J.; Lazarchick, J. Diagnosing Spindle Cell Variant of Primary Cutaneous B-Cell Lymphoma: Potential Pitfalls and Solutions. *Ann. Clin. Lab. Sci.* **2016**, *46*, 209–212.
110. Menguy, S.; Frison, E.; Prochazkova-Carlotti, M.; Dalle, S.; Dereure, O.; Boulinguez, S.; Dalac, S.; Machet, L.; Ram-Wolff, C.; Verneuil, L.; et al. Double-hit or dual expression of MYC and BCL2 in primary cutaneous large B-cell lymphomas. *Mod. Pathol.* **2018**, *31*, 1332–1342. [CrossRef]
111. Hamilton, S.N.; Wai, E.S.; Tan, K.; Alexander, C.; Gascoyne, R.D.; Connors, J.M. Treatment and outcomes in patients with pri-mary cutaneous B-cell lymphoma: The BC Cancer Agency experience. *Int. J. Radiat. Oncol. Biol Phys.* **2013**, *87*, 719–725. [CrossRef]
112. Beylot-Barry, M.; Mermin, D.; Maillard, A.; Bouabdallah, R.; Bonnet, N.; Duval-Modeste, A.-B.; Mortier, L.; Ingen-Housz-Oro, S.; Ram-Wolff, C.; Barete, S.; et al. A Single-Arm Phase II Trial of Lenalidomide in Relapsing or Refractory Primary Cutaneous Large B-Cell Lymphoma, Leg Type. *J. Investig. Dermatol.* **2018**, *138*, 1982–1989. [CrossRef]
113. Willemze, R.; Jaffe, E.S.; Burg, G.; Cerroni, L.; Berti, E.; Swerdlow, S.H.; Ralfkiaer, E.; Chimenti, S.; Diaz-Perez, J.L.; Duncan, L.M.; et al. WHO-EORTC Classification for Cutaneous Lymphomas. *Blood* **2005**, *105*, 3768–3785. [CrossRef]
114. Sica, A.; Vitiello, P.; Caccavale, S.; Sagnelli, C.; Calogero, A.; Dodaro, C.A.; Pastore, F.; Ciardiello, F.; Argenziano, G.; Reginelli, A.; et al. Primary cutaneous DLBCL non-GCB type: Challenges of a rare case. *Open Med.* **2020**, *15*, 119–125. [CrossRef] [PubMed]
115. Kodama, K.; Massone, C.; Chott, A.; Metze, D.; Kerl, H.; Cerroni, L. Primary cutaneous large B-cell lymphomas: Clinicopathologic features, classification, and prognostic factors in a large series of patients. *Blood* **2005**, *106*, 2491–2497. [CrossRef] [PubMed]
116. Jaffe, E.S. Navigating the cutaneous B-cell lymphomas: Avoiding the rocky shoals. *Mod. Pathol.* **2019**, *33*, 96–106. [CrossRef] [PubMed]
117. Ponzoni, M.; Arrigoni, G.; Gould, V.E.; Del Curto, B.; Maggioni, M.; Scapinello, A.; Paolino, S.; Cassisa, A.; Patriarca, C. Lack of CD 29 (β1 integrin) and CD 54 (ICAM-1) adhesion molecules in intravascular lymphomatosis. *Hum. Pathol.* **2000**, *31*, 220–226. [CrossRef]

118. Khalidi, H.S.; Brynes, R.K.; Browne, P.; Koo, C.H.; Battifora, H.; Medeiros, L.J. Intravascular large B-cell lymphoma: The CD5 antigen is expressed by a subset of cases. *Mod. Pathol.* **1998**, *11*, 983–988.
119. Ferreri, A.J.M.; Campo, E.; Seymour, J.F.; Willemze, R.; Ilariucci, F.; Ambrosetti, A.; Zucca, E.; Rossi, G.; López-Guillermo, A.; Pavlovsky, M.A.; et al. Intravascular lymphoma: Clinical presentation, natural history, management and prognostic factors in a series of 38 cases, with special emphasis on the 'cutaneous variant'. *Br. J. Haematol.* **2004**, *127*, 173–183. [CrossRef]
120. Dojcinov, S.D.; Venkataraman, G.; Raffeld, M.; Pittaluga, S.; Jaffe, E. EBV Positive Mucocutaneous Ulcer—A Study of 26 Cases Associated with Various Sources of Immunosuppression. *Am. J. Surg. Pathol.* **2010**, *34*, 405–417. [CrossRef]
121. Ikeda, T.; Gion, Y.; Yoshino, T.; Sato, Y. A review of EBV-positive mucocutaneous ulcers focusing on clinical and pathological aspects. *J. Clin. Exp. Hematop.* **2019**, *59*, 64–71. [CrossRef]
122. Sundram, U. Cutaneous Lymphoproliferative Disorders: What's New in the Revised 4th Edition of the World Health Organization (WHO) Classification of Lymphoid Neoplasms. *Adv. Anat. Pathol.* **2019**, *26*, 93–113. [CrossRef]
123. Zanelli, M.; Sanguedolce, F.; Palicelli, A.; Zizzo, M.; Martino, G.; Caprera, C.; Fragliasso, V.; Soriano, A.; Valle, L.; Ricci, S.; et al. EBV-Driven Lymphoproliferative Disorders and Lymphomas of the Gastrointestinal Tract: A Spectrum of Entities with a Common Denominator (Part 1). *Cancers* **2021**, *13*, 4578. [CrossRef]

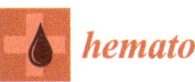

Review

The NKL- and TALE-Codes Represent Hematopoietic Gene Signatures to Evaluate Deregulated Homeobox Genes in Hodgkin Lymphoma

Stefan Nagel

Department of Human and Animal Cell Lines, Leibniz-Institute DSMZ, German Collection of Microorganisms and Cell Cultures, 38124 Braunschweig, Germany; sna@dsmz.de

Abstract: Homeobox genes encode transcription factors which control basic processes in development and differentiation. Concerning the sequence conservation in their homeobox, these genes are arranged into particular groups sharing evolutionary ancestry and resembling in function. We have recently described the physiological expression patterns of two homeobox gene groups, NKL and TALE, in early hematopoiesis and subsequent lymphopoiesis. The hematopoietic activities of eleven NKL and nine TALE homeobox genes have been termed as NKL- and TALE-codes, respectively. Due to the developmental impact of homeobox genes, these expression data indicate a key role for their activity in normal hematopoietic differentiation processes, including B-cell development. On the other hand, aberrant expression of NKL- and TALE-code members or ectopic activation of non-code members have been frequently reported in lymphoid malignancies, demonstrating their oncogenic potential in the hematopoietic compartment. Here, we provide an overview of the established NKL- and TALE-codes in normal lymphopoiesis and of deregulated homeobox genes in Hodgkin lymphoma, demonstrating the capability of gene codes to identify homeo-oncogenes in lymphoid malignancies.

Keywords: EBV; HLX; HOXB9; NFIB; PBX1; STAT3; TLX2

Citation: Nagel, S. The NKL- and TALE-Codes Represent Hematopoietic Gene Signatures to Evaluate Deregulated Homeobox Genes in Hodgkin Lymphoma. *Hemato* **2022**, *3*, 122–130. https://doi.org/10.3390/hemato3010011

Academic Editors: Alina Nicolae and Antonino Carbone

Received: 22 December 2021
Accepted: 26 January 2022
Published: 2 February 2022

Publisher's Note: MDPI stays neutral with regard to jurisdictional claims in published maps and institutional affiliations.

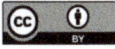

Copyright: © 2022 by the author. Licensee MDPI, Basel, Switzerland. This article is an open access article distributed under the terms and conditions of the Creative Commons Attribution (CC BY) license (https://creativecommons.org/licenses/by/4.0/).

1. Hematopoiesis and B-Cell Development

In the course of hematopoiesis, all of the blood and immune cells are produced. Today, developing and mature hematopoietic cells are extensively defined even at the molecular level, allowing for the retracement of underlying mechanisms of cell differentiation [1]. Hematopoietic stem cells (HSCs) are located in the bone marrow and generate common progenitors, which represent the starting points for the myeloid and lymphoid cell lineages. The common lymphoid progenitor (CLP) generates all of the types of lymphocytes, comprising B-cells, T-cells, natural killer (NK)-cells, and innate lymphoid cells (ILC). The process of B-cell development begins with the CLP-derived B-cell progenitor (BCP) and includes the rearrangements of B-cell receptor genes encoding the immunoglobulin chains. BCPs differentiate via the pro-B-cell and pre-B-cell stages into naïve B-cells. Early T-cell progenitors migrate into the thymus to complete their differentiation. In contrast, for the final differentiation steps to memory B-cells and plasma cells via the stage of germinal center (GC) B-cells, naïve B-cells migrate into lymph nodes, the spleen, and other lymphoid tissues. In these compartments, additional molecular alterations occur, such as somatic hypermutation and class switching of the B-cell receptor genes. These alterations are operated at the DNA level and prone to generate oncogenic gene rearrangements and mutations.

The main steps of lymphopoiesis including B-cell development are controlled at the transcriptional level [2,3]. Accordingly, several transcription factors (TFs), such as BCL6, EBF1, MYB, PAX5, PRDM1, SPIB, and TCF3 are members of a B-cell specific regulatory network, which orchestrates basic differentiation processes [4–7]. TCF3 plays a prominent role for the development of all types of lymphocytes, while EBF1 and PAX5 are basic factors of the B-cell lineage [3,8]. BCL6 and PRDM1 inhibit each other and are involved in differentiation processes taking place in the GC [9]. Provoked by aberrant chromosomal rearrangements or gene mutations, deregulations of these developmental TFs are reported to contribute to the generation of B-cell malignancies [10,11]. Therefore, the knowledge of physiological activities of developmental TFs supports the understanding of both the normal and abnormal processes in B-cell differentiation.

2. Classification of Homeobox Genes

Homeobox genes encode TFs, which mainly control development and cell/tissue differentiation [12]. They represent the second strongest group of TFs in humans [13]. Their conserved homeobox encodes the homeodomain, which forms a 3D-structure classified as helix–turn–helix. The homeodomain is about 60 amino acid residues long and consists of three helices. Helix 3 shows the strongest sequence conformance, fits into the major groove of the DNA, and performs sequence–specific interactions [14]. Accordingly, helix 3 has been termed as a recognition helix. Moreover, the homeodomain mediates contacts with chromatin and cofactors, thus representing the operating basis of these TFs [12].

With regards to the similarities in their homeobox sequences, these genes are arranged in classes and subclasses. Overall, eleven classes have been recognized, comprising ANTP, CERS, CUT, HNF, LIM, POU, PRD, PROS, SINE, TALE, and ZF [15]. The largest classes are antennapedia (ANTP) and paired (PRD). The ANTP class contains the subclasses HOX-like (HOXL) and NK-like (NKL). This established scheme reflects the evolutionary history of these genes, which have been detected in all of the eukaryotes and expanded in Metazoa [16]. The human genome contains 235 homeobox genes [15]. The process of gene duplication has generated gene clusters, which subsequently diversified and separated, but are still present for the HOX genes and to some extent, for the NKL genes [17]. The human genome contains four HOX gene clusters, called HOXA, HOXB, HOXC, and HOXD, showing an evolutionary conserved arrangement and colinear activities in the embryonal development. Furthermore, the human genome contains 48 NKL subclass members. For instance, NKL homeobox genes TLX3, NKX2-5, and MSX2 are distant neighbors and located at chromosomal position 5q35, displaying their evolutionary history as part of an ancient and more comprehensive NKL gene cluster [15,17].

The basic impact of homeobox genes in developmental processes is evident by nominating several members as master genes. NKL homeobox gene NKX2-3 has been described as a fundamental regulator of spleen development. Knockdown of this gene in embryonal mice results in asplenic animals [18]. Furthermore, NKX2-3 is hematopoietically expressed in human HSCs and silenced in the following stages of differentiation, indicating functional roles at the stem cell level [19]. NKX2-5 is involved in the development of both the spleen and heart [20,21]. Its role in heart development is evolutionary conserved in vertebrates and insects, highlighting the profound developmental impact of homeobox genes. Finally, PAX5 is a member of the PRD class of homeobox genes and controls the differentiation of B-cells [22]. Loss of PAX5 activity in the hematopoietic compartment disturbs the B-cell development in mice [23]. Therefore, these master genes regulate fundamental steps in the differentiation of specific cells, tissues, and organs.

3. Homeobox Gene Signatures: Lymphoid NKL- and TALE-Codes

Homeobox gene codes have been described for the first time for the clustered HOX genes expressed in the developing fruit fly *Drosophila* and later in vertebrate embryos [24]. Regarding their genomic arrangement, these genes display a colinear anterio–posterio expression pattern in the embryonic head region of mice, which has been called HOX-code [25]. The DLX-code describes a dorso–ventral expression pattern of DLX homeobox genes in the developing pharyngeal region [26]. Therefore, these gene codes represent the expression signatures of related homeobox genes for particular tissues or body regions.

Recently, we have created the NKL-code, which describes the expression of particular NKL homeobox genes in the course of hematopoiesis, including early stem cell stages, lymphopoiesis, myelopoiesis, and mature lymphoid and myeloid cells [19,27,28]. This code encompasses eleven NKL homeobox genes, showing a specific expression pattern in stem and progenitor cells, as well as mature blood and immune cells [29]. The lymphoid NKL-code is depicted in Figure 1. With regards to this code, the expression of NKX2-3 and NANOG is restricted to hematopoietic stem/progenitor cells, while HHEX and HLX are active in developing and mature lymphocytes. The activity of NKL homeobox genes is downregulated in the final differentiation stages of T-cells, ILC1, and ILC2. In B-cell development, HLX is silenced after the stage of B-cell progenitors, while HHEX and NKX6-3 contribute to the differentiation of memory B-cells and plasma cells, respectively.

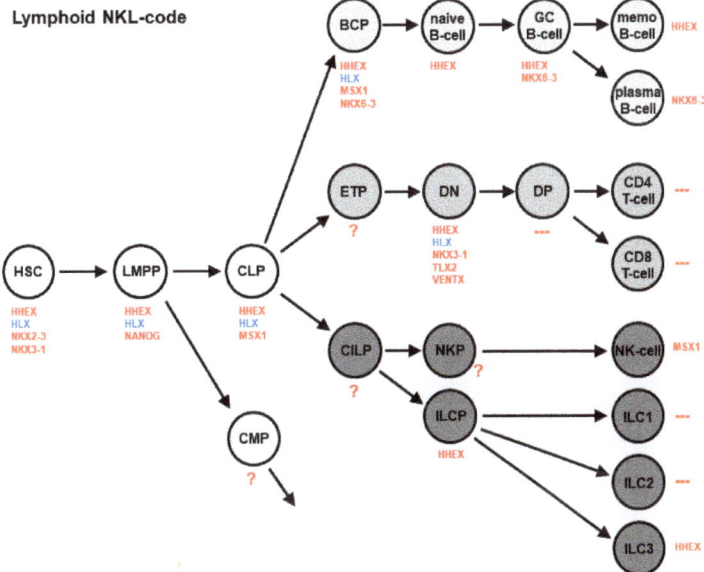

Figure 1. The lymphoid NKL-code describes activities of NKL homeobox genes (red) in stages and cell types of early hematopoiesis and lymphopoiesis, including developing B-cells, T-cells, NK-cells, and ILCs. NKL homeobox gene HLX is highlighted in blue. BCP: B-cell progenitor; CILP: Common innate lymphoid cell progenitor; CLP: Common lymphoid progenitor; CMP: Common myeloid progenitor; DN: Double negative thymocytes; DP: Double positive thymocytes; ETP: Early T-cell progenitor; GC: Germinal center; HSC: Hematopoietic stem cell; ILC: Innate lymphoid cells; LMPP: Lymphoid and myeloid primed progenitor; memo: Memory; NKP: NK-cell progenitor; ?: Cell types with unknown NKL gene activities; —: Cell types with absent NKL gene activities.

TALE genes represent a conspicuous homeobox gene class [12,30]. All of the members contain a three amino acid loop extension between helix 1 and 2, abbreviated as TALE. This very ancient group of homeobox genes encodes TFs, which are able to cooperate with other TALE or with particular HOX proteins to regulate target genes. Regarding the generation of the NKL-code, we have created the lymphoid TALE-code [31]. This gene signature includes 11 of the 20 genes of the strong TALE homeobox gene class, expressed in early hematopoiesis and lymphopoiesis (Figure 2).

Each stage in lymphopoiesis expresses between one (ILC1) and eight (for example, naïve B-cells) TALE homeobox genes. TGF1 is expressed in all of the analyzed cell types, while PBX1, for example, is restricted to stem and progenitor cells. Thereafter, PBX1 is silenced in the course of B-cell development [31,32], indicating a suppressive function in lymphoid maturation.

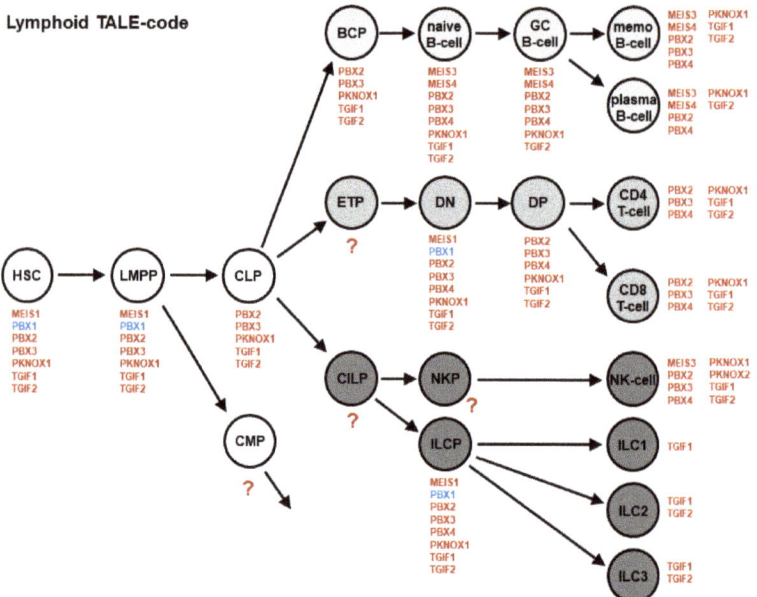

Figure 2. The lymphoid TALE-code describes the activities for TALE homeobox genes (red) in stages and cell types of early hematopoiesis and lymphopoiesis, including developing B-cells, T-cells, NK-cells, and ILCs. TALE homeobox gene PBX1 is highlighted in blue. BCP: B-cell progenitor; CILP: Common innate lymphoid cell progenitor; CLP: Common lymphoid progenitor; CMP: Common myeloid progenitor; DN: Double negative thymocytes; DP: Double positive thymocytes; ETP: Early T-cell progenitor; GC: Germinal center; HSC: Hematopoietic stem cell; ILC: Innate lymphoid cells; LMPP: Lymphoid and myeloid primed progenitor; memo: Memory; NKP: NK-cell progenitor; ?: Cell types with unknown TALE gene activities.

4. Deregulated Homeobox Genes in Hodgkin Lymphoma

4.1. Hodgkin Lymphoma

Hodgkin lymphoma (HL) is a GC-derived B-cell malignancy, although rare cases with T-cell origin have been described [33]. With regards to the histological and phenotypical characteristics, this tumor type is classified into two main groups, classical HL and nodular lymphocyte predominant HL (NLPHL). Classical HL is further divided into the subtypes nodular sclerosis, mixed cellularity, lymphocyte-rich, and lymphocyte-depleted. The typical large tumor cells are called Hodgkin Reed Sternberg (HRS) and lymphocyte predominant (LP) cells, respectively for the classical HL and NLPHL groups, occurring rarely in infiltrated lymph nodes. Therefore, most of the cells of the tumor mass represent reactive lymphocytes, macrophages, dendritic cells, and granulocytes [34].

The specific phenotype and rareness of HRS and LP cells complicate their analysis. However, established bona fide HL cell lines may serve as suitable models to investigate their molecular abnormalities [35]. HL has a long and intense background of causal research revealing several hallmarks, including aberrant receptor-signaling, inhibition of apoptosis, activated NFkB-pathway, loss of B-cell associated TFs, EBV infection, and immune escape [34,36]. HL is one of the most frequent lymphomas in the Western world. In addition, the current chemotherapeutic and radiation protocols have substantially improved the prognosis [34].

In HL, several deregulated homeobox genes have been reported, belonging to different classes/subclasses: ANTP/HOXL (HOXB9, MNX1/HLXB9), ANTP/NKL (DLX1, EMX2, HLX, NKX2-2, NKX3-2, TLX2), POU (POU2AF1/BOB1, POU2F2/OCT2), PRD (HOPX, PAX5, MIXL1, OTX1, OTX2), SINE (SIX1), TALE (IRX3, IRX4, MEIS1, MEIS3, PBX1, PBX4, TGIF1), and ZF (ZHX2) [29,31,37–46]. Downregulation of B-cell associated homeobox gene activities has been described for PAX5, POU2AF1/BOB1, POU2F2/OCT2, and ZHX2, basically contributing to the generation of this malignancy by disturbed B-cell differentiation [41,46]. The remaining deregulated homeobox genes are aberrantly overexpressed or ectopically activated. Recently, we have systematically analyzed the groups of NKL and TALE homeobox genes in hematopoiesis and revealed aberrant activities of two members in HL, which are detailed in the following section [30,36].

4.2. Deregulated NKL Homeobox Gene HLX in HL

A systematic screening for deregulated NKL homeobox genes in HL revealed six members [27]. A subsequent comparison of lymphoid NKL-code members with HL patient data demonstrated aberrant overexpression of HLX in about 8% of patients [37]. HL cell line L-540 showed conspicuously high HLX expression levels and served as a model to investigate the upstream and downstream factors. Expression profiling analysis, knockdown and inhibitor experiments, reporter gene assays, in addition to chromatin immunoprecipitation data showed that STAT3 directly activates HLX in L-540. Furthermore, analyses of the subcellular localization of STAT3 indicated that deacetylation of STAT3 protein supports nuclear translocation and the subsequent activation of HLX expression [37]. Consistently, Kube et al. have reported that STAT3 represents an aberrantly activated TF in HL [47]. Analyses of HLX target genes revealed the inhibition of differentiation factors BCL11A, MSX1 and SPIB, and of pro-apoptotic factor BCL2L11 [37]. Therefore, HLX impacts the HL hallmark processes B-cell differentiation and apoptosis. The deregulated activity and oncogenic function of HLX in HL cells is summarized in Figure 3.

The activator role of STAT3 for HLX expression has also been shown in the pathological contexts of anaplastic large cell lymphoma (ALCL) and EBV-positive diffuse large B-cell lymphoma (DLBCL). In ALCL, STAT3 is overexpressed, mutated, and aberrantly activated, representing a hallmark oncogene for this disease [48,49]. Using ALCL cell lines as models, we have demonstrated that STAT3 in addition to STAT3-activators and STAT3-target genes including HLX are overexpressed and targeted by copy number gains. Moreover, the oncogenic fusion protein NPM1–ALK activates STAT3, which can in turn drive HLX expression in ALCL cell lines [50].

Infection with Epstein–Barr virus (EBV) plays a pathognomonic role in B-cell lymphomas, including HL and DLBCL [51]. EBV-encoded proteins deregulate the activity of several signaling pathways, including JAK–STAT [52–54]. Accordingly, isolated EBV-positive and EBV-negative cell populations of DLBCL cell line DOHH-2 were used to demonstrate that EBV-factors LMP1 and LMP2A mediate STAT3 activation, which can in turn drive HLX expression in this malignancy [55]. Therefore, aberrant HLX activation by STAT3 is a general oncogenic transaction, playing a role in HL, ALCL, and DLBCL.

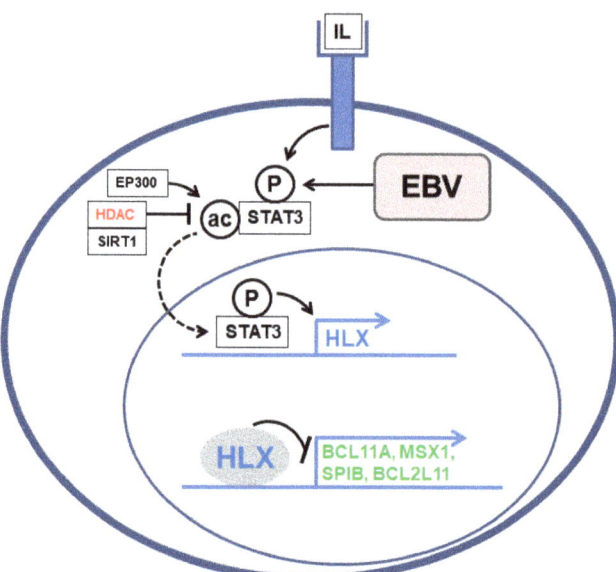

Figure 3. This diagram shows the regulation and function of aberrantly expressed NKL homeobox gene HLX. STAT3 is activated by interleukin (IL)-receptor-signaling or EBV-infection resulting in phosphorylation (P). The subcellular localization of STAT3 is regulated by acetylation (ac). EP300 mediates acetylation, while SIRT1 and overexpressed histone deacetylases (HDACs, red) perform deacetylation. Phosphorylated and deacetylated STAT3 translocate into the nucleus (dashed arrow) to activate its target gene HLX. HLX can in turn operate as a repressor to inhibit the target genes BCL11A, MSX1, SPIB, and BCL2L11 (green).

4.3. Deregulated TALE Homeobox Gene PBX1 in HL

Screening for deregulated TALE homeobox genes in HL patients revealed seven class members, including PBX1 [31]. The HL cell line SUP-HD1 expressed elevated PBX1 levels and served as a model to analyze upstream and downstream factors of this TALE homeobox gene. Genomic analysis demonstrated a copy number gain for PBX1 at 1q23 in SUP-HD1, which may underlie its upregulation. Target gene analysis revealed that PBX1 activated the differentiation factor NFIB and NKL homeobox gene TLX2. Of note, aberrant overexpression of NFIB in addition to NFIA, NFIC, and NFIX may indicate that this family of developmental TFs plays a substantial role in the pathogenesis of HL [31].

TALE homeodomain factors are described to interact with homeodomain factors of the TALE class or of the HOXL subclass [56]. This feature may represent a very ancient function of TALE factors [30]. Recently, we have found by a combination of PCR-screens the use of degenerate oligonucleotides and expression profiling analysis overexpression of HOXL subclass member HOXB9 in HL cell lines. HOXB9 is normally silent in hematopoietic cells, indicating ectopic activation. Therefore, once again, a copy number gain may underlie elevated HOXB9 expression in HL [39]. Additional analyses of the identified PBX1-target genes demonstrated that TLX2 is coregulated by PBX1 and HOXB9, while NFIB and TNFRSF9 are regulated by PBX1 or HOXB9, respectively. Deregulation of NFIB and TLX2 may impact B-cell differentiation, while TNFRSF9 has been implicated in immune escape [31,57,58]. Furthermore, TLX2 was shown to inhibit apoptosis via TBX15 and BCL2L11 (Figure 4). Therefore, PBX1 and HOXB9 support several oncogenic hallmark processes in HL.

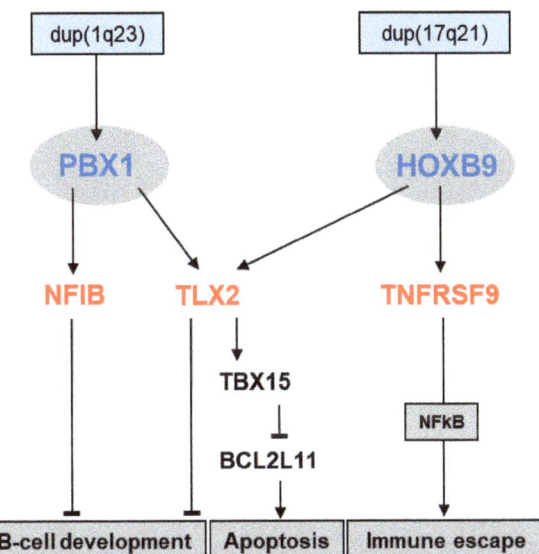

Figure 4. This diagram shows the activation and function of aberrantly expressed TALE homeobox gene PBX1 and HOXL homeobox gene HOXB9 in HL. Both genes are targeted by genomic copy number gains. PBX1 activates NFIB and TLX2, while HOXB9 activates TLX2 and TNFRSF9. NFIB and TLX2 mediate the inhibition of B-cell development, and TLX2 inhibits apoptosis via TBX15 and BCL2L11. TNFRSF9 supports aberrant immune escape via NFkB-signaling.

5. Conclusions

In conclusion, homeobox genes encode basic TFs with oncogenic functions, in the case that they are deregulated. Homeobox gene codes serve to describe the physiological differentiation processes and to identify and evaluate aberrant homeobox gene activities in coresponding tumor entities. Deregulated NKL- and TALE-code members HLX and PBX1 play important pathogenic roles in HL, and may thus have diagnostic and/or therapeutic potentials.

Funding: This research received no external funding.

Acknowledgments: I would like to thank Corinna Meyer for excellent technical support.

Conflicts of Interest: The author declares no conflict of interest.

References

1. Liggett, L.A.; Sankaran, V.G. Unraveling hematopoiesis through the lens of genomics. *Cell* **2020**, *182*, 1384–1400. [CrossRef] [PubMed]
2. Boller, S.; Grosschedl, R. The regulatory network of B-cell differentiation: A focused view of early B-cell factor 1 function. *Immunol. Rev.* **2014**, *261*, 102–115. [CrossRef] [PubMed]
3. Rothenberg, E.V. Transcriptional control of early T and B cell developmental choices. *Annu. Rev. Immunol.* **2014**, *32*, 283–321. [CrossRef] [PubMed]
4. Méndez, A.; Mendoza, L. A network model to describe the terminal differentiation of B cells. *PLoS Comput. Biol.* **2016**, *12*, e1004696. [CrossRef] [PubMed]
5. Smith, E.; Sigvardsson, M. The roles of transcription factors in B lymphocyte commitment, development, and transformation. *J. Leukoc. Biol.* **2004**, *75*, 973–981. [CrossRef] [PubMed]
6. Nutt, S.L.; Kee, B.L. The transcriptional regulation of B cell lineage commitment. *Immunity* **2007**, *26*, 715–725. [CrossRef]
7. Sokalski, K.M.; Li, S.K.; Welch, I.; Cadieux-Pitre, H.A.; Gruca, M.R.; DeKoter, R.P. Deletion of genes encoding PU.1 and Spi-B in B cells impairs differentiation and induces pre-B cell acute lymphoblastic leukemia. *Blood* **2011**, *118*, 2801–2808. [CrossRef]
8. Kucinski, I.; Wilson, N.K.; Hannah, R.; Kinston, S.J.; Cauchy, P.; Lenaerts, A.; Grosschedl, R.; Göttgens, B. Interactions between lineage-associated transcription factors govern haematopoietic progenitor states. *EMBO J.* **2020**, *39*, e104983. [CrossRef]

9. Shaffer, A.L.; Yu, X.; He, Y.; Boldrick, J.; Chan, E.P.; Staudt, L.M. BCL-6 represses genes that function in lymphocyte differentiation, inflammation, and cell cycle control. *Immunity* 2000, *13*, 199–212. [CrossRef]
10. Ma, E.S. Recurrent cytogenetic abnormalities in Non-Hodgkin's lymphoma and chronic lymphocytic leukemia. *Methods Mol. Biol.* 2017, *1541*, 279–293.
11. Bödör, C.; Reiniger, L. Catalog of genetic progression of human cancers: Non-Hodgkin lymphoma. *Cancer Metastasis Rev.* 2016, *35*, 109–127. [CrossRef] [PubMed]
12. Bürglin, T.R. Homeodomain subtypes and functional diversity. *Subcell Biochem.* 2011, *52*, 95–122. [PubMed]
13. Vaquerizas, J.M.; Kummerfeld, S.K.; Teichmann, S.A.; Luscombe, N.M. A census of human transcription factors: Function, expression and evolution. *Nat. Rev. Genet.* 2009, *10*, 252–263. [CrossRef] [PubMed]
14. Gehring, W.J.; Müller, M.; Affolter, M.; Percival-Smith, A.; Billeter, M.; Qian, Y.Q.; Otting, G.; Wüthrich, K. The structure of the homeodomain and its functional implications. *Trends Genet.* 1990, *6*, 323–329. [CrossRef]
15. Holland, P.W.; Booth, H.A.; Bruford, E.A. Classification and nomenclature of all human homeobox genes. *BMC Biol.* 2007, *5*, 47. [CrossRef] [PubMed]
16. Weirauch, M.T.; Hughes, T.R. A catalogue of eukaryotic transcription factor types, their evolutionary origin, and species distribution. *Subcell Biochem.* 2011, *52*, 25–73.
17. Pollard, S.L.; Holland, P.W. Evidence for 14 homeobox gene clusters in human genome ancestry. *Curr. Biol.* 2000, *10*, 1059–1062. [CrossRef]
18. Pabst, O.; Zweigerdt, R.; Arnold, H.H. Targeted disruption of the homeobox transcription factor Nkx2-3 in mice results in postnatal lethality and abnormal development of small intestine and spleen. *Development* 1999, *126*, 2215–2225. [CrossRef]
19. Nagel, S.; Pommerenke, C.; Scherr, M.; Meyer, C.; Kaufmann, M.; Battmer, K.; MacLeod, R.A.; Drexler, H.G. NKL homeobox gene activities in hematopoietic stem cells, T-cell development and T-cell leukemia. *PLoS ONE* 2017, *12*, e0171164. [CrossRef]
20. Lints, T.J.; Parsons, L.M.; Hartley, L.; Lyons, I.; Harvey, R.P. Nkx-2.5: A novel murine homeobox gene expressed in early heart progenitor cells and their myogenic descendants. *Development* 1993, *119*, 419–431. [CrossRef]
21. Brendolan, A.; Ferretti, E.; Salsi, V.; Moses, K.; Quaggin, S.; Blasi, F.; Cleary, M.L.; Selleri, L. A Pbx1-dependent genetic and transcriptional network regulates spleen ontogeny. *Development* 2005, *132*, 3113–3126. [CrossRef] [PubMed]
22. Cobaleda, C.; Schebesta, A.; Delogu, A.; Busslinger, M. Pax5: The guardian of B cell identity and function. *Nat. Immunol.* 2007, *8*, 463–470. [CrossRef] [PubMed]
23. Urbánek, P.; Wang, Z.Q.; Fetka, I.; Wagner, E.F.; Busslinger, M. Complete block of early B cell differentiation and altered patterning of the posterior midbrain in mice lacking Pax5/BSAP. *Cell* 1994, *79*, 901–912. [CrossRef]
24. Lewis, E.B. A gene complex controlling segmentation in Drosophila. *Nature* 1978, *276*, 565–570. [CrossRef] [PubMed]
25. Hunt, P.; Gulisano, M.; Cook, M.; Sham, M.H.; Faiella, A.; Wilkinson, D.; Boncinelli, E.; Krumlauf, R. A distinct Hox code for the branchial region of the vertebrate head. *Nature* 1991, *353*, 861–864. [CrossRef] [PubMed]
26. Depew, M.J.; Simpson, C.A.; Morasso, M.; Rubenstein, J.L. Reassessing the Dlx code: The genetic regulation of branchial arch skeletal pattern and development. *J. Anat.* 2005, *207*, 501–561. [CrossRef]
27. Nagel, S.; MacLeod, R.A.F.; Meyer, C.; Kaufmann, M.; Drexler, H.G. NKL homeobox gene activities in B-cell development and lymphomas. *PLoS ONE* 2018, *13*, e0205537. [CrossRef]
28. Nagel, S.; Scherr, M.; MacLeod, R.A.F.; Pommerenke, C.; Koeppel, M.; Meyer, C.; Kaufmann, M.; Dallmann, I.; Drexler, H.G. NKL homeobox gene activities in normal and malignant myeloid cells. *PLoS ONE* 2019, *14*, e0226212. [CrossRef]
29. Nagel, S. NKL-Code in normal and aberrant hematopoiesis. *Cancers* 2021, *13*, 1961. [CrossRef]
30. Mukherjee, K.; Bürglin, T.R. Comprehensive analysis of animal TALE homeobox genes: New conserved motifs and cases of accelerated evolution. *J. Mol. Evol.* 2007, *65*, 137–153. [CrossRef]
31. Nagel, S.; Pommerenke, C.; Meyer, C.; MacLeod, R.A.F.; Drexler, H.G. Establishment of the TALE-code reveals aberrantly activated homeobox gene PBX1 in Hodgkin lymphoma. *PLoS ONE* 2021, *16*, e0246603. [CrossRef] [PubMed]
32. Sanyal, M.; Tung, J.W.; Karsunky, H.; Zeng, H.; Selleri, L.; Weissman, I.L.; Herzenberg, L.A.; Cleary, M.L. B-cell development fails in the absence of the Pbx1 proto-oncogene. *Blood* 2007, *109*, 4191–4199. [CrossRef] [PubMed]
33. Küppers, R. The biology of Hodgkin's lymphoma. *Nat. Rev. Cancer* 2009, *9*, 15–27. [CrossRef] [PubMed]
34. Küppers, R.; Engert, A.; Hansmann, M.L. Hodgkin lymphoma. *J. Clin. Invest.* 2012, *122*, 3439–3447. [CrossRef] [PubMed]
35. Drexler, H.G.; Pommerenke, C.; Eberth, S.; Nagel, S. Hodgkin lymphoma cell lines: To separate the wheat from the chaff. *Biol. Chem.* 2018, *399*, 511–523. [CrossRef] [PubMed]
36. Weniger, M.A.; Küppers, R. Molecular biology of Hodgkin lymphoma. *Leukemia* 2021, *35*, 968–981. [CrossRef] [PubMed]
37. Nagel, S.; Pommerenke, C.; Meyer, C.; Kaufmann, M.; MacLeod, R.A.F.; Drexler, H.G. Aberrant expression of NKL homeobox gene HLX in Hodgkin lymphoma. *Oncotarget* 2018, *9*, 14338–14353. [CrossRef]
38. Nagel, S.; MacLeod, R.A.F.; Pommerenke, C.; Meyer, C.; Kaufmann, M.; Drexler, H.G. NKL homeobox gene NKX2-2 is aberrantly expressed in Hodgkin lymphoma. *Oncotarget* 2018, *9*, 37480–37496. [CrossRef]
39. Nagel, S.; Burek, C.; Venturini, L.; Scherr, M.; Quentmeier, H.; Meyer, C.; Rosenwald, A.; Drexler, H.G.; MacLeod, R.A. Comprehensive analysis of homeobox genes in Hodgkin lymphoma cell lines identifies dysregulated expression of HOXB9 mediated via ERK5 signaling and BMI1. *Blood* 2007, *109*, 3015–3023. [CrossRef]
40. Nagel, S.; Scherr, M.; Quentmeier, H.; Kaufmann, M.; Zaborski, M.; Drexler, H.G.; MacLeod, R.A. HLXB9 activates IL6 in Hodgkin lymphoma cell lines and is regulated by PI3K signalling involving E2F3. *Leukemia* 2005, *19*, 841–846. [CrossRef]

41. Stein, H.; Marafioti, T.; Foss, H.D.; Laumen, H.; Hummel, M.; Anagnostopoulos, I.; Wirth, T.; Demel, G.; Falini, B. Down-regulation of BOB.1/OBF.1 and Oct2 in classical Hodgkin disease but not in lymphocyte predominant Hodgkin disease correlates with immunoglobulin transcription. *Blood* **2001**, *97*, 496–501. [CrossRef] [PubMed]
42. Krenacs, L.; Himmelmann, A.W.; Quintanilla-Martinez, L.; Fest, T.; Riva, A.; Wellmann, A.; Bagdi, E.; Kehrl, J.H.; Jaffe, E.S.; Raffeld, M. Transcription factor B-cell-specific activator protein (BSAP) is differentially expressed in B cells and in subsets of B-cell lymphomas. *Blood* **1998**, *92*, 1308–1316. [CrossRef] [PubMed]
43. Drakos, E.; Rassidakis, G.Z.; Leventaki, V.; Guo, W.; Medeiros, L.J.; Nagarajan, L. Differential expression of the human MIXL1 gene product in non-Hodgkin and Hodgkin lymphomas. *Hum. Pathol.* **2007**, *38*, 500–507. [CrossRef] [PubMed]
44. Nagel, S.; Ehrentraut, S.; Meyer, C.; Kaufmann, M.; Drexler, H.G.; MacLeod, R.A. Aberrantly Eexpressed OTX homeobox genes deregulate B-Cell differentiation in Hodgkin lymphoma. *PLoS ONE* **2015**, *10*, e0138416. [CrossRef]
45. Nagel, S.; Meyer, C.; Kaufmann, M.; Drexler, H.G.; MacLeod, R.A. Aberrant expression of homeobox gene SIX1 in Hodgkin lymphoma. *Oncotarget* **2015**, *6*, 40112–40126. [CrossRef]
46. Nagel, S.; Schneider, B.; Rosenwald, A.; Meyer, C.; Kaufmann, M.; Drexler, H.G.; MacLeod, R.A. t(4;8)(q27;q24) in Hodgkin lymphoma cells targets phosphodiesterase PDE5A and homeobox gene ZHX2. *Genes Chromosomes Cancer* **2011**, *50*, 996–1009. [CrossRef]
47. Kube, D.; Holtick, U.; Vockerodt, M.; Ahmadi, T.; Haier, B.; Behrmann, I.; Heinrich, P.C.; Diehl, V.; Tesch, H. STAT3 is constitutively activated in Hodgkin cell lines. *Blood* **2001**, *98*, 762–770. [CrossRef]
48. Zamo, A.; Chiarle, R.; Piva, R.; Howes, J.; Fan, Y.; Chilosi, M.; Levy, D.E.; Inghirami, G. Anaplastic lymphoma kinase (ALK) activates Stat3 and protects hematopoietic cells from cell death. *Oncogene* **2002**, *21*, 1038–1047. [CrossRef]
49. Crescenzo, R.; Abate, F.; Lasorsa, E.; Tabbo, F.; Gaudiano, M.; Chiesa, N.; Di Giacomo, F.; Spaccarotella, E.; Barbarossa, L.; Ercole, E.; et al. Convergent mutations and kinase fusions lead to oncogenic STAT3 activation in anaplastic large cell lymphoma. *Cancer Cell.* **2015**, *27*, 516–532. [CrossRef]
50. Nagel, S.; Pommerenke, C.; MacLeod, R.A.F.; Meyer, C.; Kaufmann, M.; Drexler, H.G. The NKL-code for innate lymphoid cells reveals deregulated expression of NKL homeobox genes HHEX and HLX in anaplastic large cell lymphoma (ALCL). *Oncotarget* **2020**, *11*, 3208–3226. [CrossRef]
51. Shannon-Lowe, C.; Rickinson, A.B.; Bell, A.I. Epstein-Barr virus-associated lymphomas. *Philos. Trans. R. Soc. Lond. B Biol. Sci.* **2017**, *372*, 20160271. [CrossRef] [PubMed]
52. Kato, H.; Karube, K.; Yamamoto, K.; Takizawa, J.; Tsuzuki, S.; Yatabe, Y.; Kanda, T.; Katayama, M.; Ozawa, Y.; Ishitsuka, K. Gene expression profiling of Epstein-Barr virus-positive diffuse large B-cell lymphoma of the elderly reveals alterations of characteristic oncogenetic pathways. *Cancer Sci.* **2014**, *105*, 537–544. [CrossRef] [PubMed]
53. Kung, C.P.; Raab-Traub, N. Epstein-Barr virus latent membrane protein 1 induces expression of the epidermal growth factor receptor through effects on Bcl-3 and STAT3. *J. Virol.* **2008**, *82*, 5486–5493. [CrossRef] [PubMed]
54. Incrocci, R.; Barse, L.; Stone, A.; Vagvala, S.; Montesano, M.; Subramaniam, V.; Swanson-Mungerson, M. Epstein-Barr Virus Latent Membrane Protein 2A (LMP2A) enhances IL-10 production through the activation of Bruton's tyrosine kinase and STAT3. *Virology* **2017**, *500*, 96–102. [CrossRef] [PubMed]
55. Nagel, S.; Uphoff, C.C.; Dirks, W.G.; Pommerenke, C.; Meyer, C.; Drexler, H.G. Epstein-Barr virus (EBV) activates NKL homeobox gene HLX in DLBCL. *PLoS ONE* **2019**, *14*, e0216898. [CrossRef] [PubMed]
56. Selleri, L.; Zappavigna, V.; Ferretti, E. "Building a perfect body": Control of vertebrate organogenesis by PBX-dependent regulatory networks. *Genes Dev.* **2019**, *33*, 258–275. [CrossRef] [PubMed]
57. Chen, K.S.; Lim, J.W.C.; Richards, L.J.; Bunt, J. The convergent roles of the nuclear factor I transcription factors in development and cancer. *Cancer Lett.* **2017**, *410*, 124–138. [CrossRef] [PubMed]
58. Ho, W.T.; Pang, W.L.; Chong, S.M.; Castella, A.; Al-Salam, S.; Tan, T.E.; Moh, M.C.; Koh, L.K.; Gan, S.U.; Cheng, C.K.; et al. Expression of CD137 on Hodgkin and Reed-Sternberg cells inhibits T-cell activation by eliminating CD137 ligand expression. *Cancer Res.* **2013**, *73*, 652–661. [CrossRef]

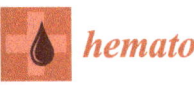 hemato

Article

Burkitt Lymphoma Incidence in Five Continents

Sam M. Mbulaiteye * and Susan S. Devesa

Infections and Immunoepidemiology Branch, Division of Cancer Epidemiology and Genetics, National Cancer Institute, Bethesda, MD 20892, USA; devesas@nci.nih.gov
* Correspondence: mbulaits@mail.nih.gov; Tel.: +1-240-276-7108

Abstract: Burkitt lymphoma (BL) is a rare non-Hodgkin lymphoma first described in 1958 by Denis Burkitt in African children. BL occurs as three types, endemic, which occurs in Africa and is causally attributed to Epstein-Barr virus and *P. falciparum* infections; sporadic, which occurs in temperate areas, but the cause is obscure; and immunodeficiency-type, which is associated with immunosuppression. All BL cases carry *IG::MYC* chromosomal translocations, which are necessary but insufficient to cause BL. We report a comprehensive study of the geographic, sex, and age-specific patterns of BL among 15,122 cases from Cancer Incidence in Five Continents Volume XI for 2008–2012 and the African Cancer Registry Network for 2018. Age-standardized BL rates were high (>4 cases per million people) in Uganda in Africa, and Switzerland and Estonia in Europe. Rates were intermediate (2–3.9) in the remaining countries in Europe, North America, and Oceania, and low (<2) in Asia. Rates in India were 1/20th those in Uganda. BL rates varied within and between regions, without showing a threshold to define BL as endemic or sporadic. BL rates were twice as high among males as females and showed a bimodal age pattern with pediatric and elderly peaks in all regions. Multi-regional transdisciplinary research is needed to elucidate the epidemiological patterns of BL.

Keywords: Burkitt lymphoma; epidemiology; *Plasmodium falciparum*; Epstein Barr virus; registry studies; multimodal cancer; non-Hodgkin lymphoma; HIV/AIDS

1. Introduction

Burkitt lymphoma (BL) is an aggressive B-cell non-Hodgkin lymphoma of germinal center B cells [1], first described as a jaw sarcoma in Ugandan children by Denis Burkitt in 1958 [2]. The pathology of BL was defined as a diffuse infiltration of medium-sized lymphoid cells, with pale staining macrophages giving a "starry-sky" appearance under the microscope [3,4]. This pathology definition enabled the epidemiology and clinical behavior of BL cases to be studied worldwide [5–8], at different anatomic sites [4,9,10], and from periods predating Burkitt's report [11]. The World Health Organization (WHO) introduced the eponym "Burkitt tumor" to standardize the classification of BL cases worldwide and to recognize Burkitt's seminal contribution [12].

The early study of BL revealed a comparatively high incidence of BL cases in warm, wet, low-lying areas, particularly in Africa, and a low incidence of BL cases in temperate or arid areas [13]. This simple distribution was used to classify BL cases as endemic or sporadic, and provided a useful insight about possible causal factors, notably that BL was caused by a virus [14,15] or parasite, such as malaria, vectored by insects in Africa [16]. Discovery of Epstein-Barr virus (EBV), by electron microscopy in tumor samples obtained from an African child [17], appeared to confirm the virus hypothesis. EBV DNA was detected in ~95% of endemic BL cases, consistent with this hypothesis. However, EBV DNA was detected in only 10–20% of sporadic BL cases, suggesting that EBV was not necessary for development of BL. EBV also did not satisfy the "insect-vector transmission mode" of the hypothesis because it was transmitted by saliva [18,19] and was equally prevalent in areas with endemic and sporadic BL. The insect-vector hypothesis was satisfied by holoendemic

Plasmodium falciparum, which is transmitted by female *Anopheline* mosquitoes and is co-endemic with BL [20,21]. Thus, the hypothesis was modified to suggest that interactions between EBV and *P. falciparum* infection promote BL risk, with *P. falciparum* promoting B-cell proliferation through chronic stimulation of the reticulo-endothelial system [21] and increasing EBV burden [22]. The hypothesis that EBV and *P. falciparum* cooperate in BL development is one of the earliest examples of polymicrobial etiology of cancer [23]. Subsequently, the identification of BL in previously healthy young homosexual men in the US in the early 1980s [24] led to recognition of the acquired immunodeficiency syndrome (AIDS) [25] and focused attention on immunosuppression as a co-factor in BL etiology. For a short time, BL was used as a sentinel condition in the surveillance of AIDS as one of the AIDS-defining cancers [26].

Molecular studies showing consistent detection of *IG::MYC* translocations [27,28] confirmed common pathology of BL reported in diverse settings. The translocation is believed to be an early, possibly initiating event, in all forms of BL. Clinical studies, demonstrating similar responses to chemotherapy for endemic cases in Africa [29–31] and sporadic cases in the US and elsewhere [32,33], reinforced the notion that BL cases diagnosed in different settings shared common pathology. Research on BL marks a watershed moment in cancer research, which gave birth to new specialties, including discovery of tumor viruses, elucidation of biology, re-focusing research on chemotherapy to combination regimens with intent to cure cancer, and increased interest in global oncology [34]. The excitement triggered by BL prompted Joseph Burchenal to declare in 1966 [35] that geographic studies of BL would reveal new principles in cancer research. These new principles include six human tumor viruses that have been discovered [36] and now are linked to ~1 million cancers worldwide (about one-sixth of the cancer burden) [37] that are prime targets for cancer prevention.

However, our understanding of the worldwide epidemiology of BL is incomplete because current research of BL does not have a global coverage [15,38]. Our understanding is also limited by the pathology definition established six decades ago, which did not codify a gold standard [39,40]. For example, the pathology definition recognized variant pathology features, such as differences in cell size, shape, degree of differentiation, amount of stroma and number of histocytes. BL cases with variant pathology have been described as atypical BL or Burkitt-like [41], and were classified and coded with BL until 2008 [42,43]. Thus, it is difficult to compare BL data from single countries [44–48] or in limited geographical regions [15,49–53] because the variant BL cases may be treated differently and the results are difficult to generalize. For example, the incidence rate of BL in the US increased steeply (~7% per year) between 1973 and 2005 and exhibited pediatric, adult, and elderly age-specific peaks [46,47]. While the adult patterns could be attributed to the underlying HIV epidemic in the US [47], this explanation was difficult to reconcile with the lack of corresponding increases in BL in Africa, one of the regions with many cases of AIDS [54], or in India and China, which also have a substantial burden of HIV [55–57]. An attempt to resolve this issue by analyzing BL data for cases diagnosed in four continents between 1963–2002 [58] confirmed the temporal patterns of BL and the multiple age-specific peaks but not the correlation between BL and regional HIV prevalence. Data in this study were sparse or not available for sub-Saharan Africa, North Africa, the Middle East, and the Caribbean.

We conducted an epidemiological analysis of 15, 122 BL cases diagnosed worldwide using data reported to the International Agency for Research on Cancer (IARC) Cancer Incidence in Five Continents Volume XI (CI5(XI)) for 2008–2012 [59] and estimated by the African Cancer Registry Network (AFRCN) for 2018 [50].

2. Materials and Methods

The CI5(XI) data [59] were compiled from cancer registries in 65 countries (details in Supplementary Table S1). The cancer coverage was sub-national in most countries, except for nineteen that have national coverage (36 countries had a single registry and twenty-nine had multiple registries). The CI5(XI) report represents about 15% of the worldwide population. The lowest coverage is in Africa (1%), Central and South America (8%), and Asia (7%), while near half or higher are in Europe (46%), Oceania (77%), and the highest in North America (98%).

Cancer data were available for the 5-year period 2008–2012 in most countries, but only for shorter periods (four or three years, Supplementary Table S1) in a few. BL was defined as cases with International Classification of Diseases, 10th edition (ICD10) code = C83.7 [60]. BL data were downloaded by registry as case counts and person-years by gender and 5-year age group (Supplementary Table S2). Burkitt cell leukemia (BCL), which is coded as C91.8 (mature B-cell leukemia, Burkitt type) was not coded with BL in CI5(XI). Data are presented by country. Data from multiple registries in a country were aggregated to calculate country-specific estimates. US data were available for white and black people as well as overall. To minimize the impact of sparse data on the rates, we restricted analyses to countries with a minimum of total cases. Specifically, 30 total cases for geographic analyses of overall rates (38 countries), 60 total cases for sex-specific analyses (28 countries), and 100 total cases for age-specific analyses (18 countries), referred to as the 30/60/100 criteria. Because cancer data cover only 1% of people in Africa, we supplemented the African data with estimates published by AFRCN for 2018 [60]. AFRCN estimated BL rates by calculating the proportions of NHL (ICD10 codes C82–86, C96) in GLOBOCAN 2018 within 5 broad sex-specific age groups that were attributed to BL [50]. The calculated proportions were applied to the estimated number of NHL cases (by sex and age) in GLOBOCAN 2018 for the African countries (Supplementary Table S3). Countries that have no registries were included by using the mean of the proportions (within age–sex groups) from the nearest neighboring countries with cancer registries. We filtered these data using 30/60/100 total case criteria to include data for 27 countries for the geographic patterns, 16 countries for sex-specific patterns, and 10 countries for age-specific patterns (Supplementary Table S3).

2.1. Age-Standardized Incidence Rates

Age-standardized incidence rates (ASR) of BL per million person-years were calculated by country using the CI5(XI) data, adjusted to the World Standard Population of Segi and Doll [61]. The available AFRCN data were age-adjusted using the same standard. The overall BL ASRs were plotted on the world map to discern geographic patterns. The sex-specific rates were plotted on horizontal bar charts, sorted in descending order by the rates among males by region and within region to discern regional patterns. Male-to-female incidence rate ratios were calculated and tabulated.

2.2. Age-Specific Incidence Rates

Age-adjusted age-specific BL rates were calculated for 5 age groups (0–14, 15–34, 35–54, 55–74, 75+). Our goal was to confirm or refute the multimodal patterns hypothesized based on previous reports in the US [46,47,62] and data from four continents but not Africa [58]. Rates based on $\geq$10 cases were plotted on a log scale on the y-axis and age intervals on the x-axis on a linear interval scale (Supplementary Table S4). We compared age-specific incidence rate ratios (IRRs) for BL in different countries versus rates among US white people, which we selected as the referent because it was the largest group in the dataset. The IRR results were plotted as horizontal bar charts to discern patterns.

3. Results

3.1. Worldwide Geographic Patterns of BL

We downloaded data for 11,743 BL cases from the CI5(XI) report during 2008–2012 (Supplementary Table S2) and retained for geographic analysis 11,446 BL cases from 38 countries with ≥30 total BL cases (1 in Africa, 5 in Central or South America, the US and Canada in North America, 9 in Asia, 19 in Europe, and 2 in Oceania). Five countries accounted for 67.9% of BL cases (Table 1): US (47.2%) in North America; United Kingdom (8.3%), and Germany (5.9%) in Europe; South Korea (3.3%) in Asia, and Australia in Oceania (3.2%).

Table 1. Burkitt lymphoma incidence by region and country for both sexes combined, sorted by rate within region, based on data from Cancer Incidence in Five Continents Volume XI [CI5(XI)] 2008–2012 and the African Cancer Registry Network (AFRCN) 2018.

Region	Country [1]	Total Cases [2]	Total Rate [3]	Incidence Rate Ratio [4]
International CI5(XI) data for 2008–2012:				
Africa				
	Uganda	124	9.28	2.91
Central/South America				
	Colombia	60	3.19	1.00
	Puerto Rico	60	3.13	0.98
	Uruguay	48	2.82	0.88
	Brazil	41	2.23	0.70
	Ecuador	33	1.15	0.36
North America				
	US white people (referent)	4482	3.19	1.00
	United States (US)	5405	3.09	0.97
	US black people	611	2.68	0.84
	Canada	194	1.47	0.46
Asia				
	Israel	143	3.77	1.18
	Saudi Arabia: Saudi	54	2.41	0.76
	Turkey	115	2.30	0.72
	Republic of Korea	376	1.72	0.54
	Japan	276	1.55	0.49
	Jordan: Jordanians	39	1.17	0.37
	Thailand	44	0.88	0.28
	India	128	0.59	0.18
	China	120	0.45	0.14
Europe				
	Estonia	35	5.67	1.78
	Switzerland	96	4.12	1.29
	Belgium	199	3.72	1.16
	Norway	90	3.49	1.10
	Spain	153	3.34	1.05
	Italy	347	3.23	1.01

Table 1. *Cont.*

Region	Country [1]	Total Cases [2]	Total Rate [3]	Incidence Rate Ratio [4]
	The Netherlands	265	3.16	0.99
	France	172	3.13	0.98
	Lithuania	37	3.00	0.94
	Denmark	77	2.92	0.91
	United Kingdom	950	2.68	0.84
	Ireland	67	2.64	0.83
	Austria	99	2.44	0.77
	Germany	676	2.43	0.76
	Czech Republic	91	1.97	0.62
	Belarus	70	1.96	0.61
	Ukraine	252	1.52	0.48
	Poland	37	0.88	0.27
	Russian Federation	30	0.72	0.22
Oceania				
	New Zealand	80	3.21	1.01
	Australia	363	3.12	0.98
African AFRCN data for 2018:				
Eastern Africa				
	Malawi	521	19.3	6.05
	Uganda	307	4.8	1.50
	Zambia	105	4.2	1.32
	Rwanda	42	3.5	1.10
	Burundi	37	3.4	1.07
	South Sudan	39	2.5	0.78
	Tanzania	171	2.2	0.69
	Madagascar	71	2.1	0.66
	Kenya	102	1.7	0.53
	Mozambique	72	1.7	0.53
	Ethiopia	56	0.4	0.13
Middle Africa				
	Cameroon	251	8.0	2.51
	Congo, Democratic People Republic of	261	2.9	0.91
	Angola	86	2.1	0.66
	Chad	38	1.7	0.53
Northern Africa				
	Sudan	90	2.0	0.63
	Egypt	178	1.7	0.53
	Morocco	55	1.7	0.53
	Algeria	37	0.9	0.28
Southern Africa				
	South Africa	94	1.6	0.50

Table 1. *Cont.*

Region	Country [1]	Total Cases [2]	Total Rate [3]	Incidence Rate Ratio [4]
Western Africa				
	Cote d'Ivoire	138	4.6	1.44
	Nigeria	647	2.8	0.88
	Ghana	86	2.4	0.75
	Senegal	48	2.4	0.75
	Burkina Faso	58	2.2	0.69
	Mali	41	1.4	0.44
	Niger	45	1.2	0.38

[1] In the CI5(XI) data, Uganda and Saudi Arabia each had 1 sub-national registry, Colombia and the Russian Federation had 4, Ecuador and Poland had 5, Brazil had 6, Thailand had 7, Turkey had 8, Japan, Switzerland, and Germany had 9, Canada had 12, Spain had 14, France had 15, India had 16, China and Italy had 36. [2] Includes countries with at least 30 total cases. [3] Rates per million person-years, age-adjusted using the 1960 Segi world standard. [4] Incidence rate ratio compared to rates of US white people.

Figure 1a and Table 1 show the geographic distribution of BL worldwide. Using CI5(XI) data, we observed a 20-fold range between Uganda (the country with the highest BL ASR) and China (the country with the lowest BL rate). In addition, BL rates varied 2–8-fold within and between regions. To simplify reporting, the rates were categorized descriptively and arbitrarily as "high", defined as ≥4 cases per million person-years, "intermediate", defined as 2–3.9 cases per million, and "low", defined as <2 cases per million. All regions included countries with high, intermediate, or low BL rates. In CI5(XI) data, BL rates were high in Uganda (9.28 per million), Switzerland, and Estonia, with 4.12 and 5.67 cases per million, respectively. BL rates were intermediate in the US in North America and in Central/South America; in Israel, Saudi Arabia, and Turkey in Asia; and in most countries in Europe. BL rates were low in most countries in Asia and the Czech Republic, Belarus, Ukraine, Poland, and the Russian Federation in Europe. Worldwide, BL rates were lowest in China (0.45) and India (0.59). The BL incidence rate ratio (IRR), relative to the rate among white people in the US, was about three for Uganda and less than 0.2 for China and India.

The AFRCN dataset included 3899 estimated BL cases in 54 African countries in 2018 (Supplementary Table S3) and 3676 BL cases from 27 countries with ≥30 cases (Table 1, Figure 1, inset map for Africa). Five countries accounted for 54.0% of the cases: Nigeria (17.6%), Malawi (14.2%), Uganda (8.4%), Democratic Republic of Congo (7.1%), and Cameroon (6.8%). While the CI5(XI) data from Uganda only appeared to suggest a threshold in the BL rates that could be used to classify cases in Africa (based on Uganda only) as endemic and those diagnosed elsewhere as sporadic BL, this apparent threshold was an artifact of sparse data. No threshold was evident when we used the AFRCN data, which showed a mosaic pattern with various countries in Africa having high, intermediate, or low BL rates. The highest and lowest BL rates were in East Africa where the Malawi rate of 19.3 was 48 times that of 0.4 in Ethiopia. BL rates were high (≥4) in five countries (Malawi, Cameroon, Uganda, Cote d'Ivoire, and Zambia) in low-lying regions in the Congo-Nile basin [15]. This pattern also corresponds to regions that are most prone to *P. falciparum* transmission (Figure 1b). BL rates were intermediate (2.0–3.9) in Eastern Africa in Rwanda, Burundi, South Sudan, Tanzania, and Madagascar; in Middle Africa in the Democratic Republic of Congo and Angola; in Western Africa in Nigeria, Ghana, Senegal, and Burkina Faso; and in Northern Africa in Sudan. BL rates were low (<2.0) in Eastern Africa in Kenya, Mozambique, and Ethiopia; in Middle Africa in Chad; in Northern Africa in Egypt, Morocco, and Algeria; in Western Africa in Niger and Mali; and in South Africa in Southern Africa.

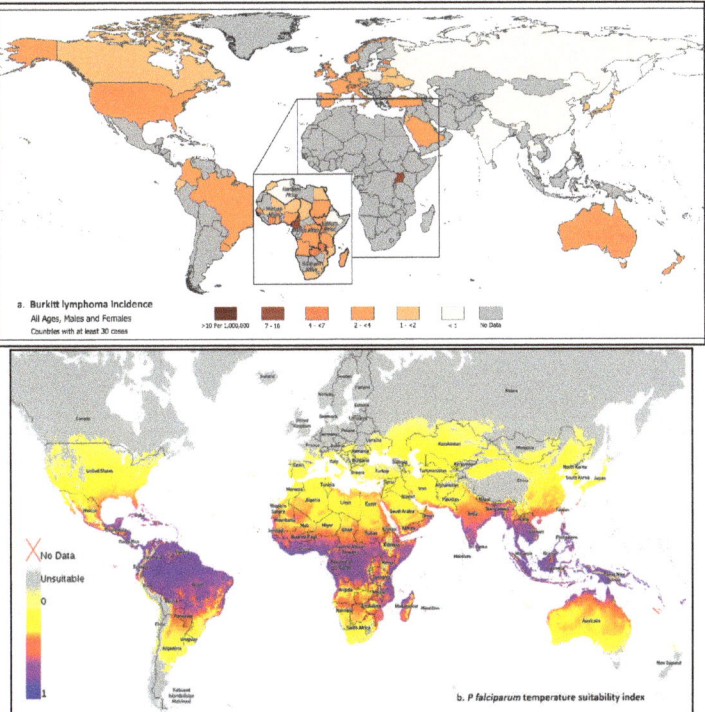

Figure 1. (**a**) Age-standardized Burkitt lymphoma rates per million person-years (world standard) for males and females combined in 38 countries with at least 30 cases during 2008–2012, using data from CI5(XI). Inset shows data for Africa in 27 countries with at least 30 cases during 2018 from the AFRCN. (**b**) World map showing *P. falciparum* temperature suitability index for *P. falciparum* transmission 2010 (data from the Malaria Atlas Project: https://malariaatlas.org/explorer/#/; accessed on 9 June 2022).

Table 2 and Figure 2a,b show the sex-specific BL rates in the CI5(XI) and AFRCN data for countries with at least 60 total cases. BL rates were higher in males than females in all countries. The male-to-female ratio exceeded 2.00 in most countries and 4.00 in seven countries. By far, BL rates were highest among males and females in Uganda and Malawi, followed by Cameroon. The lowest rates among both males and females (<1.0) were in India and China. The sex-specific rates showed within and between regional variation.

Table 2. Burkitt lymphoma incidence by region and country by sex, sorted by male rate within region, based on data from Cancer Incidence in Five Continents Volume XI [CI5(XI)] 2008–2012 and the African Cancer Registry Network (AFRCN) 2018.

		MALES		FEMALES		
Region	Country [1]	Cases [2]	Rate [3]	Cases [2]	Rate [3]	Male-to-Female Rate Ratio [4]
International CI5(XI) data for 2008–2012:						
Africa						
	Uganda	71	11.74	53	7.05	1.67
Central/South America						
	Puerto Rico	49	5.32	11	1.03	5.14
	Colombia	47	5.10	13	1.38	3.71

Table 2. Cont.

Region	Country [1]	MALES		FEMALES		Male-to-Female Rate Ratio [4]
		Cases [2]	Rate [3]	Cases [2]	Rate [3]	
North America						
	US white people	3344	4.94	1138	1.45	3.41
	United States (US)	3997	4.75	1408	1.46	3.25
	US black people	433	4.04	178	1.45	2.79
	Canada	151	2.35	43	0.58	4.02
Asia						
	Israel	99	5.36	44	2.17	2.47
	Turkey	87	3.42	28	1.12	3.07
	Republic of Korea	289	2.71	87	0.70	3.86
	Japan	205	2.54	71	0.57	4.45
	India	80	0.70	48	0.47	1.47
	China	77	0.55	43	0.34	1.63
Europe						
	Switzerland	71	6.63	25	1.54	4.31
	Norway	69	5.53	21	1.37	4.03
	Belgium	129	5.16	70	2.26	2.28
	The Netherlands	202	5.02	63	1.25	4.02
	Italy	255	5.02	92	1.38	3.65
	Spain	108	4.89	45	1.72	2.84
	France	122	4.70	50	1.56	3.02
	Denmark	57	4.56	20	1.23	3.72
	United Kingdom	695	4.12	255	1.25	3.30
	Austria	76	4.10	23	0.75	5.47
	Ireland	48	3.98	19	1.29	3.09
	Germany	485	3.75	191	1.09	3.43
	Czech Republic	66	3.06	25	0.84	3.65
	Belarus	47	3.00	23	0.87	3.47
	Ukraine	166	2.22	86	0.78	2.84
Oceania						
	New Zealand	60	4.94	20	1.52	3.25
	Australia	279	4.90	84	1.33	3.70
African AFRCN data for 2018:						
Eastern Africa						
	Malawi	405	29.7	116	8.7	3.41
	Zambia	84	6.6	21	1.7	3.88
	Uganda	201	5.9	106	3.7	1.59
	Tanzania	114	2.8	57	1.5	1.87
	Madagascar	39	2.3	32	1.9	1.21
	Kenya	67	2.2	35	1.2	1.83
	Mozambique	36	1.7	36	1.7	1.00

Table 2. Cont.

Region	Country [1]	MALES		FEMALES		Male-to-Female Rate Ratio [4]
		Cases [2]	Rate [3]	Cases [2]	Rate [3]	
Middle Africa						
	Cameroon	159	10.4	92	5.6	1.86
	Congo, Democratic People Republic of	179	4.3	82	1.5	2.87
	Angola	68	3.2	18	0.9	3.56
Northern Africa						
	Sudan	63	2.7	27	1.3	2.08
	Egypt	137	2.5	41	0.8	3.13
Southern Africa						
	South Africa	52	1.9	42	1.4	1.36
Western Africa						
	Cote d'Ivoire	76	5.2	62	3.9	1.33
	Ghana	68	3.7	18	1.0	3.70
	Nigeria	379	3.0	268	2.5	1.20

[1] In the CI5(XI) data, Uganda had 1 sub-national registry, Colombia had 4, Turkey had 8, Japan, Switzerland, and Germany had 9, Canada had 12, Spain had 14, France had 15, India had 16, China and Italy had 36. [2] Includes countries with at least 60 total cases. [3] Rates per million person-years, age-adjusted using the 1960 Segi world standard. [4] Incidence Rate Ratio, Male Rate relative to Female Rate.

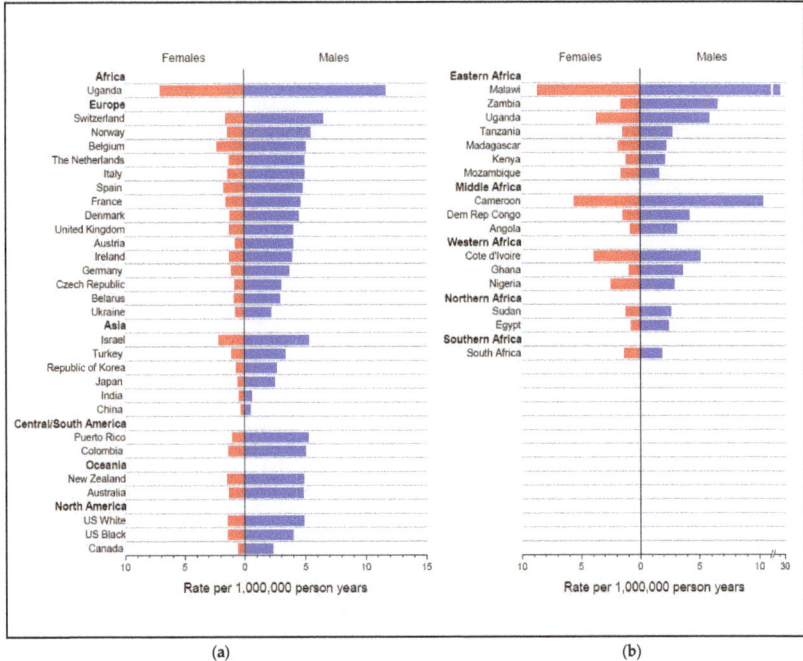

Figure 2. Age-standardized Burkitt lymphoma rates per million person-years (world) for males and females for countries with at least 60 cases total: (**a**) for 28 countries included in CI5(XI) and (**b**) for 16 countries included in the AFRCN data. The x-axis scale for Malawi is broken to accommodate the higher male BL rate in that country.

The proportion of BL cases aged 0–14 years was ~13% in the US, ~50% in Israel and Turkey, ~62% of cases in the Democratic Republic of Congo, 75% in Uganda, and 100% in Malawi and Zambia (Supplementary Table S4). BL incidence exhibited a bimodal pattern, with an early peak in the pediatric (0–14 years) age group and a second peak in the adult/elderly (55+) age groups (Figure 3). BL rates were lower for ages 15–54 years than the pediatric and elderly rates, representing the trough of a U-shape age-specific incidence curve. This shape of the age-specific BL rates was observed in all regions, except among US white people, US black people, and Australia where rates among adults were higher than the pediatric rates but lower than the elderly rates. The BL rates in one age group were correlated with rates in the other age groups, suggesting that when BL rates were intermediate in one age group, they were intermediate in the other age groups as well.

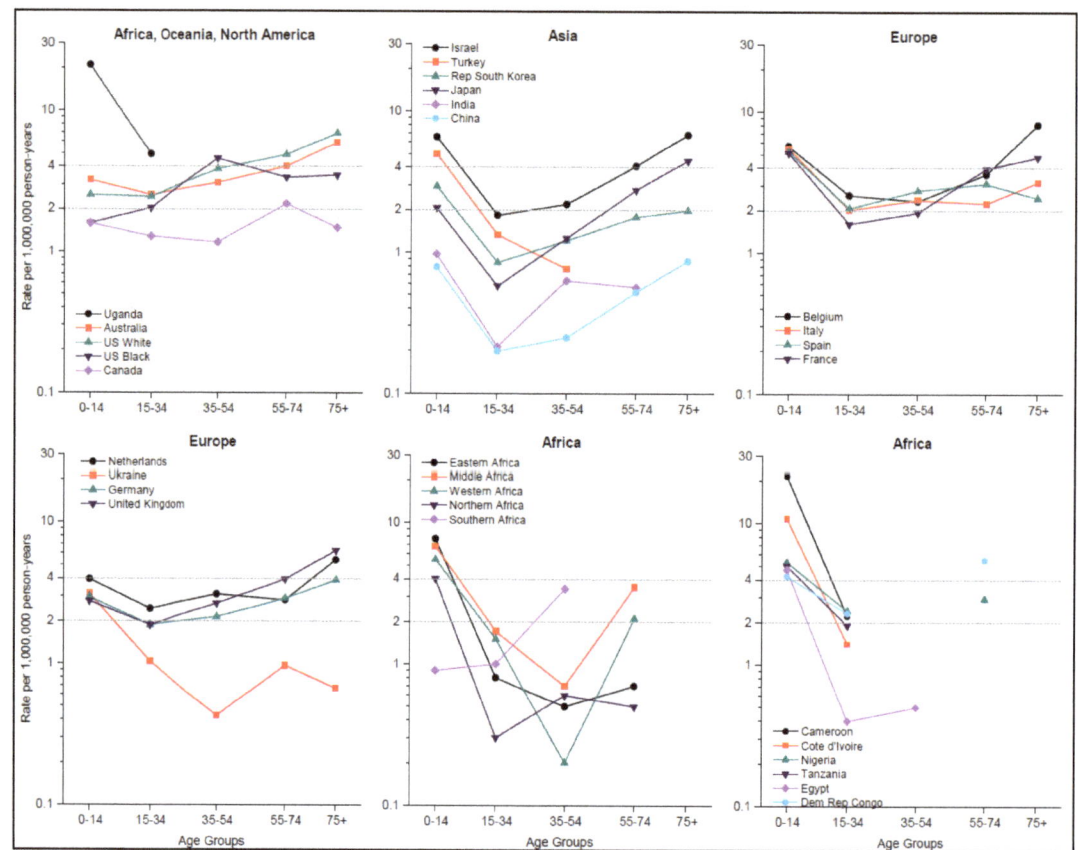

Figure 3. Burkitt lymphoma incidence rates for five age groups for countries with ≥100 total cases: Rates for 18 countries in five continents are based on CI5(XI) data for 2008–2012, and rates for Africa are supplemented with data reported to the AFRCN for 2018 by region and separately for six countries with cases in both 0–14 and 15–34 age groups. Rates based on <10 cases are not shown. Horizontal lines for BL rates = 2 and 4 cases per million divide the graph space into three areas corresponding to low, intermediate, and high BL rates (see results).

While country-specific data were sparse at ages ≥35 years, making it difficult to discern patterns at older ages for most African countries, bimodal patterns were observed in data aggregated by region. The exception was South Africa whose pattern resembled that in US white and black people, Australia, and the UK.

3.2. Age-Specific Incidence Rates Relative to BL Rates in US White Individuals

Figure 4 shows geographic variation in age-specific IRR as compared to US white people rates as the referent group (Supplementary Table S4). Among children aged 0–14 years, the IRRs ranged between 2.0–3.0 in Israel, Belgium, Italy, Spain, and France, and exceeded 8.0 in Uganda, in contrast to IRRs <0.5 in India and China. Among adults aged ≥55 years, IRRs were <0.5 in Canada, Korea, and Italy, and ≤0.2 in India, China, and Ukraine. Among those aged ≥75, IRRs were close to 1.0 only in Israel, Belgium, and the United Kingdom. Among US black individuals, all the IRRs were <0.85 except 35–54 where it was 1.2. Rates among US white adults aged 35 and older were the highest among all groups except US black people aged 35–54, those aged 75+ in Belgium, and those aged 55–74 in the Democratic Republic of Congo. Among the 10 countries in Africa, the IRRs for those aged 0–14 ranged from 1.6 to 2.0 in four countries, from 2.1 to 5.6 in four countries, to 8.5 in Cameroon and 24.6 in Malawi.

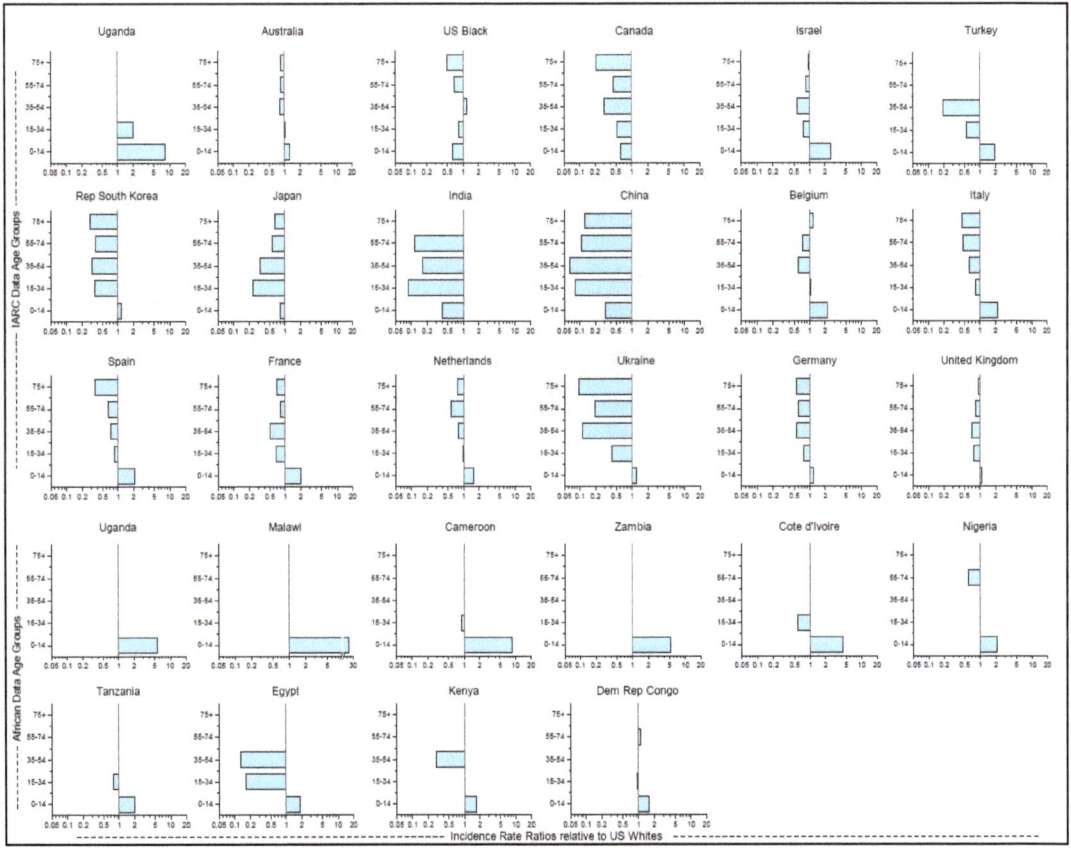

Figure 4. Age-specific Incidence Rate Ratios (IRR) of Burkitt lymphoma with the rate for US white individuals as the reference group. IRRs are plotted as horizontal bars along on the x-axis and the age groups on the y-axis. The first three rows are IRR using CI5(XI) data, while the bottom two rows use AFRCN data.

4. Discussion

Our report presents the most complete descriptive analysis of population profiles of BL, based on 15,122 BL cases diagnosed in 64 counties in five continents, including 26 from Africa. The results reveal three key insights. First, that there is no quantitative threshold for classifying all BL cases from Africa as endemic and all cases from elsewhere as sporadic. Rather, the geographic patterns describe a mosaic pattern with countries with high, intermediate, and low BL rates scattered in all continents, except in Asia, and North, South and Central America where none of the countries reached the threshold for high BL rate. This pattern suggests that there might be multiple risk factors that influence the within- and between-regional variation of BL rates. Because BL has a multi-factorial etiology, including EBV [63,64], *P. falciparum* [65], HIV [25], and immune dysregulation, including from genetic or nutritional factors [66], the mosaic pattern observed here provides an epidemiological framework, as did the endemic/sporadic classification, for discovery of etiological factors that vary regionally, leading to pockets of high or deficit BL rates. Second, we confirm that BL predominates in males, including in countries that reported only pediatric cases. Finally, we show that BL risk is bimodal in all populations, and the proportions of pediatric versus adult-type BL vary geographically.

Our finding that BL rates were highest in Eastern (Malawi and Uganda) and Middle Africa (Cameroon) agrees with historical data [67]. This pattern is attributed to climatic co-factors favoring *P. falciparum* transmission [68]. Exposure to holoendemic *P. falciparum* for >6 months per annum [69,70] is the strongest geographic co-factor responsible for this pattern (Figure 1b). BL rates were intermediate or low in countries where climate is unfavorable to transmission of *P. falciparum* [69,71]. Thus, the rate in Malawi was 11 times that in Kenya and 48 times that in Ethiopia, which lie at a high elevation (>5000 ft); 11–14 times those in Chad and Mali, which have a dry or arid climate (<20 inches of rainfall per year); and 11 times that in South Africa with a temperate climate (<16 °C) [70]. However, our finding that geographic patterns of BL rates vary across countries with apparently similar climate might be due to contribution of other etiological factors [72]. These factors could be related to micro-geographical variation in patterns of genetic complexity of *P. falciparum* infection (number of different clones capable of causing an infection at the same time) [73–75] or parasites with distinct genetic profiles or strains [76,77]. Entomological factors, including type of mosquitoes, biting habits (night or day), host preference, and niche factors (where mosquitoes live) could also lead to subtle variation in BL rates [78]. Although not usually considered, other infections that are spread by mosquitoes could contribute [65]. Finally, the role of EBV variants [63,64], nutritional deficiencies, such as dietary selenium [79] or magnesium [66], are exposures that could modify geographical patterns of BL.

We confirm that BL from all regions is multimodal. The clearest evidence of multimodality was first reported in US data [46,47,58], but the results were not generalizable. Multimodality is an epidemiological manifestation of biologic heterogeneity [80,81]. Multi-modal patterns were reported in a small series of HIV-negative BL cases from France that were diagnosed carefully [62], reducing concern that multimodality is due to diagnostic misclassification and increasing support for age-related biologic heterogeneity. Recent molecular studies of BL support the hypothesis of biological heterogeneity with age. A study of 162 well-diagnosed sporadic BL cases in Germany reported that the proportion of EBV + BL cases increased with the age at BL diagnosis [82]. Because EBV + BL is characterized by fewer somatic mutations in driver genes, particularly those in the apoptotic pathway, than EBV—BL [83], this finding suggests that EBV could be a biological marker of age-related heterogeneity in BL. This idea was also supported by findings that somatic mutations in *ID3, TCF3, CCND3,* and *SOX11* genes were detected more frequently in pediatric BL patients than adult cases [82], which agrees with the EBV data discussed above. Independent support for this idea has been reported in a study of 230 BL cases from Africa, the US, Germany, and Brazil, which showed distinct somatic mutations in pediatric cases (*ARID1A*) versus adult cases (*TET2*) [84]. A promising area of research is to elucidate the molecular basis of multimodality of BL in regional and global datasets.

We confirm the male predominance of BL, which was previously based on limited datasets [46,73,85], with worldwide BL data, including from countries with only pediatric cases. Sex patterns may suggest a role of reproductive factors or social factors related to gender, but these explanations are implausible because this pattern is observed in all countries with only pediatric or both pediatric and adult cases, and in countries with different socioeconomic statuses. The simplest explanation may be a role of recessive genetic factors on sex chromosomes [86]. Thus, females who carry one allele of a predisposing recessive genetic variant on the X-chromosome could experience lower risk of BL because the random lyonization of alleles could lead to escape from X-inactivation of the tumor-suppressor gene (abbreviated as EXITS) [87]. This idea is supported by recent findings of somatic mutations in *DDX3X* on the X-chromosome [88] and sex determining region Y-box transcription factor 11 (*SOX11*) in BL tumors [82]. However, germline studies are needed to confirm the population level effects of this hypothesis.

Our findings that BL rates in India and China are 1/20th those in Uganda and 1/6th the rate in US white people is puzzling given the role of *P. falciparum* and EBV as risk factors for BL. Climate is suitable for *P. falciparum* transmission in India (Figure 1b) [89] and China, although transmission has recently been eliminated in China [90]. EBV infection is prevalent in Asia and its epidemiology is similar to that in Africa more than that in the US or Europe [91,92]. While underdiagnosis and/or underascertainment of BL are possible explanations for the discrepant low BL rates in Asia, that explanation is inconsistent with the high rates for nasopharyngeal cancer [93] and extra-nodal NK/T-cell lymphomas [94], both associated with EBV, in Asia. The low BL rates could be an epidemiological manifestation indicating that EBV strains circulating in Asia have a lower population attributable risk for BL than EBV in Africa [63]. EBV phylogenetic data have confirmed that EBV in Asia is genetically distinct from EBV in Africa [63,95–97]. Moreover, the EBV in US/Europe is phylogenetically closer to that in Africa [63,96], which is intriguing given that BL rates in US/Europe intermediate to those in Africa versus Asia. Molecular analysis of EBV variants in regions with different BL rates could lead to discovery of EBV variants with differential risk for BL.

Our findings that BL is multimodal raise several questions. First, could it be that adult cases are missed in those countries where only or mostly pediatric cases were reported? If so, why are adult cases missed? Second, the observation that compared to US white people, pediatric BL rates were twice as high in five European countries (Belgium, Netherlands, France, Italy, and Spain) and in two Asian countries (Israel and Turkey) was unexpected because both regions are thought to have a comparable risk profile for EBV and *P. falciparum*. Similarly, the observation that adult BL rates were lower in most countries than rates among US white people is puzzling. It is difficult to explain why pediatric and adult BL rates vary. While it is theoretically possible that differences in case ascertainment, diagnosis, and registration of BL contribute, it is difficult to imagine how under-ascertainment could lead to different patterns for pediatric versus adult cases. As we noted in the Methods, BL might be coded differently. It was identified using ICD10 code C83.7, which is in the non-Hodgkin lymphoma range. BCL, a mature B-cell leukemia, Burkitt type that is assigned code C91.8 was, per IARC practice, not included with BL in CI5(XI). The US Surveillance, Epidemiology, and End Results (SEER) Program, includes the BCL ICD-0-3 morphology code 9826 with the BL morphology code 9687 to calculate BL rates, which increases US SEER BL cases by up to 15% [46,88]. Researchers need to be cognizant of these differences in handling of BL and BCL types when making comparisons in rates between our CI5 data and those reported using national registries or over time. However, this would not explain why pediatric versus adult rates would vary geographically as noted above.

The interpretation of BL rates assumes accurate and reliable diagnosis, classification, and registration [83,98–101]. However, BL data are clouded with uncertainty because a gold standard has not been established. The WHO has devoted efforts to improving and standardizing BL diagnosis through successive revisions of the Classification of Hematopoietic and Lymphoid Tissues, but the impact on global BL data is unknown. In 2008 [42], the WHO recommended that diagnosis of Burkitt-like lymphoma (BLL) be reclassified to B-cell lymphoma unclassifiable (BCL-U) with features intermediate between BL and diffuse large B-cell lymphoma (DLBCL). In 2016 [43], the WHO further recommended that cases still diagnosed as BLL based on having features like BL but with multiple chromosomal translocations, e.g., *MYC/BCL6*, or *BCL2*, be assigned a new name called high-grade B-cell lymphoma (HGBL) with double-hit or triple-hit lymphoma, or not otherwise specified (NOS). However, BL cases with features like BL that lacked *MYC* rearrangement but with 11q alterations (gain in 11q23.2-23.3 and losses of 11q24.1-ter) were assigned a new name BLL-11q. These cases, although technically not BL, are still coded along with BL morphology code 9687 in ICD-O3, highlighting the difficulties that still surround the definition, the accuracy, and reliability of BL data [43,102–104]. The 5th edition classification of haematolymphoid tumors leaves the definition of BL unchanged but stresses EBV as a marker of discrete biologic groups (EBV-positive versus EBV-negative BL) based on consistent findings of common molecular features regardless of epidemiologic context and geographic location. Thus, EBV status should supersede epidemiological subtypes of endemic, sporadic, and immunodeficiency-associated [105]. While consensus guidelines should improve the reliability of diagnosis, accuracy is at the mercy of pathologists who diagnose cases and the quality of their experience, which is likely variable because BL is rare, and at the mercy of data abstractors and coders who translate technical diagnoses into classification codes that may be ambiguous [42,106,107]. The quality of these services likely varies between poorer [108] and richer areas based on better access to adequate tumor material, appropriate test equipment, reagents, and pathology referral support [41,109–111]. We performed a limited evaluation of NHL data (C82-86, C96) versus BL to assess to what extent quality of data (underascertainment or incomplete data) contributes versus variation in risk factors for five countries with most variable BL rates, namely, the US, Uganda, Hong Kong, China, and India. Focusing on NHL and BL rates in males, where number of BL cases are reasonably large, we observed that male NHL rates were highest in the US, for both white and black individuals, then in Uganda and Hong Kong, and then lower in other parts of China and India. The rates ranged from 1.8 to 7.6 per million in China, with a median of about 4.0. The rates ranged from 1.2 to 5.3 per million in India, with a median of about 3.0. The ratio of the BL to the NHL rate was 1.65 for Uganda, 0.34–0.43 in the US, and 0.14 in China and 0.23 in India. These patterns suggested to us that there is considerable geographic variation in both the BL and NHL rates, with the relative variation greater for BL than for NHL. We infer from this limited comparison that the differences in case identification and real differences in risk are playing a role in the observed patterns of BL. While issues of differences in case identification and registration might be greater in poorer countries, they may occur in richer countries based on whether patients access health care through private or single payer systems [112,113].

We believe uncertainty about the validity of BL diagnoses in different regions has reduced the enthusiasm to conduct BL research, particularly in poorer countries. Thus, almost all high-impact research on BL, such as using molecular methods to define BL [98–102], testing novel treatments [105], and developing? prognostic indices? [114–116] has been conducted in richer countries. The exclusion of poorer countries from BL research is ironic given that Denis Burkitt's epoch-making report was based on cases seen in Africa [12]. Burkitt's report is one of the most important epidemiological cancer discoveries of the last century, ranking close to the "two-hit hypothesis" by Alfred Knudson based on analysis of retinoblastoma data [117] and the hereditary cancer predisposition syndrome by Drs. Frederick Li and Joseph Fraumeni [118]. Those reports have inspired coordinated multidisciplinary global research [119] establishing retinoblastoma and the LFS as epidemiological models for discovery of genetic cancer predisposition and biology [120,121]. While the seminal discoveries in viral oncology, cancer chemotherapy, and characterization of the tumor lysis syndrome resulting from BL research showed its potential as a disease model for discovery [122], subsequent research has been less revealing because it is conducted in limited geographical and disciplinary settings [123], which limits the type of questions that can be answered. The unanswered questions include a reliable definition of the gold standard of BL diagnosis, BL subtypes, the multimodal patterns, discovery of EBV variants and predisposition to BL, development of simpler diagnostic methods, and better therapies.

Our analysis shows that thousands of BL cases occur globally. These cases confirm the feasibility of conducting BL research globally to answer questions identified here. One mechanism could be modeled along the framework of the International Collaboration for Cancer Classification and Research (IC^{3}R) under the World Health Organization. International research on BL could boost access to BL expertise in poorer countries, enable the recruitment of diverse BL cases for research to answer outstanding questions and support development of novel technology, such as liquid biopsy [124] and telepathology [111] to support BL research and care. International research on BL could deliver on the promise of BL envisioned six decades ago by Joseph Burchenal.

5. Conclusions

To summarize, we report the first epidemiological analysis of BL diagnosed worldwide. BL rates were highest in countries in Africa, intermediate in North America, Europe, and South/Central America, and lowest in Asia. BL rates varied within and between regions. BL rates in Asia, particularly India and China, were 1/20th of those in Africa. The deficit of rates in Asia could be due to underascertainment of cases in that region or could be an epidemiological clue that EBV variants circulating in Asia are associated with lower virulence for BL. We observed that BL predominates in males in all countries, including those with only pediatric cases. This pattern may be due to recessive genetic factors on sex chromosomes that influence the risk for BL. Our results show that BL is multimodal in all regions, providing epidemiological evidence for biologic heterogeneity of BL cases. Given the concerns about data quality discussed above, it will be important to repeat comprehensive epidemiological analyses of worldwide cases at reasonable intervals to reevaluate and update the patterns as the quality of the underlying data improves over time. The number of BL cases reported worldwide support the feasibility of conducting international transdisciplinary collaborative research on BL.

Supplementary Materials: The following supporting information can be downloaded at: https://www.mdpi.com/article/10.3390/hemato3030030/s1. Table S1: List of the CI5 (XI) registries and how the data were combined to estimate country-specific estimates. Table S2: Table showing BL counts and rates overall and by gender for all the countries whose data were downloaded from Cancer Incidence in Five Continents (XI) report IARC Scientific Publications No. 166 registries. Data are sorted by total case count within region. Only countries with $\geq$30 cases were included in the geographic analysis, those with $\geq$60 cases were included in the sex-specific analysis, while those with $\geq$100 cases were included in the age-specific analyses. Table S3: Table showing BL counts and rates overall and by gender for all the countries whose data were downloaded from the African Cancer Registry Network. Only countries with $\geq$30 cases were included in the geographic analysis, those with $\geq$60 cases were included in the sex-specific analysis, while those with $\geq$100 cases were included in the age-specific analyses. Table S4: Table showing age-specific counts, rates, and incidence rate ratios in CI5 (XI) and AFRCN countries with $\geq$100 cases

Author Contributions: S.M.M. conceived the study, guided the analysis, interpreted the data, and drafted the manuscript. S.S.D. analyzed the data, interpreted the data, and edited the paper. All authors have read and agreed to the published version of the manuscript.

Funding: This research was funded by the Intramural Research Program of the Division of Cancer Epidemiology and Genetics, National Cancer Institute, National Institutes of Health, Department of Health, and Human Services Contracts HHSN261201100063C and HHSN261201100007I.

Institutional Review Board Statement: Ethical review and approval were not applicable because we analyzed anonymized data available via public datasets.

Informed Consent Statement: Not applicable for studies not involving humans.

Data Availability Statement: The datasets used and/or analyzed during the current study can be downloaded from the CI5-XI website (https://ci5.iarc.fr/CI5-XI/Default.aspx; accessed on 21 August 2021) using the Help/Download option or requested from AFCRN secretariat (https://afcrn.org/index.php/research/researches-andcollaborations; accessed on 22 October 2021).

Acknowledgments: We thank Jacques Ferlay of the International Agency for Research on Cancer for granting access to data files. We thank Maxwell D. Parkin, Biying Liu, and all of the registries, members of the African Cancer Registry Network (AFRCN) (http://afcrn.org/index.php/membership/membership-list; accessed on 22 October 2021), for giving us their BL data from Africa for 2018. We thank Marianne Hyer, Emily Carver, and Jeremy Lyman of Information Management Systems (Rockville, Maryland) for preparing the files for analysis, drawing the maps and bar charts, and David Check of the Division of Cancer Epidemiology and Genetics, National Cancer Institute (Bethesda, Maryland) for drawing age-specific graphs and incidence rate ratio graphs as well as polishing other figures. This article is dedicated to Elaine S. Jaffe who has dedicated her service to using pathology to help the definition and discovery in lymphoma.

Conflicts of Interest: The authors declare no conflict of interest. The funders had no role in the design of the study; in the collection, analyses, or interpretation of data; in the writing of the manuscript, or in the decision to publish the results.

References

1. Basso, K.; Dalla-Favera, R. Germinal centres and B cell lymphomagenesis. *Nat. Rev. Immunol.* **2015**, *15*, 172–184. [CrossRef] [PubMed]
2. Burkitt, D. A sarcoma involving the jaws in African children. *Br. J. Surg.* **1958**, *46*, 218–223. [CrossRef] [PubMed]
3. Hutt, M.S.; Wright, D.H. Central African lymphomas. *Lancet* **1963**, *1*, 109–110. [CrossRef]
4. Wright, D.H. Cytology and histochemistry of the Burkitt lymphoma. *Br. J. Cancer* **1963**, *17*, 50–55. [CrossRef]
5. Dorfman, R.F. Childhood Lymphosarcoma in St. Louis, Missouri, Clinically and Histologically Resembling Burkitt's Tumor. *Cancer* **1965**, *18*, 418–430. [CrossRef]
6. Burkitt, D. Burkitt's lymphoma outside the known endemic areas of Africa and New Guinea. *Int. J. Cancer* **1967**, *2*, 562–565. [CrossRef]
7. Wright, D.H. Burkitt's tumour in England. A comparison with childhood lymphosarcoma. *Int. J. Cancer* **1966**, *1*, 503–514. [CrossRef]
8. Booth, K.; Burkitt, D.P.; Bassett, D.J.; Cooke, R.A.; Biddulph, J. Burkitt Lymphoma in Papua New Guinea. *Br. J. Cancer* **1967**, *21*, 657. [CrossRef]
9. O'Conor, G.T.; Davies, J.N. Malignant tumors in African children. With special reference to malignant lymphoma. *J. Pediatr.* **1960**, *56*, 526–535. [CrossRef]
10. O'Conor, G.T. Malignant lymphoma in African children. II. A pathological entity. *Cancer* **1961**, *14*, 270–283. [CrossRef]
11. Brown, J.B.; O'Keefe, C.D. Sarcoma of the ovary with unusual oral metastases. *Ann. Surg.* **1928**, *87*, 467–471. [CrossRef]
12. Berard, C. Histopathological definition of Burkitt's tumour. *Bull World Health Organ* **1969**, *40*, 601–607.
13. Burkitt, D. A tumour syndrome affecting children in tropical Africa. *Postgrad. Med. J.* **1962**, *38*, 71–79. [CrossRef]
14. Burkitt, D. A Children's Cancer with Geographical Limitations. *Cancer Prog.* **1963**, *92*, 102–113. [PubMed]
15. Burkitt, D. A "tumour safari" in East and Central Africa. *Br. J. Cancer* **1962**, *16*, 379–386. [CrossRef] [PubMed]
16. Dalldorf, G.; Linsell, C.A.; Barnhart, F.E.; Martyn, R. An Epidemiologic Approach to the Lymphomas of African Children and Burkitt's Sacroma of the Jaws. *Perspect. Biol. Med.* **1964**, *7*, 435–449. [CrossRef] [PubMed]
17. Epstein, M.A.; Achong, B.G.; Barr, Y.M. Virus Particles in Cultured Lymphoblasts from Burkitt's Lymphoma. *Lancet* **1964**, *1*, 702–703. [CrossRef]
18. Henle, G.; Henle, W.; Diehl, V. Relation of Burkitt's tumor-associated herpes-ytpe virus to infectious mononucleosis. *Proc. Natl. Acad. Sci. USA* **1968**, *59*, 94–101. [CrossRef]
19. Geser, A.; Brubaker, G.; Olwit, G.W. The frequency of Epstein-Barr virus infection and Burkitt's lymphoma at high and low altitudes in East Africa. *Rev. Epidemiol. Sante Publique* **1980**, *28*, 307–321.
20. Bouvard, V.; Baan, R.A.; Grosse, Y.; Lauby-Secretan, B.; El Ghissassi, F.; Benbrahim-Tallaa, L.; Guha, N.; Straif, K. Carcinogenicity of malaria and of some polyomaviruses. *Lancet Oncol.* **2012**, *13*, 339–340. [CrossRef]
21. Burkitt, D.P. Etiology of Burkitt's lymphoma—An alternative hypothesis to a vectored virus. *J. Natl. Cancer Inst.* **1969**, *42*, 19–28. [PubMed]
22. Torgbor, C.; Awuah, P.; Deitsch, K.; Kalantari, P.; Duca, K.A.; Thorley-Lawson, D.A. A multifactorial role for P. falciparum malaria in endemic Burkitt's lymphoma pathogenesis. *PLoS Pathog.* **2014**, *10*, e1004170. [CrossRef] [PubMed]
23. DiMaio, D.; Emu, B.; Goodman, A.L.; Mothes, W.; Justice, A. Cancer Microbiology. *J. Natl. Cancer Inst.* **2021**, *114*, 651–663. [CrossRef] [PubMed]
24. Ziegler, J.L.; Drew, W.L.; Miner, R.C.; Mintz, L.; Rosenbaum, E.; Gershow, J.; Lennette, E.T.; Greenspan, J.; Shillitoe, E.; Beckstead, J.; et al. Outbreak of Burkitt's-like lymphoma in homosexual men. *Lancet* **1982**, *2*, 631–633. [CrossRef]
25. Centers for Disease Control. Diffuse, undifferentiated non-Hodgkins lymphoma among homosexual males—United States. *MMWR Morb Mortal Wkly Rep.* **1982**, *31*, 277–279.

26. Castro, K.G.; John, W.M.D.; Ward, M.D.; Slutsker, M.D.L.; James, W.M.P.H.; Buehler, M.D.; Jaffe, M.D.H.W.; Berkelman, M.D.R.L. 1993 revised classification system for HIV infection and expanded surveillance case definition for AIDS among adolescents and adults. *MMWR Recomm. Rep.* **1992**, *41*, 1–19. [CrossRef]
27. Manolov, G.; Manolova, Y. Marker band in one chromosome 14 from Burkitt lymphomas. *Nature* **1972**, *237*, 33–34. [CrossRef]
28. Dalla-Favera, R.; Bregni, M.; Erikson, J.; Patterson, D.; Gallo, R.C.; Croce, C.M. Human c-myc onc gene is located on the region of chromosome 8 that is translocated in Burkitt lymphoma cells. *Proc. Natl. Acad. Sci. USA* **1982**, *79*, 7824–7827. [CrossRef]
29. Oettgen, H.F.; Clifford, P.; Burkitt, D. Malignant Lymphoma Involving the Jaw in African Children—Treatment with Alkylating Agents and Actinomycin-D. *Cancer Chemother. Rep.* **1963**, *28*, 25–34.
30. Oettgen, H.F.; Burkitt, D.; Burchenal, J.H. Malignant lymphoma involving the jaw in African children: Treatment with Methotrexate. *Cancer* **1963**, *16*, 616–623. [CrossRef]
31. Burkitt, D.; Hutt, M.S.; Wright, D.H. The African Lymphoma: Preliminary Observations on Response to Therapy. *Cancer* **1965**, *18*, 399–410. [CrossRef]
32. Cohen, M.H.; Bennett, J.M.; Berard, C.W.; Ziegler, J.L.; Vogel, C.L.; Sheagren, J.N.; Carbone, P.P. Burkitt's tumor in the United States. *Cancer* **1969**, *23*, 1259–1272. [CrossRef]
33. Ziegler, J.L. Treatment results of 54 American patients with Burkitt's lymphoma are similar to the African experience. *N. Engl. J. Med.* **1977**, *297*, 75–80. [CrossRef] [PubMed]
34. Ziegler, J.L. Research projects in Burkitt's lymphoma. *JAMA* **1972**, *222*, 1167. [CrossRef]
35. Burchenal, J.H. Geographic chemotherapy–Burkitt's tumor as a stalking horse for leukemia: Presidential address. *Cancer Res.* **1966**, *26*, 2393–2405.
36. Risks to Humans. Epstein-Barr Virus and Kaposi's Sarcoma Herpesvirus/Human Herpesvirus 8. In Proceedings of the IARC Working Group on the Evaluation of Carcinogenic, Lyon, France, 17–24 June 1997; Volume 70, pp. 1–492.
37. de Martel, C.; Georges, D.; Bray, F.; Ferlay, J.; Clifford, G.M. Global burden of cancer attributable to infections in 2018: A worldwide incidence analysis. *Lancet Glob. Health* **2020**, *8*, e180–e190. [CrossRef]
38. Burkitt, D.P. Observations on the geography of malignant lymphoma. *E. Afr. Med. J.* **1961**, *38*, 511–514.
39. Wright, D.H. Burkitt's Tumour. A Post-Mortem Study of 50 Cases. *Br. J. Surg.* **1964**, *51*, 245–251. [CrossRef]
40. O'Conor, G.T.; Rappaport, H.; Smith, E.B. Childhood Lymphoma Resembling "Burkitt Tumor" in the United States. *Cancer* **1965**, *18*, 411–417. [CrossRef]
41. Ogwang, M.D.; Zhao, W.; Ayers, L.W.; Mbulaiteye, S.M. Accuracy of Burkitt lymphoma diagnosis in constrained pathology settings: Importance to epidemiology. *Arch. Pathol. Lab. Med.* **2011**, *135*, 445–450. [CrossRef]
42. Leoncini, L.; Raphael, M.; Stein, H.; Harris, N.L.; Jaffe, E.S.; Kluin, P.M. *Burkitt Lymphoma*, 4th ed.; International Agency for Research on Cancer (IARC): Lyon, France, 2008; pp. 262–264.
43. Swerdlow, S.H.; Campo, E.; Pileri, S.A.; Harris, N.L.; Stein, H.; Siebert, R.; Advani, R.; Ghielmini, M.; Salles, G.A.; Zelenetz, A.D.; et al. The 2016 revision of the World Health Organization classification of lymphoid neoplasms. *Blood* **2016**, *127*, 2375–2390. [CrossRef]
44. Roy, S.F.; Ghazawi, F.M.; Le, M.; Lagace, F.; Roy, C.F.; Rahme, E.; Savin, E.; Zubarev, A.; Sasseville, D.; Popradi, G.; et al. Epidemiology of adult and pediatric Burkitt lymphoma in Canada: Sequelae of the HIV epidemic. *Curr. Oncol.* **2020**, *27*, 83–89. [CrossRef] [PubMed]
45. Caetano Dos Santos, F.L.; Michalek, I.M.; Wojciechowska, U.; Didkowska, J.; Walewski, J. Improved survival of Burkitt lymphoma/leukemia patients: Observations from Poland, 1999–2020. *Ann. Hematol.* **2022**, *101*, 1059–1065. [CrossRef] [PubMed]
46. Mbulaiteye, S.M.; Anderson, W.F.; Bhatia, K.; Rosenberg, P.S.; Linet, M.S.; Devesa, S.S. Trimodal age-specific incidence patterns for Burkitt lymphoma in the United States, 1973–2005. *Int. J. Cancer* **2010**, *126*, 1732–1739. [CrossRef]
47. Guech-Ongey, M.; Simard, E.P.; Anderson, W.F.; Engels, E.A.; Bhatia, K.; Devesa, S.S.; Mbulaiteye, S.M. AIDS-related Burkitt lymphoma in the United States: What do age and CD4 lymphocyte patterns tell us about etiology and/or biology? *Blood* **2010**, *116*, 5600–5604. [CrossRef]
48. Boerma, E.G.; van Imhoff, G.W.; Appel, I.M.; Veeger, N.J.; Kluin, P.M.; Kluin-Nelemans, J.C. Gender and age-related differences in Burkitt lymphoma–epidemiological and clinical data from The Netherlands. *Eur. J. Cancer* **2004**, *40*, 2781–2787. [CrossRef]
49. Orem, J.; Mbidde, E.K.; Lambert, B.; de Sanjose, S.; Weiderpass, E. Burkitt's lymphoma in Africa, a review of the epidemiology and etiology. *Afr. Health Sci.* **2007**, *7*, 166–175. [PubMed]
50. Hammerl, L.; Colombet, M.; Rochford, R.; Ogwang, D.M.; Parkin, D.M. The burden of Burkitt lymphoma in Africa. *Infect. Agents Cancer* **2019**, *14*, 17. [CrossRef] [PubMed]
51. de-The, G. Is Burkitt's lymphoma related to perinatal infection by Epstein-Barr virus? *Lancet* **1977**, *1*, 335–338. [CrossRef]
52. Mwanda, O.W.; Rochford, R.; Moormann, A.M.; Macneil, A.; Whalen, C.; Wilson, M.L. Burkitt's lymphoma in Kenya: Geographical, age, gender and ethnic distribution. *East Afr. Med. J.* **2004**, S68–S77. [CrossRef]
53. Burkitt, D.P. Epidemiology of Brukitts Lymphoma. *Proc. R. Soc. Med. Lond.* **1971**, *64*, 909.
54. Muchengeti, M.; Bartels, L.; Olago, V.; Dhokotera, T.; Chen, W.C.; Spoerri, A.; Rohner, E.; Bütikofer, L.; Ruffieux, Y.; Singh, E.; et al. Cohort profile: The South African HIV Cancer Match (SAM) Study, a national population-based cohort. *BMJ Open* **2022**, *12*, e053460. [CrossRef] [PubMed]
55. Mbulaiteye, S.M.; Katabira, E.T.; Wabinga, H.; Parkin, D.M.; Virgo, P.; Ochai, R.; Workneh, M.; Coutinho, A.; Engels, E.A. Spectrum of cancers among HIV-infected persons in Africa: The Uganda AIDS-Cancer Registry Match Study. *Int. J. Cancer* **2006**, *118*, 985–990. [CrossRef]

56. Akarolo-Anthony, S.N.; Maso, L.D.; Igbinoba, F.; Mbulaiteye, S.M.; Adebamowo, C.A. Cancer burden among HIV-positive persons in Nigeria: Preliminary findings from the Nigerian AIDS-cancer match study. *Infect. Agent. Cancer* **2014**, *9*, 1. [CrossRef]
57. Godbole, S.V.; Nandy, K.; Gauniyal, M.; Nalawade, P.; Sane, S.; Koyande, S.; Toyama, J.; Hegde, A.; Virgo, P.; Bhatia, K.; et al. HIV and cancer registry linkage identifies a substantial burden of cancers in persons with HIV in India. *Medicine* **2016**, *95*, e4850. [CrossRef] [PubMed]
58. Mbulaiteye, S.M.; Anderson, W.F.; Ferlay, J.; Bhatia, K.; Chang, C.; Rosenberg, P.S.; Devesa, S.S.; Parkin, D.M. Pediatric, elderly, and emerging adult-onset peaks in Burkitt's lymphoma incidence diagnosed in four continents, excluding Africa. *Am. J. Hematol.* **2012**, *87*, 573–578. [CrossRef]
59. Bray, F.C.M.; Mery, L.; Piñeros, M.; Znaor, A.; Zanetti, R.; Ferlay, J. (Eds.) *Cancer Incidence in Five Continents, Vol. XI (Electronic Version)*; International Agency for Research on Cancer: Lyon, France, 2017.
60. *International Statistical Classification of Diseases and Related Health Problem*, 10th ed.; World Health Organization: Geneva, The Switzerland, 1992.
61. Doll, R.; Payne, P.; Waterhouse, J.A.H. *Cancer Incidence In Five Continents*; Union Internationale Contre le Cancer: Geneva, The Switzerland, 1966; Volume 1.
62. Mbulaiteye, S.M.; Anderson, W.F. Age-related heterogeneity of Burkitt lymphoma. *Br. J. Haematol.* **2018**, *180*, 153–155. [CrossRef] [PubMed]
63. Liao, H.-M.; Liu, H.; Chin, P.-J.; Li, B.; Hung, G.-C.; Tsai, S.; Otim, I.; Legason, I.D.; Ogwang, M.D.; Reynolds, S.J.; et al. Epstein-Barr Virus in Burkitt Lymphoma in Africa Reveals a Limited Set of Whole Genome and LMP-1 Sequence Patterns: Analysis of Archival Datasets and Field Samples From Uganda, Tanzania, and Kenya. *Front. Oncol.* **2022**, *12*, 812224. [CrossRef]
64. van den Bosch, C.A. Is endemic Burkitt's lymphoma an alliance between three infections and a tumour promoter? *Lancet Oncol.* **2004**, *5*, 738–746. [CrossRef]
65. Aka, P.; Vila, M.C.; Jariwala, A.; Nkrumah, F.; Emmanuel, B.; Yagi, M.; Palacpac, N.M.; Periago, M.V.; Neequaye, J.; Kiruthu, C.; et al. Endemic Burkitt lymphoma is associated with strength and diversity of Plasmodium falciparum malaria stage-specific antigen antibody response. *Blood* **2013**, *122*, 629–635. [CrossRef]
66. Ravell, J.; Otim, I.; Nabalende, H.; Legason, I.D.; Reynolds, S.J.; Ogwang, M.D.; Ndugwa, C.M.; Marshall, V.; Whitby, D.; Goedert, J.J.; et al. Plasma magnesium is inversely associated with Epstein-Barr virus load in peripheral blood and Burkitt lymphoma in Uganda. *Cancer Epidemiol.* **2018**, *52*, 70–74. [PubMed]
67. Linet, M.S.; Brown, L.M.; Mbulaiteye, S.M.; Check, D.; Ostroumova, E.; Landgren, A.; Devesa, S.S. International long-term trends and recent patterns in the incidence of leukemias and lymphomas among children and adolescents ages 0–19 years. *Int. J. Cancer* **2016**, *138*, 1862–1874. [CrossRef] [PubMed]
68. Burkitt, D. A children's cancer dependent on climatic factors. *Nature* **1962**, *194*, 232–234. [CrossRef] [PubMed]
69. Kafuko, G.W.; Burkitt, D.P. Burkitt's lymphoma and malaria. *Int. J. Cancer* **1970**, *6*, 1–9. [CrossRef]
70. Craig, M.H.; Snow, R.W.; le Sueur, D. A climate-based distribution model of malaria transmission in sub-Saharan Africa. *Parasitol. Today* **1999**, *15*, 105–111. [CrossRef]
71. Burkitt, D.; Wright, D. Geographical and tribal distribution of the African lymphoma in Uganda. *Br. Med. J.* **1966**, *1*, 569–573. [CrossRef]
72. Mbulaiteye, S.M. Burkitt Lymphoma: Beyond discoveries. *Infect. Agent. Cancer* **2013**, *8*, 35. [CrossRef]
73. Emmanuel, B.; Kawira, E.; Ogwang, M.D.; Wabinga, H.; Magatti, J.; Nkrumah, F.; Neequaye, J.; Bhatia, K.; Brubaker, G.; Biggar, R.J.; et al. African Burkitt Lymphoma: Age-Specific Risk and Correlations with Malaria Biomarkers. *Am. J. Trop. Med. Hyg.* **2011**, *84*, 397–401. [CrossRef]
74. Arisue, N.; Chagaluka, G.; Palacpac, N.M.Q.; Johnston, W.T.; Mutalima, N.; Peprah, S.; Bhatia, K.; Borgstein, E.; Liomba, G.N.; Kamiza, S.; et al. Assessment of Mixed Plasmodium falciparumsera5 Infection in Endemic Burkitt Lymphoma: A Case-Control Study in Malawi. *Cancers* **2021**, *13*, 1692. [CrossRef]
75. Johnston, W.T.; Mutalima, N.; Sun, D.; Emmanuel, B.; Bhatia, K.; Aka, P.; Wu, X.; Borgstein, E.; Liomba, G.N.; Kamiza, S.; et al. Relationship between Plasmodium falciparum malaria prevalence, genetic diversity and endemic Burkitt lymphoma in Malawi. *Sci. Rep.* **2014**, *4*, 3741. [CrossRef]
76. Band, G.; Leffler, E.M.; Jallow, M.; Sisay-Joof, F.; Ndila, C.M.; Macharia, A.W.; Hubbart, C.; Jeffreys, A.E.; Rowlands, K.; Nguyen, T.; et al. Malaria protection due to sickle haemoglobin depends on parasite genotype. *Nature* **2022**, *602*, 106–111. [CrossRef] [PubMed]
77. Gomez-Diaz, E.; Ranford-Cartwright, L. Evolutionary race: Malaria evolves to evade sickle cell protection. *Cell Host Microbe* **2022**, *30*, 139–141. [CrossRef]
78. Ellwanger, J.H.; Cardoso, J.D.C.; Chies, J.A.B. Variability in human attractiveness to mosquitoes. *Curr. Res. Parasitol. Vector Borne Dis.* **2021**, *1*, 100058. [CrossRef] [PubMed]
79. Sumba, P.O.; Kabiru, E.W.; Namuyenga, E.; Fiore, N.; Otieno, R.O.; Moormann, A.M.; Orago, A.S.; Rosenbaum, P.F.; Rochford, R. Microgeographic variations in Burkitt's lymphoma incidence correlate with differences in malnutrition, malaria and Epstein-Barr virus. *Br. J. Cancer* **2010**, *103*, 1736–1741. [CrossRef]
80. Macmahon, B. Epidemiological evidence of the nature of Hodgkin's disease. *Cancer* **1957**, *10*, 1045–1054. [CrossRef]
81. Ries, L.A.G.; Devesa, S.S. Cancer incidence, mortality, and patient survival in the United States. In *Cancer Epidemiology and Prevention*, 3rd ed.; Schottenfeld, D., Fraumeni, J.F., Jr., Eds.; Oxford University Press: New York, NY, USA, 2006; pp. 139–167.

82. Richter, J.; John, K.; Staiger, A.M.; Rosenwald, A.; Kurz, K.; Michgehl, U.; Ott, G.; Franzenburg, S.; Kohler, C.; Finger, J.; et al. Epstein-Barr virus status of sporadic Burkitt lymphoma is associated with patient age and mutational features. *Br. J. Haematol.* **2022**, *196*, 681–689. [CrossRef]
83. Grande, B.M.; Gerhard, D.S.; Jiang, A.; Griner, N.B.; Abramson, J.S.; Alexander, T.B.; Allen, H.; Ayers, L.W.; Bethony, J.M.; Bhatia, K.; et al. Genome-wide discovery of somatic coding and noncoding mutations in pediatric endemic and sporadic Burkitt lymphoma. *Blood* **2019**, *133*, 1313–1324. [CrossRef] [PubMed]
84. Thomas, N.; Dreval, K.; Gerhard, D.S.; Hilton, L.K.; Abramson, J.S.; Bartlett, N.L.; Bethony, J.; Bowen, J.; Bryan, A.C.; Casper, C.; et al. Genetic Subgroups Inform on Pathobiology in Adult and Pediatric Burkitt Lymphoma. *Medrxiv* **2021**. [CrossRef]
85. Mbulaiteye, S.M.; Biggar, R.J.; Bhatia, K.; Linet, M.S.; Devesa, S.S. Sporadic childhood Burkitt lymphoma incidence in the United States during 1992-2005. *Pediatr. Blood Cancer* **2009**, *53*, 366–370. [CrossRef]
86. Osunkoya, B.O. Burkitt's Lymphoma. In *Critical Reviews in Tropical Medicine: Volume 1*; Chandra, R.K., Ed.; Springer: Boston, MA, USA, 1982; pp. 367–393.
87. Dunford, A.; Weinstock, D.M.; Savova, V.; Schumacher, S.E.; Cleary, J.P.; Yoda, A.; Sullivan, T.J.; Hess, J.M.; Gimelbrant, A.A.; Beroukhim, R.; et al. Tumor-suppressor genes that escape from X-inactivation contribute to cancer sex bias. *Nat. Genet.* **2017**, *49*, 10–16. [CrossRef] [PubMed]
88. Zhou, P.; Blain, A.E.; Newman, A.M.; Zaka, M.; Chagaluka, G.; Adlar, F.R.; Offor, U.T.; Broadbent, C.; Chaytor, L.; Whitehead, A.; et al. Sporadic and endemic Burkitt lymphoma have frequent FOXO1 mutations but distinct hotspots in the AKT recognition motif. *Blood Adv.* **2019**, *3*, 2118–2127. [CrossRef] [PubMed]
89. Weiss, D.J.; Lucas, T.C.D.; Nguyen, M.; Nandi, A.K.; Bisanzio, D.; Battle, K.E.; Cameron, E.; Twohig, K.A.; Pfeffer, D.A.; Rozier, J.A.; et al. Mapping the global prevalence, incidence, and mortality of Plasmodium falciparum, 2000–2017: A spatial and temporal modelling study. *Lancet* **2019**, *394*, 322–331. [CrossRef]
90. Wang, Z.; Liu, Y.; Li, Y.; Wang, G.; Lourenco, J.; Kraemer, M.; He, Q.; Cazelles, B.; Li, Y.; Wang, R.; et al. The relationship between rising temperatures and malaria incidence in Hainan, China, from 1984 to 2010: A longitudinal cohort study. *Lancet Planet Health* **2022**, *6*, e350–e358. [CrossRef]
91. de-The, G.; Day, N.E.; Geser, A.; Lavoue, M.F.; Ho, J.H.; Simons, M.J.; Sohier, R.; Tukei, P.; Vonka, V.; Zavadova, H. Sero-epidemiology of the Epstein-Barr virus: Preliminary analysis of an international study—A review. *IARC Sci. Publ.* **1975**, *11*, 3–16.
92. de-The, G.; Lavoue, M.F.; Muenz, L. Differences in EBV antibody titres of patients with nasopharyngeal carcinoma originating from high, intermediate and low incidence areas. *IARC Sci. Publ.* **1978**, *20*, 471–481.
93. Yu, M.C. Nasopharyngeal carcinoma: Epidemiology and dietary factors. *IARC Sci. Publ.* **1991**, *105*, 39–47.
94. Wong, Y.; Meehan, M.T.; Burrows, S.R.; Doolan, D.L.; Miles, J.J. Estimating the global burden of Epstein-Barr virus-related cancers. *J. Cancer Res. Clin. Oncol* **2022**, *148*, 31–46. [CrossRef]
95. Zanella, L.; Riquelme, I.; Buchegger, K.; Abanto, M.; Ili, C.; Brebi, P. A reliable Epstein-Barr Virus classification based on phylogenomic and population analyses. *Sci. Rep.* **2019**, *9*, 9829. [CrossRef]
96. Bridges, R.; Correia, S.; Wegner, F.; Venturini, C.; Palser, A.; White, R.E.; Kellam, P.; Breuer, J.; Farrell, P.J. Essential role of inverted repeat in Epstein-Barr virus IR-1 in B cell transformation; geographical variation of the viral genome. *Philos. Trans. R. Soc. Lond. B Biol. Sci.* **2019**, *374*, 20180299. [CrossRef]
97. Correia, S.; Bridges, R.; Wegner, F.; Venturini, C.; Palser, A.; Middeldorp, J.M.; Cohen, J.I.; Lorenzetti, M.A.; Bassano, I.; White, R.E.; et al. Sequence Variation of Epstein-Barr Virus: Viral Types, Geography, Codon Usage, and Diseases. *J. Virol.* **2018**, *92*, e01132-18. [CrossRef]
98. Dave, S.S.; Fu, K.; Wright, G.W.; Lam, L.T.; Kluin, P.; Boerma, E.J.; Greiner, T.C.; Weisenburger, D.D.; Rosenwald, A.; Ott, G.; et al. Molecular diagnosis of Burkitt's lymphoma. *N. Engl. J. Med.* **2006**, *354*, 2431–2442. [CrossRef] [PubMed]
99. Schmitz, R.; Young, R.M.; Ceribelli, M.; Jhavar, S.; Xiao, W.; Zhang, M.; Wright, G.; Shaffer, A.L.; Hodson, D.J.; Buras, E.; et al. Burkitt lymphoma pathogenesis and therapeutic targets from structural and functional genomics. *Nature* **2012**, *490*, 116–120. [CrossRef]
100. Richter, J.; Schlesner, M.; Hoffmann, S.; Kreuz, M.; Leich, E.; Burkhardt, B.; Rosolowski, M.; Ammerpohl, O.; Wagener, R.; Bernhart, S.H.; et al. Recurrent mutation of the ID3 gene in Burkitt lymphoma identified by integrated genome, exome and transcriptome sequencing. *Nat. Genet.* **2012**, *44*, 1316–1320. [PubMed]
101. Dunleavy, K.; Pittaluga, S.; Shovlin, M.; Steinberg, S.M.; Cole, D.; Grant, C.; Wiedemann, B.; Staudt, L.M.; Jaffe, E.S.; Little, R.F.; et al. Low-intensity therapy in adults with Burkitt's lymphoma. *N. Engl. J. Med.* **2013**, *369*, 1915–1925. [CrossRef]
102. Campo, E.; Swerdlow, S.H.; Harris, N.L.; Pileri, S.; Stein, H.; Jaffe, E.S. The 2008 WHO classification of lymphoid neoplasms and beyond: Evolving concepts and practical applications. *Blood* **2011**, *117*, 5019–5032. [CrossRef] [PubMed]
103. Harris, N.L.; Jaffe, E.S.; Diebold, J.; Flandrin, G.; Muller-Hermelink, H.K.; Vardiman, J.; Lister, T.A.; Bloomfield, C.D. The World Health Organization classification of neoplastic diseases of the hematopoietic and lymphoid tissues. Report of the Clinical Advisory Committee meeting, Airlie House, Virginia, November, 1997. *Ann. Oncol.* **1999**, *10*, 1419–1432. [CrossRef] [PubMed]
104. Harris, N.L.; Jaffe, E.S.; Stein, H.; Banks, P.M.; Chan, J.K.; Cleary, M.L.; Delsol, G.; De Wolf-Peeters, C.; Falini, B.; Gatter, K.C.; et al. A revised European-American classification of lymphoid neoplasms: A proposal from the International Lymphoma Study Group. *Blood* **1994**, *84*, 1361–1392. [CrossRef]

105. Alaggio, R.; Amador, C.; Anagnostopoulos, I.; Attygalle, A.D.; Araujo, I.B.d.O.; Berti, E.; Bhagat, G.; Borges, A.M.; Boyer, D.; Calaminici, M.; et al. The 5th edition of the World Health Organization Classification of Haematolymphoid Tumours: Lymphoid Neoplasms. *Leukemia* **2022**, *36*, 1720–1748. [CrossRef]
106. Jaffe, E.S.; Harris, N.L.; Diebold, J.; Muller-Hermelink, H.K. World Health Organization classification of neoplastic diseases of the hematopoietic and lymphoid tissues. A progress report. *Am. J. Clin. Pathol.* **1999**, *111*, S8–S12.
107. Swerdlow, S.H.; Cook, J.R. As the world turns, evolving lymphoma classifications-past, present and future. *Hum. Pathol.* **2020**, *95*, 55–77. [CrossRef]
108. Nathwani, B.N.; Sasu, S.J.; Ahsanuddin, A.N.; Hernandez, A.M.; Drachenberg, M.R. The critical role of histology in an era of genomics and proteomics: A commentary and reflection. *Adv. Anat. Pathol.* **2007**, *14*, 375–400. [CrossRef] [PubMed]
109. Naresh, K.N.; Ibrahim, H.A.H.; Lazzi, S.; Rince, P.; Onorati, M.; Ambrosio, M.R.; Bilhou-Nabera, C.; Amen, F.; Reid, A.; Mawanda, M.; et al. Diagnosis of Burkitt lymphoma using an algorithmic approach—Applicable in both resource-poor and resource-rich countries. *Br. J. Haematol.* **2011**, *154*, 770–776. [CrossRef] [PubMed]
110. Orem, J.; Sandin, S.; Weibull, C.E.; Odida, M.; Wabinga, H.; Mbidde, E.; Wabwire-Mangen, F.; Meijer, C.J.; Middeldorp, J.M.; Weiderpass, E. Agreement between diagnoses of childhood lymphoma assigned in Uganda and by an international reference laboratory. *Clin. Epidemiol.* **2012**, *4*, 339–347. [PubMed]
111. Westmoreland, K.D.; Montgomery, N.D.; Stanley, C.C.; El-Mallawany, N.K.; Wasswa, P.; van der Gronde, T.; Mtete, I.; Butia, M.; Itimu, S.; Chasela, C.; et al. Plasma Epstein-Barr virus DNA for pediatric Burkitt lymphoma diagnosis, prognosis and response assessment in Malawi. *Int. J. Cancer* **2017**, *140*, 2509–2516. [CrossRef] [PubMed]
112. Morrow, R.H., Jr.; Levine, P.H.; Ziegler, J.L.; Berard, C. Letter: What is Burkitt's lymphoma? *Lancet* **1974**, *2*, 1268–1269. [CrossRef]
113. Wright, D.H. What is Burkitt's lymphoma and when is it endemic? *Blood* **1999**, *93*, 758. [CrossRef]
114. Alderuccio, J.P.; Olszewski, A.J.; Evens, A.M.; Collins, G.P.; Danilov, A.V.; Bower, M.; Jagadeesh, D.; Zhu, C.; Sperling, A.; Kim, S.H.; et al. HIV-associated Burkitt lymphoma: Outcomes from a US-UK collaborative analysis. *Blood Adv.* **2021**, *5*, 2852–2862. [CrossRef]
115. Olszewski, A.J.; Jakobsen, L.H.; Collins, G.P.; Cwynarski, K.; Bachanova, V.; Blum, K.A.; Boughan, K.M.; Bower, M.; Dalla Pria, A.; Danilov, A.; et al. Burkitt Lymphoma International Prognostic Index. *J. Clin. Oncol.* **2021**, *39*, 1129–1138. [CrossRef]
116. Evens, A.M.; Danilov, A.; Jagadeesh, D.; Sperling, A.; Kim, S.H.; Vaca, R.; Wei, C.; Rector, D.; Sundaram, S.; Reddy, N.; et al. Burkitt lymphoma in the modern era: Real-world outcomes and prognostication across 30 US cancer centers. *Blood* **2021**, *137*, 374–386. [CrossRef]
117. Knudson, A.G., Jr. Heredity and human cancer. *Am. J. Pathol.* **1974**, *77*, 77–84.
118. Li, F.P.; Fraumeni, J.F., Jr. Rhabdomyosarcoma in children: Epidemiologic study and identification of a familial cancer syndrome. *J. Natl. Cancer Inst.* **1969**, *43*, 1365–1373. [PubMed]
119. Global Retinoblastoma Study, G.; Fabian, I.D.; Abdallah, E.; Abdullahi, S.U.; Abdulqader, R.A.; Adamou Boubacar, S.; Ademola-Popoola, D.S.; Adio, A.; Afshar, A.R.; Aggarwal, P.; et al. Global Retinoblastoma Presentation and Analysis by National Income Level. *JAMA Oncol.* **2020**, *6*, 685–695. [CrossRef] [PubMed]
120. Srivastava, S.; Zou, Z.Q.; Pirollo, K.; Blattner, W.; Chang, E.H. Germ-line transmission of a mutated p53 gene in a cancer-prone family with Li-Fraumeni syndrome. *Nature* **1990**, *348*, 747–749. [CrossRef] [PubMed]
121. Malkin, D.; Li, F.P.; Strong, L.C.; Fraumeni, J.F., Jr.; Nelson, C.E.; Kim, D.H.; Kassel, J.; Gryka, M.A.; Bischoff, F.Z.; Tainsky, M.A.; et al. Germ line p53 mutations in a familial syndrome of breast cancer, sarcomas, and other neoplasms. *Science* **1990**, *250*, 1233–1238. [CrossRef]
122. Ablin, A.; Stephens, B.G.; Hirata, T.; Wilson, K.; Williams, H.E. Nephropathy, xanthinuria, and orotic aciduria complicating Burkitt's lymphoma treated with chemotherapy and allopurinol. *Metabolism* **1972**, *21*, 771–778. [CrossRef]
123. Mbulaiteye, S.M.; Talisuna, A.O.; Ogwang, M.D.; McKenzie, F.E.; Ziegler, J.L.; Parkin, D.M. African Burkitt's lymphoma: Could collaboration with HIV-1 and malaria programmes reduce the high mortality rate? *Lancet* **2010**, *375*, 1661–1663. [CrossRef]
124. Xian, R.R.; Kinyera, T.; Otim, I.; Sampson, J.N.; Nabalende, H.; Legason, I.D.; Stone, J.; Ogwang, M.D.; Reynolds, S.J.; Kerchan, P.; et al. Plasma EBV DNA: A Promising Diagnostic Marker for Endemic Burkitt Lymphoma. *Front. Oncol.* **2021**, *11*, 804083. [CrossRef]

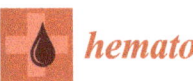

Review

Lymphomas in People Living with HIV

Emanuela Vaccher [1], Annunziata Gloghini [2], Chiara C. Volpi [2] and Antonino Carbone [3,*]

[1] Medical Oncology and Immune-Related Tumours, Centro di Riferimento Oncologico (CRO), IRCCS, National Cancer Institute, Via F. Gallini 2, I-33081 Aviano, Italy
[2] Department of Pathology and Laboratory Medicine, Fondazione IRCCS Istituto Nazionale dei Tumori, Via Venezian 1, I-20133 Milano, Italy
[3] Department of Pathology, Centro di Riferimento Oncologico (CRO), IRCCS, National Cancer Institute, Via F. Gallini 2, I-33081 Aviano, Italy
* Correspondence: acarbone@cro.it; Tel.: +39-0434-659085

Abstract: Lymphomas in people living with HIV (PLWH) are associated with Epstein Barr virus (EBV) and Kaposi-sarcoma-associated herpesvirus (KSHV). They include primary effusion lymphoma, large B-cell lymphoma arising in multicentric Castleman disease, plasmablastic lymphoma, Burkitt lymphoma, diffuse large B-cell lymphoma, and Hodgkin lymphoma (HL). Inclusion of these lymphomas in the WHO classification of tumors of hematopoietic and lymphoid tissues and the increasing recognition of these disorders have resulted in established clinical management that has led to improved outcomes. In this review, we report on the current management in lymphomas occurring in PLWH with an emphasis on KSHV-associated disorders and EBV-related HL. We also report on the simultaneous occurrence of KSHV- and EBV-associated disorders and highlight preventive measures that have been planned for tumor prevention in PLWH. In conclusion, it is recommended that treatment choice for PLWH affected by lymphoma, and receiving effective combined antiretroviral therapy (cART), should not be influenced by HIV status. Moreover, there is an urgent need (1) to reduce the current large disparities in health care between HIV-infected and HIV-uninfected populations, (2) to disseminate effective treatment, and (3) to implement preventive strategies for PLWH.

Keywords: lymphomas; people living with HIV; management; tumor prevention in people living with HIV; EBV; KSHV

1. Introduction

Before the development of effective combination antiretroviral therapy (cART), the relative risk for non-Hodgkin lymphoma (NHL) in people living with HIV (PLWH) was estimated as 60–200 fold compared to the general population [1–3]. Despite the introduction of cART, the incidence of lymphoma in PLWH is increasing compared to the general population [4,5].

Lymphomas occurring in PLWH are characterized by advanced stage, extranodal involvement at presentation, an aggressive clinical course, and are usually associated with Epstein Barr virus (EBV) and/or Kaposi-sarcoma-associated herpesvirus (KSHV) [4,6,7]. They include those KSHV- and EBV-related entities that are particularly concentrated in this population at high risk of infection-related cancers, i.e., primary effusion lymphoma (PEL), large B-cell lymphoma arising in multicentric Castleman disease (MCD), and plasmablastic lymphoma (PBL) [4,8]. There are probably no tumors that occur uniquely in PLWH, even if they are much more frequent and cluster highly in this group. Lymphomas that develop in the absence of HIV infection, i.e., Burkitt lymphoma (BL), diffuse large B-cell lymphoma (DLBCL), and Hodgkin lymphoma (HL), occur in PLWH with increased incidence compared to the HIV negative population [8]. Despite the introduction of cART DLBCL remains a leading malignancy, the incidence of BL, PEL, and PBL remains stable, while the incidence of HL- and KSHV-associated MCD is increasing [4,5]. Importantly, all KSHV-associated lymphoid proliferations have been also detected in HIV-negative individuals [9]. The increasing recognition of these disorders and their clear inclusion in the WHO classification [10] have resulted in established clinical management and consensus treatment protocols that have led to improvement in outcomes.

It is well known that the HIV pandemic remains a critical health problem, even though modern cART has changed the infection into a chronic manageable disease. Today, malignant tumors represent an important risk of death in PLWH, justifying and enhancing the role that hematologists and oncologists have, alongside infectious disease skills, in the effective management of PLWH with lymphoma and other tumors.

Significant gaps remain between PLWH and the general cancer population, particularly in cancer care. It is mandatory to close this gap to improve treatment outcomes. Clinical trials of immunotherapeutic strategies to simultaneously eradicate cancer and persistent HIV infection are warranted [11].

In this review, we report on the current management of HIV-related hematologic malignancies with emphasis on KSHV-associated disorders [12] and EBV-related HL [7]. We also highlight preventive measures that have been planned to avoid a second tumor and, in general, to prevent tumor development, including virus-related and unrelated cancers.

2. Pathologic and Virologic Features

The majority of lymphoid proliferations in PLWH are associated with tumor cell infection by EBV (DLBCL, 25–100%; BL, 60%; PEL, 80–100%; PBL, 70%; HL, 80–100%). The minority of lymphoid proliferations in PLWH are associated with infection by KSHV; PEL, 100%; MCD-associated large B-cell lymphoma (LBCL), 100%; and MCD, 100%. Only PEL is associated with the infection by both herpesviruses [4,6,7].

DLBCL in PLWH display either centroblastic or immunoblastic morphology (Figure 1A) showing a GC B-cell like profile (CD20+, CD10− or +, BCL6− or +, MUM1/IRF4−, and CD138−) or the activated B-cell-like profile (CD20+, CD10−, BCL6−, MUM1/IRF4+, CD138+, and CD38+), respectively. BL in PLWH displays a proliferation of medium-sized tumor cells, often demonstrating a starry sky appearance (Figure 1B). BL tumor cells express B-cell germinal center antigens (CD20+, CD10+, BCL6+, and BCL2−) and high proliferative rates (Ki67+ 100%).

PEL in PLWH express a plasma cell profile (CD138+, CD38+, and MUM1/IRF4, B-cell markers-, and T-cell markers-). Immunohistochemical staining for ORF73/LANA1 reveals KSHV infection in all cases (Figure 2). PEL tumor cells are also often positive for EBV-encoded small RNA (EBER). PBL in PLWH consists of tumor cells displaying plasma cell differentiation (CD138+, CD38+, MUM1/IRF4+), and are often positive for EBV infection.

In classic HL occurring in PLWH, Hodgkin and Reed–Sternberg cells (HRS) express the typical diagnostic profile (CD15+, CD30+, CD40+, and MUM1/IRF4+). As shown in Figure 3, HRS cells typically express positivity for EBER and LMP1 (EBV-type II latency). Table 1 lists lymphoproliferative disorders showing EBV positivity. In contrast with classic HL, these lymphoproliferative disorders lack typical/diagnostic HRS cells [5].

Images were taken using a Nikon Eclipse 80i microscope (Nikon, Tokyo, Japan) with a Pan Fluor 40×/0.75 objective and Nikon digital sight DS-Fi1 camera equipped with control unit-DS-L2 (Nikon). Images were processed using Adobe Photoshop 6 (Adobe Systems).

In MCD KSHV positive plasmablasts in the mantle zones of expanded follicles are the diagnostic marker (Figure 4). Plasmablasts in MCD typically express cytoplasmic monotypic lambda light chain, IgM, CD19, and MYC, CD38, CD45, and CD79a, while they are usually negative for CD10, CD20, CD30, CD138, BCL6, PAX5, T-cell antigens, and EBV infection. KSHV-MCD is commonly associated with other disorders and malignancies either at presentation or in the course of the disease (see below). Table 2 lists disorders and malignancies concurrent with KSHV-MCD [12].

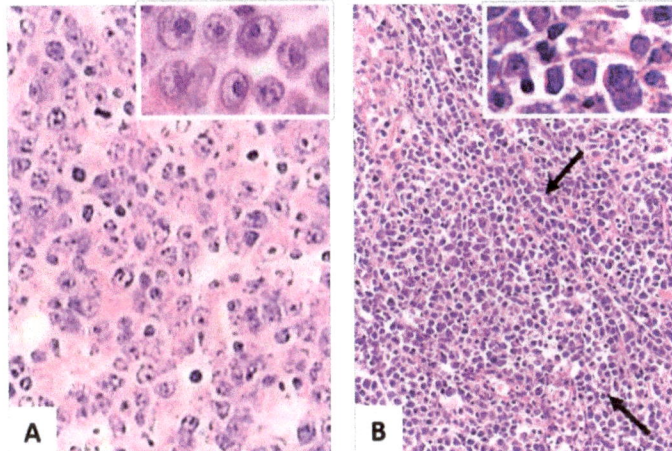

Figure 1. (**A**) Diffuse large B-cell lymphoma (DLBCL) with immunoblastic-plasmacytoid features in an individual infected by HIV. Most tumor cells have plentiful cytoplasm and round or oval nuclei with large nucleoli. The inset shows that the morphology of tumor cells is immunoblastic. (**B**) Burkitt lymphoma in an individual infected by HIV. A homogeneous proliferation of medium-sized tumor cells displaying cohesive and starry sky (arrows) patterns. In the inset, tumor cells show round nuclei, multiple nucleoli, and small cytoplasms. H&E, hematoxylin–eosin stain. Original magnification ×400 (A, B inset); ×200 (**B**). Images were taken using a Nikon Eclipse 80i microscope (Nikon, Tokyo, Japan) with Pan Fluor 20×/0.75 and Pan Fluor 40×/0.75 objectives and Nikon digital sight DS-Fi1 camera equipped with control unit-DS-L2 (Nikon). Images were processed using Adobe Photoshop CS2 V9.0 (Adobe Systems).

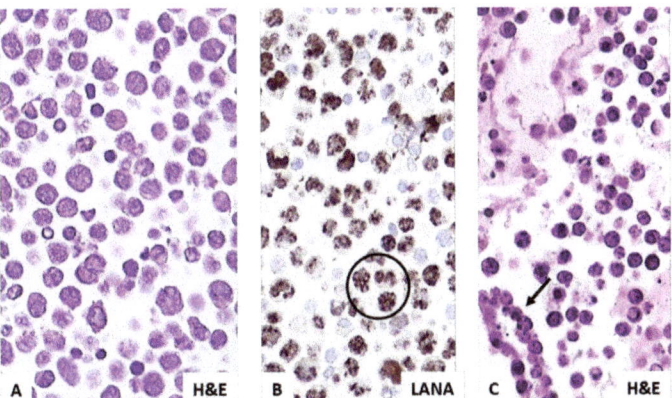

Figure 2. Primary effusion lymphoma (PEL) in individuals infected by HIV. (**A**) In a cell line derived from a classic PEL, tumor cells display features resembling anaplastic large lymphoma cells. (**B**) Immunohistochemical staining for ORF73/LANA1 detects evidence of KSHV infection. Typically, the staining pattern is speckled, more evident in circled cells. (**C**) In a cell block derived from a classic PEL, tumor cells display features of blastic medium-sized lymphoma. Benign mesothelial cells are also recognizable (arrow). H&E, hematoxylin–eosin stain; ORF73/LANA1, hematoxylin counterstain. Original magnification ×400. Images were taken using a Nikon Eclipse 80i microscope (Nikon, Tokyo, Japan) with a Pan Fluor 40×/0.75 objective and Nikon digital sight DS-Fi1 camera equipped with control unit-DS-L2 (Nikon). Images were processed using Adobe Photoshop CS2 V9.0 (Adobe Systems).

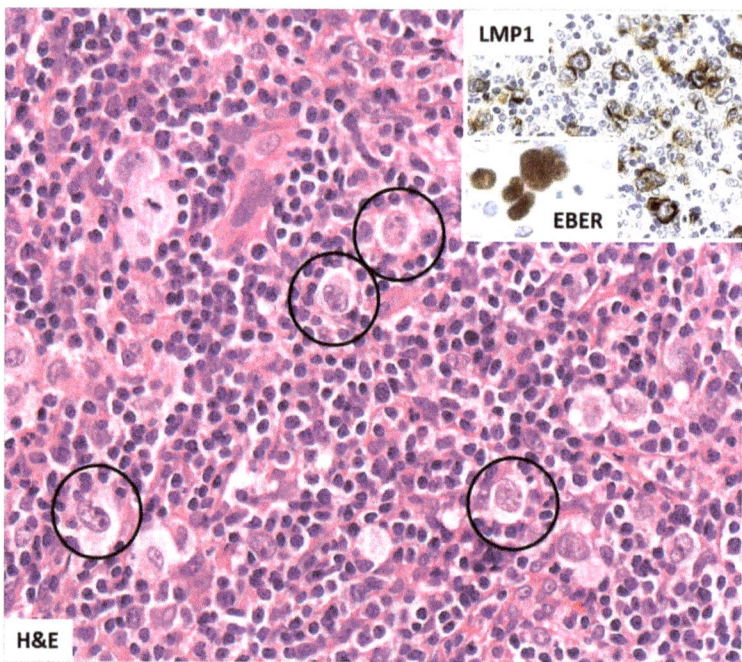

Figure 3. Hodgkin lymphoma (HL) in individuals infected by HIV. Hodgkin and Reed–Sternberg (HRS) cells are seen within a mixed inflammatory microenvironment. Several circled cells are mononuclear Hodgkin cells. In the inset, EBV-infected tumor cells are demonstrated by EBER in situ hybridization and LMP1 immunostaining. H&E, hematoxylin–eosin stain; EBER, in situ hybridization; LMP1, immunohistochemistry, hematoxylin counterstain. Original magnification ×400.

Table 1. Hodgkin lymphoma and other lymphoproliferative disorders in which proliferative or malignant cells can demonstrate EBV positivity *.

Categories	Lymphomas and Lymphoproliferative Disorders
B-cell malignancies	Hodgkin lymphoma Diffuse large B-cell lymphoma Burkitt lymphoma Plasmablastic lymphoma
NK- and T-cell malignancies	Angioimmunoblastic T-cell lymphoma [#] Follicular T-cell lymphoma [#] Peripheral T-cell lymphomas Extranodal NK/T cell lymphoma, nasal type
Immunodeficiency related	Post-transplant lymphoproliferative disorders HIV-related

* Modified and adapted from Toner et al. [7]. [#] B-cells are EBV positive.

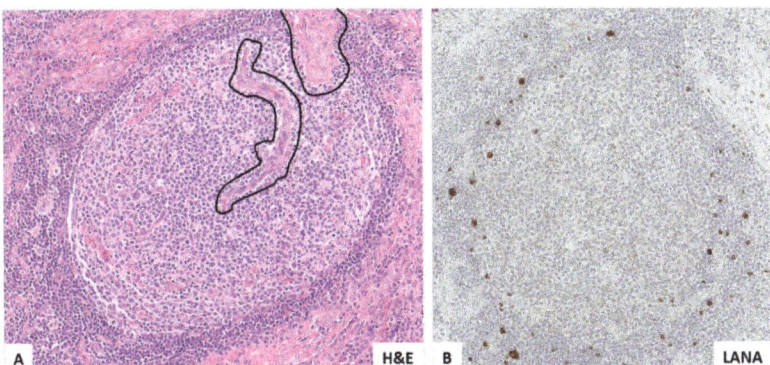

Figure 4. KSHV-associated multicentric Castleman disease (MCD). (**A**) An expanded lymphoid follicle shows a large germinal center. Vascular structures are present within the germinal center and around the follicle (demonstrated by dark outline). (**B**) KSHV-infected LANA-stained cells are found predominantly in the mantle zone of the follicle but are also seen scattered as single cells at the border of the interfollicular area. H&E, hematoxylin–eosin stain; ORF73/LANA1, immunohistochemistry, hematoxylin counterstain. Original magnification ×200.

Table 2. Disorders and malignancies concurrent with KSHV-MCD *.

KSHV-Associated Disorders	Kaposi Sarcoma
	Primary effusion lymphoma
	MCD-associated large B-cell lymphoma
	KSHV-positive germinotropic lymphoproliferative disorder

* Modified and adapted from Carbone et al. [12].

Images were taken using a Nikon Eclipse 80i microscope (Nikon, Tokyo, Japan) with a Pan Fluor 20×/0.75 objective and Nikon digital sight DS-Fi1 camera equipped with control unit-DS-L2 (Nikon). Images were processed using Adobe Photoshop CS2 V9.0 (Adobe Systems).

Other lymphomas that can develop in PLWH include primary central nervous system lymphomas, high grade B-cell lymphomas, lymphomas of the marginal zone, polymorphic B-cell lymphoma PTLD-like, plasmacytoma, myeloma, and peripheral T-cell lymphoma [13].

3. Simultaneous Occurrence of KSHV- and EBV-Associated Disorders in PLWH

KSHV-MCD occurring in PLWH may be found in association with other malignancies including Kaposi sarcoma (KS) (Figures 5 and 6) and B-cell lymphomas (PEL), that are consistently associated with KSHV, and frequently with EBV infection (PEL). MCD-associated LBCL is a new lymphoma category that usually arises in association with HIV infection. The tumor cells display plasmablastic features are usually positive for CD45 and CD20, and express terminal B-cell differentiation markers, including MUM1/IRF4, and are often negative for EBV.

In KSHV-positive germinotropic lymphoproliferative disorder (usually benign), patients present with localized lymphadenopathy without immunodeficiency. Plasmablasts, confined to expanded germinal centers, are positive for cytoplasmic monotypic light chain, CD38, MUM1, viral IL6, LANA1, and EBV [14].

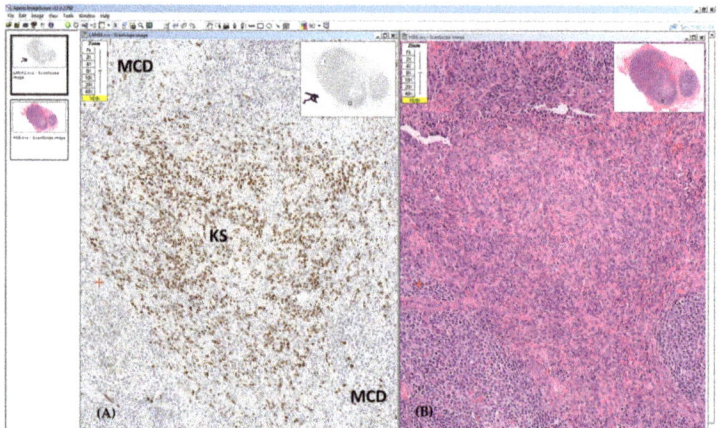

Figure 5. Synchronized images. (**A**) LANA1 staining reveals a micro area of Kaposi sarcoma (KS) placed between two follicles featuring multicentric Castleman disease (MCD). The lesion is vascular and the positive LANA1 cells have a spindle morphology. In the follicular mantle zone, plasmablasts are also positive for LANA1. (**B**) Hematoxylin–eosin stain shows interfollicular, endothelial proliferation consistent with KS.

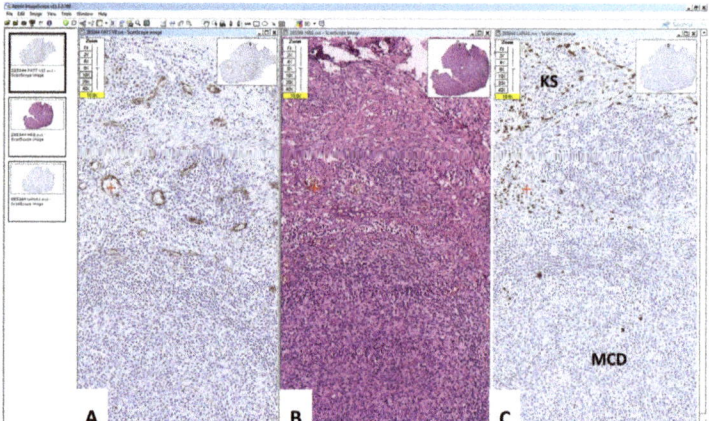

Figure 6. Triple synchronized images. The Figure shows a small Kaposi sarcoma (KS) lesion in a lymph node (top) and a follicle with the typical features observed in multicentric Castleman disease (MCD) (bottom). The KS lesion located in the context of the lymph node is revealed by immunohistological stain for Factor VII (**A**) and is synchronized with hematoxylin and eosin stain (**B**) and immuno-histological stain for LANA1 (**C**).

Other disorders concurrent with KSHV-MCD include HIV-associated disorders and EBV-associated disorders. For example, in HIV-infected persons, and in other immunosuppressed patients, the so-called EBV positive hyperplastic (plasmacytic/plasmoblastic) B-cell lymphoproliferative lesion may occur (Figure 7) [15].

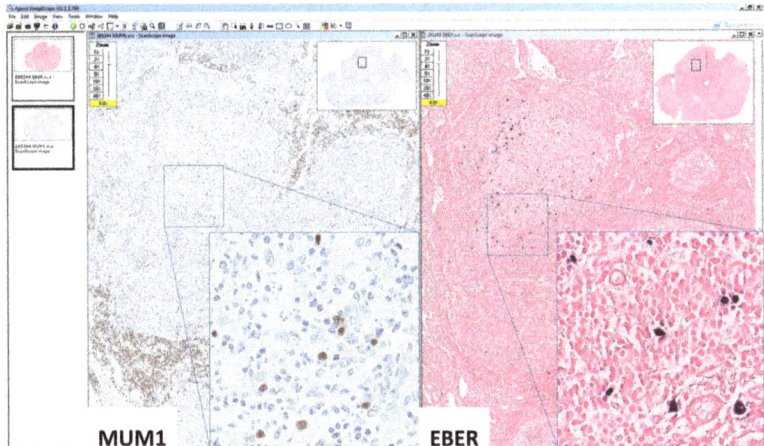

Figure 7. Synchronized images of a small lymphoproliferative lesion with the LANA1-, EBV+, MUM1+ profile. In the same lymph node of Figure 6, two areas containing EBV-positive cells (inset) which were LANA1 negative (not shown) and were located in areas containing MUM1 expressing cells (inset).

4. Treatment Strategies

Treatment of lymphomas in PLWH has evolved over time in tandem with improved control of HIV infection and immune function restoration by cART [4,16–18]. In the pre-cART era, outcomes were poor regardless of the treatment used, including low-dose chemotherapy, risk-adjusted intensive chemotherapy, and infusional chemotherapy [13].

The combination of cART with chemoimmunotherapy significantly improved the outcomes of the lymphomas in PLWH, with 5-year survival increasing from 13% in the pre-cART era (1986–1995) to 70–80% in the late cART era (2005–2015) [19]. Aggressive lymphomas remain the main cause of death in PLWH [20]. Prognosis depends on lymphoma-related characteristics that are incorporated into the age-adjusted International Prognostic Index (IPI) or Burkitt's lymphoma IPI score, as well as by the lack of a complete response (CR) to therapy rather than on HIV-specific factors [4,21]. Importantly, PLWH with cancer are commonly excluded from innovative clinical trials [4,22].

Treatment choice for PLWH affected by lymphoma receiving effective cART should not be influenced by HIV status. Nevertheless, in PLWH affected by lymphomas there are special considerations that must be considered in the antineoplastic treatment, such as the presence of HIV and the comorbidity of other coinfections including oncogenic viruses. Concurrent administration of cART with chemotherapy has been associated with improved CR rates and improved immune recovery. Side effects due to drug–drug interactions may occur with CYP3A4 inhibitors such as ritonavir and cobicistat-based antiretroviral regimens. Integrase strand-transfer inhibitors (INSTIs) without cobicistat (raltegravir, dolutegravir, and bictegravir) have advantages in drug–drug interactions and result in a more rapid decline in HIV viremia. All PLWH with cancer must receive cART during antineoplastic treatment, preferably with INSTI-based regimens. In addition, maximizing supportive care, especially prophylaxis for opportunistic infections, is essential in high-risk patients [4].

The development of second primary cancers (SPC) is now an important cause of morbidity and mortality in HIV-positive lymphoma survivors, arguing for the need for regular monitoring and surveillance programs [23–27]. Therefore, there is an urgent need (1) to reduce the current large disparities in health care between HIV-infected and HIV-uninfected populations, (2) to disseminate effective treatment, and (3) to implement prevention strategies for PLWH.

5. Front-Line Treatment for Non-Hodgkin Lymphoma

Non-Hodgkin lymphomas (NHLs) in PLWH are aggressive diseases that require immediate treatment. The most common up-front treatment for DLBCL is rituximab (R) and chemotherapy in PLWH, although an initial randomized phase 2 trial indicated safety issues particularly in patients with low CD4 counts ($\leq 50/\mu L$) and in those who received rituximab "maintenance" [28], which has not been shown to be beneficial in HIV-negative NHL. Subsequent phase 2 trials with R-CHOP (cyclophosphamide, doxorubicin, vincristine, and prednisone), R-CDE (cyclophosphamide, doxorubicin, and etoposide), or dose adjusted (DA)-EPOCH-R (etoposide, prednisone, vincristine, and doxorubicin-cyclophosphamide at a dose adjusted for CD4 count) plus rituximab resulted in complete response (CR) rates of 69–91% and 2-year survival rates of 62–77%, with a low infectious mortality rate (<10%) [29,30] (Table 3) [28–34]. In a pooled analysis, the combination of rituximab and chemotherapy showed a significant benefit for all CD20-positive HIV-NHL patients compared to chemotherapy alone (higher CR rates and better progression-free survival (PFS) and overall survival), supporting its use in HIV-DLBCL [35]. Notably, prophylaxis of opportunistic infections in high-risk patients must be maximized according to current HIV management guidelines (https://aidsinfo.nih.gov/guidelines/html/4/adult (accessed on 26 July 2022) and adolescent.oi-prevention and treatment guidelines).

Table 3. Major clinical trials with rituximab (R) and chemotherapy in HIV-associated aggressive B-cell Non-Hodgkin lymphomas.

	Patients N°	Study Design	CD4 Count /μL	DLBCL %	aa-IPI ≥ 2 %	CR Rate %	PFS	Overall Survival	Infectious Death %
R-CHOP-R vs. CHOP (Kaplan et al., 2005 [28])	150	Phase 3	130	81	43	58 vs. 47	11.3 vs. 9.5 mos	28 vs. 35 mos	14 °° vs. 2 *
R-CHOP (Bouè et al., 2006 [31])	61	Phase 2	172	72	48	77	69% (2 yr)	75% (2 yr)	2
R-CHOP (Ribera et al., 2008 [32])	95	Phase 2	158	81	58	69	NA	56% (3 yr)	7
R-CDE (Spina et al., 2005 [33])	74	Phase 2 *	161	72	57	70	52% EFS (2 yr)	64% (2 yr)	7
R-EPOCH (Sparano et al., 2010 [29])	106	Randomized phase 2: R-EPOCH vs. EPOCH-R	194	80	64	73 vs. 55	66 vs. 63% (2 yr)	70 vs. 67% (2 yr)	10 °° vs. 7
SC-EPOCH-RR (Dunleavy et al., 2010 [30])	33	Phase 2	208	100	76	91	84% (5yr)	68% (5yr)	0
VORINOSTAT-R °-EPOCH (Ramos 2020 [34])	90	Randomized Phase 2	54 % (<200)	71	66	68 vs. 74	63 vs. 69% EFS (3 yr)	70 vs. 77% (3 yr)	NA

R, rituximab; CHOP, Cyclophosphamide, Doxorubicin, Vincristine, Prednisone; R-CDE, 96 h continuous infusion (ci) Cyclophosphamide, Doxorubicin, Etoposide; R-EPOCH, 96 h ci Etoposide, Prednisone, Vincristine, Cyclophosphamide dose adjusted to CD4 count and Doxorubicin; SC-EPOCH-RR, short course (median 3 cycles, range 3–5) EPOCH plus dose-dense (days 1,5) Rituximab; DLBCL, Diffuse Large B Cell Lymphoma; aa-IPI, age-adjusted international Prognostic Score; CR, complete remission; PFS, progression-free survival; EFS, event-free survival; OS, overall survival; * $p < 0.005$; °° majority of patients with CD4 count < 50/μL and without combination antiretroviral therapy. R °, rituximab in CD20-positive NHL.

A pooled analysis by the AIDS Malignacy Consortium (AMC) suggests that infusional R-EPOCH may be more effective than bolus treatment with R-CHOP in patients with HIV-associated aggressive B-cell NHLs. However, in a randomized prospective trial in immunocompetent patients with DLBCL, DA-R-EPOCH, and R-CHOP were found to be equally effective [36].

Recently, the AMC-075 trial (Table 3) reported that the addition of the oncolytic vorinostat to EPOCH+/− rituximab had no benefit on treatment outcomes or HIV reservoir. Only Myc protein expression was significantly associated with worse outcomes, with 3-year event-free survival (EFS) of 44% in Myc-positive compared with 83% in Myc-negative DLBCL [34].

To date, the best therapy for HIV-associated BL remains unclear. Several retrospective studies suggest that dose-intensive up-front therapies may be better than R-CHOP, as in the general population. A phase 2 trial with a modified CODOX-M/IVAC regimen (cyclophosphamide, doxorubicin, vincristine, methotrexate, etoposide, ifofosfamide, and cytarabine) in combination with rituximab resulted in a 2-year survival rate of 69%, with favorable toxicity compared with the parent regimen [37].

The risk-adapted strategy DA-EPOCH proved effective for BL patients without CNS involvement (4 years EFS 85%), regardless of HIV status [38,39]. A large retrospective international study in the late cART era showed better outcomes with the CODOX-M/IVAC chemotherapy, with longer PFS (hazard ratio (HR) 0.45, $p = 0.005$) and longer overall survival (HR 0.44, $p = 0.007$) compared to the other regimens. The highest treatment-related mortality (TRM) was observed with hyperCVAD/MA (hyperfractionated cyclophosphamide, vincristine, doxorubicin, and dexamethasone, followed by high-dose methotrexate) (18%), followed by DA-EPOCH (13%) and CODOX-M/IVAC (7%). DA-EPOCH-R, on the other hand, resulted in a higher 3-year CNS recurrence (HR 2.52, $p = 0.03$) compared to the other regimens, with no TRM benefit [40].

In the cART era, the prognosis of PBL and PEL remains dismal, with a median overall survival of less than one year [4], although long-term survival can be achieved in selected cases [41]. Of note, in the AMC-075 trial, patients with PBL or PEL treated with DA-EPOCH with/without vorinostat, had 3-year EFS of 60% and 71%, respectively, which compares favorably with poor outcomes in retrospective series [34].

Clinical trials using combined treatment approaches with chemotherapy and targeted therapies such as bortezomib, lenalidomide, or daratumumab are currently in progress.

6. Treatment of Relapsed or Refractory Lymphoma

Since 2000, several prospective studies have demonstrated the safety and the efficacy of HD-chemotherapy with an autologous stem cell transplantation (HDC/ASCT) strategy in relapsed/refractory lymphomas of PLWH, with 3 yr overall survival ranging from 61% to 85% and low treatment-related mortality ($\leq$5%) (Table 4) [42–50]. In retrospective case–control studies, outcomes between PLWH patients and controls were not statistically different [48,51,52]. However, data on long-term PLWH survivors affected by relapsed/refractory lymphoma undergoing HD/ASCT support the need of active surveillance of opportunistic infections (35%) early after HD/ASCT and second cancers (19%) later from ASCT [49].

Table 4. Major prospective and retrospective studies on autologous hematopoietic stem cell transplantation in relapsed/refractory HIV lymphomas. *

References	Patients N°	Study (s) Design	Conditioning Regimen	Follow-Up Median, mos	PFS %	Overall Survival %	TRM %
Gabarre et al., 2004 [50]	14	Prospective Phase 2	BEAM, TBI-based, Bu/Cy	32	NA	5 pts alive	0
Krishnan et al., 2005 [45]	20	Retrospective Case–control s	CBV, TBI/CyEto	32	85	85	5
Serrano et al., 2005 [46]	33	Prospective phase 2	BEAM, BEAC, TBI-based	58	53	61	0
Spitzer et al., 2008 [47]	20	Prospective phase 2	Low dose Bu/Cy	6	49	74	5
Re et al., 2003 [42]	27	Prospective phase 2 s	BEAM	44	76	75	0
Balsalobre et al., 2009 [48]	68	Retrospective multicentric s	BEAM, TBI-based	32	56	61	4
Zanet et al., 2015 [49]	26 CR	Retrospective Single-centric s	BEAM	72	86 (10 yr)	91 (10 yr)	0
Alvarnas et al., 2016 [44]	40	Prospective	BEAM	25	80	82	5

* 166 patients with diffuse large B-cell lymphoma and 82 with Hodgkin lymphoma. PFS: progression free survival; TRM: treatment-related mortality; BEAM: carmustine, etoposide, cytarabine, melphalan; TBI: total body irradiation; Bu/Cy: busulfan/cyclophosphamide; NA: not available; CBV: cyclophosphamide, carmustine, etoposide; CyEto: cytarabine, etoposide; BEAC: carmustine, etoposide, cytarabine, cyclophosphamide; CR: complete response.

Allogenic hematopoietic cell transplant (alloHCT) is an emerging treatment modality for selected PLWH patients with different hematological disorders including refractory lymphomas [53–55]. In one small phase II study, the 1 yr non relapsed mortality rate was 12%, the 1 yr overall survival 59%, and complete donor chimerism was 69% at 6 months. However, alloHCT was limited by the risk of graft-versus-host disease (grade 2–4 44%), severe infectious complications (47%), or unexpected adverse events (82%) [54]. It is noteworthy that there have been two cases of a virological cure of HIV after alloHCT using CCR5Δ32 homozygous donors [53,56].

Chimeric antigen receptor (CAR) T-cell therapy, originally studied as an HIV eradication therapy without significant efficacy, is an alternative for the treatment of highly refractory lymphomas in the general population. To date, severe toxicity and logistical problems limit its use in HIV-lymphoma patients [57]. Notably, bispecific CAR (duoCAR T cells) reduced cellular HIV infection in a humanized mouse model by 97% [58]. Future studies should investigate the role of multitarget CAR T cells in HIV-lymphoma patients.

7. Hodgkin Lymphoma

It has been reported that HL incidence was growing among PLWH patients on cART, specifically during immune reconstitution inflammatory syndrome [59–61]. However, recent reports have shown stabilizing/slightly declining rates of HL in PLWH [62,63]. Patients typically present moderate immune deficiency, B symptoms, and advanced stages involving bone marrow, liver, and spleen [13]. Involvement of bone marrow by HL at diagnosis (i.e., primary bone marrow HL) was found in 3–14% of cases and was characterized by an aggressive clinical course [64]. Noteworthy involvement of bone marrow by HL at diagnosis was found in 61% of cases in an HIV endemic setting [65].

A stage-adopted pretreatment approach is the current therapy for HL regardless of HIV status. Treatment with ABVD regimen (doxorubicin, bleomycin, vinblastine, dacarbazine) has been shown to be safe and effective (CR rate 74%, 5-year overall survival 81%) in PLWH with HL. Good results have also been reported with BEACOP (bleomycin, etoposide, doxorubicin, cyclophosphamide, vincristine, procarbazine, and prednisolone) with a CR rate of 86% and 2-year overall survival of 91% in PLWH with advanced HL. However, BEACOPP is rarely used in frontline therapy because of its high toxicity (dose reduction/delay > 50%, TMR 6%) [5,66].

Risk-adjusted therapy on the basis of baseline fluorodeoxyglucose position emission tomography (FDG-PET) may be an appropriate standardized approach in patients with HIV-HL as in the general population. Preliminary data suggest that a negative interim PET (after two chemotherapy courses) may be predictive of higher PFS in HIV-HL patients but needs confirmation [67,68]. Recently, in a large series of PLWH with HL with a homogeneous management, a high total metabolic tumor volume (TMTV > 527 cm^3) on baseline FDG-PET was the only parameter associated with a poorer PFS (2-year PFS 71% vs. 91% in patients with TMTV $\leq$ 527) [69].

Patients with relapsed/refractory HL on effective cART should be treated with salvage chemotherapy followed by ASCT. In a phase 2 trial the combination of brentuximab vedotin and AVD (doxorubicin, vinblastine, and dacarbazine) was safe and effective, with 2-year PFS 86% and 2-year overall survival 92%. There are only limited data on immune checkpoint inhibitors (ICIs) in HIV-HL patients since they have been excluded from all clinical trials in the general population [5]. The results of two clinical trials support the safety and efficacy on ICIs in PWLH with advanced cancers, without a negative impact on HIV viremia and CD4 cell count [70,71].

8. Multicentric Castleman Disease

KSHV-MCD is a remitting B-cell lymphoid disorder, usually occurring in PLWH on cART, that if untreated is usually fatal. The disease is characterized by an elevated KSHV viral load and increased serum levels of cytokines including viral IL-6, systemic inflammatory symptoms, multiple lymphadenopathies, organomegaly, and laboratory abnormalities. KSHV-MCD simultaneously occurs together with other KSHV- and EBV- associated disorders (see above).

Rituximab-based therapy is the standard of care, resulting in a 5-year overall survival rate of 90% and an 11-fold lower risk of developing lymphoma. Patients with concurrent KS and MCD require rituximab plus pegylated liposomal doxorubicin because KS can be reactivated by rituximab [12]. Recently, a series of 62 PLWH with KSHV-MCD reported long-term survival with 10-year survival rates of 73% and 81% for patients without and with KS, respectively. Notably, patients who received rituximab plus doxorubicin followed by maintenance therapy with high-dose zidovudine and valganciclovir or alpha-IFN had the best 5-year PFS (89%) [4,72]. To date, the overall benefit of maintenance therapy remains unclear. Intermittent rituximab therapy for relapsed disease may be a reasonable alternative strategy for prolonged disease management. A multidimensional approach is needed in this complex disease.

9. Preventive Measures

Early cART access and maintenance of immune recovery in PLWH is still the key strategy to prevent infectious-related malignancies, including lymphoma [73]. This benefit may be linked to CD4 cell recovery as well as to different mechanisms impacting coinfections with oncogenic viruses [73,74].

Today the survival of many PLWH with cancer is approaching that of the general population. Surveillance programs should be carried out in cancer survivors because they are at increased risk for SPC, probably due to persistence of the etiological agents as well as the immunosuppressive/carcinogenic effects of treatments [23–26]. Population-based linkage studies found that 9% of all HIV-associated cancers in the United States and Europe were second or subsequent cancers, a similar proportion but with higher incidence than in the general population [24,27]. From 1990 to 2010, the standardized incidence ratio (SIR) for SPCs was elevated for Kaposi's sarcoma (28.0), anal cancer (17.0), NHL (11.1), HL (5.4), and liver cancer (3.6) in the US-population-based linkage study [24]. Of note, the pattern of SPCs differs by first primary cancer and by sex [25,27,75]. A large linkage study (1996–2015) found an increased risk of second primary non-lymphoid cancers after lymphoid malignancy, particularly myeloid malignancies, Kaposi's sarcoma, and HPV-associated cancers, including anal, vaginal/vulvar, and rectal squamous cell carcinomas [25]. In a population-based cancer registry study in the United States, anal cancer risk was particularly high in DLBCL survivors with HIV (SIR 68) compared with survivors without HIV (SIR 2.09) [75]. Long-term persistence of HPV, particularly high-risk HPV, is more common in PWLH than in the general population and correlates with low CD4 count [76].

To date, there is a lack of appropriate prevention and screening programs for SPCs. Nevertheless, preventive measures such as immunization (HPV and HBV vaccination), antiviral therapy (HCV), and early disease detection through screening programs (Table 5) should be recommended for all PLWH including cancer survivors [13,77] (https://aidsinfo.nih.gov/guidelines/html/4/adult and adolescent.oi-prevention and treatment guidelines (accessed on 26 July 2022); www.nccn.org (accessed on 26 July 2022)).

At present, the new SARS-CoV-2 and COVID-19 pandemic represent a global public health crisis. Large cohort studies have shown that patients with cancer, especially hematological malignancies, are at high risk for COVID-19-associated complications [78].

International guidelines recommend three doses of mRNA vaccines plus additional booster doses for PWLH with advanced HIV infection and/or cancers. Pre-exposure prevention with monoclonal antibodies (tikagevimab plus cilgavimab) is recommended for immunocompromised patients (www.nccn.org (accessed on 26 July 2022)). Close vigilance and monitoring during antineoplastic treatment and persistent HIV care are mandatory.

Table 5. Prevention and screening programs for common solid tumors in persons living with HIV (PLWH).

Cancer	Prevention	Patients at Risk	Screening Methods	Screening Frequency
Cervical cancer	HPV vaccination *	-Sexually active women -Age ≥ 21 yrs	Pap Testing (PT) Co-testing (Pap Testing+HPV Testing) Colposcopy (C)	-Age < 30 yrs: baseline, every 12 mos until 3 normal PTs, then every 3 yrs -Age ≥ 30 yrs: baseline, every 12 mos until 3 normal PTs, then every 3 yrs or every 3 yrs if normal co-testing -Annualy co-testing if normal PT and positive HR-HPV testing -Performed C if abnormal PT or positive HR-HPV testing
Anal cancer	HPV vaccination *	-All PLWHs -MSM -All PLWHs with a history of anogenital condylomas -Women with abnormal genital histology	-Visual inspection of perianal region plus digital rectal examination Anal Pap Testing (aPT) -HRA **	-Annually -Baseline and annually, every 3–6 mos if abnormal aPT -Performed HRA if abnormal aPT (ASCUS, LSIL, HSIL)
Liver cancer	-HBV vaccination -HBV/HCV therapy -Alcohol cessation	-HCV/HIV with cirrhosis -HBV/HIV resistant to antiviral therapy	Abdominal ultrasonography+/-AFP testing	-Every 6–12 mos
Lung cancer	Smoking cessation	-Smokers > 20 pack-year -Current or former smokers who quit smoking within 10 yrs and age > 40 yrs	Low-dose chest CT	Annually
Skin cancer	Reduction/protection sun exposure	-Fair skin -White/non-Hispanic ethnicity	Skin examination	Annually

* The WHO recommends vaccination of preadolescent girls and boys long before HIV infection; the CDC recommends three doses of HPV vaccine in all women ≤ 26 years, in all men ≤ 21 years, and in MSM or individuals with a compromised immune system (including HIV) through age 26 years if not received earlier. ** in MSM, the highest anal cancer risk group, the most cost-effective screening modality is primary HRA. Abbreviations: AFP, a-fetoprotein; ASCUS, atypical squamous cells of undetermined significance; HBV hepatitis B virus; HCV, hepatitis C virus; HPV, Human Papilloma virus; HRA, high resolution anoscopy; HSIL, high-grade squamous intraepithelial lesion; LSIL, low-grade intraepithelial lesion; MSM, men who have sex with men; Pap, Papanicolaou cytology.

10. Concluding Remarks

Lymphomas occurring in PLWH have been included in "The International Consensus Classification of Mature Lymphoid Neoplasms" [10]. Their clear inclusion will result in consensus treatment protocols leading to further improvements in outcomes. Moreover, novel therapeutic strategies targeting EBV and KSHV will be further investigated in pre-clinical research. As multiple KSHV-associated malignancies and EBV-associated disorders may be present in PLWH, careful pathological review, using suitable immunohistochemical panels, is critical for the correct diagnosis, thus, ensuring optimal treatment and outcomes for patients with KSHV-MCD. Importantly, it is recommended that the treatment choice for PLWH affected by lymphoma, and receiving effective cART, should not be influenced by HIV status.

Author Contributions: A.C. designed the work, wrote the manuscript. E.V., A.G. and C.C.V. wrote the manuscript. All authors have read and agreed to the published version of the manuscript.

Funding: This research received no external funding.

Institutional Review Board statement: Not applicable.

Informed consent statement: Not applicable.

Data availability statement: Not applicable.

Conflicts of Interest: The authors declare no conflict of interest.

References

1. Polesel, J.; Clifford, G.M.; Rickenbach, M.; Dal Maso, L.; Battegay, M.; Bouchardy, C.; Furrer, H.; Hasse, B.; Levi, F.; Probst-Hensch, N.M.; et al. Non-Hodgkin lymphoma incidence in the Swiss HIV Cohort Study before and after highly active antiretroviral therapy. *AIDS* **2008**, *22*, 301–306. [CrossRef] [PubMed]
2. Simard, E.P.; Pfeiffer, R.M.; Engels, E.A. Cumulative incidence of cancer among individuals with acquired immunodeficiency syndrome in the United States. *Cancer* **2011**, *117*, 1089–1096. [CrossRef] [PubMed]

3. Han, X.; Jemal, A.; Hulland, E.; Simard, E.P.; Nastoupil, L.; Ward, E.; Flowers, C.R. HIV Infection and Survival of Lymphoma Patients in the Era of Highly Active Antiretroviral Therapy. *Cancer Epidemiol. Biomark. Prev.* **2017**, *26*, 303–311. [CrossRef]
4. Carbone, A.; Vaccher, E.; Gloghini, A. Hematologic cancers in individuals infected by HIV. *Blood* **2022**, *139*, 995–1012. [CrossRef] [PubMed]
5. Carbone, A.; Gloghini, A.; Serraino, D.; Spina, M.; Tirelli, U.; Vaccher, E. Immunodeficiency-associated Hodgkin lymphoma. *Expert Rev. Hematol.* **2021**, *14*, 547–559. [CrossRef]
6. Cesarman, E.; Chadburn, A.; Rubinstein, P.G. KSHV/HHV8-mediated hematologic diseases. *Blood* **2022**, *139*, 1013–1025. [CrossRef]
7. Toner, K.; Bollard, C.M. EBV+ lymphoproliferative diseases: Opportunities for leveraging EBV as a therapeutic target. *Blood* **2022**, *139*, 983–994. [CrossRef]
8. Said, J.; Cesarman, E.; Rosenwald, A.; Harris, N. Lymphomas associated with HIV infection. In *WHO Classification of Tumours of Haematopoietic and Lymphoid Tissues*; Swerdlow, S.H., Campo, E., Harris, N.L., Jaffe, E.S., Stein, H., Arber, D.A., Hasserjian, R.P., Beau, L., et al., Eds.; International Agency for Research on Cancer: Lyon, France, 2017; pp. 449–452.
9. Bower, M.; Carbone, A. KSHV/HHV8-Associated Lymphoproliferative Disorders: Lessons Learnt from People Living with HIV. *Hemato* **2021**, *2*, 703–712. [CrossRef]
10. Campo, E.; Jaffe, E.S.; Cook, J.R.; Quintanilla-Martinez, L.; Swerdlow, S.H.; Anderson, K.C.; Brousset, P.; Cerroni, L.; de Leval, L.; Dirnhofer, S.; et al. The International Consensus Classification of Mature Lymphoid Neoplasms: A Report from the Clinical Advisory Committee. *Blood* **2022**. [CrossRef]
11. Chen, X.; Jia, L.; Zhang, X.; Zhang, T.; Zhang, Y. One arrow for two targets: Potential co-treatment regimens for lymphoma and HIV. *Blood Rev.* **2022**, 100965. [CrossRef]
12. Carbone, A.; Borok, M.; Damania, B.; Gloghini, A.; Polizzotto, M.N.; Jayanthan, R.K.; Fajgenbaum, D.C.; Bower, M. Castleman disease. *Nat. Rev. Dis. Primers* **2021**, *7*, 84. [CrossRef] [PubMed]
13. Carbone, A.; Vaccher, E.; Gloghini, A.; Pantanowitz, L.; Abayomi, A.; de Paoli, P.; Franceschi, S. Diagnosis and management of lymphomas and other cancers in HIV-infected patients. *Nat. Rev. Clin. Oncol.* **2014**, *11*, 223–238. [CrossRef] [PubMed]
14. Du, M.Q.; Diss, T.C.; Liu, H.; Ye, H.; Hamoudi, R.A.; Cabeçadas, J.; Dong, H.Y.; Harris, N.L.; Chan, J.K.; Rees, J.W.; et al. KSHV- and EBV-associated germinotropic lymphoproliferative disorder. *Blood* **2002**, *100*, 3415–3418. [CrossRef] [PubMed]
15. Natkunam, Y.; Gratzinger, D.; Chadburn, A.; Goodlad, J.R.; Chan, J.K.C.; Said, J.; Jaffe, E.S.; de Jong, D. Immunodeficiency-associated lymphoproliferative disorders: Time for reappraisal? *Blood* **2018**, *132*, 1871–1878. [CrossRef]
16. Gopal, S.; Patel, M.R.; Yanik, E.L.; Cole, S.R.; Achenbach, C.J.; Napravnik, S.; Burkholder, G.A.; Reid, E.G.; Rodriguez, B.; Deeks, S.G.; et al. Temporal trends in presentation and survival for HIV-associated lymphoma in the antiretroviral therapy era. *J. Natl. Cancer Inst.* **2013**, *105*, 1221–1229. [CrossRef]
17. Yarchoan, R.; Uldrick, T.S. HIV-Associated Cancers and Related Diseases. *N. Engl. J. Med.* **2018**, *378*, 1029–1041. [CrossRef]
18. Noy, A. Optimizing treatment of HIV-associated lymphoma. *Blood* **2019**, *134*, 1385–1394. [CrossRef]
19. Ramaswami, R.; Chia, G.; Dalla Pria, A.; Pinato, D.J.; Parker, K.; Nelson, M.; Bower, M. Evolution of HIV-Associated Lymphoma Over 3 Decades. *J. Acquir. Immune Defic. Syndr.* **2016**, *72*, 177–183. [CrossRef]
20. Horner, M.J.; Shiels, M.S.; Pfeiffer, R.M.; Engels, E.A. Deaths Attributable to Cancer in the US Human Immunodeficiency Virus Population During 2001–2015. *Clin. Infect. Dis.* **2021**, *72*, e224–e231. [CrossRef]
21. Olszewski, A.J.; Jakobsen, L.H.; Collins, G.P.; Cwynarski, K.; Bachanova, V.; Blum, K.A.; Boughan, K.M.; Bower, M.; Dalla Pria, A.; Danilov, A.; et al. Burkitt Lymphoma International Prognostic Index. *J. Clin. Oncol.* **2021**, *39*, 1129–1138. [CrossRef]
22. Yarchoan, R.; Ramaswami, R.; Lurain, K. HIV-associated malignancies at 40: Much accomplished but much to do. *Glob. Health Med.* **2021**, *3*, 184–186. [CrossRef] [PubMed]
23. Mukhtar, F.; Ilozumba, M.; Utuama, O.; Cimenler, O. Change in Pattern of Secondary Cancers After Kaposi Sarcoma in the Era of Antiretroviral Therapy. *JAMA Oncol.* **2018**, *4*, 48–53. [CrossRef] [PubMed]
24. Hessol, N.A.; Whittemore, H.; Vittinghoff, E.; Hsu, L.C.; Ma, D.; Scheer, S.; Schwarcz, S.K. Incidence of first and second primary cancers diagnosed among people with HIV, 1985-2013: A population-based, registry linkage study. *Lancet HIV* **2018**, *5*, e647–e655. [CrossRef]
25. Mahale, P.; Ugoji, C.; Engels, E.A.; Shiels, M.S.; Peprah, S.; Morton, L.M. Cancer risk following lymphoid malignancies among HIV-infected people. *AIDS* **2020**, *34*, 1237–1245. [CrossRef]
26. Abrahão, R.; Li, Q.W.; Malogolowkin, M.H.; Alvarez, E.M.; Ribeiro, R.C.; Wun, T.; Keegan, T.H.M. Chronic medical conditions and late effects following non-Hodgkin lymphoma in HIV-uninfected and HIV-infected adolescents and young adults: A population-based study. *Br. J. Haematol.* **2020**, *190*, 371–384. [CrossRef]
27. Poizot-Martin, I.; Lions, C.; Delpierre, C.; Makinson, A.; Allavena, C.; Fresard, A.; Brégigeon, S.; Rojas Rojas, T.; Delobel, P.; Group The Dat, A.S. Prevalence and Spectrum of Second Primary Malignancies among People Living with HIV in the French Dat'AIDS Cohort. *Cancers* **2022**, *14*, 401. [CrossRef]
28. Kaplan, L.D.; Lee, J.Y.; Ambinder, R.F.; Sparano, J.A.; Cesarman, E.; Chadburn, A.; Levine, A.M.; Scadden, D.T. Rituximab does not improve clinical outcome in a randomized phase 3 trial of CHOP with or without rituximab in patients with HIV-associated non-Hodgkin lymphoma: AIDS-Malignancies Consortium Trial 010. *Blood* **2005**, *106*, 1538–1543. [CrossRef]

29. Sparano, J.A.; Lee, J.Y.; Kaplan, L.D.; Levine, A.M.; Ramos, J.C.; Ambinder, R.F.; Wachsman, W.; Aboulafia, D.; Noy, A.; Henry, D.H.; et al. Rituximab plus concurrent infusional EPOCH chemotherapy is highly effective in HIV-associated B-cell non-Hodgkin lymphoma. *Blood* **2010**, *115*, 3008–3016. [CrossRef]
30. Dunleavy, K.; Little, R.F.; Pittaluga, S.; Grant, N.; Wayne, A.S.; Carrasquillo, J.A.; Steinberg, S.M.; Yarchoan, R.; Jaffe, E.S.; Wilson, W.H. The role of tumor histogenesis, FDG-PET, and short-course EPOCH with dose-dense rituximab (SC-EPOCH-RR) in HIV-associated diffuse large B-cell lymphoma. *Blood* **2010**, *115*, 3017–3024. [CrossRef]
31. Boué, F.; Gabarre, J.; Gisselbrecht, C.; Reynes, J.; Cheret, A.; Bonnet, F.; Billaud, E.; Raphael, M.; Lancar, R.; Costagliola, D. Phase II trial of CHOP plus rituximab in patients with HIV-associated non-Hodgkin's lymphoma. *J. Clin. Oncol.* **2006**, *24*, 4123–4128. [CrossRef]
32. Ribera, J.M.; Oriol, A.; Morgades, M.; González-Barca, E.; Miralles, P.; López-Guillermo, A.; Gardella, S.; López, A.; Abella, E.; García, M. Safety and efficacy of cyclophosphamide, adriamycin, vincristine, prednisone and rituximab in patients with human immunodeficiency virus-associated diffuse large B-cell lymphoma: Results of a phase II trial. *Br. J. Haematol.* **2008**, *140*, 411–419. [CrossRef] [PubMed]
33. Spina, M.; Jaeger, U.; Sparano, J.A.; Talamini, R.; Simonelli, C.; Michieli, M.; Rossi, G.; Nigra, E.; Berretta, M.; Cattaneo, C.; et al. Rituximab plus infusional cyclophosphamide, doxorubicin, and etoposide in HIV-associated non-Hodgkin lymphoma: Pooled results from 3 phase 2 trials. *Blood* **2005**, *105*, 1891–1897. [CrossRef] [PubMed]
34. Ramos, J.C.; Sparano, J.A.; Chadburn, A.; Reid, E.G.; Ambinder, R.F.; Siegel, E.R.; Moore, P.C.; Rubinstein, P.G.; Durand, C.M.; Cesarman, E.; et al. Impact of Myc in HIV-associated non-Hodgkin lymphomas treated with EPOCH and outcomes with vorinostat (AMC-075 trial). *Blood* **2020**, *136*, 1284–1297. [CrossRef] [PubMed]
35. Barta, S.K.; Xue, X.; Wang, D.; Tamari, R.; Lee, J.Y.; Mounier, N.; Kaplan, L.D.; Ribera, J.M.; Spina, M.; Tirelli, U.; et al. Treatment factors affecting outcomes in HIV-associated non-Hodgkin lymphomas: A pooled analysis of 1546 patients. *Blood* **2013**, *122*, 3251–3262. [CrossRef]
36. Bartlett, N.L.; Wilson, W.H.; Jung, S.H.; Hsi, E.D.; Maurer, M.J.; Pederson, L.D.; Polley, M.C.; Pitcher, B.N.; Cheson, B.D.; Kahl, B.S.; et al. Dose-Adjusted EPOCH-R Compared With R-CHOP as Frontline Therapy for Diffuse Large B-Cell Lymphoma: Clinical Outcomes of the Phase III Intergroup Trial Alliance/CALGB 50303. *J. Clin. Oncol.* **2019**, *37*, 1790–1799. [CrossRef]
37. Ramos, J.C.; Sparano, J.A.; Rudek, M.A.; Moore, P.C.; Cesarman, E.; Reid, E.G.; Henry, D.; Ratner, L.; Aboulafia, D.; Lee, J.Y.; et al. Safety and Preliminary Efficacy of Vorinostat With R-EPOCH in High-risk HIV-associated Non-Hodgkin's Lymphoma (AMC-075). *Clin. Lymphoma Myeloma Leuk.* **2018**, *18*, 180–190.e182. [CrossRef]
38. Dunleavy, K.; Pittaluga, S.; Shovlin, M.; Steinberg, S.M.; Cole, D.; Grant, C.; Widemann, B.; Staudt, L.M.; Jaffe, E.S.; Little, R.F.; et al. Low-intensity therapy in adults with Burkitt's lymphoma. *N. Engl. J. Med.* **2013**, *369*, 1915–1925. [CrossRef]
39. Roschewski, M.; Dunleavy, K.; Abramson, J.S.; Powell, B.L.; Link, B.K.; Patel, P.; Bierman, P.J.; Jagadeesh, D.; Mitsuyasu, R.T.; Peace, D.; et al. Multicenter Study of Risk-Adapted Therapy With Dose-Adjusted EPOCH-R in Adults With Untreated Burkitt Lymphoma. *J. Clin. Oncol.* **2020**, *38*, 2519–2529. [CrossRef]
40. Alderuccio, J.P.; Olszewski, A.J.; Evens, A.M.; Collins, G.P.; Danilov, A.V.; Bower, M.; Jagadeesh, D.; Zhu, C.; Sperling, A.; Kim, S.H.; et al. HIV-associated Burkitt lymphoma: Outcomes from a US-UK collaborative analysis. *Blood Adv.* **2021**, *5*, 2852–2862. [CrossRef]
41. Vaccher, E.; Carbone, A. Simultaneous occurrence of KSHV-associated malignancies in a patient affected by HIV. *Blood* **2021**, *137*, 3149. [CrossRef]
42. Re, A.; Cattaneo, C.; Michieli, M.; Casari, S.; Spina, M.; Rupolo, M.; Allione, B.; Nosari, A.; Schiantarelli, C.; Vigano, M.; et al. High-dose therapy and autologous peripheral-blood stem-cell transplantation as salvage treatment for HIV-associated lymphoma in patients receiving highly active antiretroviral therapy. *J. Clin. Oncol.* **2003**, *21*, 4423–4427. [CrossRef] [PubMed]
43. Michieli, M.; Mazzucato, M.; Tirelli, U.; De Paoli, P. Stem cell transplantation for lymphoma patients with HIV infection. *Cell Transpl.* **2011**, *20*, 351–370. [CrossRef] [PubMed]
44. Alvarnas, J.C.; Le Rademacher, J.; Wang, Y.; Little, R.F.; Akpek, G.; Ayala, E.; Devine, S.; Baiocchi, R.; Lozanski, G.; Kaplan, L.; et al. Autologous hematopoietic cell transplantation for HIV-related lymphoma: Results of the BMT CTN 0803/AMC 071 trial. *Blood* **2016**, *128*, 1050–1058. [CrossRef]
45. Krishnan, A.; Molina, A.; Zaia, J.; Smith, D.; Vasquez, D.; Kogut, N.; Falk, P.M.; Rosenthal, J.; Alvarnas, J.; Forman, S.J. Durable remissions with autologous stem cell transplantation for high-risk HIV-associated lymphomas. *Blood* **2005**, *105*, 874–878. [CrossRef] [PubMed]
46. Serrano, D.; Carrión, R.; Balsalobre, P.; Miralles, P.; Berenguer, J.; Buño, I.; Gómez-Pineda, A.; Ribera, J.M.; Conde, E.; Díez-Martín, J.L. HIV-associated lymphoma successfully treated with peripheral blood stem cell transplantation. *Exp. Hematol.* **2005**, *33*, 487–494. [CrossRef] [PubMed]
47. Spitzer, T.R.; Ambinder, R.F.; Lee, J.Y.; Kaplan, L.D.; Wachsman, W.; Straus, D.J.; Aboulafia, D.M.; Scadden, D.T. Dose-reduced busulfan, cyclophosphamide, and autologous stem cell transplantation for human immunodeficiency virus-associated lymphoma: AIDS Malignancy Consortium study 020. *Biol. Blood Marrow Transpl.* **2008**, *14*, 59–66. [CrossRef] [PubMed]
48. Balsalobre, P.; Díez-Martín, J.L.; Re, A.; Michieli, M.; Ribera, J.M.; Canals, C.; Rosselet, A.; Conde, E.; Varela, R.; Cwynarski, K.; et al. Autologous stem-cell transplantation in patients with HIV-related lymphoma. *J. Clin. Oncol.* **2009**, *27*, 2192–2198. [CrossRef]

49. Zanet, E.; Taborelli, M.; Rupolo, M.; Durante, C.; Mazzucato, M.; Zanussi, S.; De Paoli, P.; Serraino, D.; Tirelli, U.; Lleshi, A.; et al. Postautologous stem cell transplantation long-term outcomes in 26 HIV-positive patients affected by relapsed/refractory lymphoma. *AIDS* **2015**, *29*, 2303–2308. [CrossRef]
50. Gabarre, J.; Marcelin, A.G.; Azar, N.; Choquet, S.; Lévy, V.; Lévy, Y.; Tubiana, R.; Charlotte, F.; Norol, F.; Calvez, V.; et al. High-dose therapy plus autologous hematopoietic stem cell transplantation for human immunodeficiency virus (HIV)-related lymphoma: Results and impact on HIV disease. *Haematologica* **2004**, *89*, 1100–1108.
51. Díez-Martín, J.L.; Balsalobre, P.; Re, A.; Michieli, M.; Ribera, J.M.; Canals, C.; Conde, E.; Rosselet, A.; Gabriel, I.; Varela, R.; et al. Comparable survival between HIV+ and HIV- non-Hodgkin and Hodgkin lymphoma patients undergoing autologous peripheral blood stem cell transplantation. *Blood* **2009**, *113*, 6011–6014. [CrossRef]
52. Krishnan, A.; Palmer, J.M.; Zaia, J.A.; Tsai, N.C.; Alvarnas, J.; Forman, S.J. HIV status does not affect the outcome of autologous stem cell transplantation (ASCT) for non-Hodgkin lymphoma (NHL). *Biol. Blood Marrow Transpl.* **2010**, *16*, 1302–1308. [CrossRef] [PubMed]
53. Gupta, R.K.; Abdul-Jawad, S.; McCoy, L.E.; Mok, H.P.; Peppa, D.; Salgado, M.; Martinez-Picado, J.; Nijhuis, M.; Wensing, A.M.J.; Lee, H.; et al. HIV-1 remission following CCR5Δ32/Δ32 haematopoietic stem-cell transplantation. *Nature* **2019**, *568*, 244–248. [CrossRef] [PubMed]
54. Ambinder, R.F.; Wu, J.; Logan, B.; Durand, C.M.; Shields, R.; Popat, U.R.; Little, R.F.; McMahon, D.K.; Cyktor, J.; Mellors, J.W.; et al. Allogeneic Hematopoietic Cell Transplant for HIV Patients with Hematologic Malignancies: The BMT CTN-0903/AMC-080 Trial. *Biol. Blood Marrow Transpl.* **2019**, *25*, 2160–2166. [CrossRef]
55. Kwon, M.; Bailén, R.; Balsalobre, P.; Jurado, M.; Bermudez, A.; Badiola, J.; Esquirol, A.; Miralles, P.; López-Fernández, E.; Sanz, J.; et al. Allogeneic stem-cell transplantation in HIV-1-infected patients with high-risk hematological disorders. *AIDS* **2019**, *33*, 1441–1447. [CrossRef] [PubMed]
56. Allers, K.; Hütter, G.; Hofmann, J.; Loddenkemper, C.; Rieger, K.; Thiel, E.; Schneider, T. Evidence for the cure of HIV infection by CCR5Δ32/Δ32 stem cell transplantation. *Blood* **2011**, *117*, 2791–2799. [CrossRef] [PubMed]
57. Rust, B.J.; Kiem, H.P.; Uldrick, T.S. CAR T-cell therapy for cancer and HIV through novel approaches to HIV-associated haematological malignancies. *Lancet Haematol.* **2020**, *7*, e690–e696. [CrossRef]
58. Anthony-Gonda, K.; Bardhi, A.; Ray, A.; Flerin, N.; Li, M.; Chen, W.; Ochsenbauer, C.; Kappes, J.C.; Krueger, W.; Worden, A.; et al. Multispecific anti-HIV duoCAR-T cells display broad in vitro antiviral activity and potent in vivo elimination of HIV-infected cells in a humanized mouse model. *Sci. Transl. Med.* **2019**, *11*, eaav5685. [CrossRef]
59. Bohlius, J.; Schmidlin, K.; Boué, F.; Fätkenheuer, G.; May, M.; Caro-Murillo, A.M.; Mocroft, A.; Bonnet, F.; Clifford, G.; Paparizos, V.; et al. HIV-1-related Hodgkin lymphoma in the era of combination antiretroviral therapy: Incidence and evolution of CD4[+] T-cell lymphocytes. *Blood* **2011**, *117*, 6100–6108. [CrossRef]
60. Goedert, J.J.; Bower, M. Impact of highly effective antiretroviral therapy on the risk for Hodgkin lymphoma among people with human immunodeficiency virus infection. *Curr. Opin. Oncol.* **2012**, *24*, 531–536. [CrossRef]
61. Kowalkowski, M.A.; Mims, M.P.; Amiran, E.S.; Lulla, P.; Chiao, E.Y. Effect of immune reconstitution on the incidence of HIV-related Hodgkin lymphoma. *PLoS ONE* **2013**, *8*, e77409. [CrossRef]
62. Shiels, M.S.; Islam, J.Y.; Rosenberg, P.S.; Hall, H.I.; Jacobson, E.; Engels, E.A. Projected Cancer Incidence Rates and Burden of Incident Cancer Cases in HIV-Infected Adults in the United States Through 2030. *Ann. Intern. Med.* **2018**, *168*, 866–873. [CrossRef] [PubMed]
63. Kimani, S.M.; Painschab, M.S.; Horner, M.J.; Muchengeti, M.; Fedoriw, Y.; Shiels, M.S.; Gopal, S. Epidemiology of haematological malignancies in people living with HIV. *Lancet HIV* **2020**, *7*, e641–e651. [CrossRef]
64. Martis, N.; Mounier, N. Hodgkin lymphoma in patients with HIV infection: A review. *Curr. Hematol. Malig. Rep.* **2012**, *7*, 228–234. [CrossRef] [PubMed]
65. Swart, L.; Novitzky, N.; Mohamed, Z.; Opie, J. Hodgkin lymphoma at Groote Schuur Hospital, South Africa: The effect of HIV and bone marrow infiltration. *Ann. Hematol.* **2019**, *98*, 381–389. [CrossRef] [PubMed]
66. Moahi, K.; Ralefala, T.; Nkele, I.; Triedman, S.; Sohani, A.; Musimar, Z.; Efstathiou, J.; Armand, P.; Lockman, S.; Dryden-Peterson, S. HIV and Hodgkin Lymphoma Survival: A Prospective Study in Botswana. *JCO Glob. Oncol.* **2022**, *8*, e2100163. [CrossRef]
67. Okosun, J.; Warbey, V.; Shaw, K.; Montoto, S.; Fields, P.; Marcus, R.; Virchis, A.; McNamara, C.; Bower, M.; Cwynarski, K. Interim fluoro-2-deoxy-D-glucose-PET predicts response and progression-free survival in patients with Hodgkin lymphoma and HIV infection. *AIDS* **2012**, *26*, 861–865. [CrossRef]
68. Danilov, A.V.; Li, H.; Press, O.W.; Shapira, I.; Swinnen, L.J.; Noy, A.; Reid, E.; Smith, S.M.; Friedberg, J.W. Feasibility of interim positron emission tomography (PET)-adapted therapy in HIV-positive patients with advanced Hodgkin lymphoma (HL): A sub-analysis of SWOG S0816 Phase 2 trial. *Leuk. Lymphoma* **2017**, *58*, 461–465. [CrossRef]
69. Louarn, N.; Galicier, L.; Bertinchamp, R.; Lussato, D.; Montravers, F.; Oksenhendler, É.; Merlet, P.; Gérard, L.; Vercellino, L. First Extensive Analysis of (18)F-Labeled Fluorodeoxyglucose Positron Emission Tomography-Computed Tomography in a Large Cohort of Patients With HIV-Associated Hodgkin Lymphoma: Baseline Total Metabolic Tumor Volume Affects Prognosis. *J. Clin. Oncol.* **2022**, *40*, 1346–1355. [CrossRef]
70. Uldrick, T.S.; Gonçalves, P.H.; Abdul-Hay, M.; Claeys, A.J.; Emu, B.; Ernstoff, M.S.; Fling, S.P.; Fong, L.; Kaiser, J.C.; Lacroix, A.M.; et al. Assessment of the Safety of Pembrolizumab in Patients With HIV and Advanced Cancer-A Phase 1 Study. *JAMA Oncol.* **2019**, *5*, 1332–1339. [CrossRef]

71. Gonzalez-Cao, M.; Morán, T.; Dalmau, J.; Garcia-Corbacho, J.; Bracht, J.W.P.; Bernabe, R.; Juan, O.; de Castro, J.; Blanco, R.; Drozdowskyj, A.; et al. Assessment of the Feasibility and Safety of Durvalumab for Treatment of Solid Tumors in Patients With HIV-1 Infection: The Phase 2 DURVAST Study. *JAMA Oncol.* **2020**, *6*, 1063–1067. [CrossRef]
72. Ramaswami, R.; Lurain, K.; Polizzotto, M.N.; Ekwede, I.; Waldon, K.; Steinberg, S.M.; Mangusan, R.; Widell, A.; Rupert, A.; George, J.; et al. Characteristics and outcomes of KSHV-associated multicentric Castleman disease with or without other KSHV diseases. *Blood Adv.* **2021**, *5*, 1660–1670. [CrossRef] [PubMed]
73. Borges, Á.H.; Neuhaus, J.; Babiker, A.G.; Henry, K.; Jain, M.K.; Palfreeman, A.; Mugyenyi, P.; Domingo, P.; Hoffmann, C.; Read, T.R.; et al. Immediate Antiretroviral Therapy Reduces Risk of Infection-Related Cancer During Early HIV Infection. *Clin. Infect. Dis.* **2016**, *63*, 1668–1676. [CrossRef] [PubMed]
74. Lundgren, J.D.; Babiker, A.G.; Gordin, F.; Emery, S.; Grund, B.; Sharma, S.; Avihingsanon, A.; Cooper, D.A.; Fätkenheuer, G.; Llibre, J.M.; et al. Initiation of Antiretroviral Therapy in Early Asymptomatic HIV Infection. *N. Engl. J. Med.* **2015**, *373*, 795–807. [CrossRef] [PubMed]
75. Herr, M.M.; Schonfeld, S.J.; Dores, G.M.; Engels, E.A.; Tucker, M.A.; Curtis, R.E.; Morton, L.M. Risk for malignancies of infectious etiology among adult survivors of specific non-Hodgkin lymphoma subtypes. *Blood Adv.* **2019**, *3*, 1961–1969. [CrossRef]
76. Pérez-González, A.; Cachay, E.; Ocampo, A.; Poveda, E. Update on the Epidemiological Features and Clinical Implications of Human Papillomavirus Infection (HPV) and Human Immunodeficiency Virus (HIV) Coinfection. *Microorganisms* **2022**, *10*, 1047. [CrossRef]
77. Osarogiagbon, R.U.; Liao, W.; Faris, N.R.; Meadows-Taylor, M.; Fehnel, C.; Lane, J.; Williams, S.C.; Patel, A.A.; Akinbobola, O.A.; Pacheco, A.; et al. Lung Cancer Diagnosed Through Screening, Lung Nodule, and Neither Program: A Prospective Observational Study of the Detecting Early Lung Cancer (DELUGE) in the Mississippi Delta Cohort. *J. Clin. Oncol.* **2022**, *40*, 2094–2105. [CrossRef]
78. Lee, L.Y.; Cazier, J.B.; Angelis, V.; Arnold, R.; Bisht, V.; Campton, N.A.; Chackathayil, J.; Cheng, V.W.; Curley, H.M.; Fittall, M.W.; et al. COVID-19 mortality in patients with cancer on chemotherapy or other anticancer treatments: A prospective cohort study. *Lancet* **2020**, *395*, 1919–1926. [CrossRef]

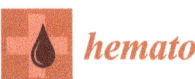

Review

KSHV/HHV8-Associated Lymphoproliferative Disorders: Lessons Learnt from People Living with HIV

Mark Bower [1] and Antonino Carbone [2,*]

[1] Department of Oncology and National Centre for HIV Malignancy, Chelsea & Westminster Hospital, London SW10 9NH, UK; m.bower@imperial.ac.uk
[2] Department of Pathology, Centro di Riferimento Oncologico di Aviano (CRO), Istituto di Ricovero e Cura a Carattere Scientifico (IRCCS), Via F. Gallini 2, I-33081 Aviano, Italy
* Correspondence: acarbone@cro.it

Abstract: In 1992, Kaposi sarcoma herpesvirus (KSHV/HHV8) was discovered and identified as the causative agent for Kaposi sarcoma. Subsequently, the presence of this virus has been detected in a number of lymphoproliferative disorders in people living with HIV (PLWH), including: KSHV-associated multicentric Castleman disease, primary effusion lymphoma, KSHV-positive diffuse large B-cell lymphoma, and germinotropic lymphoproliferative disorder. Each of these rare entities has subsequently been diagnosed in HIV-negative individuals. The recognition of some of these KSHV/HHV8-associated lymphoproliferative disorders has led to their inclusion in the WHO classification of lymphomas in 2008 and the revision of 2016; however, further revision is under way to update the classification. The relatively recent recognition of these lymphoproliferative disorders and their low incidence, particularly in the HIV-negative population, means that there is little published evidence and consensus on their clinical features and management. The publication of a new WHO classification of lymphomas should yield diagnostic clarity, providing an impetus for retrospective case series and prospective clinical trials in these KSHV/HHV8-associated lymphoproliferative disorders.

Keywords: lymphomas in PLWH; KSHV/HHV8; EBV; lymphoma classification; management; cART

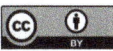

1. Introduction

On 5 June 1981, a report in the Mortality Morbidity Weekly Report (MMWR) of clusters of Pneumocystis pneumonia heralded the AIDS epidemic. Just one month later, on 3 July, a headline on the front page of the New York Times read "Rare cancer seen in 41 homosexuals". It subsequently became apparent that the incidence of Kaposi sarcoma (KS) was increased many thousands of times amongst people living with HIV (PLWH). An epidemiological investigation of Kaposi sarcoma amongst PLWH by Dame Valerie Beral and Harold Jaffe in 1990 pointed to a sexually transmitted infection [1]. In 1994, the novel oncogenic herpes virus known as Kaposi sarcoma herpesvirus (KSHV), or Human herpesvirus 8 (HHV8), was discovered by Yuan Chang and her husband Patrick Moore [2]. Thus, the search for and discovery of this novel oncogenic herpesvirus was led by the clinical observation and scientific analysis of the distribution of KS amongst PLWH.

The evidence that KSHV/HHV8 plays a causal role in the pathogenesis of KS followed shortly after its discovery. Firstly, KSHV/HHV8 is detectable in the malignant spindle cells of all forms of KS, whether associated with HIV infection, allograft recipients, or classical or endemic forms of KS. Secondly, molecular evaluation revealed that KSHV/HHV8 is monoclonal in KS lesions, indicating that KSHV/HHV8 infection precedes the clonal expansion of KS spindle cells [3]. Thirdly, an elegant study demonstrated that the presence of KSHV/HHV8 in the blood of PLWH, prior to the introduction of combination antiretroviral therapy, predicts the subsequent development of KS [4]. Fourthly, the global distribution of KSHV/HHV8 mirrors the prevalence of KS. Finally, the KSHV/HHV8 genome encodes around 90 genes, along with multiple non-coding RNAs, including microRNAs. Several of these viral genes have been pirated from host cells over millennia of co-evolution and possess potentially oncogenic functions.

Following the identification of a causal role for KSHV/HHV8 in KS, the virus was linked to a number of lymphoproliferative diseases. In 1995, the presence of KSHV/HHV8 was detected in a form of plasmablastic multicentric Castleman disease, seen most frequently in PLWH [5]. Similarly, and around the same time, KSHV/HHV8—often in combination with Epstein Barr virus (EBV)—was linked to primary effusion lymphoma (PEL), which was also known as body cavity lymphoma [6,7]. Recent iterations of the WHO classification of haematological malignancy have included KSHV/HHV8-associated diffuse large B-cell lymphomas, which have frequently arisen on a background of KSHV/HHV8-associated multicentric Castleman disease. More recently, in 2002, KSHV/HHV8—along with EBV— was identified in the rare entity germinotropic lymphoproliferative disorder (GLPD) [8]. Interestingly, whilst most KSHV/HHV8-associated lymphoproliferative disorders occur more frequently in PLWH, solid organ allograft recipients, and those from KSHV/HHV8 endemic areas, GLPD is most commonly seen in immunocompetent individuals.

Without the HIV pandemic, the discovery of KSHV/HHV8 would almost certainly have been delayed and the recognition of these KSHV/HHV8-associated lymphoproliferations would undoubtedly have been postponed; although, it is noteworthy that all forms of KSHV/HHV8-associated lymphoproliferations have been described in HIV-negative individuals. The purpose of the review is to analyse KSHV/HHV8-associated lymphoproliferations, considering how oncogenic herpesviruses contribute to the development of lymphomas. Based on the knowledge of these entities, the WHO classification of lymphomas considered the immunodeficiency-related lymphoproliferations and included the spectrum of KSHV/HHV8- and EBV-related disorders in PLWH, as well as in HIV-negative individuals.

2. Pathological and Clinical Features

Tables 1 and 2 show the immunophenotypic markers, virologic associations, and genetic markers of these lymphoproliferative disorders (MCD, PEL, KSHV+DLBCL, and GLPD). Co-infection of KSHV/HHV8 with EBV in tumour cells is present in only two lymphoproliferative disorders, namely PEL and GLPD. These disorders are very different from each other in terms of malignancy (malignant PEL, non-malignant GLPD), aggressiveness, and type of affected people (immunocompromised PEL, immunocompetent GLPD). KSHV/HHV8-related diseases in HIV-positive and HIV-negative subjects are morphologically indistinguishable, but their incidence is higher in PLWH than in the general population.

Table 1. Pathologic spectrum and immunophenotypic markers in KSHV/HHV8-MCD, PEL, KSHV/HHV8-DLBCL, and GLPD.

	CD20	IRF4/MUM1	CD138	Other Positive Cell Markers
Classic PEL	Negative	Positive	Positive	CD30, CD31, CD71, EMA
Solid PEL	Negative	Positive	Positive	CD30, EMA
KSHV/HHV8-MCD-DLBCL	Positive (may be lost)	Positive	Positive	Lambda light chain, CD45
KSHV/HHV8-MCD	Negative	Positive	Negative	CD38, IgM, Lambda light chain
GLPD	Negative	Positive	Positive (may be lost)	Monotypic light chain

Abbreviations: DLBCL—diffuse large B-cell lymphoma; NOS; PEL—primary effusion lymphoma; MCD—multicentric Castleman disease; GLPD—germinotropic lymphoproliferative disorder. Modified and adapted from Carbone et al. [9,10].

Table 2. Virologic association, and genetic features in KSHV/HHV8-MCD, PEL, KSHV/HHV8-DLBCL, and GLPD.

	EBV Infection (Frequency)	KSHV/HHV8 Infection	Genetic Features
Classic PEL	Positive (80–100%)	Positive (100%)	Complex karyotype, no recurrent translocation, *Tp53* and *RAS* rarely mutated
Solid PEL	Positive (80–100%)	Positive (100%)	Occasional p53 positive cells
KSHV/HHV8-MCD-DLBCL	Negative	Positive (100%)	*Myc* rearrangement, *TP53* point mutation
KSHV/HHV8-MCD	Negative	Positive (100%)	
GLPD	Positive (100%)	Positive (100%)	

Abbreviations: DLBCL—diffuse large B-cell lymphoma; PEL—primary effusion lymphoma; MCD—multicentric Castleman disease; GLPD—germinotropic lymphoproliferative disorder; EBV—Epstein Barr Virus; KSHV/HHV8—Kaposi sarcoma-associated herpesvirus. Modified and adapted from Carbone et al. [9,10].

2.1. KSHV/HHV8-Associated Multicentric Castleman Disease (KSHV/HHV8-MCD)

MCD is a generalized lymphoproliferative disease [11] which may display in the lymphoid tissues' interfollicular plasmacytosis or rich intrafollicular or perifollicular vascularity, with hyalinization. KSHV/HHV8-MCD is a plasmablastic variant of MCD (Figure 1) [12,13].

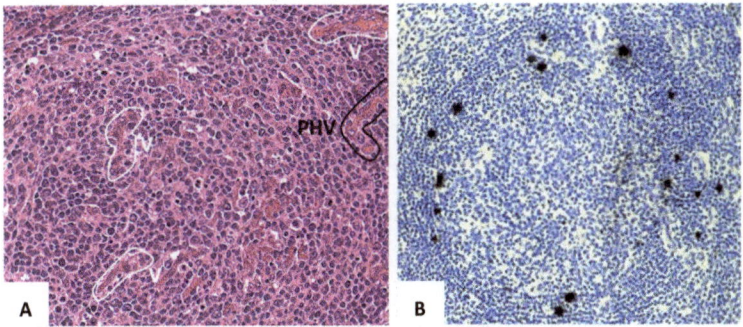

Figure 1. KSHV/HHV8-associated MCD. (**A**) There is a marked intrafollicular vascular proliferation (V). The lymphoid follicle also has typical penetrating hyalinised vessels (PHV). (**B**) In the follicular mantle, some large atypical cells, consistent with plasmablasts, are positive for KSHV/HHV8 viral IL-6. Magnification ×20 (**A**,**B**).

Disorders that morphologically overlap with MCD include follicular hyperplasia, NOS, HIV-associated lymphadenopathy, autoimmune disorders, HL, and plasmacytoma [14].

Patients with KSHV/HHV8-MCD present with marked constitutional symptoms, generalised lymphadenopathy, and splenomegaly. Fever, night sweats, and weight loss are common and up to half the patients have cutaneous or lymph node Kaposi sarcoma. Autoimmune haemolytic anaemia and thrombocytopenia are frequent, alongside hypergammaglobulinemia and hypoalbuminemia. Approximately 10% have features of haemophagocytosis and 10% have pulmonary involvement with ground-glass pneumonitis. KSHV/HHV8-MCD is a relapsing and remitting illness and two clinical criteria have been devised for establishing a diagnosis of active MCD, one from the French ANRS (Agence Nationale de Recherche sur le SIDA) 117 CastlemaB trial group and one from the National Cancer Institute (NCI) [15,16] (see Table 3). The French ANRS definition requires the following: raised serum C-reactive protein (CRP) (in the absence of any other cause), pyrexia, and at least 3 of 12 clinical features [15]. The National Cancer Institute (NCI) scheme requires the following: raised serum CRP, at least one clinical symptom, and one laboratory abnormality probably or definitely attributed to MCD [16]. The serum CRP cut-off is higher in the French (>20 mg/L) than in the US (>3 mg/L) scheme. Although the two systems have been compared in an independent patient population of 75 cases [17], one of the simplest and most reliable laboratory markers of active KSHV/HHV8-MCD is a markedly elevated blood KSVH level.

Table 3. Comparison of French ANRS (Agence Nationale de Recherche sur le SIDA) 117 CastlemaB trial group and the National Cancer Institute (NCI) criteria used to define a flare of KSHV-associated multicentric Castelman disease [15,16].

ANRS Criteria	NCI Criteria
Fever	Fatigue CTAE grade > 1
C-reactive protein > 20 mg/L in the absence of any other aetiology	Fever or night sweats
Peripheral lymphadenopathy	Weight loss
Enlarged spleen	Respiratory symptoms
Oedema	Gastrointestinal symptoms
Pleural effusion	Neurological symptoms
Ascites	Oedema or effusion
Cough	Xerostomia
Nasal obstruction	Rash
Xerostomia	
Rash	
Central neurologic symptoms	Anaemia (Hb < 12 g/dL)
Jaundice	Thrombocytopenia (<100 × 10^9/L)
Autoimmune haemolytic anaemia	Hypoalbuminemia (<35 g/L)
	Serum CRP > 3 mg/L

2.2. Primary Effusion Lymphoma (PEL), Classic, and Solid Variants

PEL is an AIDS-a disease and one third of patients have coincidental Kaposi sarcoma. There is a pathological or clinical overlap between PEL, KSHV/HHV8-MCD, and KSHV/HHV8 inflammatory cytokine syndrome (KICS). KICS is a condition characterized by elevated levels of viral proteins and cytokines, such as MCD. However, KICS is not associated with lymphadenopathy. PEL tumour cells, both in classic form and in solid variant, display a plasmablastic or anaplastic morphology, are positive for latency-associated nuclear antigen 1 (LANA1) (Figure 2), and are often positive for EBV/EBER. They are frequently positive for CD45, CD38, CD138, BLIMP1, VSc38, MUM1, CD30, and EMA.

PEL was first described in 1989 in the context of PLWH [18] and the link with KSHV/HHV8 was discovered in 1995 [6]. As originally defined, PEL is a large B-cell lymphoma presenting in pleural, peritoneal, or pericardial effusions. These effusions are not usually associated with lymphoma masses; although, up to a third of patients have co-existing Kaposi sarcoma. In the early case series of PEL among PLWH, patients were usually young men who have sex with men (MSM) with low CD4 cell counts and the PEL lymphoma cells were co-infected with both KSHV/HHV8 and EBV [19]. Subsequently, PEL was described in solid organ transplant recipients [20] as well as elderly HIV-negative individuals who live in areas of high KSHV/HHV8 prevalence [21,22].

A decade after the original description of PEL, the category was expanded to include extra-cavity solid lymphomas with the same morphology, immunophenotype, and virology [23,24]. These solid PEL have been described in both PLWH and HIV-negative individuals and often present with extra-nodal disease.

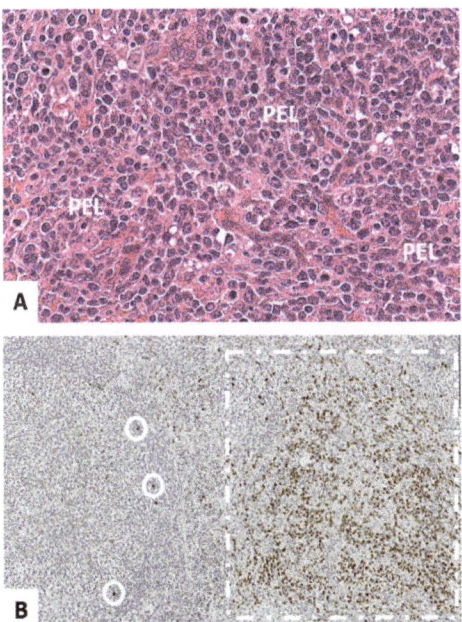

Figure 2. KSHV/HHV8-associated MCD and solid PEL. (**A**) The figure shows large atypical lymphoid cells with plasmablastic morphology, consistent with solid PEL. The tumour cells are negative for CD20 and variably positive for CD138 and CD30 (not shown). (**B**) This lymphoma is involving the lymph node in the interfollicular zone of the lymph node (dashed). Neoplastic cells are positive for LANA. In the follicular mantle, some large, atypical cells, consistent with plasmablasts, are also positive for LANA (circled). Magnification ×40 (**A**), ×20 (**B**).

A recent meta-analysis included 301 cases of whom 181 (63%) occurred in PLWH [25]. Over 90% PEL cases occurred in men, including 85% in HIV-negative individuals and the median age was 55 years (43 years in PLWH and 73 years in HIV-negative individuals). Almost half the cases involved the pleural cavity followed by abdominal cavity (14%) and pericardium (8%) and 28% had involvement of multiple body cavities.

KSHV/HHV8-positive diffuse B-large cell lymphoma, NOS.

KSHV/HHV8-positive diffuse large B-cell lymphoma, NOS is a relatively new lymphoma category, usually arising in association with MCD and HIV infection. The tumour cells display plasmablastic features and are usually positive for CD45 or CD20 and express terminal B-cell differentiation markers, including MUM1. They are often negative for EBV/EBER.

Many of these lymphomas arise in the context of KSHV/HHV8-MCD in PLWH. The risk of lymphoma in patients with KSHV/HHV8-MCD is extremely high and may affect up to one in five patients [26,27], and in one series, lymphoma was the most frequent cause of death [28]. In many cases, the lymphomas were positive for KSVH and most frequently were classified as primary effusion lymphomas and large B-cell lymphomas (KSHV/HHV8-positive DLBCL or NOS in the 2016 WHO classification), both with poor prognoses. KSHV/HHV8-DLBCL is most commonly present with lymphadenopathy and splenomegaly; although, extra-nodal involvement does occur uncommonly. The limited number of cases reported and (to some extent) the relatively recent recognition of this sub-classification means that not only is the optimal therapy uncertain, but the prognosis is also unclear; although, it is a widely held view that the prognosis is worse than KSHV/HHV8-negative DLBCL in the same HIV-positive population.

2.3. KSHV/HHV8-Positive Germinotropic Lymphoproliferative Disorder (GLPD)

GLPD usually presents with localized lymphadenopathy, often without immunodeficiency. A plasmablastic proliferation is confined to expanded germinal centres, which are positive for cytoplasmic monotypic light chain, CD38, MUM1, KSHV/HHV8 viral IL6, LANA1, and EBV/EBER (Figures 3 and 4).

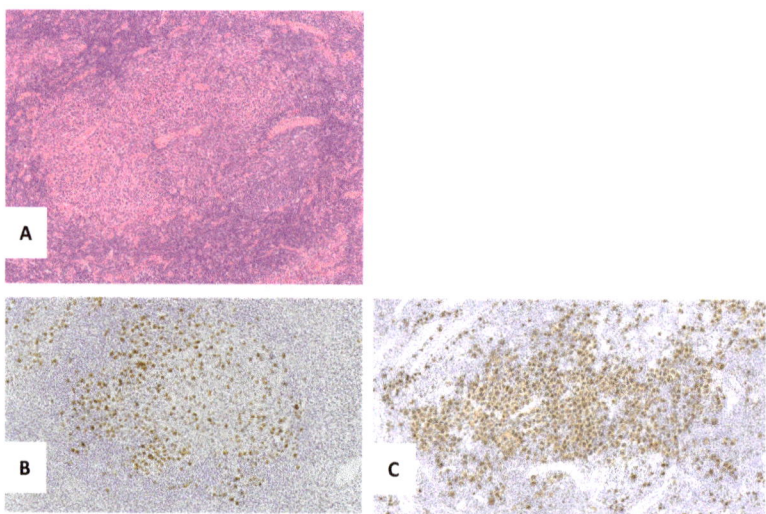

Figure 3. Germinotropic lymphoproliferative disorder. (**A**) The Hematoxylin and Eosin stain shows aggregates of plasmablasts with the involved germinal centres. (**B**) Plasmablasts are positive for MUM1. (**C**) In situ hybridization for EBV-encoded RNA (EBER) shows EBV infection.

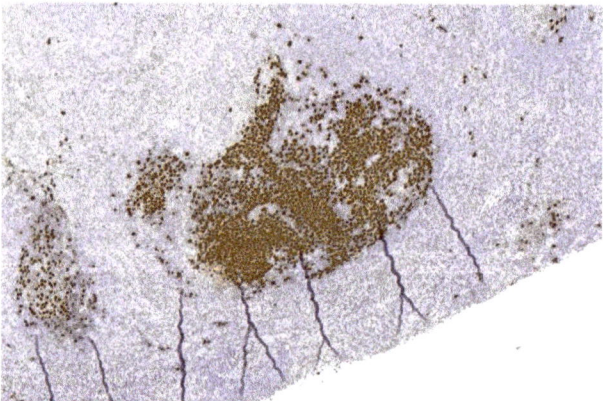

Figure 4. Germinotropic lymphoproliferative disorder. Immunohistochemical stain for KSHV/HHV8-encoded LANA shows co-infection of KSHV/HHV8 in the plasmablasts, within the involved germinal centres.

GLPD is a very rare disease with an indolent clinical course. A systematic review of the published literature in 2020 only identified 19 cases [29], only 5 of which were those of HIV-seropositive individuals. The described cases occurred mostly in middle aged men (68% male, mean age 58) and all presented with nodal involvement. Lymphadenopathy was present in all cases but fewer than half had constitutional symptoms and most of those who did were PLWH.

3. Treatment and Outcome

3.1. KSHV/HHV8-MCD

The clinical care of PLWH who developed KSHV/HHV8-MCD was revolutionised in 2007 by the publication of two prospective open-label phase 2 clinical studies, that established the efficacy of rituximab [15,30]. Subsequently, it was established that for patients with life-threatening organ failure or the presence of concurrent Kaposi sarcoma (KS), the addition of chemotherapy to rituximab was required. In general etoposide is the additional drug of choice for patients with life-threating disease, whilst pegylated liposomal doxorubicin is usually added to rituximab if there is concurrent KS. Three large European cohort studies have described the medium-term outcomes of this approach using rituximab-based immunochemotherapy in a total of 249 patients, yielding 5 year overall survival in excess of 90% [26,28,31]. Despite the high response rates and good long-term survival following rituximab-based treatment, relapse is frequent and can usually be salvaged with a further course of rituximab [28].

Even though rituximab-based therapy is highly successful in KSHV/HHV8-MCD, other management strategies have been investigated, including the use of anti-herpes virus therapies. Anti-herpes virus drugs target viral replication, and for this reason have very limited success in KS where the majority of KSVH is latent. However, in KSHV/HHV8-MCD there are high levels of lytic replication of KSHV/HHV8 and this makes the approach with anti-herpes agents attractive. Several small studies using anti-virals have reported efficacy in KSHV/HHV8-MCD, but in most cases the responses were brief [32–36]. A combination of valganciclovir and zidovudine has been most widely studied with a recent publication reporting 5 year progression-free survival (PFS) of just 26% as first line therapy but a more promising 87% 5 year PFS, when used as maintenance after rituximab-based immunochemotherapy for 10 patients, compared with a figure of 62% for 16 patients who did not receive maintenance [37]. It is thought that KSHV/HHV8 encoded vIL-6, an early lytic gene of KSHV/HHV8, contributes to the pathogenesis of KSHV/HHV8-MCD. This virokine binds to the gp80 subunit of the IL-6 receptor, which is the target of the monoclonal antibody tocilizumab. However, single agent tocilizumab achieved only transient responses in just 5 of 8 HIV patients with KSHV/HHV8-MCD [38].

3.2. PEL

The treatment of PEL in both PLWH and HIV-negative individuals is not based on clinical trial evidence. Nevertheless, there is a general consensus that patients should be treated with multi-agent chemotherapy, along with combination antiretroviral therapy, opportunistic infection prophylaxis, and careful consideration of the potential pharmacological interactions (if HIV seropositive) [39]. The most widely employed regimens are dose-adjusted EPOCH (etoposide, prednisolone, vincristine, cyclophosphamide, doxorubicin) or CHOP (cyclophosphamide, doxorubicin, vincristine, prednisolone). Rituximab may be added to these regimens if the tumour expresses CD20, although this is uncommon. The prognosis is pretty poor, with fewer than 50% alive at 1 year [40,41]; although, earlier series reported an even worse prognosis [42,43]. In a meta-analysis of 301 patients from the literature, systemic chemotherapy was associated with an improved median survival (8 months vs 1.8 m). Furthermore, in this analysis, peritoneal involvement and elevated serum LDH were associated with worse prognosis, whilst pericardial involvement carried a lower risk of death. Interestingly, HIV status did not influence prognosis [25].

The poor outcomes have led investigators to explore the roles of molecular-targeting therapies in PEL, including immunomodulatory drugs (thalidomide, lenalidomide, pomalidomide), proteosome inhibitors (bortezomib), and monoclonal antibodies targeting CD30 (brentuximab) and CD38 (daratumumab), but with limited success [44].

3.3. KSHV/HHV8-Associated DLBCL

Again, there is no consensus regarding optimal treatment of these tumours and prognosis is poor [45]. Either CODOX-M/IVAC (as used for Burkitt lymphoma and leukaemia) or dose-adjusted EPOCH are frequently used, whilst CHOP chemotherapy is generally considered inadequate [39].

3.4. GLPD

With so few cases described in the literature it is impossible to be clear about the optimal therapeutic strategies in GLPD. Combination chemotherapy with CHOP or EPOCH has been administered to seven patients and five have achieved remission. However, a less aggressive approach was taken in ten patients with monitoring, surgery, or radiotherapy but no systemic anticancer therapy. The very limited data suggests that GLPD may be a more indolent disorder than other KSHV/HHV8-associated lymphoproliferations [8,29,46].

4. Conclusions

Following the discovery of KSHV/HHV8, it was quickly identified in MCD and subsequently in PEL, some PBL, and in the rare cases of these diseases that occur in HIV-negative individuals. The pathogenetic role of KSHV/HHV8 in these lymphoproliferations is uncertain; although, the virus encodes many potential oncogenes and tumour suppressor genes, which could contribute, though many are lytic antigens. The increasing recognition of these KSHV/HHV8 lymphoproliferative disorders and their clear identification in the WHO classification has driven forward knowledge of their clinical behaviour and treatment. Thus, the recognition of KSHV/HHV8-MCD has resulted in established clinical criteria, clinical management trials, and consensus treatment protocols that have led to improvements in survival. To a lesser extent, these advances have also been seen for PEL, which was first included in the WHO classification in 2001. It is hoped that the inclusion of KSHV/HHV8-associated DLBCL in the 2016 revision and the inclusion of GLPD in future classifications will similarly lead to greater recognition, better treatments, and survival benefits for patients.

Funding: This research received no external funding.

Conflicts of Interest: The authors declare no conflict of interest.

References

1. Beral, V.; Peterman, T.A.; Berkelman, R.L.; Jaffe, H.W. Kaposi's sarcoma among persons with AIDS: A sexually transmitted infection? *Lancet* **1990**, *335*, 123–128. [CrossRef]
2. Chang, Y.; Cesarman, E.; Pessin, M.S.; Lee, F.; Culpepper, J.; Knowles, D.M.; Moore, P.S. Identification of herpesvirus-like DNA sequences in AIDS-associated Kaposi's sarcoma. *Science* **1994**, *266*, 1865–1869. [CrossRef] [PubMed]
3. Judde, J.G.; Lacoste, V.; Briere, J.; Kassa-Kelembho, E.; Clyti, E.; Couppié, P.; Buchrieser, C.; Tulliez, M.; Morvan, J.; Gessain, A. Monoclonality or oligoclonality of human herpesvirus 8 terminal repeat sequences in Kaposi's sarcoma and other diseases. *J. Natl. Cancer Inst.* **2000**, *92*, 729–736. [CrossRef] [PubMed]
4. Whitby, D.; Boshoff, C.; Hatzioannou, T.; Weiss, R.A.; Schulz, T.F.; Howard, M.R.; Brink, N.S.; Tedder, R.S.; Tenant-Flowers, M.; Copas, A. Detection of Kaposi's sarcoma-associated herpesvirus (KSHV) in peripheral blood of HIV-infected individuals predicts progression to Kaposi's sarcoma. *Lancet* **1995**, *364*, 799–802. [CrossRef]
5. Soulier, J.; Grollet, L.; Oksenhendler, E.; Cacoub, P.; Cazals-Hatem, D.; Babinet, P.; d'Agay, M.F.; Clauvel, J.P.; Raphael, M.; Degos, L. Kaposi's sarcoma-associated herpesvirus-like DNA sequences in multicentric Castleman's disease. *Blood* **1995**, *86*, 1276–1280. [CrossRef] [PubMed]
6. Cesarman, E.; Chang, Y.; Moore, P.S.; Said, J.W.; Knowles, D.M. Kaposi's sarcoma-associated herpesvirus-like DNA sequences in AIDS-related body-cavity-based lymphomas. *N. Engl. J. Med.* **1995**, *332*, 1186–1191. [CrossRef] [PubMed]
7. Nador, R.G.; Cesarman, E.; Chadburn, A.; Dawson, D.B.; Ansari, M.Q.; Sald, J.; Knowles, D.M. Primary effusion lymphoma: A distinct clinicopathologic entity associated with the Kaposi's sarcoma-associated herpes virus. *Blood* **1996**, *88*, 645–656. [CrossRef] [PubMed]
8. Du, M.-Q.; Diss, T.C.; Liu, H.; Ye, H.; Hamoudi, R.A.; Cabeçadas, J.; Dong, H.Y.; Harris, N.L.; Chan, J.K.C.; Rees, J.W.; et al. KSHV- and EBV-associated germinotropic lymphoproliferative disorder. *Blood* **2002**, *100*, 3415–3418. [CrossRef] [PubMed]
9. Carbone, A.; Vaccher, E.; Gloghini, A.; Pantanowitz, L.; Abayomi, A.; de Paoli, P.; Franceschi, S. Diagnosis and management of lymphomas and other cancers in HIV-infected patients. *Nat. Rev. Clin. Oncol.* **2014**, *11*, 223–238. [CrossRef]
10. Carbone, A.; Vaccher, E.; Gloghini, A. Hematological cancers in individuals infected by HIV. *Blood* **2021**. [CrossRef]
11. Kessler, E. Multicentric giant lymph node hyperplasia. A report of seven cases. *Cancer* **1985**, *56*, 2446–2451. [CrossRef]

12. Van Rhee, F.; Oksenhendler, E.; Srkalovic, G.; Voorhees, P.; Lim, M.; Dispenzieri, A.; Ide, M.; Parente, S.; Schey, S.; Streetly, M.; et al. International evidence-based consensus diagnostic and treatment guidelines for unicentric Castleman disease. *Blood Adv.* **2020**, *4*, 6039–6050. [CrossRef] [PubMed]
13. Wang, H.-W.; Pittaluga, S.; Jaffe, E.S. Multicentric Castleman disease: Where are we now? *Semin. Diagn. Pathol.* **2016**, *33*, 294–306. [CrossRef] [PubMed]
14. Vega, F.; Miranda, R.N.; Medeiros, L.J. KSHV/HHV8-positive large B-cell lymphomas and associated diseases: A heterogeneous group of lymphoproliferative processes with significant clinicopathological overlap. *Mod. Pathol.* **2019**, *33*, 18–28. [CrossRef] [PubMed]
15. Gérard, L.; Bérezné, A.; Galicier, L.; Meignin, V.; Obadia, M.; de Castro, N.; Jacomet, C.; Verdon, R.; Madelaine-Chambrin, I.; Boulanger, E. Prospective Study of Rituximab in Chemotherapy-Dependent Human Immunodeficiency Virus Associated Multicentric Castleman's Disease: ANRS 117 CastlemaB Trial. *J. Clin. Oncol.* **2007**, *25*, 3350–3356. [CrossRef] [PubMed]
16. Uldrick, T.S.; Polizzotto, M.; Yarchoan, R. Recent advances in Kaposi sarcoma herpesvirus-associated multicentric Castleman disease. *Curr. Opin. Oncol.* **2012**, *24*, 495–505. [CrossRef] [PubMed]
17. Bower, M.; Pria, A.D.; Coyle, C.; Nelson, M.; Naresh, K. Diagnostic Criteria Schemes for Multicentric Castleman Disease in 75 Cases. *JAIDS J. Acquir. Immune Defic. Syndr.* **2014**, *65*, e80–e82. [CrossRef]
18. Knowles, D.M.; Inghirami, G.; Ubriaco, A.; Dalla-Favera, R. Molecular genetic analysis of three AIDS-associated neo-plasms of uncertain lineage demonstrates their B-cell derivation and the possible pathogenetic role of the Epstein-Barr virus. *Blood* **1989**, *73*, 792–799. [CrossRef] [PubMed]
19. Simonelli, C.; Spina, M.; Cinelli, R.; Talamini, R.; Tedeschi, R.; Gloghini, A.; Vaccer, E.; Carbone, A.; Tirelli, U. Clinical features and outcome of primary effusion lymphoma in HIV-infected patients: A single-institution study. *J. Clin. Oncol.* **2003**, *21*, 3948–3954. [CrossRef]
20. Riva, G.; Luppi, M.; Barozzi, P.; Forghieri, F.; Potenza, L. How I treat HHV8/KSHV-related diseases in posttransplant patients. *Blood* **2012**, *120*, 4150–4159. [CrossRef]
21. Said, J.W.; Tasaka, T.; Takeuchi, S.; Asou, H.; de Vos, S.; Cesarman, E.; Knowles, D.M.; Koeffler, H.P. Primary effusion lymphoma in women: Report of two cases of Kaposi's sarcoma herpes virus-associated effusion-based lymphoma in human immunodeficiency virus-negative women. *Blood* **1996**, *88*, 3124–3128. [CrossRef]
22. Ascoli, V.; Scalzo, C.C.; Danese, C.; Vacca, K.; Pistilli, A.; Coco, F.L. Human herpes virus-8 associated primary effusion lymphoma of the pleural cavity in HIV-negative elderly men. *Eur. Respir. J.* **1999**, *14*, 1231–1234. [CrossRef] [PubMed]
23. Chadburn, A.; Hyjek, E.; Mathew, S.; Cesarman, E.; Said, J.; Knowles, D.M. KSHV-Positive solid lymphomas represent an extra-cavitary variant of primary effusion lymphoma. *Am. J. Surg. Pathol.* **2004**, *28*, 1401–1416. [CrossRef]
24. Carbone, A.; Gloghini, A.; Vaccer, E.; Marchetti, G.; Gaidano, G.; Tirelli, U. KSHV/HHV-8 associated lymph node based lymphomas in HIV seronegative subjects. Report of two cases with anaplastic large cell morphology and plasmablastic immunophenotype. *J. Clin. Pathol.* **2005**, *58*, 1039–1045. [CrossRef]
25. Aguilar, C.; Laberiano, C.; Beltran, B.; Diaz, C.; Taype-Rondan, A.; Castillo, J.J. Clinicopathologic characteristics and survival of patients with primary effusion lymphoma. *Leuk. Lymphoma* **2020**, *61*, 2093–2102. [CrossRef] [PubMed]
26. Gérard, L.; Michot, J.M.; Burcheri, S.; Fieschi, C.; Longuet, P.; Delcey, V.; Meignin, V.; Agbalika, F.; Chevret, S.; Oksenhendler, E. Rituximab decreases the risk of lymphoma in patients with HIV-associated multicentric Castleman disease. *Blood* **2012**, *119*, 2228–2233. [CrossRef] [PubMed]
27. Oksenhendler, E.; Boulanger, E.; Galicier, L.; Du, M.Q.; Dupin, N.; Diss, T.C.; Hamoudi, R.; Daniel, M.T.; Agbalika, F.; Boshoff, C.; et al. High incidence of Kaposi sarcoma-associated herpesvirus-related non-Hodgkin lym-phoma in patients with HIV infection and multicentric Castleman disease. *Blood* **2002**, *99*, 2331–2336. [CrossRef]
28. Pria, A.D.; Pinato, D.; Roe, J.; Naresh, K.; Nelson, M.; Bower, M. Relapse of HHV8-positive multicentric Castleman disease following rituximab-based therapy in HIV-positive patients. *Blood* **2017**, *129*, 2143–2147. [CrossRef]
29. Zanelli, M.; Zizzo, M.; Bisagni, A.; Froio, E.; de Marco, L.; Valli, R.; Filosa, A.; Luminari, S.; Martino, G.; Massaro, F.; et al. Germinotropic lymphoproliferative disorder: A systematic review. *Ann. Hematol.* **2020**, *99*, 2243–2253. [CrossRef]
30. Bower, M.; Powles, T.; Williams, S.; Davis, T.N.; Atkins, M.; Montoto, S.; Orkin, C.; Webb, A.; Fisher, M.; Nelson, M.; et al. Brief Communication: Rituximab in HIV-Associated Multicentric Castleman Disease. *Ann. Intern. Med.* **2007**, *147*, 836–839. [CrossRef] [PubMed]
31. Hoffmann, C.; Schmid, H.; Müller, M.; Teutsch, C.; van Lunzen, J.; Esser, S.; Wolf, T.; Wyen, C.; Sabranski, M.; Horst, H.-A.; et al. Improved outcome with rituximab in patients with HIV-associated multicentric Castleman disease. *Blood* **2011**, *118*, 3499–3503. [CrossRef] [PubMed]
32. Uldrick, T.S.; Polizzotto, M.; Aleman, K.; O'Mahony, D.; Wyvill, K.M.; Wang, V.; Marshall, V.; Pittaluga, S.; Steinberg, S.M.; Tosato, G.; et al. High-dose zidovudine plus valganciclovir for Kaposi sarcoma herpesvirus-associated multicentric Castleman disease: A pilot study of virus-activated cytotoxic therapy. *Blood* **2011**, *117*, 6977–6986. [CrossRef] [PubMed]
33. Casper, C.; Nichols, W.G.; Huang, M.L.; Corey, L.; Wald, A. Remission of HHV-8 and HIV-associated multi-centric Castleman disease with ganciclovir treatment. *Blood* **2004**, *103*, 1632–1634. [CrossRef] [PubMed]
34. Oksenhendler, E.; Duarte, M.; Soulier, J.; Cacoub, P.; Welker, Y.; Cadranel, J.; Cazals-Hatem, D.; Autran, B.; Clauvel, J.P.; Raphael, M. Multicentric Castleman's disease in HIV infection: A clinical and pathological study of 20 patients. *AIDS* **1996**, *10*, 61–67. [CrossRef] [PubMed]

35. Berezne, A.; Agbalika, F.; Oksenhendler, E. Failure of cidofovir in HIV-associated multicentric Castleman disease. *Blood* **2004**, *103*, 4368–4369. [CrossRef]
36. Senanayake, S.; Kelly, J.; Lloyd, A.; Waliuzzaman, Z.; Goldstein, D.; Rawlinson, W. Multicentric Castleman's disease treated with antivirals and immunosuppressants. *J. Med. Virol.* **2003**, *71*, 399–403. [CrossRef]
37. Ramaswami, R.; Lurain, K.; Polizzotto, M.N.; Ekwede, I.; Waldon, K.; Steinberg, S.M.; Mangusan, R.; Widell, A.; Rupert, A.; George, J.; et al. Characteristics and outcomes of KSHV-associated multicentric Castleman disease with or without other KSHV diseases. *Blood Adv.* **2021**, *5*, 1660–1670. [CrossRef]
38. Ramaswami, R.; Lurain, K.; Peer, C.J.; Serquiña, A.; Wang, V.Y.; Widell, A.; Goncalves, P.; Steinberg, S.M.; Marshall, V.; George, J.; et al. Tocilizumab in patients with symptomatic Kaposi sarcoma herpesvirus–associated multicentric Castleman disease. *Blood* **2020**, *135*, 2316–2319. [CrossRef]
39. Writing Group; Bower, M.; Palfreeman, A.; Alfa-Wali, M.; Bunker, C.; Burns, F.; Churchill, D.; Collins, S.; Cwynarski, K.; Edwards, S.; et al. British HIV Association guidelines for HIV-associated malignancies 2014. *HIV Med.* **2014**, *15*, 1–92. [CrossRef]
40. Guillet, S.; Gérard, L.; Meignin, V.; Agbalika, F.; Cuccini, W.; Denis, B.; Katlama, C.; Galicier, L.; Oksenhendler, E. Classic and extracavitary primary effusion lymphoma in 51 HIV-infected patients from a single institution. *Am. J. Hematol.* **2016**, *91*, 233–237. [CrossRef]
41. Lurain, K.; Polizzotto, M.N.; Aleman, K.; Bhutani, M.; Wyvill, K.M.; Gonçalves, P.H.; Ramaswami, R.; Marshall, V.A.; Miley, W.; Steinberg, S.M.; et al. Viral, immunologic, and clinical features of primary effusion lymphoma. *Blood* **2019**, *133*, 1753–1761. [CrossRef] [PubMed]
42. Olszewski, A.J.; Fallah, J.; Castillo, J.J. Human immunodeficiency virus-associated lymphomas in the antiretroviral therapy era: Analysis of the National Cancer Data Base. *Cancer* **2016**, *122*, 2689–2697. [CrossRef] [PubMed]
43. El-Fattah, M.A. Clinical characteristics and survival outcome of primary effusion lymphoma: A review of 105 patients. *Hematol. Oncol.* **2017**, *35*, 878–883. [CrossRef] [PubMed]
44. Shimada, K.; Hayakawa, F.; Kiyoi, H. Biology and management of primary effusion lymphoma. *Blood* **2018**, *132*, 1879–1888. [CrossRef] [PubMed]
45. Castillo, J.J.; Winer, E.S.; Stachurski, D.; Perez, K.; Jabbour, M.; Milani, C.; Colvin, G.; Butera, J.N. Prognostic Factors in Chemotherapy-Treated Patients with HIV-Associated Plasmablastic Lymphoma. *Oncology* **2010**, *15*, 293–299. [CrossRef] [PubMed]
46. Ronaghy, A.; Wang, H.-Y.; Thorson, J.A.; Medeiros, L.J.; Xie, Y.; Zhang, X.; Sheikh-Fayyaz, S. PD-L1 and Notch1 expression in KSHV/HHV-8 and EBV associated germinotropic lymphoproliferative disorder: Case report and review of the literature. *Pathology* **2017**, *49*, 430–435. [CrossRef]

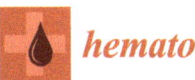

Review

Indolent T- and NK-Cell Lymphoproliferative Disorders of the Gastrointestinal Tract: Current Understanding and Outstanding Questions

Craig R. Soderquist * and Govind Bhagat *

Department of Pathology and Cell Biology, Columbia University Irving Medical Center, 630 West 168th Street, New York, NY 10032, USA
* Correspondence: crs2130@cumc.columbia.edu (C.R.S.); gb96@cumc.columbia.edu (G.B.)

Abstract: Indolent T- and NK-cell lymphoproliferative disorders of the gastrointestinal tract are uncommon clonal neoplasms that have a protracted clinical course and limited response to therapy. In recent years, advances in the immunophenotypic, genetic, and clinical characterization of these disorders have led to increased awareness and a better understanding of disease pathogenesis. However, many questions remain unanswered, including those concerning the cell(s) of origin, inciting immune or environmental factors, and the molecular pathways underlying disease progression and transformation. In this review, we discuss recent findings regarding the immunophenotypic and genomic spectrum of these lymphoproliferative disorders and highlight unresolved issues.

Keywords: indolent; T-cell; NK-cell; lymphoproliferative disorder; gastrointestinal tract; genetics; cell of origin

Citation: Soderquist, C.R.; Bhagat, G. Indolent T- and NK-Cell Lymphoproliferative Disorders of the Gastrointestinal Tract: Current Understanding and Outstanding Questions. *Hemato* 2022, 3, 219–231. https://doi.org/10.3390/hemato3010018

Academic Editors: Antonino Carbone and Alina Nicolae

Received: 1 February 2022
Accepted: 8 March 2022
Published: 10 March 2022

Publisher's Note: MDPI stays neutral with regard to jurisdictional claims in published maps and institutional affiliations.

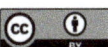

Copyright: © 2022 by the authors. Licensee MDPI, Basel, Switzerland. This article is an open access article distributed under the terms and conditions of the Creative Commons Attribution (CC BY) license (https://creativecommons.org/licenses/by/4.0/).

1. Introduction

Accumulating evidence over the past two decades has led to the recognition of rare indolent T- and NK-cell lymphoproliferative disorders (LPDs) occurring in the gastrointestinal (GI) tract and rarely other organs that have unique clinical, morphologic, immunophenotypic, and genetic features. Carbonnel et al. reported the first case of "low grade" small intestinal T-cell lymphoma in 1994 involving the duodenum of a 28 year-old man with a 7-year history of diarrhea and weight loss [1]. Since then, over 70 additional cases have been reported in a variety of GI sites, all showing similar patterns of mucosal infiltration by bland appearing small-sized lymphocytes (Figure 1A,B,D,E; Table 1), indolent clinical behavior, and poor response to chemotherapy [2–29]. The vast majority of these LPDs persisted as organ-confined disease for years, at times with regional lymph node involvement; however, dissemination outside the GI tract has been documented in some cases, and transformation to aggressive lymphomas has rarely been observed. Although early series described predominantly CD4+ cases (Figure 1C), many subsequent studies have reported CD8+ cases (Figure 1F), and less commonly CD4−/CD8− and CD4+/CD8+ LPDs. The clonal nature of these diseases was established and confirmed by investigators from the 1990s through the early 2010s, but no recurrent chromosomal changes were identified. In recent years, high throughput DNA- and RNA-based sequencing approaches have provided greater insights into the genetic bases of these LPDs and recurrent alterations in multiple gene classes and pathways are now recognized. The knowledge gained thus far has led to the inclusion of these diseases within a provisional category in the 2017 revised 4th edition of the WHO classification of lymphoid neoplasms, termed "indolent T-cell LPD of the GI tract" (ITLPD-GI) [30].

In addition to LPDs of T-cell lineage, indolent LPDs of natural killer (NK) cells also occur in the GI tract. The first case ("atypical NK-cell proliferation of the gastrointestinal tract") was reported by Vega et al. in 2006 [31], followed by two series from the United States and Japan describing morphologically similar lymphoproliferations, albeit with distinct clinical presentations and sites of involvement, designated "NK-cell enteropathy" (NKCE) and "lymphomatoid gastropathy" [32,33]. Over the years, nearly 50 cases of indolent NK-cell LPDs have been reported, as isolated case reports or small series [34–46], further refining the clinical, morphologic, and immunophenotypic features of these diseases, which are currently considered to represent a single entity, referred to as NKCE in this manuscript. In contrast to ITLPD-GI, the lesional cells of NKCE are medium- to large-sized and show mild pleomorphism (Figure 1J,K; Table 1) but lack the histopathologic features of extranodal NK/T-cell lymphomas, i.e., angioinvasion/angiodestruction and EBV infection [31–46]. Until recently, it wasn't clear whether NKCE represented reactive or neoplastic proliferations, in part due to the challenges associated with demonstrating clonality of NK-cells; however, a recent study identified recurrent mutations in a small number of cases [46], supporting the neoplastic character of at least some if not all cases of NKCE.

Despite advances in our understanding of the pathobiology of ITLPD-GI and NKCE, many questions remain. The cell(s) of origin of these lymphoid proliferations have not been established and the (micro)environmental and immunological factors associated with disease initiation as well as those related to disease progression and transformation are unknown. Alterations of molecular pathways and signaling networks, as a consequence of mutations and structural genetic alterations, remain to be deciphered, and optimal strategies for disease monitoring need to be defined. Here we review recent progress in the immunophenotypic and genetic characterization of ITLPD-GI and NKCE and call attention to some of the lingering questions.

2. Indolent T-Cell Lymphoproliferative Disorder of the Gastrointestinal Tract (ITLPD-GI)

2.1. Immunophenotype

ITLPD-GI encompasses immunophenotypically heterogeneous diseases. Of the >70 cases reported to date, 34 are $CD4^+$ [2,3,5,8,10,14,16,17,22–24,26–28], 29 are $CD8^+$ [4–6,10–13,15,18,19,25,27,29], 5 are $CD4^-/CD8^-$ ("double-negative", DN) [7,10,25,27], and 3 are $CD4^+/CD8^+$ ("double-positive," DP) [5,9,27] (Table 1). Comprehensive immunophenotypic analyses have not been performed in all cases; however, virtually all cases express CD2 and CD3, and partial downregulation or loss of CD5 and/or CD7 has been reported in ~25% of cases. CD103 is generally negative, though variable expression has been described in 2 $CD4^+$ cases [14,17] and 3 $CD8^+$ cases [10,27] and partial weak CD56 expression has been observed in one $CD8^+$ case [27]. T-cell receptor (TCR) αβ or βF1 is positive in all analyzed cases and T-follicular helper cell (TFH) markers (CD10, BCL6, PD1, CXCL13) are usually negative, although weak positivity for CD10 and CXCL13 was reported in one DN case [10] and PD1 expression in two cases, each exhibiting DN and DP phenotypes [27]. Expression of the regulatory T-cell (Treg) marker FOXP3 was negative in all cases tested [21,27]. The cytotoxic marker TIA1 is frequently expressed by $CD8^+$ cases, and $CD8^+$ and DN cases display variable granzyme B and perforin expression [4–8,10,12,15,18,19,21,25,27]. Aberrant CD20 expression has been reported in five cases (2 $CD4^+$, 1 $CD8^+$, 2 DN) [7,10,15,16]. Epstein–Barr virus (EBV)-encoded RNA (EBER) is negative in the T-cells, though rare admixed EBV^+ cells, probably B-cells, have been reported in two cases [2,10]. The Ki-67 proliferation index is inherently low (usually <5%). CD30 and/or MUM1 expression has been reported in transformed cases, but not during the indolent phase of disease [5,21,22].

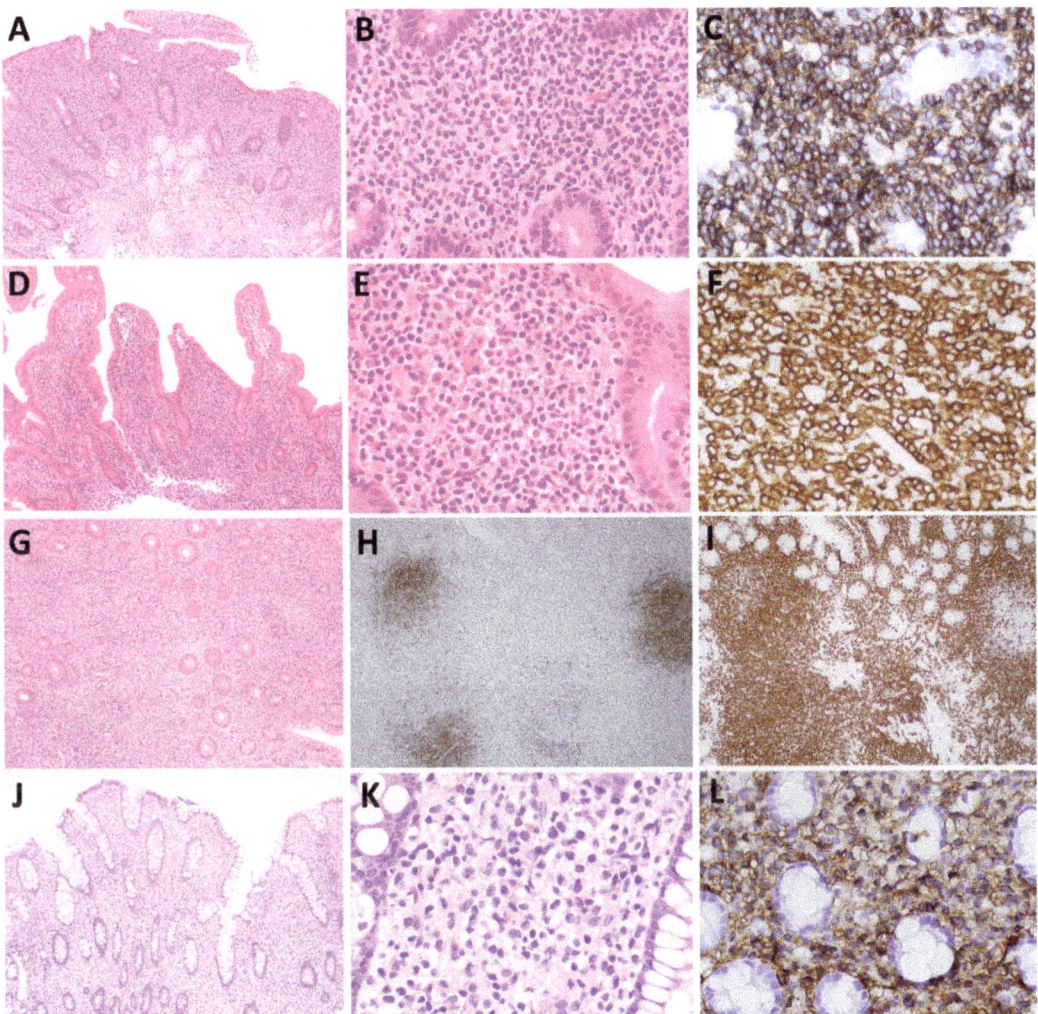

Figure 1. Histopathologic and immunophenotypic features of ITLPD-GI and NKCE. (A–C) CD4+ ITLPD-GI: (A) A duodenal biopsy shows expansion of the lamina propria by a dense lymphocytic infiltrate that extends into the submucosa, accompanied by villous atrophy and crypt hyperplasia. (B) The lymphocytes are small and have round or mildly irregular nuclei, condensed chromatin, inconspicuous nucleoli, and scant cytoplasm. (C) The vast majority of lymphocytes express CD4. (D–F) CD8+ ITLPD-GI: (D) The lymphocytic infiltrate within the lamina propria mildly distends the lower portions of the villi; no villous atrophy or crypt hyperplasia is evident. (E) The lymphocytes are small and mature appearing and do not show significant atypia. (F) In this case, the lymphocytes are CD8-positive. (G–I) **Reactive B-cell follicles:** (G) Scattered, small lymphoid follicles can be seen in some cases, which are comprised of (H) B-cells (CD20+) and surrounded by neoplastic (I) T-cells (CD3+). (J–L) **NKCE:** (J) A colonic biopsy shows an infiltrate of lymphoid cells within the lamina propria that displaces the crypts. (K) The lymphoid cells are medium- to large-sized and have ovoid or irregular nuclei, fine chromatin, indistinct or small nucleoli, and moderate or abundant cytoplasm. (L) The cells express CD56.

2.2. Cell(s) of Origin

Lamina propria (LP) helper T-cells (Th) are believed to be the cell of origin of CD4$^+$ ITLPD-GI. CD4$^+$ T-cells comprise the largest LP T-lymphocyte subset (~70%) [47] and they represent a diverse family, including Th type 1 and 2 (Th1, Th2) cells, T-follicular helper (TFH) cells, and regulatory T-cells (Tregs), amongst others [48,49]. Absence of TFH and Treg markers by CD4$^+$ ITLPD-GI argues against their derivation from these T-cell lineages. By immunohistochemistry, CD4$^+$ cases show heterogeneous expression of T-bet (TBX21) and GATA3 [27], which are master transcription factors governing Th1 vs. Th2 cell development [50]. Th1, Th2, and hybrid Th1/2 profiles have each been observed (Figure 2A,B), and in one case with longitudinal data, a phenotypic shift from a Th1/Th2 to Th2 profile was noted over time [27]. The etiology and significance of this phenotypic variability is unknown. Studies have shown that Th cells, both within and outside the GI tract, are not restricted to singular fates and can display phenotypic plasticity even after lineage specification [50]. It is presently unclear whether T-bet$^+$/GATA3$^+$ ITLPD-GI derive from bifunctional Th1/2 cells that develop directly from naïve T-cells in certain immune/inflammatory conditions [51] or committed Th subsets, which have been reprogrammed to adopt a mixed Th1/Th2 phenotype [52]. Inter-tumoral differences in the frequency of T-bet and GATA3 expression favors the latter supposition. The impact of lineage-specific transcription factor co-expression on cellular identity and function, however, remains poorly understood. Importantly, since RORγt (transcriptional regulator of Th17 differentiation) can be co-expressed with either T-bet or GATA3 in certain pathological conditions, induction of a Th17 program by some CD4$^+$ ITLPD-GI cannot be ruled out (Figure 2A,B).

CD8$^+$ ITLPD-GI are favored to originate from lamina propria CD8$^+$ T-cells, which constitute a smaller subset of lamina propria T-cells (~30%) [47]. Similar to their CD4$^+$ counterparts, LP CD8$^+$ T-cells are subclassified based on their cytokine expression profiles into type 1 effector (Tc1) and type 2 effector (Tc2) T-cells. Immunohistochemical analysis has shown that most CD8$^+$ ITLPD-GI express GATA3, suggesting an origin from Tc2 T-cells [27,53] (Figure 2A,B).

The cellular derivation of the DN and DP ITLPD-GI cases is not known. DN and DP T-cells represent uncommon GI mucosal T-cell subsets, and most of the knowledge regarding origin, differentiation, and function of these cells is inferred from their peripheral blood (PB) counterparts or from murine studies. LP DN T-cells have not been functionally characterized, but PB DN T-cells have been shown to derive from activated CD4$^+$ or CD8$^+$ T-cell subsets, which have downregulated these antigens due to chronic antigenic stimulation in response to infectious agents or in autoimmune/inflammatory conditions [54,55] (Figure 2A,B). LP DP T-cells have also not been characterized in humans; however in rhesus macaques (*Macaca mulatta*), LP DP T-cells have been shown to represent terminally differentiated effector memory T-cells with innate cytotoxic activity [56], which are inferred to play roles in viral immune responses, similar to human PB DP T-cells [57] (Figure 2A,B). It remains to be determined whether DN and DP ITLPD-GI arise from CD4$^+$ or CD8$^+$ T-cell subsets that have silenced or upregulated CD4 or CD8 expression (Figure 2A,B). In one reported DN case, the authors hypothesized that CD4 expression had been lost during disease progression; however, this supposition was not confirmed by TCR clonality analysis of early and late samples [22]. The lineage of the DN case expressing two TFH antigens (CD10 and CXCL13) is unclear, given the co-expression of TIA1 and perforin [10]. Expression of PD-1 by DN and DP ITLPDs (in the absence of other TFH markers) could be a manifestation of an "exhausted" cell state due to chronic activation/antigen stimulation [58].

Interrogation of gene expression programs and chromatin accessibility states of ITLPD-GI by transcriptome (e.g., RNA-seq [59]) and chromatin profiling (e.g., ATAC-seq [60]), and comparisons with normal mucosal and/or PB T-cell subsets, could help delineate the cell(s) of origin of the different immunophenotypic subtypes and unravel the transcriptional and epigenetic mechanisms responsible for disease heterogeneity.

2.3. Genetics

2.3.1. Clonality, Karyotyping, and Chromosome Microarray Analyses

All cases analyzed demonstrate clonal T-cell receptor gene (*TR*) rearrangements [2–10,12,14,15,17,19–29]. Karyotype analysis of isolated cases has identified a few non-recurrent chromosome abnormalities [2,13,27]. In a CD4$^+$ case, Carbonnel et al. detected a translocation t(4q27; 16p13) involving the interleukin-2 (*IL2*) gene on chromosome 4q27 and TNF Receptor Superfamily Member 17 (*TNFRSF17*), also known as B-cell maturation antigen (BCMA), on chromosome 16p13 [1,2,61]. In another CD4$^+$ case, a bone marrow sample showed a balanced translocation t(9;17)(p24;q21) that later was shown to represent a *STAT3-JAK2* fusion [27]. Chromosome microarray studies have revealed a multitude of non-recurrent copy number changes in 10 of the 13 analyzed cases [21,26]. Large segmental chromosomal gains and losses were seen in some cases, encompassing numerous genes, and no minimal commonly altered region has been uncovered till now. Of interest, however, some of the altered loci (1p13, 4q27, 16p13, 17q21) harbor genes with potential relevance to ITLPD-GI pathogenesis, which might be deregulated as a consequence of the copy number aberrations, e.g., loss of *SOCS1*, *TNIP3*, and *CD58*, and gain of *STAT3*.

2.3.2. Next-Generation Sequencing (NGS)

JAK/STAT Pathway Alterations

Recent RNA- and DNA-based sequencing studies identified frequent genetic abnormalities in ITLPD-GI, with an enrichment of alterations involving the JAK/STAT pathway (Figure 2D). Recurrent *STAT3-JAK2* rearrangements were observed in 5/11 (45%) CD4$^+$ cases, but not in any CD8$^+$ (0/12, 0%), DN (0/3, 0%), or DP (0/2, 0%) cases (one case listed in the EAHP workshop report by Montes-Moreno et al. was included in the study of Soderquist et al.) [5,10,27]. The rearrangements generate fusion transcripts joining the first 21 coding exons of *STAT3* with the last 9 exons of *JAK2*. The resultant protein retains many key functional domains of *STAT3*, including the Src homology 2 (SH2) domain, and *JAK2*, including the JAK homology 1 (JH1) tyrosine kinase domain, and activates STAT5.

In some cases lacking *STAT3-JAK2* rearrangements, genetic alterations in other components of the JAK/STAT pathway were detected. Specifically, activating *STAT3* point mutations were seen in 3 cases; 1/4 (25%) CD4$^+$ cases, 1/1 (100%) DP case, and 1/2 (50%) DN cases, but in none of the 10 CD8$^+$ cases assessed [6,10,25,27]. The reported *STAT3* mutations, D661Y and S614R, are well-characterized SH2 domain hotspot mutations, which enhance dimerization, nuclear transport, and activation of the STAT3 transcription factor, leading to heightened JAK/STAT signaling in response to cytokine stimulation [62,63]. Deletion of *SOCS1*, a negative regulator of the JAK family proteins [64], was also reported in one CD4$^+$ case [27].

IL2 Structural Alterations

Rearrangements or deletions involving the 3' untranslated region (UTR) of the *IL2* gene, which encodes an important T-cell cytokine that signals via multiple pathways, including the JAK/STAT pathway [65], have been identified in two CD8$^+$ cases (2/4, 50%), but not in any CD4$^+$ (0/4, 0%), DP 0/1 (%), or DN (0/1, 05) cases [27]. Mapping of these structural alterations showed that they result in loss of most or all of the 3' UTR AU-rich regulatory elements (AREs) which serve as binding sites for components of the mRNA degradation machinery and play a key role in mRNA stability [66]. In cultured T-cells, deletion of certain *IL2* 3' UTR AREs resulted in longer mRNA half-life [67], demonstrating a potential mechanism wherein 3' UTR alterations could modulate turnover and concentration of *IL2* transcripts. The functional significance of these structural abnormalities (genes and signaling pathways impacted) in ITLPD-GI, however, is not clear.

Other Altered Genes and Pathways

Beyond JAK/STAT signaling, other pathways/gene classes are also altered in ITLPD-GI. Putative loss-of-function mutations in epigenetic modifier genes, including genes involved in DNA methylation (*TET2*, *DNMT3A*) and histone modification (*KMT2D*, *EZH2*), have been identified in five cases, including 3/5 (60%) CD4$^+$ cases, 1/1 (100%) double-negative case, and 1/1 (100%) double-positive case, but not in five CD8$^+$ cases analyzed [6,10,27]. While these specific variants have not been functionally characterized, mutations in epigenetic modifiers are pervasive in hematopoietic neoplasia and are known to disrupt CpG methylation, chromatin structure, and gene expression. Additionally, non-recurrent alterations have been observed in genes affecting NF-κB signaling. One CD4$^+$ case harbored a frameshift *TNFAIP3* mutation and one CD8$^+$ case demonstrated a small inversion disrupting *TNIP3* (also known as TNFAIP3 Interacting Protein 3). Since both TNFAIP3 and TNIP are negative regulators of NF-κB signaling, these presumed loss-of-function mutations are predicted to result in aberrant NF-κB activation.

2.3.3. Genetic Stability and Evolution

Longitudinal genetic data have only been reported for five cases to date [27]. Four of those five cases, including two with JAK/STAT pathway and epigenetic modifier mutations, showed stable genomic profiles for many years, which tracked the indolent disease course. In contrast, the ITLPD of one patient treated with multiple chemotherapeutic regimens over the years, including antimetabolite drugs, which eventually transformed to aggressive lymphoma, demonstrated genetic evolution over time.

Mutations targeting epigenetic modifiers and the JAK/STAT pathway likely represent early events in ITLPD-GI pathogenesis, as has been proposed in other hematopoietic neoplasms [68–70], whereas mutations targeting other pathways, particularly those predisposing to genomic instability, e.g., *TP53*, may be late events. The implications of the sequence of acquisition and interplay of somatic lesions, as well as the role of chemotherapy, in fostering clonal evolution and disease progression await clarification.

2.4. *Environmental and Immunologic Factors*

To date, no inherited, environmental, or immunologic factors have been definitively linked to ITLPD-GI and disease-specific triggers are unknown. Some observations, however, suggest a potential role of chronic antigenic stimulation and/or immune dysregulation. An underrecognized histologic feature of ITLPD-GI is the presence of reactive lymphoid follicles (Figure 1G–I). Whether these structures are related to disease pathogenesis or represent epiphenomenon ("reactive") change, is not known. Prior and/or concurrent inflammatory or autoimmune diseases, including Crohn's disease, ulcerative colitis, autoimmune enteropathy, and rheumatoid arthritis have been reported in a few patients [6,12,22,25–27], and viral infections, either gastrointestinal (e.g., HHV6), extra-intestinal (e.g., HSV), or systemic (e.g., HTLV-1) have also been described [25,26].

The contributions of immune dysregulation and/or suppression in triggering or modifying the course of ITLPD-GI is not known, since many patients have been treated with a variety of immunomodulatory agents, including TNF inhibitors (infliximab, adalimumab, and certolizumab), mycophenolate mofetil, methotrexate, and 6-mercaptopurine, either before or after ITLPD-GI diagnosis [6,12,19,22,25,27]. Two ITLPD-GI cases were also reported following solid organ transplant (liver and kidney) [12,17].

It is possible that persistent antigenic stimulation amplifies signaling cascades normally utilized by mucosal immune subsets, resulting in augmented survival and proliferation, which can increase the likelihood of incurring genetic lesions. It is unclear whether some immunomodulatory agents have mutagenic effects in addition to impairing tumor immunosurveillance, which allows the unrestrained expansion of neoplastic T-cell clones.

Table 1. Pathologic and genetic characteristics of ITLPD-GI and NKCE.

	ITLPD-GI	NKCE
Site of involvement	**GI tract:** Small intestine (84%, 53/63), colon (48%, 30/63), stomach (38%, 24/63), oral cavity (5 cases), esophagus (2 cases) **Abdominal lymph nodes:** enlarged (47%, 22/47), biopsy confirmed involvement (12 cases) **Other:** Bone marrow (9 cases), blood, liver, peripheral lymph nodes	**GI tract:** Stomach (73%, 35/48), small intestine (31%, 15/48), colon (27%, 13/48) **Other:** Gallbladder, cystic duct lymph node, esophagus, vagina *
Cytomorphology	Small size, round, oval or mildly irregular nuclei, condensed chromatin, inconspicuous nucleoli, scant/moderate cytoplasm	Medium/large size, ovoid or irregular nuclei, fine chromatin, inconspicuous nucleoli, moderate pale cytoplasm with occasional azurophilic granules
Immunophenotype	**CD4$^+$:** 48% (34/71), **CD8$^+$:** 41% (29/71), **DN:** 7% (5/71), **DP:** 4% (3/71) **Typical:** CD2$^+$, CD3$^+$, CD5$^+$, CD7$^+$, TCR$\alpha\beta^+$, CD103$^-$, CD10$^-$, BCL6$^-$, PD1$^-$, CXCL13$^-$, FOXP3$^-$, CD30$^-$, MUM1$^-$, MATK$^-$ **Variant:** CD5$^-$ (14%, 6/42), CD7$^-$ (24%, 9/38), CD103$^+$ (5 cases), CD20$^+$ (5 cases), CD56$^+$ (1 case), PD1$^+$ (2 cases), CXCL13$^+$ and CD10$^+$ (1 case) **Cytotoxic markers:** **CD8:** TIA1$^+$ (96%), GrzB$^+$ (30%) **CD4:** TIA$^+$ (0%), GrzB$^+$ (0%) **Ki-67 index:** <10%	**Typical:** sCD3$^-$, cCD3$^+$, CD5$^-$, CD2$^+$, CD7$^+$, CD56$^+$, CD4$^-$, CD8$^-$, TIA1$^+$, GrzB$^+$ **Variant:** CD2$^-$ (30%, 7/23), CD7$^-$ (1 case), CD8$^+$ (11%, 5/46) **Ki-67 index:** <40%
Other histopathologic features	**Typical:** Diffuse or nodular infiltrate largely confined to the lamina propria **Other:** Small clusters of lymphocytes infiltrating crypt or villous epithelium, scattered B-cell follicles, and occasionally granulomas	Well-circumscribed infiltrate within the lamina propria, often surrounded by a rim of polymorphous inflammatory cells Absence of angioinvasion/angiodestruction
Chromosome/ genomic structural alterations	**CD4** **Translocations:** *STAT3-JAK2* (45%, 5/11) *IL2-TNFRSF17* **Gains/Losses:** **Gains:** Chr: 1p, 1q, 8q, 13q, 15q, 17q, 19q, X **Losses:** Chr: 1p, 3q, 4q, 7q, 9p, 10p, 15q, 16p, 19p, 19q, 20q, X **CD8** **Structural alterations:** *IL2 3'UTR-RHOH* *IL2 3' UTR del/IL2-TNIP3* †	None reported
Mutations	**CD4** **JAK/STAT pathway:** *STAT3, SOCS1* del **Epigenetics:** *TET2, KMT2D, EZH2* **Other:** *TNFAIP3, DIS3* **CD8** **JAK/STAT pathway:** None reported **Other:** *MCM5*	**JAK/STAT pathway:** *JAK3* (27%, 3/11) **Other:** *PTPRS, AURKB, AXL, ERBB4, IGF1R, PIK3CB, CUL3, CHEK2, RUNX1T1, CIC, SMARCB1, SETD5*

DN: double-negative (CD4$^-$/CD8$^-$); DP: double-positive (CD4$^+$/CD8$^+$); GI: gastrointestinal; GrzB: granzyme B. * Indolent NK-cell proliferations can occasionally be seen outside the GI tract. † Two *IL2* alterations were observed in one case: a deletion spanning the majority of the 3' UTR ("*IL2 3' UTR del*") and an inversion involving *IL2* and *TNIP3* ("*IL2-TNIP3*").

3. NK-Cell Enteropathy (NKCE)

3.1. Immunophenotype

The neoplastic cells demonstrate a phenotype typical of NK-cells: CD3(cytoplasmic)$^+$, CD3(surface)$^-$, CD7$^+$, CD5$^-$, and CD56$^+$ (Figure 1L, Table 1), with variable downregulation/loss of CD2. They often express one or more cytotoxic granule proteins (TIA1, granzyme-B, and/or perforin) and usually lack CD4 and CD8 expression; however, four CD8$^+$ cases have been reported [31–46]. The Ki-67 labeling index is generally <40%, but higher proliferation indices (up to 90%) have been reported in a few cases. In situ hybridization for EBER is always negative.

3.2. Cell of Origin

It is not known whether mucosal tissue-resident or circulating NK-cells are the normal counterparts of NKCE (Figure 2C). Mucosal NK-cells normally account for a small fraction of lymphoid cells in the GI tract [71–74]. Various subpopulations of cells with NK attributes reside within the LP, including conventional NK-cells, tissue-resident NK-cells, and NK-like innate lymphoid cells; however, knowledge of the function and distribution of these populations is limited [71–74]. These cells are believed to play roles in combatting viruses and other intracellular pathogens via secretion of cytotoxic proteins and IFN-γ [72,74]. The occurrence of two cases of indolent NK-cell LPDs in the gallbladder, one in a cystic duct lymph node and one in the vagina [38,43,45,75], suggests that either extra-intestinal (and rarely extra-GI sites) harbor unique tissue-specific NK-cell populations or provide a microenvironment conducive to the growth and proliferation of NK-cells that traffic to these locations.

3.3. Genetics

Until recently, there was no evidence that NKCE represented a clonal or neoplastic disorder. In keeping with NK-cell derivation, the LPDs show an absence of clonal *TR* gene rearrangements [31–35,40–42,45]. Heterogeneous killer-cell immunoglobulin-like receptor (KIR) expression was reported in a single case [31]. In 2019, Xiao et al. identified identical somatic *JAK3* K563_C565del mutations in 3 out of 10 (30%) NKCE cases [46] (Figure 2D, Table 1). This in-frame deletion of three amino acids is predicted to disrupt a portion of the JH2 pseudokinase domain responsible for modulating inhibitory feedback and suppression of JAK kinase activity. While the K563_C565del mutation has not been functionally characterized, similar mutations in the JH2 domain in other lymphoid neoplasms have been shown to result in upregulation of JAK activity [76]. Immunohistochemical analysis showed p-STAT5 staining in all NKCE cases tested, irrespective of *JAK3* mutations, suggesting ubiquitous activation of the JAK/STAT pathway in NKCE [46]. In addition, an assortment of non-recurrent somatic variants were identified, but their pathogenic significance is presently uncertain [46].

3.4. Environmental and Immunologic Factors

No instigating factors for NKCE are known, though similar to ITLPD-GI, chronic antigenic stimulation and dysregulated immune signaling have been implicated. In cases from Japan, many of the gastric cases had co-existing *H. pylori* infection, and a history of gastric cancer was noted in others; however, no definitive causal links between NKCE and these diseases have been identified [33,34,36,39,41,42,45,46]. In two cases, anti-gliadin antibodies were reported in the absence of histologic evidence of celiac disease [31,43].

4. Disease Monitoring of ITLPD-GI and NKCE

While the majority of ITLPD-GI persist for years without evidence of disease dissemination outside the GI tract, imaging reveals enlarged abdominal lymph nodes in ~50% of cases [2,4,13,16,17,19,23–28], and biopsy-confirmed nodal involvement has been reported in ~15% of cases [2,10,13,26,27] (Table 1). Spread to bone marrow and peripheral blood, amongst other sites, is considered uncommon [2,4,7,13,19,21,22,24,26,27]. NKCE can also persist for years to decades, sometimes showing a relapsing/remitting course, though unlike ITLPD-GI, disease dissemination outside the GI tract has not been documented [31–46]. It is important to note, however, that either systemic evaluation was not documented in many studies of ITLPD-GI and NKCE or information regarding the assays used to investigate presence of disease outside the GI tract was not provided.

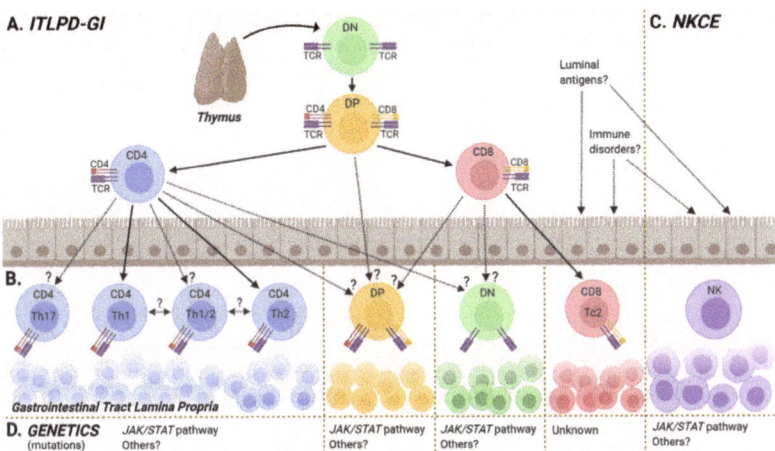

Figure 2. Pathogenetic aspects of ITLPD-GI and NKCE: (**A**) During "normal" T-cell development, immature double-negative ("DN") thymocytes give rise to double-positive ("DP") thymocytes in the thymus, which subsequently express either CD4 or CD8 following positive and negative selection. (**B**) Mature T-cells migrate to the gastrointestinal tract lamina propria. CD4$^+$ ITLPD-GI manifest Th1, Th2, or hybrid Th1/2 profiles; acquisition of a Th17 fate has not been excluded. CD8$^+$ cases predominantly display a Tc2 profile. It is not known whether the rare DP cases derive from DP thymocytes, which migrate directly to the intestinal mucosa, or from single-positive T-cells which up-regulate CD4$^+$ or CD8$^+$. DN ITLPD-GI may derive from activated CD4$^+$ or CD8$^+$ T-cells that have downregulated the T-cell co-receptors. (**C**) The cell of origin of NKCE (tissue-resident or circulating NK-cells) is unclear. The inciting factors for ITLPD-GI and NKCE (local or systemic) have not been elucidated. (**D**) Genetic alterations in the JAK/STAT signaling pathway have been identified in most immunophenotypic subsets of ITLPD-GI and in NKCE.

Currently, the optimal strategies and frequency of testing for extra-GI disease in these indolent LPDs are unclear. When present, the burden of ITLPD-GI in the peripheral blood is generally low, therefore high analytic sensitivity of the assay is paramount. Multiplex polymerase chain reaction (PCR) analysis for *TR* rearrangement, which has utility in the evaluation of ITLPD-GI but not NKCE, shows a limit of detection (LOD) of ~5% of T-cells (range 1–10%), though comparison with involved GI biopsy results can improve confidence at the lower end [77]. NGS-based clonality methods are more sensitive (LOD ~2.5%) and can more accurately identify and track disease-associated clonotypes, as well as distinguish them from background non-neoplastic clonal expansions due to other etiologies [78]. Flow cytometry can detect immunophenotypically aberrant T- and NK-cell populations, but a substantial proportion of ITLPD-GI and NKCE do not harbor overt immunophenotypic abnormalities. Finally, targeted NGS analysis of PB circulating DNA to detect disease-associated mutations ("liquid biopsy"), although not yet attempted in ITLPD-GI or NKCE, has been reported to be equally or more sensitive than standard PCR analysis in other lymphoid malignancies harboring mutations [79]. Periodic imaging is recommended, and bone marrow biopsy may also be considered; however, invasive procedures should perhaps be used more sparingly (e.g., at initial diagnosis or on suspicion of disease progression). For each of these modalities, additional studies are required to establish the appropriate assessment intervals.

5. Summary

Progress in the clinicopathologic, immunophenotypic, and molecular characterization of ITLPD-GI and NKCE has increased awareness of these rare and underrecognized disorders, furthered our understanding of disease pathogenesis, and confirmed their neoplastic nature; however, many questions remain. While targeted genomic profiling studies have identified recurrent alterations in many cases of ITLPD-GI and NKCE, unbiased whole exome or genome sequencing analyses are required to delineate the genetic landscape of these diseases and decipher their clonal architecture. The etiology of the different immunophenotypic subsets of ITLPD-GI is still a mystery and it remains to be seen whether similar diseases in some animals can serve as surrogates for human ITLPD-GI and provide clues about disease-initiating factors [80]. The use of newer multi-omic approaches integrating genetic, epigenetic, transcriptomic, and metabolomic data may unmask novel therapeutic targets. Finally, it is hoped that incorporation of newer disease monitoring tools will allow a better understanding of the natural course of indolent T- and NK-cell LPDs.

Author Contributions: C.R.S. and G.B.: conceptualization, methodology, formal analysis, investigation, data curation, writing—original draft preparation, writing—review and editing. All authors have read and agreed to the published version of the manuscript.

Funding: This research received no external funding.

Conflicts of Interest: Neither author has any conflict of interest to disclose.

References

1. Carbonnel, F.; Lavergne, A.; Messing, B.; Tsapis, A.; Berger, R.; Galian, A.; Nemeth, J.; Brouet, J.C.; Rambaud, J.C. Extensive small intestinal T-cell lymphoma of low-grade malignancy associated with a new chromosomal translocation. *Cancer* **1994**, *73*, 1286–1291. [CrossRef]
2. Carbonnel, F.; D'Almagne, H.; Lavergne, A.; Matuchansky, C.; Brouet, J.C.; Sigaux, F.; Beaugerie, L.; Nemeth, J.; Coffin, B.; Cosnes, J.; et al. The clinicopathological features of extensive small intestinal CD4 T cell infiltration. *Gut* **1999**, *45*, 662–667. [CrossRef] [PubMed]
3. Egawa, N.; Fukayama, M.; Kawaguchi, K.; Hishima, T.; Hayashi, Y.; Funata, N.; Ibuka, T.; Koike, M.; Miyashita, H.; Tajima, T. Relapsing oral and colonic ulcers with monoclonal T-cell infiltration. A low grade mucosal T-lymphoproliferative disease of the digestive tract. *Cancer* **1995**, *75*, 1728–1733. [CrossRef]
4. Leventaki, V.; Manning, J.T.; Luthra, R.; Mehta, P.; Oki, Y.; Romaguera, J.E.; Medeiros, L.J.; Vega, F. Indolent peripheral T-cell lymphoma involving the gastrointestinal tract. *Hum. Pathol.* **2014**, *45*, 421–426. [CrossRef] [PubMed]
5. Sharma, A.; Oishi, N.; Boddicker, R.L.; Hu, G.; Benson, H.K.; Ketterling, R.P.; Greipp, P.T.; Knutson, D.L.; Kloft-Nelson, S.M.; He, R.; et al. Recurrent STAT3-JAK2 fusions in indolent T-cell lymphoproliferative disorder of the gastrointestinal tract. *Blood* **2018**, *131*, 2262. [CrossRef]
6. Edison, N.; Belhanes-Peled, H.; Eitan, Y.; Guthmann, Y.; Yeremenko, Y.; Raffeld, M.; Elmalah, I.; Trougouboff, P. Indolent T-cell lymphoproliferative disease of the gastrointestinal tract after treatment with adalimumab in resistant Crohn's colitis. *Hum. Pathol.* **2016**, *57*, 45–50. [CrossRef]
7. Wang, X.; Ng, C.-S.; Chen, C.; Yu, G.; Yin, W. An unusual case report of indolent T-cell lymphoproliferative disorder with aberrant CD20 expression involving the gastrointestinal tract and bone marrow. *Diagn. Pathol.* **2018**, *13*, 82. [CrossRef]
8. Zanelli, M.; Zizzo, M.; Sanguedolce, F.; Martino, G.; Soriano, A.; Ricci, S.; Ruiz, C.C.; Annessi, V.; Ascani, S. Indolent T-cell lymphoproliferative disorder of the gastrointestinal tract: A tricky diagnosis of a gastric case. *BMC Gastroenterol.* **2020**, *20*, 336. [CrossRef]
9. Guo, L.; Wen, Z.; Su, X.; Xiao, S.; Wang, Y. Indolent T-cell lymphoproliferative disease with synchronous diffuse large B-cell lymphoma. *Medicine* **2019**, *98*, e15323. [CrossRef]
10. Montes-Moreno, S.; King, R.L.; Oschlies, I.; Ponzoni, M.; Goodlad, J.R.; Dotlic, S.; Traverse-Glehen, A.; Ott, G.; Ferry, J.A.; Calaminici, M. Update on lymphoproliferative disorders of the gastrointestinal tract: Disease spectrum from indolent lymphoproliferations to aggressive lymphomas. *Virchows Arch.* **2020**, *476*, 667–681. [CrossRef]
11. Kohri, M.; Tsukasaki, K.; Akuzawa, Y.; Tanae, K.; Takahashi, N.; Saeki, T.; Okamura, D.; Ishikawa, M.; Maeda, T.; Kawai, N.; et al. Peripheral T-cell lymphoma with gastrointestinal involvement and indolent T-lymphoproliferative disorders of the gastrointestinal tract. *Leuk. Res.* **2020**, *91*, 106336. [CrossRef] [PubMed]
12. Soon, G.; Wang, S. Indolent T-cell lymphoproliferative disease of the gastrointestinal tract in a renal transplant patient: Diagnostic pitfalls and clinical challenges. *Pathology* **2017**, *49*, 547–550. [CrossRef] [PubMed]
13. Lee, J.; Park, K.; Kim, K.H.; Bang, H.I.; Yoon, S.Y.; Choi, I.H. Diagnostic challenges of indolent peripheral T cell lymphoma: A case report and literature review. *Medicine* **2020**, *99*, e22657. [CrossRef] [PubMed]
14. Hirakawa, K.; Fuchigami, T.; Nakamura, S.; Daimaru, Y.; Ohshima, K.; Sakai, Y.; Ichimura, T. Primary gastrointestinal T-cell lymphoma resembling multiple lymphomatous polyposis. *Gastroenterology* **1996**, *111*, 778–782. [CrossRef]
15. Saggini, A.; Baciorri, F.; Di Prete, M.; Zizzari, A.G.; Anemona, L. Oral manifestation of indolent T-cell lymphoproliferative disorder of the gastrointestinal tract: A potential diagnostic pitfall. *J. Cutan. Pathol.* **2020**, *47*, 494–496. [CrossRef]

16. Nagaishi, T.; Yamada, D.; Suzuki, K.; Fukuyo, R.; Saito, E.; Fukuda, M.; Watabe, T.; Tsugawa, N.; Takeuchi, K.; Yamamoto, K.; et al. Indolent T cell lymphoproliferative disorder with villous atrophy in small intestine diagnosed by single-balloon enteroscopy. *Clin. J. Gastroenterol.* **2019**, *12*, 434–440. [CrossRef]
17. Goto, R.; Kawamura, N.; Watanabe, M.; Koshizuka, Y.; Shiratori, S.; Ara, M.; Honda, S.; Mitsuhashi, T.; Matsuno, Y.; Shimamura, T.; et al. Post-transplant indolent T cell lymphoproliferative disorder in living donor liver transplantation: A case report. *Surg. Case Rep.* **2020**, *6*, 147. [CrossRef]
18. Takahashi, N.; Tsukasaki, K.; Kohri, M.; Akuzawa, Y.; Saeki, T.; Okamura, D.; Ishikawa, M.; Maeda, T.; Kawai, N.; Matsuda, A.; et al. Indolent T-cell lymphoproliferative disorder of the stomach successfully treated by radiotherapy. *J. Clin. Exp. Hematop.* **2020**, *60*, 7–10. [CrossRef]
19. Wu, J.; Li, L.-G.; Zhang, X.-Y.; Wang, L.-L.; Zhang, L.; Xiao, Y.-J.; Xing, X.-M.; Lin, D.-L. Indolent T cell lymphoproliferative disorder of the gastrointestinal tract: An uncommon case with lymph node involvement and the classic Hodgkin's lymphoma. *J. Gastrointest. Oncol.* **2020**, *11*, 812–819. [CrossRef]
20. Ranheim, E.A.; Jones, C.; Zehnder, J.L.; Warnke, R.; Yuen, A. Spontaneously relapsing clonal, mucosal cytotoxic T-cell lymphoproliferative disorder: Case report and review of the literature. *Am. J. Surg. Pathol.* **2000**, *24*, 296–301. [CrossRef]
21. Margolskee, E.; Jobanputra, V.; Lewis, S.K.; Alobeid, B.; Green, P.H.R.; Bhagat, G. Indolent Small Intestinal CD4+ T-cell Lymphoma Is a Distinct Entity with Unique Biologic and Clinical Features. *PLoS ONE* **2013**, *8*, e68343. [CrossRef] [PubMed]
22. Perry, A.M.; Bailey, N.G.; Bonnett, M.; Jaffe, E.S.; Chan, W.C. Disease Progression in a Patient With Indolent T-Cell Lymphoproliferative Disease of the Gastrointestinal Tract. *Int. J. Surg. Pathol.* **2019**, *27*, 102–107. [CrossRef] [PubMed]
23. Zivny, J.; Banner, B.F.; Agrawal, S.; Pihan, G.; Barnard, G.F. CD4+T-cell lymphoproliferative disorder of the gut clinically mimicking celiac sprue. *Dig. Dis. Sci.* **2004**, *49*, 551–555. [CrossRef] [PubMed]
24. Svrcek, M.; Garderet, L.; Sebbagh, V.; Rosenzwajg, M.; Parc, Y.; Lagrange, M.; Bennis, M.; Lavergne-Slove, A.; Fléjou, J.-F.; Fabiani, B. Small intestinal CD4+ T-cell lymphoma: A rare distinctive clinicopathological entity associated with prolonged survival. *Virchows Arch.* **2007**, *451*, 1091–1093. [CrossRef] [PubMed]
25. Perry, A.M.; Warnke, R.A.; Hu, Q.; Gaulard, P.; Copie-Bergman, C.; Alkan, S.; Wang, H.-Y.; Cheng, J.X.; Bacon, C.M.; Delabie, J.; et al. Indolent T-cell lymphoproliferative disease of the gastrointestinal tract. *Blood* **2013**, *122*, 3599–3606. [CrossRef]
26. Malamut, G.; Meresse, B.; Kaltenbach, S.; Derrieux, C.; Verkarre, V.; Macintyre, E.; Ruskone–Fourmestraux, A.; Fabiani, B.; Radford–Weiss, I.; Brousse, N.; et al. Small Intestinal CD4+ T-Cell Lymphoma Is a Heterogenous Entity With Common Pathology Features. *Clin. Gastroenterol. Hepatol.* **2014**, *12*, 599–608. [CrossRef] [PubMed]
27. Soderquist, C.R.; Patel, N.; Murty, V.V.; Betman, S.; Aggarwal, N.; Young, K.H.; Xerri, L.; Leeman-Neill, R.; Lewis, S.K.; Green, P.H.; et al. Genetic and phenotypic characterization of indolent T-cell lymphoproliferative disorders of the gastrointestinal tract. *Haematologica* **2020**, *105*, 1895–1906. [CrossRef]
28. Sena Teixeira Mendes, L.; DAttygalle, A.; Cunningham, D.; Benson, M.; Andreyev, J.; Gonzales-de-Castro, D.; Wotherspoon, A. CD4⁻positive small T-cell lymphoma of the intestine presenting with severe bile-acid malabsorption: A supportive symptom control approach. *Br. J. Haematol.* **2014**, *167*, 265–269. [CrossRef]
29. Tsutsumi, Y.; Inada, K.-I.; Morita, K.; Suzuki, T. T-cell lymphomas diffusely involving the intestine: Report of two rare cases. *Jpn. J. Clin. Oncol.* **1996**, *26*, 264–272. [CrossRef]
30. Swerdlow, S.H.; Campo, E.; Harris, N.L.; Jaffe, E.S.; Pileri, S.A.; Stein, H.; Thiele, J.; Arber, D.A.; Hasserjian, R.P.; Le Beau, M.M.; et al. (Eds.) *World Health Organization Classification of Tumours of Haematopoietic and Lymphoid Tissues*; IARC: Lyon, France, 2016.
31. Vega, F.; Chang, C.-C.; Schwartz, M.R.; Preti, H.A.; Younes, M.; Ewton, A.; Verm, R.; Jaffe, E.S. Atypical NK-cell proliferation of the gastrointestinal tract in a patient with antigliadin antibodies but not celiac disease. *Am. J. Surg. Pathol.* **2006**, *30*, 539–544. [CrossRef]
32. Mansoor, A.; Pittaluga, S.; Beck, P.L.; Wilson, W.H.; Ferry, J.A.; Jaffe, E.S. NK-cell enteropathy: A benign NK-cell lymphoproliferative disease mimicking intestinal lymphoma: Clinicopathologic features and follow-up in a unique case series. *Blood* **2011**, *117*, 1447–1452. [CrossRef] [PubMed]
33. Takeuchi, K.; Yokoyama, M.; Ishizawa, S.; Terui, Y.; Nomura, K.; Marutsuka, K.; Nunomura, M.; Fukushima, N.; Yagyuu, T.; Nakamine, H.; et al. Lymphomatoid gastropathy: A distinct clinicopathologic entity of self-limited pseudomalignant NK-cell proliferation. *Blood* **2010**, *116*, 5631–5637. [CrossRef] [PubMed]
34. Tanaka, T.; Megahed, N.; Takata, K.; Asano, N.; Niwa, Y.; Hirooka, Y.; Goto, H. A case of lymphomatoid gastropathy: An indolent CD56-positive atypical gastric lymphoid proliferation, mimicking aggressive NK/T cell lymphomas. *Pathol. Res. Pract.* **2011**, *207*, 786–789. [CrossRef] [PubMed]
35. McElroy, M.K.; Read, W.L.; Harmon, G.S.; Weidner, N. A unique case of an indolent CD56-positive T-cell lymphoproliferative disorder of the gastrointestinal tract: A lesion potentially misdiagnosed as natural killer/T-cell lymphoma. *Ann. Diagn. Pathol.* **2011**, *15*, 370–375. [CrossRef]
36. Isom, J.A.; Arroyo, M.R.; Reddy, D.; Joshi-Guske, P.; Al-Quran, S.Z.; Li, Y.; Allan, R.W. NK cell enteropathy: A case report with 10 years of indolent clinical behaviour. *Histopathology* **2018**, *73*, 345–350. [CrossRef]
37. Wang, R.; Kariappa, S.; Toon, C.W.; Varikatt, W. NK-cell enteropathy, a potential diagnostic pitfall of intestinal lymphoproliferative disease. *Pathology* **2019**, *51*, 338–340. [CrossRef]
38. Dargent, J.-L.; Tinton, N.; Trimech, M.; de Leval, L. Lymph node involvement by enteropathy-like indolent NK-cell proliferation. *Virchows Arch.* **2021**, *478*, 1197–1202. [CrossRef]

39. Terai, T.; Sugimoto, M.; Uozaki, H.; Kitagawa, T.; Kinoshita, M.; Baba, S.; Yamada, T.; Osawa, S.; Sugimoto., K. Lymphomatoidgastropathy mimicking extranodal NK/T cell lymphoma, nasal type: A case report. *World J. Gastroenterol.* **2012**, *18*, 2140–2144. [CrossRef]
40. Koh, J.; Go, H.; Lee, W.A.; Jeon, Y.K. Benign Indolent CD56-Positive NK-Cell Lymphoproliferative Lesion Involving Gastrointestinal Tract in an Adolescent. *Korean J. Pathol.* **2014**, *48*, 73. [CrossRef]
41. Ishibashi, Y.; Matsuzono, E.; Yokoyama, F.; Ohara, Y.; Sugai, N.; Seki, H.; Miura, A.; Fujita, J.; Suzuki, J.; Fujisawa, T.; et al. A case of lymphomatoid gastropathy: A self-limited pseudomalignant natural killer (NK)-cell proliferative disease mimicking NK/T-cell lymphomas. *Clin. J. Gastroenterol.* **2013**, *6*, 287–290. [CrossRef]
42. Takata, K.; Noujima-Harada, M.; Miyata-Takata, T.; Ichimura, K.; Sato, Y.; Miyata, T.; Naruse, K.; Iwamoto, T.; Tari, A.; Masunari, T.; et al. Clinicopathologic Analysis of 6 Lymphomatoid Gastropathy Cases. *Am. J. Surg. Pathol.* **2015**, *39*, 1259–1266. [CrossRef]
43. Xia, D.; A Morgan, E.; Berger, D.; Pinkus, G.S.; Ferry, J.A.; Zukerberg, L.R. NK-Cell Enteropathy and Similar Indolent Lymphoproliferative Disorders. *Am. J. Clin. Pathol.* **2018**, *151*, 75–85. [CrossRef] [PubMed]
44. Yamamoto, J.; Fujishima, F.; Ichinohasama, R.; Imatani, A.; Asano, N.; Harigae, H. A case of benign natural killer cell proliferative disorder of the stomach (gastric manifestation of natural killer cell lymphomatoid gastroenteropathy) mimicking extranodal natural killer/T-cell lymphoma. *Leuk. Lymphoma* **2011**, *52*, 1803–1805. [CrossRef] [PubMed]
45. Hwang, S.H.; Park, J.S.; Jeong, S.H.; Yim, H.; Han, J.H. Indolent NK cell proliferative lesion mimicking NK/T cell lymphoma in the gallbladder. *Hum. Pathol. Case Rep.* **2016**, *5*, 39–42. [CrossRef]
46. Xiao, W.; Gupta, G.K.; Yao, J.; Jang, Y.J.; Xi, L.; Baik, J.; Sigler, A.; Kumar, A.; Moskowitz, A.J.; Arcila, M.E.; et al. Recurrent somatic JAK3 mutations in NK-cell enteropathy. *Blood* **2019**, *134*, 986–991. [CrossRef]
47. Jahnsen, F.L.; Farstad, I.N.; Aanesen, J.P.; Brandtzaeg, P. Phenotypic distribution of T cells in human nasal mucosa differs from that in the gut. *Am. J. Respir. Cell Mol. Biol.* **1998**, *18*, 392–401. [CrossRef]
48. Gibbons, D.L.; Spencer, J. Mouse and human intestinal immunity: Same ballpark, different players; Different rules, same score. *Mucosal Immunol.* **2011**, *4*, 148–157. [CrossRef]
49. Cosorich, I.; McGuire, H.M.; Warren, J.; Danta, M.; King, C. CCR9 expressing T helper and T follicular helper cells exhibit site-specific identities during inflammatory disease. *Front. Immunol.* **2019**, *10*, 2899. [CrossRef]
50. Zhu, J.; Paul, W.E. Heterogeneity and plasticity of T helper cells. *Cell Res.* **2009**, *20*, 4–12. [CrossRef]
51. Peine, M.; Rausch, S.; Helmstetter, C.; Fröhlich, A.; Hegazy, A.N.; Kühl, A.A.; Grevelding, C.G.; Höfer, T.; Hartmann, S.; Löhning, M. Stable T-bet+GATA-3+ Th1/Th2 Hybrid Cells Arise In Vivo, Can Develop Directly from Naive Precursors, and Limit Immunopathologic Inflammation. *PLoS Biol.* **2013**, *11*, e1001633. [CrossRef]
52. Hegazy, A.N.; Peine, M.; Helmstetter, C.; Panse, I.; Fröhlich, A.; Bergthaler, A.; Flatz, L.; Pinschewer, D.D.; Radbruch, A.; Löhning, M. Interferons Direct Th2 Cell Reprogramming to Generate a Stable GATA-3+T-bet+ Cell Subset with Combined Th2 and Th1 Cell Functions. *Immunity* **2010**, *32*, 116–128. [CrossRef] [PubMed]
53. Fox, A.; Harland, K.; Kedzierska, K.; Kelso, A. Exposure of human CD8+ T cells to type-2 cytokines impairs division and differentiation and induces limited polarization. *Front. Immunol.* **2018**, *9*, 1141. [CrossRef] [PubMed]
54. Priatel, J.J.; Utting, O.; Teh, H.-S. TCR/self-antigen interactions drive double-negative T cell peripheral expansion and differentiation into suppressor cells. *J. Immunol.* **2001**, *167*, 6188–6194. [CrossRef] [PubMed]
55. Brandt, D.; Hedrich, C.M. TCRαβ+CD3+CD4−CD8− (double negative) T cells in autoimmunity. *Autoimmun. Rev.* **2018**, *17*, 422–430. [CrossRef]
56. Pahar, B.; Lackner, A.A.; Veazey, R.S. Intestinal double-positive CD4+CD8+ T cells are highly activated memory cells with an increased capacity to produce cytokines. *Eur. J. Immunol.* **2006**, *36*, 583–592. [CrossRef]
57. Nascimbeni, M.; Shin, E.-C.; Chiriboga, L.; Kleiner, D.; Rehermann, B. Peripheral CD4(+)CD8(+) T cells are differentiated effector memory cells with antiviral functions. *Blood* **2004**, *104*, 478–486. [CrossRef]
58. Keir, M.E.; Francisco, L.M.; Sharpe, A.H. PD-1 and its ligands in T-cell immunity. *Curr. Opin. Immunol.* **2007**, *19*, 309–314. [CrossRef]
59. Hrdlickova, R.; Toloue, M.; Tian, B. RNA-Seq methods for transcriptome analysis. *Wiley Interdiscip. Rev. RNA* **2017**, *8*, e1364. [CrossRef]
60. Sun, Y.; Miao, N.; Sun, T. Detect accessible chromatin using ATAC-sequencing, from principle to applications. *Hereditas* **2019**, *156*, 29. [CrossRef]
61. Laâbi, Y.; Gras, M.P.; Carbonnel, F.; Brouet, J.C.; Berger, R.; Larsen, C.J.; Tsapis, A. A new gene, BCM, on chromosome 16 is fused to the interleukin 2 gene by a t(4;16)(q26;p13) translocation in a malignant T cell lymphoma. *EMBO J.* **1992**, *11*, 3897–3904. [CrossRef]
62. Koskela, H.L.; Eldfors, S.; Ellonen, P.; Van Adrichem, A.J.; Kuusanmäki, H.; Andersson, E.; Lagström, S.; Clemente, M.J.; Olson, T.; Jalkanen, S.E.; et al. Somatic STAT3 mutations in large granular lymphocytic leukemia. *N. Engl. J. Med.* **2012**, *366*, 1905–1913. [CrossRef] [PubMed]
63. Ettersperger, J.; Montcuquet, N.; Malamut, G.; Guegan, N.; Lastra, S.L.; Gayraud, S.; Reimann, C.; Vidal, E.; Cagnard, N.; Villarese, P.; et al. Interleukin-15-Dependent T-Cell-like Innate Intraepithelial Lymphocytes Develop in the Intestine and Transform into Lymphomas in Celiac Disease. *Immunity* **2016**, *45*, 610–625. [CrossRef] [PubMed]
64. Liau, N.P.D.; Laktyushin, A.; Lucet, I.S.; Murphy, J.M.; Yao, S.; Whitlock, E.; Callaghan, K.; Nicola, N.A.; Kershaw, N.J.; Babon, J.J. The molecular basis of JAK/STAT inhibition by SOCS1. *Nat. Commun.* **2018**, *9*, 1558. [CrossRef] [PubMed]

65. Ross, S.; Cantrell, D.A. Signaling and Function of Interleukin-2 in T Lymphocytes. *Annu. Rev. Immunol.* **2018**, *36*, 411–433. [CrossRef] [PubMed]
66. Myer, V.E.; Fan, X.C.; Steitz, J.A. Identification of HuR as a protein implicated in AUUUA-mediated mRNA decay. *EMBO J.* **1997**, *16*, 2130–2139. [CrossRef]
67. Chen, C.-Y.; Del Gatto–Konczak, F.; Wu, Z.; Karin, M. Stabilization of interleukin-2 mRNA by the c-Jun NH2-terminal kinase pathway. *Science* **1998**, *280*, 1945–1949. [CrossRef]
68. Schwartz, F.H.; Cai, Q.; Fellmann, E.; Hartmann, S.; Mäyränpää, M.I.; Karjalainen-Lindsberg, M.-L.; Sundström, C.; Scholtysik, R.; Hansmann, M.-L.; Küppers, R. TET2 mutations in B cells of patients affected by angioimmunoblastic T-cell lymphoma. *J. Pathol.* **2017**, *242*, 129–133. [CrossRef]
69. Soderquist, C.R.; Lewis, S.K.; Gru, A.A.; Vlad, G.; Williams, E.S.; Hsiao, S.; Mansukhani, M.M.; Park, D.C.; Bacchi, C.E.; Alobeid, B.; et al. Immunophenotypic Spectrum and Genomic Landscape of Refractory Celiac Disease Type II. *Am. J. Surg. Pathol.* **2021**, *45*, 905–916. [CrossRef]
70. Cording, S.; Lhermitte, L.; Malamut, G.; Berrabah, S.; Trinquand, A.; Guegan, N.; Villarese, P.; Kaltenbach, S.; Meresse, B.; Khater, S.; et al. Oncogenetic landscape of lymphomagenesis in coeliac disease. *Gut* **2021**, *71*, 497–508. [CrossRef]
71. Yu, X.; Vargas, J.; Green, P.H.; Bhagat, G. Innate Lymphoid Cells and Celiac Disease: Current Perspective. *Cell. Mol. Gastroenterol. Hepatol.* **2021**, *11*, 803–814. [CrossRef]
72. Shi, F.-D.; Ljunggren, H.-G.; La Cava, A.; Van Kaer, L. Organ-specific features of natural killer cells. *Nat. Rev. Immunol.* **2011**, *11*, 658–671. [CrossRef] [PubMed]
73. Grégoire, C.; Chasson, L.; Luci, C.; Tomasello, E.; Geissmann, F.; Vivier, E.; Walzer, T. The trafficking of natural killer cells. *Immunol. Rev.* **2007**, *220*, 169–182. [CrossRef] [PubMed]
74. Panda, S.K.; Colonna, M. Innate lymphoid cells in mucosal immunity. *Front. Immunol.* **2019**, *10*, 861. [CrossRef] [PubMed]
75. Krishnan, R.; Ring, K.; Williams, E.; Portell, C.; Jaffe, E.S.; Gru, A.A. An Enteropathy-like Indolent NK-Cell Proliferation Presenting in the Female Genital Tract. *Am. J. Surg. Pathol.* **2020**, *44*, 561. [CrossRef]
76. Kiel, M.J.; Velusamy, T.; Rolland, D.; Sahasrabuddhe, A.A.; Chung, F.; Bailey, N.G.; Schrader, A.; Li, B.; Li, J.Z.; Ozel, A.B.; et al. Integrated genomic sequencing reveals mutational landscape of T-cell prolymphocytic leukemia. *Blood* **2014**, *124*, 1460–1472. [CrossRef]
77. Van Dongen, J.J.M.; Langerak, A.W.; Brüggemann, M.; Evans, P.A.S.; Hummel, M.; Lavender, F.L.; Delabesse, E.; Davi, F.; Schuuring, E.; García-Sanz, R.; et al. Design and standardization of PCR primers and protocols for detection of clonal immunoglobulin and T-cell receptor gene recombinations in suspect lymphoproliferations: Report of the BIOMED-2 Concerted Action BMH4-CT98-3936. *Leukemia* **2003**, *17*, 2257–2317. [CrossRef]
78. Van den Brand, M.; Rijntjes, J.; Möbs, M.; Steinhilber, J.; van der Klift, M.Y.; Heezen, K.C.; Kroeze, L.I.; Reigl, T.; Porc, J.; Darzentas, N.; et al. Next-Generation Sequencing–Based Clonality Assessment of Ig Gene Rearrangements: A Multicenter Validation Study by EuroClonality-NGS. *J. Mol. Diagn.* **2021**, *23*, 1105–1115. [CrossRef]
79. Rossi, D.; Spina, V.; Bruscaggin, A.; Gaidano, G. Liquid biopsy in lymphoma. *Haematologica* **2019**, *104*, 648. [CrossRef]
80. Freiche, V.; Cordonnier, N.; Paulin, M.V.; Huet, H.; Turba, M.E.; Macintyre, E.; Malamut, G.; Cerf-Bensussan, N.; Molina, T.J.; Hermine, O.; et al. Feline low-grade intestinal T cell lymphoma: A unique natural model of human indolent T cell lymphoproliferative disorder of the gastrointestinal tract. *Lab. Investig.* **2021**, *101*, 794–804. [CrossRef]

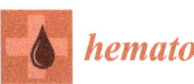

Review

Peripheral T-Cell Lymphomas of the T Follicular Helper Type: Clinical, Pathological, and Genetic Attributes

Karthik A. Ganapathi [1], Kristin H. Karner [2] and Madhu P. Menon [2,*]

1. Department of Laboratory Medicine, University of California, San Francisco, CA 94143, USA; karthik.ganapathi@ucsf.edu
2. ARUP Laboratories and Department of Pathology, University of Utah School of Medicine, Salt Lake City, UT 84108, USA; kristin.karner@aruplab.com
* Correspondence: madhu.menon@aruplab.com

Abstract: Follicular helper T-cell (TFH) lymphomas comprise a unique group of T-cell lymphomas that represent neoplastic proliferations of follicular helper T-cells and share genetic, immunophenotypic, morphologic, and clinical features. Angioimmunoblastic T-cell lymphoma (AITL) is the prototypical TFH lymphoma; in addition, the 2017 revised World Health Organization (WHO) 4th edition recognizes two other unique subtypes: follicular T-cell lymphoma (FTCL) and nodal peripheral T-cell lymphoma with the T follicular helper phenotype (PTCL-TFH). This review discusses the morphologic spectrum, immunophenotype, diagnostic mimics/pitfalls, and unique genetic attributes of this category of T-cell lymphomas.

Keywords: T follicular helper cells; TFH lymphoma; angioimmunoblastic T-cell lymphoma; follicular T-cell lymphoma; peripheral T-cell lymphoma of T-follicular helper immunophenotype; peripheral T-cell lymphoma

1. Introduction

Follicular helper T-cells (TFHs) are a specialized subset of CD4-positive helper T-cells that are essential for germinal center formation, B-cell maturation, and the development of high-affinity antibodies [1,2]. TFH differentiation from naive CD4-positive helper T-cells is a complex multistep process that is initiated by the interaction between dendritic cells (DCs) and T-cells and mediated by interleukin-6 (IL-6), inducible costimulatory (ICOS), and T-cell receptor (TCR) molecules [3]. The second stage of TFH maturation occurs during T-cell interaction with antigen-specific B-cells in the follicle or interfollicular areas. TFH and B-cell maturation in the follicle is a symbiotic process [4] and is mediated by the BCL6-IRF4-BLIMP1 transcriptional axis [5]. TFH maturation is completed in the germinal center (GC), and the majority of GC TFH cells express CD4, CXCR5, PD1, BCL6, CD10, CXCL13, and ICOS [1,6–8]. Mature TFH cells are not confined to the GC; they can exit the follicle and enter a different GC, or return to the same GC, or downregulate BCL6 and become memory TFH cells [1].

The most important function of TFH cells is GC development and function, enabling B-cell maturation and high-affinity antibody production. This critical process is exquisitely regulated and defective TFH function results in suboptimal immune responses to viral infections such as human immunodeficiency virus (HIV) [9]. TFH cells are also implicated in autoimmunity, with increased circulating TFH-like cells seen in some patients with systemic lupus erythematosus (SLE) and Sjögren's syndrome [10]. TFH cells also seem to play a role in cancer immunity, and it is postulated that they may help maintain ectopic lymphoid structures and potentially affect prognosis [11].

Understanding TFH cell maturation has also allowed the identification of these cells in normal lymphoid tissue and in neoplastic lymphoid proliferations, such as lymphomas. It is now understood that a subset of peripheral T-cell lymphomas (PTCL) represents neoplastic proliferations of TFH cells, the best-characterized of which is angioimmunoblastic T-cell lymphoma (AITL), which has unique clinical and pathologic features [12,13]. Two additional nodal T-cell lymphomas with different morphologic features than AITL, but sharing a TFH cell immunophenotype and genetic and molecular features have been described: follicular T-cell lymphoma (FTCL) and nodal peripheral T-cell lymphoma with the TFH cell phenotype (PTCL-TFH) [14–16]. Additionally, cutaneous T-cell proliferations with the TFH cell phenotype have also been described [17].

To reflect this understanding, the 2017 WHO Classification has removed FTCL and PTCL-TFH from the PTCL, not otherwise specified (PTCL, NOS) category and included them with AITL as subtypes of a new broader category, nodal lymphomas of T-follicular helper (TFH) origin (Table 1) [18]. Cutaneous TFH proliferations are not included in this category, as they do not share clinical or molecular features with nodal TFH lymphomas [19].

Table 1. 2017 WHO classification of T follicular helper cell (TFH) lymphomas.

Angioimmunoblastic T-Cell Lymphoma and Other Nodal Lymphomas of T Follicular Helper (TFH) Cell Origin
Angioimmunoblastic T-cell lymphoma
Follicular T-cell lymphoma
Nodal peripheral T-cell lymphoma with the TFH phenotype

From a practical and diagnostic standpoint, TFH lymphomas share some features. By flow cytometry, many cases show an aberrant CD3 (dim/−)/CD4+ T-cell population [20]. The most commonly used markers for identifying TFH T-cells in paraffin-embedded tissue are CD10, BCL6, PD1, CXCL13, CXCR5, ICOS, SAP, CD200, and MAF, and the recommendations for assigning a TFH phenotype include expression of at least two, ideally three TFH markers [1,6–8,12,13,18,21–24]. Given the varying sensitivities of immunohistochemical stains, utilizing a panel of markers to identify these T-cell lymphomas in routine practice is a prudent approach [25].

2. Angioimmunoblastic T-Cell Lymphoma

Angioimmunoblastic T-cell lymphoma is the prototypical member of the TFH family of PTCLs [26]. AITLs have unique clinicopathologic and pathologic features. Lymph node biopsies are characterized by a polymorphous infiltrate, effaced architecture, and expanded follicular dendritic cell (FDC) meshworks, which especially encircle the proliferating high endothelial venules (HEVs). In addition to cytogenetic abnormalities, AITLs also demonstrate a unique gene expression signature and mutational profile that is partly shared with other TFH lymphomas (discussed in detail later) [13,15,16,27–29].

2.1. Epidemiology and Clinical Features

AITL occurs usually in middle-aged and elderly patients and with a male predominance [30,31]. While it accounts for only 1–2% of non-Hodgkin's lymphoma, it is one of the more common T-cell lymphomas and constitutes 15–20% of non-cutaneous T-cell lymphomas [32,33].

Patients typically have high-stage (III-IV) disease with frequent bone marrow involvement [34]. They present with diffuse lymphadenopathy, hepatosplenomegaly, skin rashes (with or without pruritus), pleural effusion, ascites, and arthritis [30,31,35–37]. Extranodal involvement is usually seen in the liver, spleen, skin, and bone marrow, but other sites such as the lung and gastrointestinal tract can be infrequently involved [31,35,36].

Laboratory studies show polyclonal hypergammaglobulinemia, cold agglutinins, Coombs-positive hemolytic anemia, positive rheumatoid factor, anti-smooth muscle antibodies, and elevated LDH [31,38]. Complete blood counts usually show cytopenia(s) with or without eosinophilia. Patients also demonstrate immune dysfunction, immunodeficiency, and frequent EBV infection. The proliferation of EBV-positive B-cells suggest an etiologic role of EBV in this lymphoma [39,40].

Patients can have a variable clinical course, but the disease tends to be aggressive with a median survival of less than 3 y [41]. Histology or genetics do not influence the outcome [18].

2.2. Morphology and Immunophenotype

Lymph node biopsies are the most common specimens in routine practice that pathologists encounter for AITL diagnosis. An excisional biopsy is the ideal specimen, and diagnoses on small core biopsies might be challenging because of a lack of an architectural context and a paucity of tissue for ancillary tests. A diagnosis of AITL can be especially challenging in extranodal site biopsies.

Lymph node excisional biopsies generally demonstrate effacement of the architecture by a polymorphous infiltrate composed of small, atypical lymphocytes (usually with a clear cytoplasm), plasma cells, macrophages, and scattered larger cells, which appear either immunoblastic or sometimes Hodgkin's-/Reed–Sternberg cell (HRS)-like. The atypical lymphocytes are clustered especially around proliferating high endothelial venules, which are rather prominent in the biopsies. The subcapsular sinuses tend to be distended. Biopsies can also demonstrate tissue eosinophilia.

Three major patterns have been described in the context of AITL; these are sequentially named Patterns 1, 2, and 3 and are believed to be the histologic progression of the disease (Table 2). A high proportion (up to 17%) of patients present with Pattern 1 [21,42–44], which is especially challenging to diagnose because of retention of the architecture, presence of hyperplastic germinal centers, and lack of overt proliferation of high endothelial venules or polymorphous infiltration. The clues to Pattern 1 diagnosis are the absent/attenuated mantle zones surrounded by clear atypical cells, the PD1 staining pattern (circumferential perifollicular PD1 staining TFH cells as opposed to TFH cells either scattered throughout the germinal center or polarized appearing in reactive lymph nodes), and the slight branching of FDC meshworks outside of the intact germinal centers (Table 1 and Figure 1A,D,G). In addition, closer observation might identify focal expansion of the paracortex and a slight increase in HEVs. Any suspicion of a T-cell lymphoproliferative disorder should trigger a molecular or genetic analysis (see below).

Table 2. Morphologic patterns of angioimmunoblastic T-cell lymphoma.

	Pattern 1	Pattern 2	Pattern 3
Architecture	Preserved	Partially effaced	Totally effaced
Follicles	Hyperplastic germinal centers Absent/attenuated mantle zones	Atretic/regressed Castleman-like follicles	Absent or occasional compressed follicles seen at the periphery (especially highlighted with a CD20 stain)
Paracortex	Focal areas of paracortical expansion and perifollicular polymorphous infiltrate focal slight increase in HEVs	Areas with polymorphous infiltration with immunoblasts and Hodgkin's-like cells Proliferation of HEVs in the expanded areas	Marked polymorphous diffuse infiltration with immunoblasts and Hodgkin's-like cells Marked proliferation of HEVs
TFH cell	Perifollicular with occasional paracortical clustering	Paracortical aggregates spilling out of follicles with grouping around HEVs	Diffuse proliferation of TFH cells with grouping around HEVs
FDC meshworks (CD21 or CD23 IHC)	Intact with slight branching out	Partially intact with areas demonstrating expansion and encircling of HEVs	Marked expansion with encircling around HEVs

FDC, follicular dendritic cells; HEV, high endothelial venule; IHC, immunostain; TFH, follicular helper T-cells.

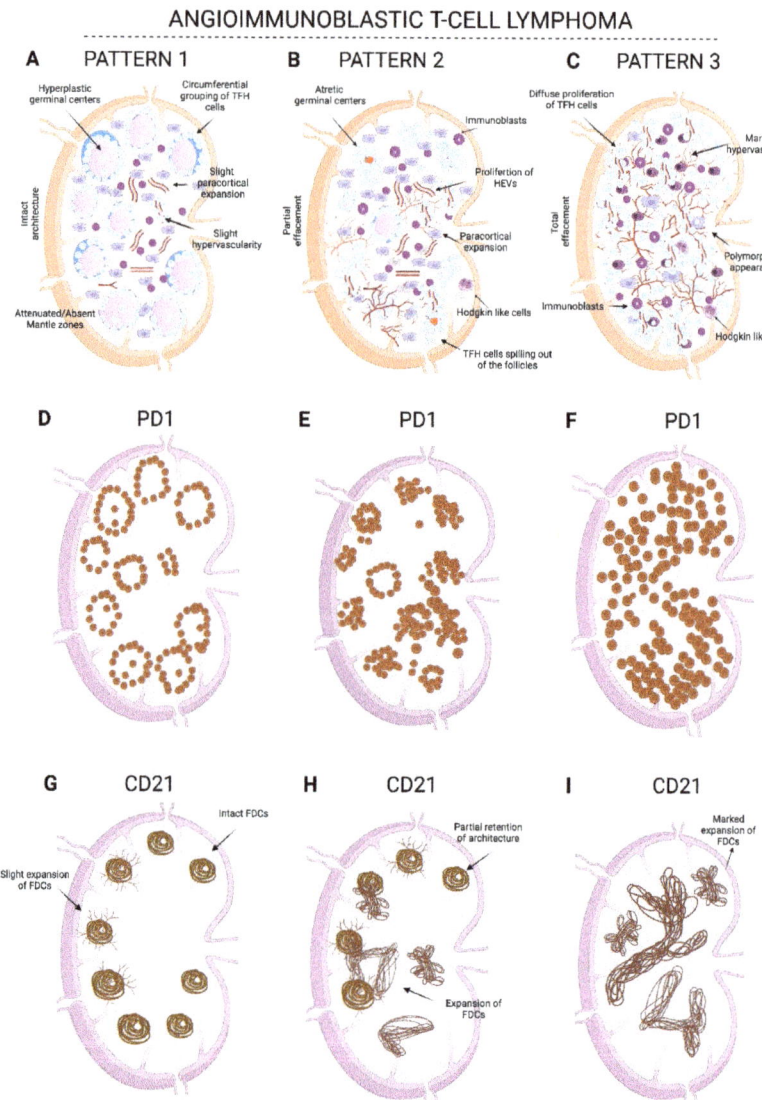

Figure 1. Morphologic patterns of AITL. Pattern 1: (**A**) intact architecture, hyperplastic germinal centers, attenuated/absent mantle zones, slight paracortical expansion, and slight proliferation of high endothelial venules; (**D**) circumferential perifollicular PD1-positive TFH cells with only occasional clustering around vessels; (**G**) intact CD21+ FDC meshworks with only slight expansion into the paracortex. Pattern 2: (**B**) Partial effacement of architecture, proliferation of HEVs, and paracortical expansion by a polymorphous infiltrate with atypical clear cells, small lymphocytes, plasma cells, macrophages, eosinophils, frequent immunoblasts, and rare Hodgkin/Reed–Sternberg-like cells; (**E**) increase in PD1-positive TFH cells extending out of the follicle into the paracortex with accumulation around the HEVs; (**H**) CD21+ FDC meshworks start expanding and encircling the HEVs. Pattern 3: (**C**) Total effacement of architecture, polymorphous infiltration with diffuse neoplastic clear-appearing T-cells, small lymphocytes, macrophages, plasma cells, eosinophils, immunoblasts, and scattered Hodgkin's-/Reed–Sternberg-like cells. Marked proliferation of HEVs is seen with neo-

plastic clear-appearing T-cells clustered around them; (**F**) PD1-positive neoplastic T-cells are diffusely present; (**I**) CD21+ FDC meshworks are markedly expanded and encircle the blood vessels. Image created in Biorender by M.M.

Pattern 2 demonstrates partial effacement/partial retention of the architecture (Figures 1B and 2A) with paracortical expansion by a polymorphous infiltrate with neoplastic clear TFH cells, small lymphocytes, plasma cells, macrophages, eosinophils, scattered immunoblasts, and Hodgkin's-/Reed-Sternberg-like cells (Figures 1B and 2C). Atretic Castleman-like follicles are also seen (Figures 1B and 2A,B). The neoplastic TFH cells are more pronounced and start spilling out of the follicles into the paracortex (Figure 1B) and encircle the HEVs; this is particularly evident with CD3 (Figure 2D) and TFH marker stains, e.g., PD1 stain (Figures 1E and 2E), CD10 (Figure 2E), and CXCL13 (Figure 2F). CD21 demonstrates partial expansion and distortion of FDC meshworks along with some areas, demonstrating retention of the architecture (Figures 1H and 2G). EBER-ish demonstrates scattered EBV+ cells, demonstrating a size range (Figure 2H).

Pattern 3 is the most recognizable pattern of AITL. Lymph nodes demonstrate complete effacement of the architecture (Figures 1C and 3A) by a polymorphous infiltrate (Figures 1C and 3B) composed of mostly atypical clear-appearing neoplastic TFH cells, macrophages, plasma cells, eosinophils, and numerous larger cells, including Hodgkin's-like cells, representing immunoblasts (Figures 1C and 3B). The neoplastic TFH cells express T-cell markers such as CD3 (Figure 3D) and TFH markers such as PD1 (Figures 1F and 3E) CD10 (Figure 3F), and CXCL13 (Figure 3G). CD21 demonstrates marked expansion and distortion of FDC meshworks (Figures 1I and 3H). CD30 is positive not only in the large HRS-like cells, but also in a subset of the smaller neoplastic TFH cells (Figure 3I). EBER-ish demonstrates scattered EBV-positive cells (Figure 3J).

Immunohistochemical studies are crucial to the diagnosis of AITL, which hinges on the demonstration of a TFH phenotype. An extensive T-cell panel, i.e., CD2, CD3, CD4, CD8, CD5, and CD7, should be used to evaluate immunophenotypic aberrancies. Aberrancies (dimness or loss) of CD3, CD5, and CD7 are most common. The vast majority of the neoplastic TFH cells are CD4-positive. As discussed above, TFH cells express several markers, i.e., CD10, BCL6, PD1, CXCL13, CXCR5, ICOS, SAP, CD200, and MAF, and the recommendations for assigning a TFH phenotype include expression of at least two, ideally three TFH markers [1,6–8,12,13,18,21–24]. Studies have also shown that, while in most cases, a four-marker panel (CD10, PD-1, CXCL13, and BCL6) is adequate, employing ICOS as an additional marker (creating a five-marker panel) greatly improves TFH phenotype detection [25]. An additional consideration is the intensity of these markers, especially PD1 and ICOS, which need to be bright to qualify as TFH markers. In addition, CD10 expression is usually variable and, in most cases, is expressed in a subset of the neoplastic TFH cells. Hence, CD10 needs to be evaluated carefully. Overall, CXCL13 and CD10 are considered most specific, while PD1 and ICOS are considered more sensitive [18]. CD21, CD23, or CD35 can be used to evaluate the FDC meshworks.

An important point worth mentioning is that AITL can relapse with a follicular T-cell lymphoma (FTCL) morphology (discussed below) and vice versa [15]. Figure 4 illustrates one such case of a patient with a previous history of AITL with a subsequent biopsy demonstrating FTCL.

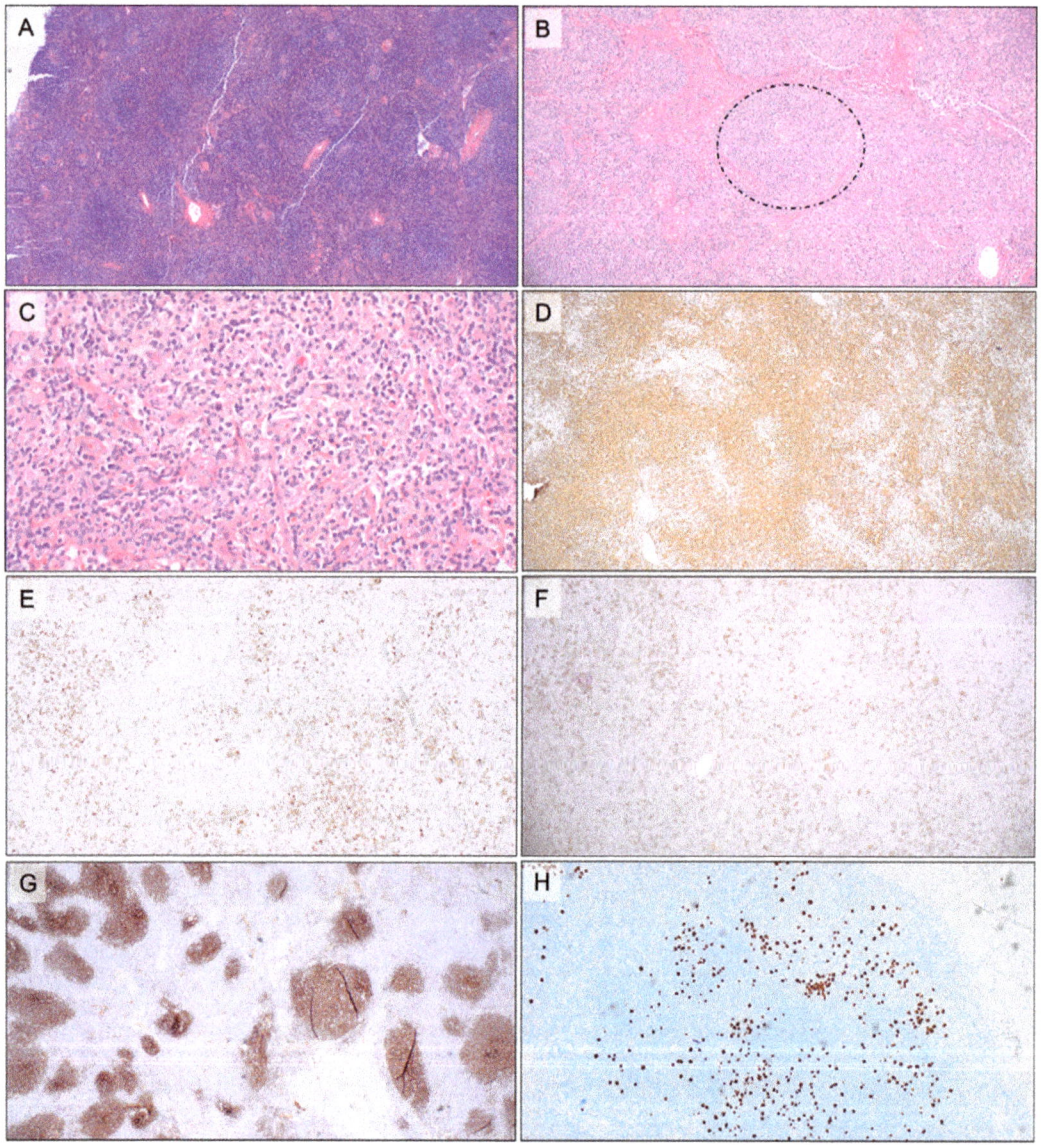

Figure 2. AITL, Pattern 2. (**A**) The lymph node architecture is partially effaced with the presence of atretic follicles, 20×; (**B**) Castleman like-follicles surrounded by atypical TFH cells, 200×; (**C**) partially effaced areas with polymorphous infiltration and the presence of neoplastic T-cells. The neoplastic T-cells are positive for (**D**) CD3, (**E**) PD1, and (**F**) CD10. (**G**) CD21 shows partial FDC meshworks (**right**) and expanded distorted FDC meshworks (**left**). (**H**) EBER-ish demonstrates scattered EBV-positive cells.

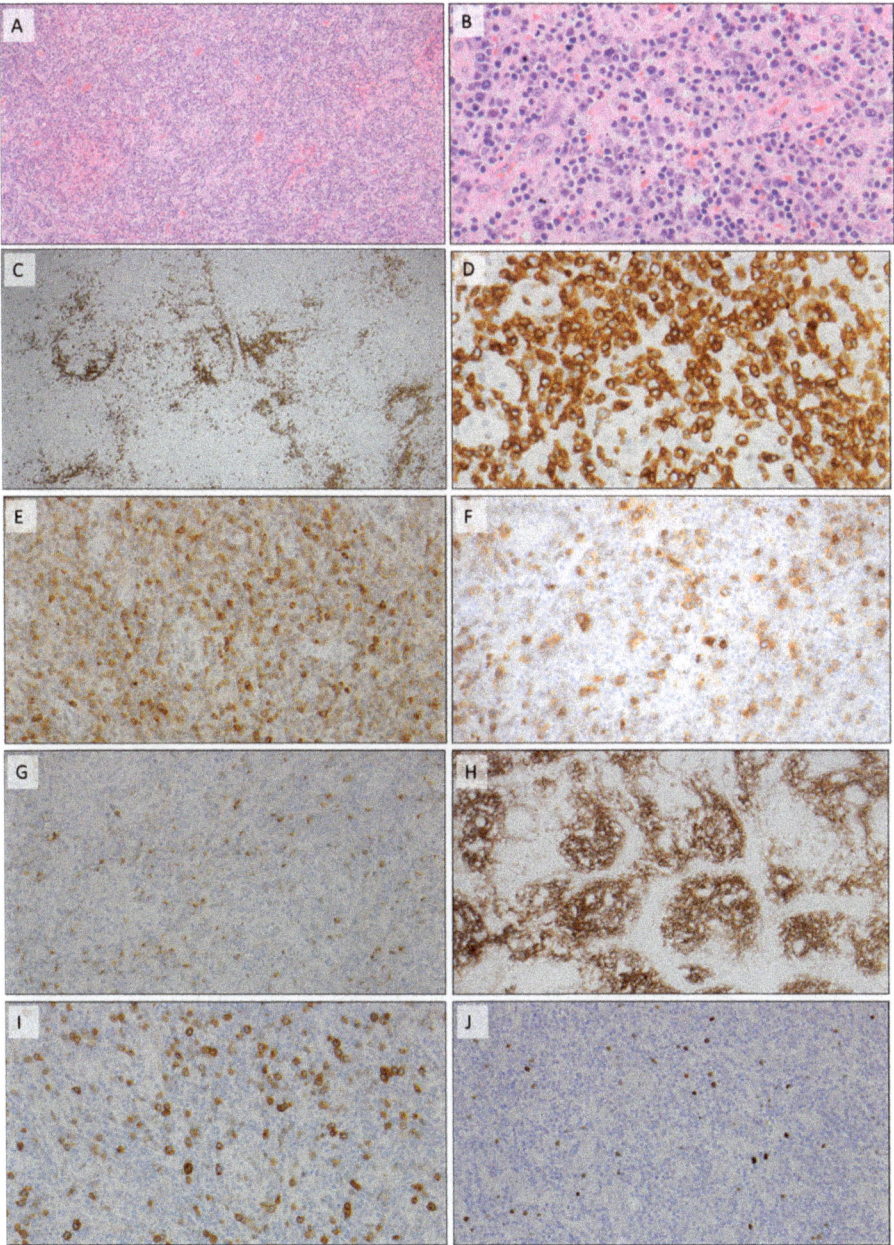

Figure 3. AITL, Pattern 3. (**A**) The lymph node architecture is completely effaced; (**B**) polymorphous infiltrate composed of neoplastic T-cells, macrophages, plasma cells, few eosinophils, and scattered immunoblasts; (**C**) CD20 demonstrates few retained B-cell areas with some follicles compressed at the periphery. The neoplastic T-cells are positive for (**D**) CD3, (**E**) PD1, (**F**) CD10, and (**G**) CXCL13. (**H**) CD21 shows expanded distorted FDC meshworks. (**I**) CD30 demonstrates positivity not only in the larger immunoblastic/Hodgkin's-like cells, but also in the surrounding smaller neoplastic T-cells. (**J**) EBER-ish demonstrates scattered EBV-positive cells.

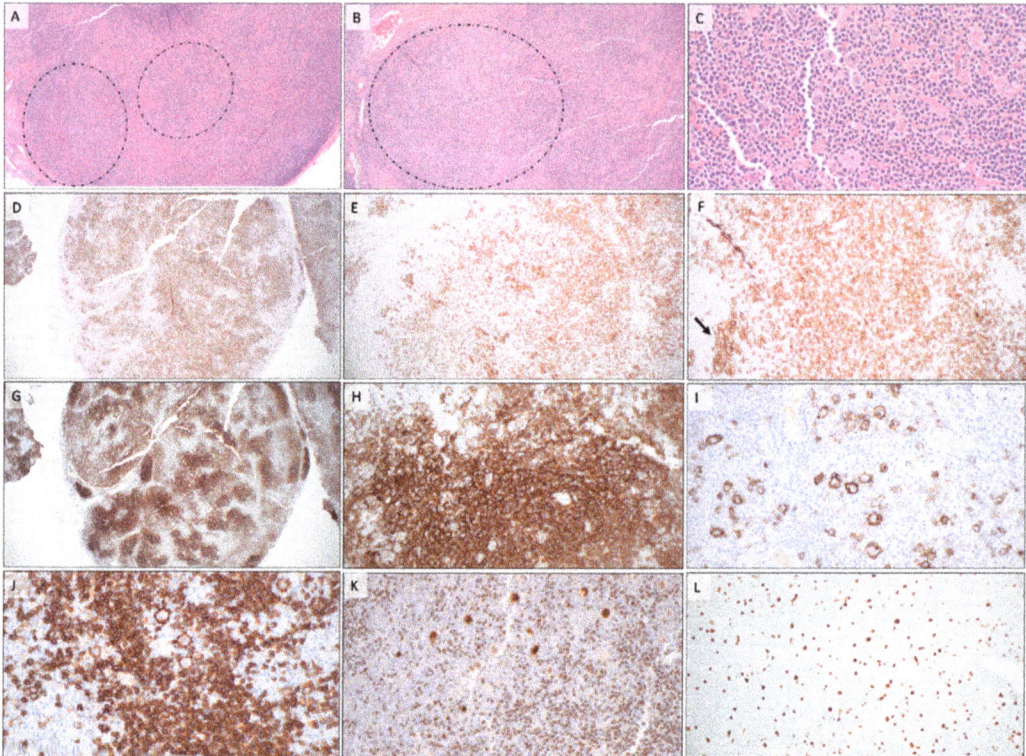

Figure 4. Follicular-T-cell-lymphoma-like relapse of AITL. (**A**) The lymph node demonstrates a nodular architecture. The nodules are composed of mostly small lymphocytes and macrophages (**B**) reminiscent of progressive transformation of germinal centers (PTGCs) and nodular lymphocyte predominant Hodgkin's lymphoma (NLPHL), with scattered larger lymphocyte predominant (LP), Hodgkin's/Reed–Sternberg-like (HRS), and immunoblasts (**C**). PD1-positive neoplastic T-cells are diffusely increased (**D**,**F**), albeit that in some of the nodules, they form rosettes around the larger cells (**E**). CD21 shows expanded distorted FDC meshworks (**G**), which also surround the HEVs (**H**). The larger HRS and LP-like cells are positive for CD30 (**I**), CD20 (**J**), and OCT2 (**K**). EBER-ish demonstrates scattered EBV-positive cells, both large and small (**L**).

2.3. EBV, B-Cell, and Plasma Cell Proliferations

B-cell and plasma cell proliferations (clonal and non-clonal) are a frequent occurrence in AITL [31]. The B-cells can appear to be either immunoblastic or HRS-like. While EBV is associated with the majority of B-cell proliferations in AITLs (more than 80%) [31,40,45], EBV-negative cases have also been reported [46]. In most cases, EBV-positive B-cells are scattered or form small clusters; however, in some cases, sheets of large B-cells are seen, which would prompt the consideration of a second diagnosis of a composite diffuse large B-cell lymphoma [45,47]. Plasmacytosis and plasma cell proliferations are a frequent occurrence in AITL, and most of these are EBV-negative. While most are polyclonal, occasional clonal plasma cell proliferations have also been reported [48,49].

2.4. Flow Cytometry

Flow cytometric studies can be a powerful ancillary tool in the diagnosis of AITL [20,50–53]. Neoplastic T-cells in AITL frequently demonstrate the downregulation or the absence of surface CD3 along with absent or diminished surface T-cell receptors

(Figure 5A,B) [53]. However, in these cases, they generally express cytoplasmic CD3 and cytoplasmic TCR-alpha/beta (Figure 5E,F). In addition, most AITL patients (as opposed to PTCL patients) also seem to demonstrate this atypical surface CD3 dim/neg population to varying extents in the peripheral blood [50,52,53]. A simple T-cell panel employing CD3, CD4, CD10, CD14, CD5, and CD45 to evaluate for surface CD3 dim/neg, CD10+, CD4+ population has been suggested to aid in AITL diagnosis, especially in bone marrow and peripheral blood [20]. Bright PD1 expression by flow cytometry has also been shown to be a useful tool for both the diagnosis and monitoring of AITL [54]. Flow cytometry studies might also demonstrate additional immunophenotypic abnormalities described in AITL, e.g., loss of CD5 or CD7.

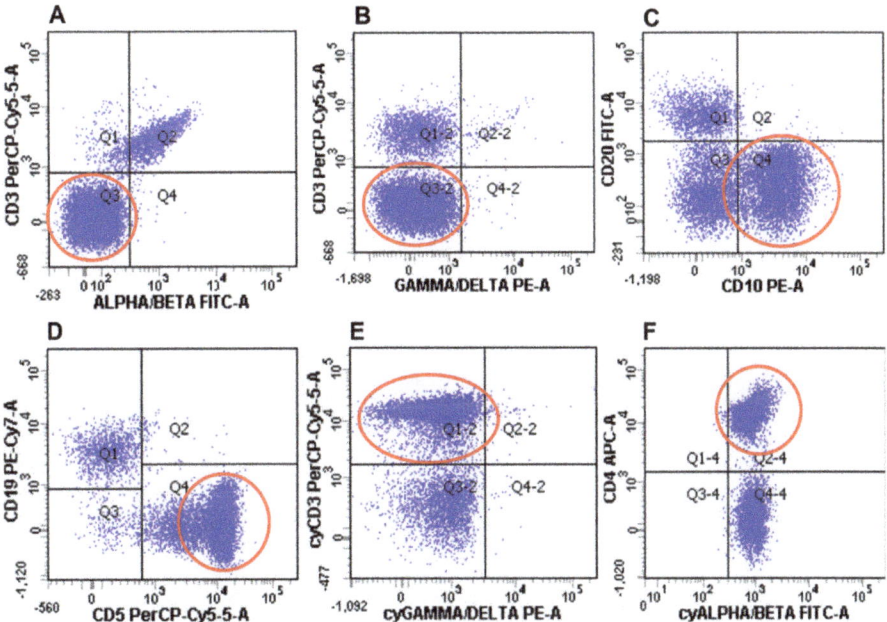

Figure 5. Flow cytometric findings in AITL The neoplastic T-cells are negative for surface CD3 and surface TCRalpha/beta (**A**) and surface TCR gamma/delta (**B**), but positive for CD10 (**C**), CD5 (**D**), cytoplasmic CD3 (**E**), cytoplasmic TCR alpha/beta (**F**), and CD4 (**F**).

2.5. Genetics

Most AITLs demonstrate clonal T-cell receptor rearrangements by PCR; in addition, they also demonstrate clonal immunoglobulin gene rearrangements in 25–30% of cases. The latter usually correspond to EBV-positive B-cell proliferations in most cases [18].

The cytogenetics and mutational spectrum of AITL, as well as the association with clonal hematopoiesis are discussed in detail in a separate section (see below).

2.6. Differential Diagnoses

While other mature T-cell lymphomas including *peripheral T-cell lymphoma NOS* should be considered in the differential diagnosis, the distinction is perhaps less critical from a treatment standpoint. As mentioned above, the diagnosis of AITL hinges on the demonstration of at least two (ideally three) TFH antigens, as well as the presence of other characteristics' findings such as a polymorphous infiltrate, aggregates of TFH cells around proliferating HEVs, and scattered EBV+ cells.

Perhaps one of the most challenging differential diagnoses of Pattern 1 AITL is *reactive lymphoid hyperplasia* [21,42–44]. Pattern 1 AITL can often be retrospectively diagnosed in a previous biopsy from a patient with a subsequent Pattern 3 AITL. The main morphologic clues in favor of a Pattern 1 AITL include absent or attenuated mantle zones, the presence of clear atypical cells surrounding the hyperplastic germinal centers (this might not be obvious), focal expansion of the paracortex, and focal increase in HEVs. This should prompt further staining with PD1, which would demonstrate the circumferential grouping of the neoplastic TFH cells and few clusters in the paracortex. CD21 would demonstrate slight branching out of the FDC meshwork. If the findings are suspicious for Pattern 1 AITL, then PCR for T-cell receptor rearrangement and next-generation sequencing studies (NGS) for IDH1, IDH2, DNMT3A, TET2, and RHOA (see below) should be ideally performed. In addition, as discussed above, flow cytometry might demonstrate a CD3dim/neg, CD4+, CD10+ population that is highly suggestive of AITL; if flow cytometry is not available on tissue, it could be attempted on peripheral blood [20,52,53]. Interestingly, several patients present at a clinically advanced stage with a Pattern 1 morphology on a biopsy; this perhaps reflects the morphologic evolution of the disease with the distinct possibility that other lymph nodes in the body might have a more evolved Pattern 3 morphology [42].

Classic Hodgkin lymphoma (CHL) can be a challenging differential diagnosis especially considering the similar polymorphous background and the presence of Hodgkin's-/Reed–Sternberg (HRS)-like cells, which is common in AITL. Adding to the difficulty is the observation that these large cells are usually CD30-positive and occasionally CD15-positive [46,55]. However, the HRS-like cells in AITL generally tend to preserve the B-cell program more often, and an extensive panel of B-cell markers, i.e., CD20, PAX5, OCT2, BOB1, and CD79a, should be employed (albeit that CD20 and PAX5 downregulation can be seen in HRS-like cells in AITL). In addition, an extensive T-cell IHC panel (CD3, CD2, CD5, CD4, CD8, CD7) should be used in challenging cases to evaluate for immunophenotypic aberrancies in T-cells. Fibrosis is unusual in AITL and is more common in CHL. Cytologic atypia in the surrounding T-cells, proliferating HEVs, FDC expansion beyond follicles, morphologic variation, pleomorphism in the larger cells, etc., would favor AITL. In addition, sheets and aggregates of PD1-positive cells beyond rosetting of HRS-like cells should raise suspicion for AITL and prompt further workup including molecular studies (PCR and NGS; see above). In addition, EBV positivity is usually restricted to the large HRS cells in CHL, while there usually is more variation in the cell size of EBV+ cells in AITL. CD30 staining in smaller lymphocytes, in addition to the larger HRS-like cells, should also prompt consideration of AITL [56]. As mentioned above, flow cytometric detection of a CD3 dim/neg, CD4+, CD10+ population can be particularly helpful in the diagnosis of AITL and other TFH lymphomas, as this population is not seen in CHL [20,50–53].

3. Follicular T-Cell Lymphoma

3.1. Epidemiology and Clinical Features

Follicular T-cell lymphoma (FTCL) was first described in 1988 [57] and is a rare entity, representing 1–2% of peripheral T-cell lymphomas. It is a disease of older individuals occurring in the sixth decade of life and slightly more common in males. Patients usually present with diffuse lymphadenopathy, and high-stage disease with extranodal and cutaneous involvement has been reported. Rare patients may show immunological abnormalities on laboratory investigations, including positive direct antibody tests (DATs) and hypergammaglobulinemia [15].

3.2. Morphology and Immunophenotype

By morphology, two distinct growth patterns are recognized: a follicular growth pattern that mimics B-cell follicular lymphoma (FL-like) and a progressive transformation of a germinal centers-like pattern (PTGC-like) (Figure 6) [18]. In cases with the FL-like pattern, the neoplastic T-cells are arranged in well-defined nodules that lack the morphological features of normal follicles. Mantle zones can either be preserved or absent. In PTGC-like cases, representing the majority of FTCL, the neoplastic T-cells are seen in small aggregates surrounded by small mantle zone B-cells arranged in large, irregular nodules. Eosinophilic infiltration is uncommon, and unlike in AITL, arborizing high endothelial venules and expanded follicular dendritic cell meshworks are not identified. The neoplastic T-cells range from small to medium with irregular nuclei, coarse to vesicular chromatin, and moderate to abundant pale cytoplasm. While the nuclear features can resemble centrocytes or centroblasts, the pale cytoplasm is a useful distinguishing feature. Scattered B-cell immunoblasts, including some resembling Hodgkin's/Reed–Sternberg cells, usually surrounded by neoplastic T-cells, are seen in a significant subset of cases.

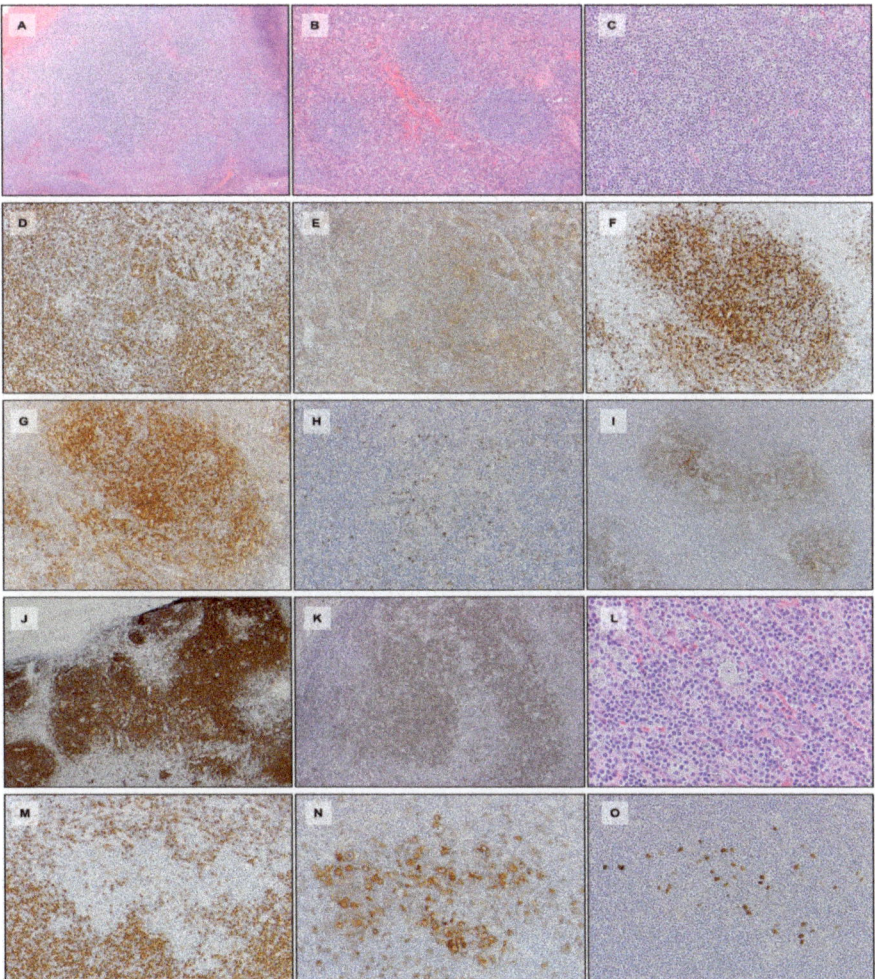

Figure 6. Follicular T-cell lymphoma with a PTGC-like pattern. (**A**) The lymph node architecture is effaced by atypical nodules containing (**B**) small mature lymphocytes resembling mantle zone cells and admixed medium-sized lymphocytes with clear cytoplasm. (**C**) Scattered Hodgkin's/Reed–Sternberg-like cells are noted. The neoplastic T-cells are positive for (**D**) CD3, (**E**) CD4, (**F**) CD10, (**G**) PD1, and (**H**) CXCL13. (**I**) CD21 shows dendritic cell meshworks within the nodules that are composed predominantly of mantle zone B-cells positive for (**J**) CD20 and (**K**) IgD. (**L**) The H/RS-like cells are positive for (**M**) PAX5 (weak), (**N**) CD30, and (**O**) EBER.

The neoplastic T-cells in FTCL express pan T-cell antigens including CD2, CD3, CD5, and CD7. An aberrant immunophenotype is seen in the majority of cases with the loss of CD7 most commonly noted [58]. They are positive for CD4 and express multiple TFH markers, with PD1 and ICOS reportedly the most sensitive, followed by CXCL13. CD10 and BCL6 are less sensitive and are expressed in fewer cases. They are negative for CD8, CD56, cytotoxic markers, and EBV. Follicular dendritic cell meshworks are limited to the nodular areas. The proliferative rate, assessed by Ki-67, is variable, with mean values approaching 50%. The transformed immunoblasts are positive for B-cell markers including CD20 and PAX5. CD30 and EBV can be expressed in a subset of cases [58].

3.3. Molecular Studies

Clonal T-cell receptor gene rearrangements are identified in the vast majority of cases; additionally, a subset of cases may show oligoclonal or clonal IgH gene rearrangements [58].

3.4. Differential Diagnoses

While it is rare, a diagnosis of FTCL should not be overlooked when evaluating a lymph node for involvement by lymphoma. FTCL with an FL-like growth pattern can mimic FL, but can be distinguished from FL by the cytologic features of the neoplastic T-cells and the expression of multiple T-cell markers by the abnormal follicles. The PTGC-like variant raises the differential diagnosis of classic Hodgkin's lymphoma, the lymphocyte-rich variant (CHL-LR), or nodular-lymphocyte-predominant Hodgkin's lymphoma (NLPHL). In cases resembling CHL or NLPHL, careful examination of the T-cells rosetting the H/RS-like cells or LP cells is mandatory, as in most FTCL cases, these T-cells are neoplastic and express multiple TFH markers, most commonly PD1, ICOS, and CD10 [59,60]. A subset of these neoplastic cells can also express CD30, which can help distinguishing them from reactive T-cells [56].

4. Peripheral T-Cell Lymphoma with TFH Phenotype

Multiple studies have shown that a significant subset of peripheral T-cell lymphomas, morphologically classified as peripheral T-cell lymphoma, not otherwise specified (PTCL, NOS), arise from TFH cells and share genomic features, but are not identical to AITL [16,28,61,62]. This relationship has also been confirmed by the evaluation of TFH marker expression in these lymphomas [14,25,63]. In recognition of these findings and to aid in better classification and therapy, the WHO 2017 Classification recommends that nodal CD4+ T-cell lymphomas be evaluated for the expression of TFH antigens and provisionally classified as peripheral T-cell lymphoma with the TFH phenotype (PTCL-TFH) if they express at least two (ideally three) TFH antigens [18]. The rates of classification as PTCL-TFH appear significantly different when using two or three TFH markers, and large-scale studies are required to help develop stringent criteria for reproducible classification [25].

Morphologically, PTCL-TFH shows diffuse effacement of the nodal architecture by neoplastic T-cells that can range in size from small to large (Figure 7). Unlike AITL, PTCL-TFH lacks the clear cell morphology, polymorphous inflammatory background, and expanded dendritic cell meshworks with high endothelial venule proliferation [14,25] (Figure 4).

PTCL-T TFH shares immunophenotypic features with AITL and FTCL with variable expression of TFH markers. PD1 and ICOS remain the most sensitive, while CXCL13, BCL6, and CD10 are expressed in fewer cases [25].

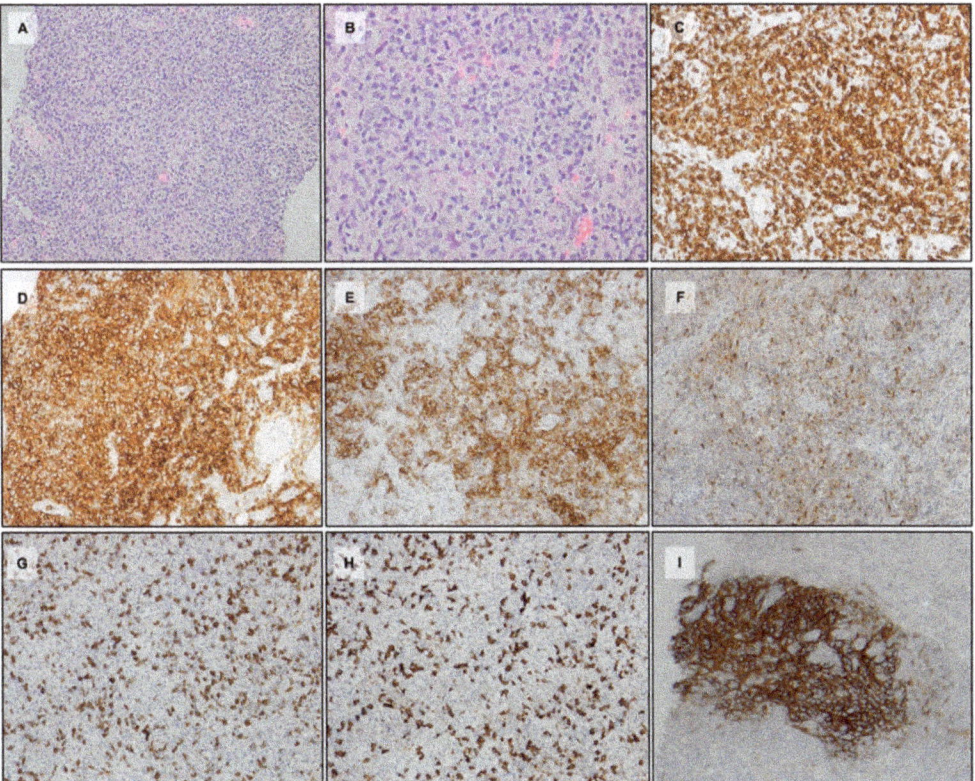

Figure 7. Peripheral T-cell lymphoma with the TFH phenotype. (**A**,**B**) The interfollicular areas are expanded by a diffuse proliferation of predominantly medium-sized cells with irregular nuclei, mature chromatin, and variable amounts of cytoplasm. The atypical cells are positive for (**C**) CD3, (**D**) CD4, (**E**) PD1, and (**F**) CXCL13 and negative for (**G**) CD7 and (**H**) CD8. (**I**) CD21 shows relatively intact dendritic cell meshworks.

5. G. Genetics of TFH Lymphomas

T-cell lymphomas of T follicular helper origin show some distinct differences from other peripheral T-cell lymphomas. Angioimmunoblastic T-cell lymphomas have a distinct gene expression profile relating to the unique microenvironment that includes a B-cell signature, angiogenesis/vascular endothelial signature, cytokine signature, and T follicular helper signature [16,29,64]. While PTCL-TFH also shares the TFH signature, it lacks the characteristic microenvironment signature of AITL. Nevertheless, the gene expression profiles of AITL, FTCL, and PTCL-TFH are similar and distinct enough to support the argument that they likely represent a continuum of a single disease [16]. Rodriguez also demonstrated that AITL, but not PTCL-TFH cases that were enriched for the B-cell signature had a more favorable prognosis [61].

Among the genetic mutations identified in T-cell lymphomas, IDH2 R172 mutations seem to be specific for AITL and have only rarely been reported in other PTCL-NOS, while they have been reported in 20–40% of AITL cases [16,29,64,65]. In one study, this mutation was significantly associated with chromosome 5 gains and upregulation of IL4, IL13, and MAPK9 [66].

TET2 mutations and, less frequently, DNMT3A mutations are also enriched in TFH lymphomas (TET2 mutations are seen in approximately 50–75% of cases). Interestingly, these mutations are not only seen in tumor cells, but are present in non-tumor hematopoietic cells as well, suggesting that these lymphomas may have a pre-malignant mutant clone (clonal hematopoiesis of indeterminate potential), much as what has been extensively described and investigated in myeloid malignancies such as myelodysplastic syndrome [16,64]. TET2 mutations have been associated with advanced-stage disease, high IPI scores, and shorter progression-free survival [67].

RHOA mutations, almost always at the G17V hotspot, are frequently identified in AITL and FTCL (60–70%) and essentially always co-occur with TET2 mutations [61,64,68]. While the TET2 mutation is found in the non-tumor hematopoietic cells, the RHOA mutation appears restricted to the tumor cells and likely occurs as a later event. The combination of the two mutations may contribute to AITL-specific pathogenesis. RHOA T19I mutations, albeit less common, have also been reported [69].

Genotype/phenotype correlations have also been described, with AITL carrying RHOA G17V mutations showing increased vasculature and prominent follicular dendritic cell meshworks [70], while those with IDH2 R172 mutations having more prominent large, clear cells and strong TFH marker expression [71].

The cytogenetic profile of AITL is considerably less abnormal than other PTCLs [66]. Chromosome 5 gains are seen in about 40% of AITL and are distinct among hematologic malignancies, which more typically show losses in chromosome 5. Cases that do not have chromosome 5 gains show enrichment of NF-KB and PI3K-AKT pathways and may have a distinct pathogenesis [66]. Additionally, ~20% of FTCL carry a recurrent translocation t(5;9)(q33;q22)(ITK-SYK). This rearrangement is not specific for FTCL and has been described in other peripheral T-cell lymphomas, including AITL [72,73].

6. TFH Lymphomas, Clonal Hematopoiesis of Indeterminate Potential, and Myeloid Neoplasms

TET2 and DNMT3A mutations are frequently noted in clonal hematopoiesis of indeterminate potential (CHIP) [74,75] and myeloid malignancies [76–78]. The subsequent discovery of TET2 and DNMT3A mutations in TFH lymphomas has prompted the investigation of the relationship between these seemingly disparate categories of hematologic malignancies. Interestingly, studies have shown that TFH lymphomas can arise from divergent clonal evolution from TET2 and DNMT3A-mutant progenitor cells upon acquisition of RHO and/or IDH2 mutations [79]. Supporting this hypothesis are reports of TFH lymphomas and myeloid malignancies (both de novo and therapy-related) co-occurring in patients and arising from TET2 and DNMT3A-mutated clonal progenitor cells [80,81]. Furthermore, the presence of two or more TET2 mutations and a mutant allele fraction > 15% appears to confer a higher risk for myeloid neoplasms in patients with TFH lymphomas [81,82]. These studies have elucidated the unique biology of TFH lymphomas and highlight the importance of the evaluation for clonal hematopoiesis in these patients, which can have important diagnostic and therapeutic implications.

7. Treatment and Conclusions

TFH lymphomas are an important subtype of peripheral T-cell lymphomas, and the last decade has seen significant advances in understanding their biology and molecular pathogenesis. The identification of shared recurrent mutations in AITL, FTCL, and PTCL-TFH has justified classifying these morphologically unique lymphomas as a single biological category. These discoveries have also provided a wealth of biomarkers for diagnosis and targets for therapy [83]. Currently, the distinction between TFH lymphomas and PTCL, NOS, has no impact on current clinical management, with most patients treated with cyclophosphamide, doxorubicin, vincristine, and prednisone (CHOP) or CHOP-like upfront therapy, but with less-than-optimal response rates. Recent studies have shown improved progression-free survival (PFS) and overall survival (OS) in patients with systemic CD30-positive T-cell lymphomas treated with CHOP-like chemotherapy regimens that replace vincristine with brentuximab vedotin, an anti-CD30 antibody drug conjugate. The majority of these patients had anaplastic large cell lymphoma (ALCL), which is characterized by diffuse and strong CD30 expression. Patients with other T-cell lymphoma subtypes expressing CD30, including AITL, were included; however, due to small sample sizes, efficacy in the non-ALCL subgroups could not be evaluated [84]. Studies evaluating the efficacy of romidepsin, a histone deacetylase inhibitor, in the treatment of TFH lymphomas have shown interesting results. Romidepsin in addition to CHOP showed marginal, but not significant beneficial effects when compared to CHOP in previously untreated patients with TFH lymphoma [85]; however, romidepsin, either alone or in combination with other drugs, had significant benefits in patients with relapsed/refractory TFH lymphoma [86]. These incongruous results warrant further investigation with larger patient cohorts. Finally, the identification of TET2, DNMT3A, and IDH mutations in TFH lymphomas has created opportunities for targeted therapy with hypomethylating agents, such as azacytidine, in combination with current therapy regimens with promising results [87,88].

Author Contributions: Conceptualization, M.P.M.; writing—original draft preparation, K.A.G., K.H.K. and M.P.M.; writing—review and editing, K.A.G. and M.P.M.; visualization, K.A.G. and M.P.M.; supervision, M.P.M. All authors have read and agreed to the published version of the manuscript.

Funding: This research received no external funding.

Institutional Review Board Statement: Not applicable.

Informed Consent Statement: Not applicable.

Data Availability Statement: Not applicable.

Conflicts of Interest: The authors declare no conflict of interest.

References

1. Crotty, S. T follicular helper cell differentiation, function, and roles in disease. *Immunity* **2014**, *41*, 529–542. [CrossRef] [PubMed]
2. Crotty, S. A brief history of t cell help to b cells. *Nat. Rev. Immunol.* **2015**, *15*, 185–189. [CrossRef] [PubMed]
3. Goenka, R.; Barnett, L.G.; Silver, J.S.; O'Neill, P.J.; Hunter, C.A.; Cancro, M.P.; Laufer, T.M. Cutting edge: Dendritic cell-restricted antigen presentation initiates the follicular helper t cell program but cannot complete ultimate effector differentiation. *J. Immunol.* **2011**, *187*, 1091–1095. [CrossRef] [PubMed]
4. Crotty, S. Follicular helper cd4 t cells (tfh). *Annu. Rev. Immunol.* **2011**, *29*, 621–663. [CrossRef]
5. Crotty, S.; Johnston, R.J.; Schoenberger, S.P. Effectors and memories: Bcl-6 and blimp-1 in t and b lymphocyte differentiation. *Nat. Immunol.* **2010**, *11*, 114–120. [CrossRef]
6. Crotty, S. T follicular helper cell biology: A decade of discovery and diseases. *Immunity* **2019**, *50*, 1132–1148. [CrossRef]
7. Suan, D.; Nguyen, A.; Moran, I.; Bourne, K.; Hermes, J.R.; Arshi, M.; Hampton, H.R.; Tomura, M.; Miwa, Y.; Kelleher, A.D.; et al. T follicular helper cells have distinct modes of migration and molecular signatures in naive and memory immune responses. *Immunity* **2015**, *42*, 704–718. [CrossRef]
8. Yu, D.; Vinuesa, C.G. The elusive identity of t follicular helper cells. *Trends Immunol.* **2010**, *31*, 377–383. [CrossRef]
9. Cubas, R.A.; Mudd, J.C.; Savoye, A.L.; Perreau, M.; van Grevenynghe, J.; Metcalf, T.; Connick, E.; Meditz, A.; Freeman, G.J.; Abesada-Terk, G., Jr.; et al. Inadequate t follicular cell help impairs b cell immunity during hiv infection. *Nat. Med.* **2013**, *19*, 494–499. [CrossRef]
10. Simpson, N.; Gatenby, P.A.; Wilson, A.; Malik, S.; Fulcher, D.A.; Tangye, S.G.; Manku, H.; Vyse, T.J.; Roncador, G.; Huttley, G.A.; et al. Expansion of circulating t cells resembling follicular helper t cells is a fixed phenotype that identifies a subset of severe systemic lupus erythematosus. *Arthritis Rheumatol.* **2010**, *62*, 234–244. [CrossRef]
11. Gu-Trantien, C.; Loi, S.; Garaud, S.; Equeter, C.; Libin, M.; de Wind, A.; Ravoet, M.; Le Buanec, H.; Sibille, C.; Manfouo-Foutsop, G.; et al. Cd4(+) follicular helper t cell infiltration predicts breast cancer survival. *J. Clin. Investig.* **2013**, *123*, 2873–2892. [CrossRef] [PubMed]
12. Grogg, K.L.; Attygalle, A.D.; Macon, W.R.; Remstein, E.D.; Kurtin, P.J.; Dogan, A. Angioimmunoblastic t-cell lymphoma: A neoplasm of germinal-center t-helper cells? *Blood* **2005**, *106*, 1501–1502. [CrossRef] [PubMed]
13. De Leval, L.; Rickman, D.S.; Thielen, C.; Reynies, A.; Huang, Y.L.; Delsol, G.; Lamant, L.; Leroy, K.; Briere, J.; Molina, T.; et al. The gene expression profile of nodal peripheral t-cell lymphoma demonstrates a molecular link between angioimmunoblastic t-cell lymphoma (aitl) and follicular helper t (tfh) cells. *Blood* **2007**, *109*, 4952–4963. [CrossRef] [PubMed]
14. Rodriguez-Pinilla, S.M.; Atienza, L.; Murillo, C.; Perez-Rodriguez, A.; Montes-Moreno, S.; Roncador, G.; Perez-Seoane, C.; Dominguez, P.; Camacho, F.I.; Piris, M.A. Peripheral t-cell lymphoma with follicular t-cell markers. *Am. J. Surg. Pathol.* **2008**, *32*, 1787–1799. [CrossRef]

15. Huang, Y.; Moreau, A.; Dupuis, J.; Streubel, B.; Petit, B.; Le Gouill, S.; Martin-Garcia, N.; Copie-Bergman, C.; Gaillard, F.; Qubaja, M.; et al. Peripheral t-cell lymphomas with a follicular growth pattern are derived from follicular helper t cells (tfh) and may show overlapping features with angioimmunoblastic t-cell lymphomas. *Am. J. Surg. Pathol.* **2009**, *33*, 682–690. [CrossRef] [PubMed]
16. Dobay, M.P.; Lemonnier, F.; Missiaglia, E.; Bastard, C.; Vallois, D.; Jais, J.P.; Scourzic, L.; Dupuy, A.; Fataccioli, V.; Pujals, A.; et al. Integrative clinicopathological and molecular analyses of angioimmunoblastic t-cell lymphoma and other nodal lymphomas of follicular helper t-cell origin. *Haematologica* **2017**, *102*, e148–e151. [CrossRef]
17. Beltraminelli, H.; Leinweber, B.; Kerl, H.; Cerroni, L. Primary cutaneous cd4+ small-/medium-sized pleomorphic t-cell lymphoma: A cutaneous nodular proliferation of pleomorphic t lymphocytes of undetermined significance? A study of 136 cases. *Am. J. Dermatopathol.* **2009**, *31*, 317–322. [CrossRef]
18. Swerdlow, S.H.; Campo, E.; Harris, N.L.; Jaffe, E.S.; Pileri, S.A.; Stein, H.; Thiele, J.; Arber, D.A.; Hasserjian, R.P.; Le Beau, M.M.; et al. *Who Classification of Tumours of Haematopoietic and Lymphoid Tissues (Revised 4th Edition)*; International Agency for Research on Cancer: Lyon, France, 2017.
19. Beltzung, F.; Ortonne, N.; Pelletier, L.; Beylot-Barry, M.; Ingen-Housz-Oro, S.; Franck, F.; Pereira, B.; Godfraind, C.; Delfau, M.H.; D'Incan, M.; et al. Primary cutaneous cd4+ small/medium t-cell lymphoproliferative disorders: A clinical, pathologic, and molecular study of 60 cases presenting with a single lesion: A multicenter study of the french cutaneous lymphoma study group. *Am. J. Surg. Pathol.* **2020**, *44*, 862–872. [CrossRef]
20. Alikhan, M.; Song, J.Y.; Sohani, A.R.; Moroch, J.; Plonquet, A.; Duffield, A.S.; Borowitz, M.J.; Jiang, L.; Bueso-Ramos, C.; Inamdar, K.; et al. Peripheral t-cell lymphomas of follicular helper t-cell type frequently display an aberrant cd3(-/dim)cd4(+) population by flow cytometry: An important clue to the diagnosis of a hodgkin lymphoma mimic. *Mod. Pathol.* **2016**, *29*, 1173–1182. [CrossRef]
21. Attygalle, A.; Al-Jehani, R.; Diss, T.C.; Munson, P.; Liu, H.; Du, M.Q.; Isaacson, P.G.; Dogan, A. Neoplastic t cells in angioimmunoblastic t-cell lymphoma express cd10. *Blood* **2002**, *99*, 627–633. [CrossRef]
22. Bisig, B.; Thielen, C.; Herens, C.; Gofflot, S.; Travert, M.; Delfau-Larue, M.H.; Boniver, J.; Gaulard, P.; de Leval, L. C-maf expression in angioimmunoblastic t-cell lymphoma reflects follicular helper t-cell derivation rather than oncogenesis. *Histopathology* **2012**, *60*, 371–376. [CrossRef] [PubMed]
23. Dorfman, D.M.; Brown, J.A.; Shahsafaei, A.; Freeman, G.J. Programmed death-1 (pd-1) is a marker of germinal center-associated t cells and angioimmunoblastic t-cell lymphoma. *Am. J. Surg. Pathol.* **2006**, *30*, 802–810. [CrossRef] [PubMed]
24. Roncador, G.; Garcia Verdes-Montenegro, J.F.; Tedoldi, S.; Paterson, J.C.; Klapper, W.; Ballabio, E.; Maestre, L.; Pileri, S.; Hansmann, M.L.; Piris, M.A.; et al. Expression of two markers of germinal center t cells (sap and pd-1) in angioimmunoblastic t-cell lymphoma. *Haematologica* **2007**, *92*, 1059–1066. [CrossRef] [PubMed]
25. Basha, B.M.; Bryant, S.C.; Rech, K.L.; Feldman, A.L.; Vrana, J.A.; Shi, M.; Reed, K.A.; King, R.L. Application of a 5 marker panel to the routine diagnosis of peripheral t-cell lymphoma with t-follicular helper phenotype. *Am. J. Surg. Pathol.* **2019**, *43*, 1282–1290. [CrossRef]
26. Dogan, A.; Attygalle, A.D.; Kyriakou, C. Angioimmunoblastic t-cell lymphoma. *Br. J. Haematol.* **2003**, *121*, 681–691. [CrossRef] [PubMed]
27. Piccaluga, P.P.; Agostinelli, C.; Califano, A.; Carbone, A.; Fantoni, L.; Ferrari, S.; Gazzola, A.; Gloghini, A.; Righi, S.; Rossi, M.; et al. Gene expression analysis of angioimmunoblastic lymphoma indicates derivation from t follicular helper cells and vascular endothelial growth factor deregulation. *Cancer Res.* **2007**, *67*, 10703–10710. [CrossRef]
28. Piccaluga, P.P.; Fuligni, F.; De Leo, A.; Bertuzzi, C.; Rossi, M.; Bacci, F.; Sabattini, E.; Agostinelli, C.; Gazzola, A.; Laginestra, M.A.; et al. Molecular profiling improves classification and prognostication of nodal peripheral t-cell lymphomas: Results of a phase iii diagnostic accuracy study. *J. Clin. Oncol.* **2013**, *31*, 3019–3025. [CrossRef]
29. Iqbal, J.; Wright, G.; Wang, C.; Rosenwald, A.; Gascoyne, R.D.; Weisenburger, D.D.; Greiner, T.C.; Smith, L.; Guo, S.; Wilcox, R.A.; et al. Gene expression signatures delineate biological and prognostic subgroups in peripheral t-cell lymphoma. *Blood* **2014**, *123*, 2915–2923. [CrossRef]
30. Mourad, N.; Mounier, N.; Briere, J.; Raffoux, E.; Delmer, A.; Feller, A.; Meijer, C.J.; Emile, J.F.; Bouabdallah, R.; Bosly, A.; et al. Clinical, biologic, and pathologic features in 157 patients with angioimmunoblastic t-cell lymphoma treated within the groupe d'etude des lymphomes de l'adulte (gela) trials. *Blood* **2008**, *111*, 4463–4470. [CrossRef]
31. Xie, Y.; Jaffe, E.S. How i diagnose angioimmunoblastic t-cell lymphoma. *Am. J. Clin. Pathol.* **2021**, *156*, 1–14. [CrossRef]
32. De Leval, L.; Gisselbrecht, C.; Gaulard, P. Advances in the understanding and management of angioimmunoblastic t-cell lymphoma. *Br. J. Haematol.* **2010**, *148*, 673–689. [CrossRef] [PubMed]
33. De Leval, L.; Parrens, M.; Le Bras, F.; Jais, J.P.; Fataccioli, V.; Martin, A.; Lamant, L.; Delarue, R.; Berger, F.; Arbion, F.; et al. Angioimmunoblastic t-cell lymphoma is the most common t-cell lymphoma in two distinct french information data sets. *Haematologica* **2015**, *100*, e361–e364. [CrossRef] [PubMed]
34. Cho, Y.U.; Chi, H.S.; Park, C.J.; Jang, S.; Seo, E.J.; Huh, J. Distinct features of angioimmunoblastic t-cell lymphoma with bone marrow involvement. *Am. J. Clin. Pathol.* **2009**, *131*, 640–646. [CrossRef] [PubMed]
35. Federico, M.; Rudiger, T.; Bellei, M.; Nathwani, B.N.; Luminari, S.; Coiffier, B.; Harris, N.L.; Jaffe, E.S.; Pileri, S.A.; Savage, K.J.; et al. Clinicopathologic characteristics of angioimmunoblastic t-cell lymphoma: Analysis of the international peripheral t-cell lymphoma project. *J. Clin. Oncol. Off. J. Am. Soc. Clin. Oncol.* **2013**, *31*, 240–246. [CrossRef] [PubMed]

36. Lachenal, F.; Berger, F.; Ghesquieres, H.; Biron, P.; Hot, A.; Callet-Bauchu, E.; Chassagne, C.; Coiffier, B.; Durieu, I.; Rousset, H.; et al. Angioimmunoblastic t-cell lymphoma: Clinical and laboratory features at diagnosis in 77 patients. *Medicine* **2007**, *86*, 282–292. [CrossRef] [PubMed]
37. Siegert, W.; Nerl, C.; Agthe, A.; Engelhard, M.; Brittinger, G.; Tiemann, M.; Lennert, K.; Huhn, D. Angioimmunoblastic lymphadenopathy (aild)-type t-cell lymphoma: Prognostic impact of clinical observations and laboratory findings at presentation. The kiel lymphoma study group. *Ann. Oncol.* **1995**, *6*, 659–664. [CrossRef]
38. Dunleavy, K.; Wilson, W.H.; Jaffe, E.S. Angioimmunoblastic t cell lymphoma: Pathobiological insights and clinical implications. *Curr. Opin. Hematol.* **2007**, *14*, 348–353. [CrossRef]
39. Anagnostopoulos, I.; Hummel, M.; Finn, T.; Tiemann, M.; Korbjuhn, P.; Dimmler, C.; Gatter, K.; Dallenbach, F.; Parwaresch, M.R.; Stein, H. Heterogeneous epstein-barr virus infection patterns in peripheral t-cell lymphoma of angioimmunoblastic lymphadenopathy type. *Blood* **1992**, *80*, 1804–1812. [CrossRef]
40. Weiss, L.M.; Jaffe, E.S.; Liu, X.F.; Chen, Y.Y.; Shibata, D.; Medeiros, L.J. Detection and localization of epstein-barr viral genomes in angioimmunoblastic lymphadenopathy and angioimmunoblastic lymphadenopathy-like lymphoma. *Blood* **1992**, *79*, 1789–1795. [CrossRef]
41. Pautier, P.; Devidas, A.; Delmer, A.; Dombret, H.; Sutton, L.; Zini, J.M.; Nedelec, G.; Molina, T.; Marolleau, J.P.; Brice, P. Angioimmunoblastic-like t-cell non hodgkin's lymphoma: Outcome after chemotherapy in 33 patients and review of the literature. *Leuk. Lymphoma* **1999**, *32*, 545–552. [CrossRef]
42. Attygalle, A.D.; Kyriakou, C.; Dupuis, J.; Grogg, K.L.; Diss, T.C.; Wotherspoon, A.C.; Chuang, S.S.; Cabecadas, J.; Isaacson, P.G.; Du, M.Q.; et al. Histologic evolution of angioimmunoblastic t-cell lymphoma in consecutive biopsies: Clinical correlation and insights into natural history and disease progression. *Am. J. Surg. Pathol.* **2007**, *31*, 1077–1088. [CrossRef]
43. Ree, H.J.; Kadin, M.E.; Kikuchi, M.; Ko, Y.H.; Go, J.H.; Suzumiya, J.; Kim, D.S. Angioimmunoblastic lymphoma (aild-type t-cell lymphoma) with hyperplastic germinal centers. *Am. J. Surg. Pathol.* **1998**, *22*, 643–655. [CrossRef]
44. Rodriguez-Justo, M.; Attygalle, A.D.; Munson, P.; Roncador, G.; Marafioti, T.; Piris, M.A. Angioimmunoblastic t-cell lymphoma with hyperplastic germinal centres: A neoplasia with origin in the outer zone of the germinal centre? Clinicopathological and immunohistochemical study of 10 cases with follicular t-cell markers. *Mod. Pathol.* **2009**, *22*, 753–761. [CrossRef] [PubMed]
45. Zettl, A.; Lee, S.S.; Rudiger, T.; Starostik, P.; Marino, M.; Kirchner, T.; Ott, M.; Muller-Hermelink, H.K.; Ott, G. Epstein-barr virus-associated b-cell lymphoproliferative disorders in angioimmunoblastic t-cell lymphoma and peripheral t-cell lymphoma, unspecified. *Am. J. Clin. Pathol.* **2002**, *117*, 368–379. [CrossRef] [PubMed]
46. Nicolae, A.; Pittaluga, S.; Venkataraman, G.; Vijnovich-Baron, A.; Xi, L.; Raffeld, M.; Jaffe, E.S. Peripheral t-cell lymphomas of follicular t-helper cell derivation with hodgkin/reed-sternberg cells of b-cell lineage: Both ebv-positive and ebv-negative variants exist. *Am. J. Surg. Pathol.* **2013**, *37*, 816–826. [CrossRef] [PubMed]
47. Willenbrock, K.; Brauninger, A.; Hansmann, M.L. Frequent occurrence of b-cell lymphomas in angioimmunoblastic t-cell lymphoma and proliferation of epstein-barr virus-infected cells in early cases. *Br. J. Haematol.* **2007**, *138*, 733–739. [CrossRef] [PubMed]
48. Balague, O.; Martinez, A.; Colomo, L.; Rosello, E.; Garcia, A.; Martinez-Bernal, M.; Palacin, A.; Fu, K.; Weisenburger, D.; Colomer, D.; et al. Epstein-barr virus negative clonal plasma cell proliferations and lymphomas in peripheral t-cell lymphomas: A phenomenon with distinctive clinicopathologic features. *Am. J. Surg. Pathol.* **2007**, *31*, 1310–1322. [CrossRef]
49. Huppmann, A.R.; Roullet, M.R.; Raffeld, M.; Jaffe, E.S. Angioimmunoblastic t-cell lymphoma partially obscured by an epstein-barr virus-negative clonal plasma cell proliferation. *J. Clin. Oncol.* **2013**, *31*, e28–e30. [CrossRef]
50. Serke, S.; van Lessen, A.; Hummel, M.; Szczepek, A.; Huhn, D.; Stein, H. Circulating cd4+ t lymphocytes with intracellular but no surface cd3 antigen in five of seven patients consecutively diagnosed with angioimmunoblastic t-cell lymphoma. *Cytometry* **2000**, *42*, 180–187. [CrossRef]
51. Stacchini, A.; Demurtas, A.; Aliberti, S.; Francia di Celle, P.; Godio, L.; Palestro, G.; Novero, D. The usefulness of flow cytometric cd10 detection in the differential diagnosis of peripheral t-cell lymphomas. *Am. J. Clin. Pathol.* **2007**, *128*, 854–864. [CrossRef]
52. Singh, A.; Schabath, R.; Ratei, R.; Stroux, A.; Klemke, C.D.; Nebe, T.; Florcken, A.; van Lessen, A.; Anagnostopoulos, I.; Dorken, B.; et al. Peripheral blood scd3(-) cd4(+) t cells: A useful diagnostic tool in angioimmunoblastic t cell lymphoma. *Hematol. Oncol.* **2014**, *32*, 16–21. [CrossRef] [PubMed]
53. Loghavi, S.; Wang, S.A.; Medeiros, L.J.; Jorgensen, J.L.; Li, X.; Xu-Monette, Z.Y.; Miranda, R.N.; Young, K.H. Immunophenotypic and diagnostic characterization of angioimmunoblastic t-cell lymphoma by advanced flow cytometric technology. *Leuk. Lymphoma* **2016**, *57*, 2804–2812. [CrossRef] [PubMed]
54. Yabe, M.; Gao, Q.; Ozkaya, N.; Huet, S.; Lewis, N.; Pichardo, J.D.; Moskowitz, A.J.; Horwitz, S.M.; Dogan, A.; Roshal, M. Bright pd-1 expression by flow cytometry is a powerful tool for diagnosis and monitoring of angioimmunoblastic t-cell lymphoma. *Blood Cancer J.* **2020**, *10*, 32. [CrossRef] [PubMed]
55. Quintanilla-Martinez, L.; Fend, F.; Moguel, L.R.; Spilove, L.; Beaty, M.W.; Kingma, D.W.; Raffeld, M.; Jaffe, E.S. Peripheral t-cell lymphoma with reed-sternberg-like cells of b-cell phenotype and genotype associated with epstein-barr virus infection. *Am. J. Surg. Pathol.* **1999**, *23*, 1233–1240. [CrossRef]
56. Hartmann, S.; Goncharova, O.; Portyanko, A.; Sabattini, E.; Meinel, J.; Kuppers, R.; Agostinelli, C.; Pileri, S.A.; Hansmann, M.L. Cd30 expression in neoplastic t cells of follicular t cell lymphoma is a helpful diagnostic tool in the differential diagnosis of hodgkin lymphoma. *Mod. Pathol.* **2019**, *32*, 37–47. [CrossRef]

57. Van den Oord, J.J.; de Wolf-Peeters, C.; O'Connor, N.T.; de Vos, R.; Tricot, G.; Desmet, V.J. Nodular t-cell lymphoma. Report of a case studied with morphologic, immunohistochemical, and DNA hybridization techniques. *Arch. Pathol. Lab. Med.* **1988**, *112*, 133–138.
58. Hu, S.; Young, K.H.; Konoplev, S.N.; Medeiros, L.J. Follicular t-cell lymphoma: A member of an emerging family of follicular helper t-cell derived t-cell lymphomas. *Hum. Pathol.* **2012**, *43*, 1789–1798. [CrossRef]
59. Sakakibara, A.; Suzuki, Y.; Kato, H.; Yamamoto, K.; Sakata-Yanagimoto, M.; Ishikawa, Y.; Furukawa, K.; Shimada, K.; Kohno, K.; Nakamura, S.; et al. Follicular t-cell lymphoma mimicking lymphocyte-rich classic hodgkin lymphoma: A case report of a diagnostic pitfall. *J. Clin. Exp. Hematop. JCEH* **2021**, *61*, 97–101. [CrossRef]
60. Moroch, J.; Copie-Bergman, C.; de Leval, L.; Plonquet, A.; Martin-Garcia, N.; Delfau-Larue, M.H.; Molinier-Frenkel, V.; Belhadj, K.; Haioun, C.; Audouin, J.; et al. Follicular peripheral t-cell lymphoma expands the spectrum of classical hodgkin lymphoma mimics. *Am. J. Surg. Pathol.* **2012**, *36*, 1636–1646. [CrossRef]
61. Rodriguez, M.; Alonso-Alonso, R.; Tomas-Roca, L.; Rodriguez-Pinilla, S.M.; Manso-Alonso, R.; Cereceda, L.; Borregon, J.; Villaescusa, T.; Cordoba, R.; Sanchez-Beato, M.; et al. Peripheral t-cell lymphoma: Molecular profiling recognizes subclasses and identifies prognostic markers. *Blood Adv.* **2021**, *5*, 5588–5598. [CrossRef]
62. Manso, R.; Gonzalez-Rincon, J.; Rodriguez-Justo, M.; Roncador, G.; Gomez, S.; Sanchez-Beato, M.; Piris, M.A.; Rodriguez-Pinilla, S.M. Overlap at the molecular and immunohistochemical levels between angioimmunoblastic t-cell lymphoma and a subgroup of peripheral t-cell lymphomas without specific morphological features. *Oncotarget* **2018**, *9*, 16124–16133. [CrossRef] [PubMed]
63. Agostinelli, C.; Hartmann, S.; Klapper, W.; Korkolopoulou, P.; Righi, S.; Marafioti, T.; Piccaluga, P.P.; Patsouris, E.; Hansmann, M.L.; Lennert, K.; et al. Peripheral t cell lymphomas with follicular t helper phenotype: A new basket or a distinct entity? Revising karl lennert's personal archive. *Histopathology* **2011**, *59*, 679–691. [CrossRef] [PubMed]
64. Attygalle, A.D. Nodal t-cell lymphomas with a t-follicular helper cell phenotype. *Diagn. Histopathol.* **2018**, *24*, 227–236. [CrossRef]
65. Cairns, R.A.; Iqbal, J.; Lemonnier, F.; Kucuk, C.; de Leval, L.; Jais, J.P.; Parrens, M.; Martin, A.; Xerri, L.; Brousset, P.; et al. Idh2 mutations are frequent in angioimmunoblastic t-cell lymphoma. *Blood* **2012**, *119*, 1901–1903. [CrossRef]
66. Heavican, T.B.; Bouska, A.; Yu, J.; Lone, W.; Amador, C.; Gong, Q.; Zhang, W.; Li, Y.; Dave, B.J.; Nairismagi, M.L.; et al. Genetic drivers of oncogenic pathways in molecular subgroups of peripheral t-cell lymphoma. *Blood* **2019**, *133*, 1664–1676. [CrossRef]
67. Lemonnier, F.; Couronne, L.; Parrens, M.; Jais, J.P.; Travert, M.; Lamant, L.; Tournillac, O.; Rousset, T.; Fabiani, B.; Cairns, R.A.; et al. Recurrent tet2 mutations in peripheral t-cell lymphomas correlate with tfh-like features and adverse clinical parameters. *Blood* **2012**, *120*, 1466–1469. [CrossRef]
68. Sakata-Yanagimoto, M.; Enami, T.; Yoshida, K.; Shiraishi, Y.; Ishii, R.; Miyake, Y.; Muto, H.; Tsuyama, N.; Sato-Otsubo, A.; Okuno, Y.; et al. Somatic rhoa mutation in angioimmunoblastic t cell lymphoma. *Nat. Genet.* **2014**, *46*, 171–175. [CrossRef]
69. Yoon, S.E.; Cho, J.; Kim, Y.J.; Ko, Y.H.; Park, W.Y.; Kim, S.J.; Kim, W.S. Comprehensive analysis of clinical, pathological, and genomic characteristics of follicular helper t-cell derived lymphomas. *Exp. Hematol. Oncol.* **2021**, *10*, 33. [CrossRef]
70. Ondrejka, S.L.; Grzywacz, B.; Bodo, J.; Makishima, H.; Polprasert, C.; Said, J.W.; Przychodzen, B.; Maciejewski, J.P.; Hsi, E.D. Angioimmunoblastic t-cell lymphomas with the rhoa p.Gly17val mutation have classic clinical and pathologic features. *Am. J. Surg. Pathol.* **2016**, *40*, 335–341. [CrossRef]
71. Steinhilber, J.; Mederake, M.; Bonzheim, I.; Serinsoz-Linke, E.; Muller, I.; Fallier-Becker, P.; Lemonnier, F.; Gaulard, P.; Fend, F.; Quintanilla-Martinez, L. The pathological features of angioimmunoblastic t-cell lymphomas with idh2(r172) mutations. *Mod. Pathol.* **2019**, *32*, 1123–1134. [CrossRef]
72. Attygalle, A.D.; Feldman, A.L.; Dogan, A. Itk/syk translocation in angioimmunoblastic t-cell lymphoma. *Am. J. Surg. Pathol.* **2013**, *37*, 1456–1457. [CrossRef] [PubMed]
73. Streubel, B.; Vinatzer, U.; Willheim, M.; Raderer, M.; Chott, A. Novel t(5;9)(q33;q22) fuses itk to syk in unspecified peripheral t-cell lymphoma. *Leukemia* **2006**, *20*, 313–318. [CrossRef] [PubMed]
74. Genovese, G.; Kahler, A.K.; Handsaker, R.E.; Lindberg, J.; Rose, S.A.; Bakhoum, S.F.; Chambert, K.; Mick, E.; Neale, B.M.; Fromer, M.; et al. Clonal hematopoiesis and blood-cancer risk inferred from blood DNA sequence. *N. Engl. J. Med.* **2014**, *371*, 2477–2487. [CrossRef]
75. Jaiswal, S.; Fontanillas, P.; Flannick, J.; Manning, A.; Grauman, P.V.; Mar, B.G.; Lindsley, R.C.; Mermel, C.H.; Burtt, N.; Chavez, A.; et al. Age-related clonal hematopoiesis associated with adverse outcomes. *N. Engl. J. Med.* **2014**, *371*, 2488–2498. [CrossRef] [PubMed]
76. Abdel-Wahab, O.; Mullally, A.; Hedvat, C.; Garcia-Manero, G.; Patel, J.; Wadleigh, M.; Malinge, S.; Yao, J.; Kilpivaara, O.; Bhat, R.; et al. Genetic characterization of tet1, tet2, and tet3 alterations in myeloid malignancies. *Blood* **2009**, *114*, 144–147. [CrossRef] [PubMed]
77. Ley, T.J.; Ding, L.; Walter, M.J.; McLellan, M.D.; Lamprecht, T.; Larson, D.E.; Kandoth, C.; Payton, J.E.; Baty, J.; Welch, J.; et al. Dnmt3a mutations in acute myeloid leukemia. *N. Engl. J. Med.* **2010**, *363*, 2424–2433. [CrossRef]
78. Papaemmanuil, E.; Gerstung, M.; Malcovati, L.; Tauro, S.; Gundem, G.; Van Loo, P.; Yoon, C.J.; Ellis, P.; Wedge, D.C.; Pellagatti, A.; et al. Clinical and biological implications of driver mutations in myelodysplastic syndromes. *Blood* **2013**, *122*, 3616–3627; quiz 3699. [CrossRef]
79. Yao, W.Q.; Wu, F.; Zhang, W.; Chuang, S.S.; Thompson, J.S.; Chen, Z.; Zhang, S.W.; Clipson, A.; Wang, M.; Liu, H.; et al. Angioimmunoblastic t-cell lymphoma contains multiple clonal t-cell populations derived from a common tet2 mutant progenitor cell. *J. Pathol.* **2020**, *250*, 346–357. [CrossRef]

80. Tiacci, E.; Venanzi, A.; Ascani, S.; Marra, A.; Cardinali, V.; Martino, G.; Codoni, V.; Schiavoni, G.; Martelli, M.P.; Falini, B. High-risk clonal hematopoiesis as the origin of aitl and npm1-mutated aml. *N. Engl. J. Med.* **2018**, *379*, 981–984. [CrossRef]
81. Lewis, N.E.; Petrova-Drus, K.; Huet, S.; Epstein-Peterson, Z.D.; Gao, Q.; Sigler, A.E.; Baik, J.; Ozkaya, N.; Moskowitz, A.J.; Kumar, A.; et al. Clonal hematopoiesis in angioimmunoblastic t-cell lymphoma with divergent evolution to myeloid neoplasms. *Blood Adv.* **2020**, *4*, 2261–2271. [CrossRef]
82. Cheng, S.; Zhang, W.; Inghirami, G.; Tam, W. Mutation analysis links angioimmunoblastic t-cell lymphoma to clonal hematopoiesis and smoking. *Elife* **2021**, *10*, e66395. [CrossRef] [PubMed]
83. Mulvey, E.; Ruan, J. Biomarker-driven management strategies for peripheral t cell lymphoma. *J. Hematol. Oncol.* **2020**, *13*, 59. [CrossRef] [PubMed]
84. Horwitz, S.; O'Connor, O.A.; Pro, B.; Illidge, T.; Fanale, M.; Advani, R.; Bartlett, N.L.; Christensen, J.H.; Morschhauser, F.; Domingo-Domenech, E.; et al. Brentuximab vedotin with chemotherapy for cd30-positive peripheral t-cell lymphoma (echelon-2): A global, double-blind, randomised, phase 3 trial. *Lancet* **2019**, *393*, 229–240. [CrossRef]
85. Bachy, E.; Camus, V.; Thieblemont, C.; Sibon, D.; Casasnovas, R.O.; Ysebaert, L.; Damaj, G.; Guidez, S.; Pica, G.M.; Kim, W.S.; et al. Romidepsin plus chop versus chop in patients with previously untreated peripheral t-cell lymphoma: Results of the ro-chop phase iii study (conducted by lysa). *J. Clin. Oncol.* **2022**, *40*, 242–251. [CrossRef] [PubMed]
86. Ghione, P.; Faruque, P.; Mehta-Shah, N.; Seshan, V.; Ozkaya, N.; Bhaskar, S.; Yeung, J.; Spinner, M.A.; Lunning, M.; Inghirami, G.; et al. T follicular helper phenotype predicts response to histone deacetylase inhibitors in relapsed/refractory peripheral t-cell lymphoma. *Blood Adv.* **2020**, *4*, 4640–4647. [CrossRef]
87. Ma, H.; O'Connor, O.A.; Marchi, E. New directions in treating peripheral t-cell lymphomas (ptcl): Leveraging epigenetic modifiers alone and in combination. *Expert Rev. Hematol.* **2019**, *12*, 137–146. [CrossRef]
88. Ma, H.; O'Connor, O.A.; Marchi, E. Management of angioimmunoblastic t-cell lymphoma (aitl) and other t follicular helper cell lymphomas (tfh ptcl). *Semin. Hematol.* **2021**, *58*, 95–102. [CrossRef]

MDPI
St. Alban-Anlage 66
4052 Basel
Switzerland
Tel. +41 61 683 77 34
Fax +41 61 302 89 18
www.mdpi.com

Hemato Editorial Office
E-mail: hemato@mdpi.com
www.mdpi.com/journal/hemato

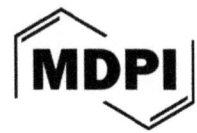

www.ingramcontent.com/pod-product-compliance
Lightning Source LLC
LaVergne TN
LVHW070442100526
838202LV00014B/1649